P9-DGV-574

Alternative Medicine
SOURCEBOOK

Health Reference Series

First Edition

Alternative Medicine
SOURCEBOOK

*Basic Consumer Health Information
about Alternatives to Conventional Medicine,
Including Acupressure, Acupuncture,
Aromatherapy, Ayurveda, Bioelectromagnetics,
Environmental Medicine, Essence Therapy,
Food and Nutrition Therapy, Herbal Therapy,
Homeopathy, Imaging, Massage, Naturopathy,
Reflexology, Relaxation and Meditation, Sound
Therapy, Vitamin and Mineral Therapy,
and Yoga, and More*

Edited by
Allan R. Cook

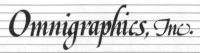

Omnigraphics, Inc.

Penobscot Building / Detroit, MI 48226

Bibliographic Note

Because this page cannot legibly accommodate all the copyright notices, the Bibliographic Note portion of the Preface constitutes an extension of the copyright notice.

Beginning with books published in 1999, each new volume of the *Health Reference Series* will be individually titled and called a "First Edition." Subsequent updates will carry sequential edition numbers. To help avoid confusion and to provide maximum flexibility in our ability to respond to informational needs, the practice of consecutively numbering each volume will be discontinued.

Edited by Allan R. Cook

Health Reference Series

Karen Bellenir, *Series Editor*
Peter D. Dresser, *Managing Editor*
Joan Margeson, *Research Associate*
Dawn Matthews, *Verification Assistant*
Margaret Mary Missar, *Research Coordinator*
Jenifer Swanson, *Research Associate*

Omnigraphics, Inc.

Matthew P. Barbour, *Vice President, Operations*
Laurie Lanzen Harris, *Vice President, Editorial Director*
Thomas J. Murphy, *Vice President, Finance and Comptroller*
Peter E. Ruffner, *Senior Vice President*
Jane J. Steele, *Marketing Consultant*

Frederick G. Ruffner, Jr., Publisher

Library of Congress Cataloging-in-Publication Data

Alternative medicine sourcebook : basic consumer information about alternatives
    to conventional medicine, including acupressure, acpuncture, aromatherapy,
    ayurveda, bioelectromagnetics, environmental medicine, essence therapy, food
    and nutrition therapy, herbal theapy, homeopathy, imaging, message,
    naturopathy, reflexology, relaxation and meditation, sound therapy, vitamin
    and mineral therapy, and yoga, and more / edited by Allan R. Cook. — 1st ed.
        p. cm. — (Health reference series)
    Includes bibliographical references (p.)
    ISBN 0-7808-0200-4 (lib. bdg. : alk. paper)
    1. Alternative medicine. I. Cook, Allan R. II. Series: Health reference
series (Unnumbered)
R733.A475 1999   99-37612
615.5—dc21   CIP

∞

This book is printed on acid-free paper meeting the ANSI Z39.48 Standard. The infinity symbol that appears above indicates that the paper in this book meets that standard.

Printed in the United States

Table of Contents

Part VII: Mind/Body Control

Part VIII: Pharmacological and Biological Treatments

Part IX: Additional Help and Information

Preface

About this Book

Traditional Western medical practices perform well in the treatment of some types of acute disease and injury. The evolution of effective surgical procedures, the discovery of bacteria, and the development of vaccines and antitoxins have produced tremendous advances in medical care. However, traditional medicine, often called biomedicine, has performed less well in the treatment of many chronic and debilitating conditions including arthritis, allergies, pain, hypertension, cancer, depression, cardiovascular disease, and digestive maladies—disorders that account for 70 percent of U.S. medical spending. The Public Health Service expects this percentage to grow as the American population ages.

Alternative and complementary medical practices offer a different perspective on treatment. Instead of relying on the traditional Western tools, they focus on the patient's natural ability and desire to heal. Alternative therapists seek to help patients achieve health by reaching a holistic balance within themselves and within society. The ways in which the many forms of alternative medicine achieve such healing vary greatly and often are not accepted fully by the scientific and medical communities.

This *Sourcebook* will help lay readers understand the issues and controversies surrounding alternative and complementary medicine. It provides an overview the major therapy families, including oriental medicine, ayurvedic medicine, homeopathy, naturopathy, and environmental medicine, and it offers in-depth descriptions of some of the most common practices, including acupuncture, acupressure, aromatherapy, bioelectromagnetics, dietary therapies, herbal therapies, manual healing, and mind/body control. A glossary and directory of additional resources provide further help and information.

How to Use this Book

This book is divided into parts and chapters. Parts focus on broad areas of interest and chapters on specific topics within those areas.

Part I: The Issues of Alternative Medicine defines the common approaches used by alternative and complementary medicine practitioners and considers the current barriers that prevent effective integration of alternative treatments into conventional medical practice.

Part II: Alternative Systems of Medical Practice identifies the most common forms of alternative therapies.

Part III: Bioelectromagnetics discusses the use of electromagnetic forces in the treatment of chronic conditions.

Part IV: Diet, Nutrition, and Lifestyle Changes examines the relationship of nutrition and exercise to health and healing.

Part V: Herbal Medicine focuses on popular herbal treatments in their many forms and considers their uses and misuses.

Part VI: Manual Healing explores the concept of healing touch and healing relief from the physical manipulation of patient's body.

Part VII: Mind / Body Control considers the interconnectedness of the mind and the body and the therapies that attribute primary importance to healing and quality of life issues.

Part VIII: Pharmacological and Biological Treatments presents an approach that uses drugs and vaccines not currently accepted by the mainstream medical profession.

Part IX: Additional Help and Information provides a glossary of important terms and a directory of resources.

Bibliographic Note

This volume contains individual documents and excerpts from periodic publications issued by the National Institutes of Health (NIH), its sister agencies and subagencies, and the Centers for Disease Control and Prevention.

It also includes copyrighted articles, reprinted with permission, from the American Academy of Family Physicians, the American Association of Critical-Care Nurses, the American Association of Occupational Nurses, American Cancer Society, *American Journal of Sports Medicine*, the American Society of Regional Anesthesia, Congressional Quarterly Inc., Elsevier Science, the Flower Essence Society, Health Affairs, *International Journal of Technology and Assessment*, *Journal of Alternative and Complementary Medicine*, *Nursing Times*, Medical Economics Publishing, Mayo Foundation for Medical Education and Research, Medical Update, *Reader's Digest*, *Remedy*, Springhouse Corporation, *Tufts University Health & Nutrition Newsletter*, *U.S. News and World Report*, Thomas Wanning, W.B. Sanders, *The Washington Times*, and Women's Health Advocate.

All copyrighted material is reprinted with permission. Document numbers where applicable and specific source citations are provided on the appropriate page of each chapter. Every effort has been made to secure all necessary rights to reprint the copyrighted material. If any omissions have been made, please contact Omnigraphics to make corrections for future editions.

Acknowledgements

Many people and organizations have contributed the material in this volume. The editor gratefully acknowledges the assistance and cooperation of Margaret Mary Missar for her patient search for the documents that make up this volume, Jennifer Swanson for gleaning the internet for the most current material, Maria Franklin for securing permission to reprint articles, Karen Bellenir for her technical assistance and advice, and Bruce the Scanman for his reinscription rectification.

Note from the Editor

This book is part of Omnigraphics' Health Reference Series. The series provides basic information about a broad range of medical concerns. It is not intended to serve as a tool for diagnosing illness, in prescribing treatments, or as a substitute for the physician/patient relationship. All persons concerned about medical symptoms or the possibility of disease are encouraged to seek professional care from an appropriate health care provider.

Our Advisory Board

The *Health Reference Series* is reviewed by an Advisory Board comprised of librarians from public, academic, and medical libraries. We would like to thank the following board members for providing guidance to the development of this series:

Nancy Bulgarelli, William Beaumont Hospital Library, Royal Oak, MI

Karen Imarasio, Bloomfield Township Library, Bloomfield Township, MI

Karen Morgan, Mardigian Library, University of Michigan, Dearborn, MI

Rosemary Orlando, St. Clair Shores Public Library, St. Clair Shores, MI

Health Reference Series *Update Policy*

The inaugural book in the *Health Reference Series* was the first edition of *Cancer Sourcebook* published in 1992. Since then, the *Series* has been enthusiastically received by librarians and in the medical community. In order to maintain the standard of providing high-quality health information for the lay person, the editorial staff at Omnigraphics felt it was necessary to implement a policy of updating volumes when warranted.

Medical researchers have been making tremendous strides, and the challenge to stay current with the most recent advances is one our editors take seriously. Each decision to update a volume will be made on an individual basis. Some of the considerations will include how much new information is available and the feedback we receive from people who use the books. If there's a topic you would like to see added to the update list, or an area of medical concern you feel has not been adequately addressed, please write to:

Editor
Health Reference Series
Omnigraphics, Inc.
2500 Penobscot Bldg.
Detroit, MI 48226

The commitment to providing on-going coverage of important medical developments has also led to some technical changes in the *Health Reference Series*. Beginning with books published in 1999, each new volume will be individually titled and called a "First Edition." Subsequent updates will carry sequential edition numbers. To help avoid confusion and to provide maximum flexibility in our ability to respond to informational needs, the practice of consecutively numbering each volume will be discontinued.

Part One

The Issues of
Alternative Medicine

Chapter 1

Classification of Alternative Medical Practices

This classification was developed by the ad hoc Advisory Panel to the Office of Alternative Medicine (OAM), National Institutes of Health (NIH) and further refined by the Workshop on Alternative Medicine as described in the report *Alternative Medicine: Expanding Medical Horizons*. This classification was designed to facilitate the grant review process and should not be considered definitive.

Diet, Nutrition, Lifestyle Changes

- Changes in Lifestyle
- Diet
- Nutritional Supplements
- Gerson Therapy
- Macrobiotics
- Megavitamin

Mind/Body Control

- Art Therapy, Relaxation Techniques
- Biofeedback
- Counseling and Prayer Therapies
- Dance Therapy
- Guided Imagery

NIH Information sheet from the Office of Alternative Medicine (OAM), June 1995.

- Humor Therapy
- Hypnotherapy
- Psychotherapy
- Sound, Music Therapy
- Support Groups
- Yoga, Meditation

Alternative Systems of Medical Practice

- Acupuncture
- Anthroposophically Extended Medicine
- Ayurveda
- Community-Based Health Care Practices
- Environmental Medicine
- Homeopathic Medicine
- Latin American Rural Practices
- Native American
- Natural Products
- Naturopathic Medicine
- Past Life Therapy
- Shamanism
- Tibetan Medicine
- Traditional Oriental Medicine

Manual Healing

- Acupressure
- Alexander Technique
- Aromatherapy
- Biofield Therapeutics
- Chiropractic Medicine
- Feldenkrais Method
- Massage Therapy
- Osteopathy
- Reflexology
- Rolfing
- Therapeutic Touch
- Trager Method
- Zone Therapy

Pharmacological and Biological Treatments

- Anti-oxidizing Agents
- Cell Treatment
- Chelation Therapy
- Metabolic Therapy
- Oxidizing Agents (Ozone, Hydrogen Peroxide)

Bioelectromagnetic Applications

- Blue Light Treatment and Artificial Lighting
- Electroacupuncture
- Electromagnetic Fields
- Electrostimulation and Neuromagnetic Stimulation Devices
- Magnetoresonance Spectroscopy

Herbal Medicine

- Echinacea (purple coneflower)
- Ginkgo Biloba extract
- Ginger rhizome
- Ginseng root
- Wild chrysanthemum flower
- Witch hazel
- Yellowdock

Chapter 2

The Nature of Alternative Medicine

The Constitution of this Republic should make special provision for Medical Freedom as well as Religious Freedom . . . To restrict the art of healing to one class of men and deny equal privileges to others will constitute the Bastille of medical science. All such laws are un-American and despotic. They are fragments of monarchy and have no place in a Republic.

—Benjamin Rush

Surgeon General of the Continental Army of the United States Signer of the Declaration of Independence

History of Medicine in the United States

Medicine in the United States has evolved from an eclectic mix of Native American, African, Eastern, and European botanical traditions. In colonial and postcolonial America, there were dozens of competing medical philosophies, each claiming to have the "divine right" to practice medicine. By the early 1800s, medical practitioners included homeopaths, naturopaths, botanics, and Thomsonians. Competition was fierce, and the practice of medicine was essentially wide open (Hogan, 1979).

Extracted from NIH Publication No. 94-066. December 1994. Due to space considerations, bibliographic data have not been reprinted in this chapter. However, to aid readers who wish to consult the original document or do further research, the in-text references have been retained.

7

However, in the mid-1800s, the medical system we now refer to as biomedicine[1] began to dominate the scene. Biomedicine was shaped by two important sets of observations made in the early 1800s: (1) specific organic entities—bacteria—were responsible for producing particular disease states and characteristic pathological damage; and (2) certain substances—antitoxins and vaccines—could improve an individual's ability to ward off the effects of these and other pathogens. Armed with this knowledge, investigators and clinicians began to conquer a myriad of devastating infectious diseases and to perfect surgical procedures. As their conquests mounted, biomedical scientists came to believe that once they found the offending pathogen, metabolic error, or chemical imbalance, all afflictions—including many mental illnesses—would eventually yield to the appropriate vaccine, antibiotic, or chemical compound (Gordon, 1980). This philosophy eventually led them to extend their purview beyond the bounds of physical and even mental disease to conditions that previously had been viewed in religious, moral, economic, or political terms. For example, births and deaths, which traditionally had taken place at home, were moved to the hospital.

During the late 1800s, the American Medical Association (AMA), which was first organized in 1847, sponsored and lobbied for enactment of State licensing laws. By 1900, every State had enacted such a law. The result was a quick decline in competition from other schools of medical practice (Starr, 1982). The ability of biomedicine to eliminate competition was further strengthened with the passage of the Pure Food and Drug Act of 1906 and the first court trial under this act in 1908 (McGinnis, 1991). In 1910, the fate of competing forms of medicine was sealed with the release of a report by Abraham Flexner, a U.S. educator and founder of the Institute for Advanced Study in Princeton, NJ. Flexner's report, *Medical Education in the United States and Canada*, was funded by the Carnegie Foundation and was instrumental in upgrading medical education. However, it also enabled medical schools with a greater orientation toward biomedicine research to receive preferential treatment from the large philanthropic foundations that were then awarding money for medical education. Indirectly, this development led to the demise of the more financially strapped alternative medical schools (King, 1984).

Although the Flexner Report is properly credited with closing many substandard medical teaching establishments, an unfortunate side effect was a complete stifling of all competing schools of thought regarding the origins of illness and the appropriateness of therapies (Coulter, 1973). This effect occurred even though Flexner had no firsthand knowledge of medicine or medical science, or of the scientific method and its potential inadequacies (King, 1984). Indeed, in the years after his report was published, Flexner became increasingly disenchanted with the rigidity of the educational standards that had become identified with his name (Starr, 1982).

With the loss of their medical schools, all but a few alternative medical systems and practices vanished into obscurity. In 1907 there were approximately 160 medical schools in the United States; by 1914, 4 years after the Flexner Report, that number had declined to around 100 (King, 1984). Thus, by the early part of this century, biomedicine had become the standard, or convention, for every facet of health and illness. As a result, for the next half century it overshadowed "less scientific" paradigms, and those who adopted and practiced it accumulated great power and prestige. Rival healing professions and perspectives gradually disappeared, were relegated to "fringe" status, or were swallowed up by the biomedical paradigm. Some alternative medicines degenerated into the stereotypical "snake oil" proprietary medicines, further eroding the credibility of legitimate alternative medicine practitioners.

Several decades ago, however, consumer confidence in conventional medicine began to show some signs of waning. Reports emerged on the side effects and inadequacies of widely used drugs, and new strains of bacteria suddenly appeared that were resistant to the first "magic bullet" antibiotics. The use of new, more powerful antibiotics eventually resulted in microbes that could thwart them, too. Meanwhile, cures for arthritis, allergies, hypertension, cancer, depression, cardiovascular disease, digestive problems, and other chronic conditions—which had replaced infectious disease as the major killers and cripplers—eluded the best minds of biomedicine. Also, the civil rights, consumer's, and women's movements raised serious questions about the availability and equity of the allocation of health care resources under this system (Gordon, 1980).

As a result, many Americans began to look outside conventional medicine for relief. Indeed, according to a recent survey conducted by Dr. David Eisenberg of the Harvard School of Medicine and Ronald Kessler of the Survey Research Center, so-called alternative therapies appear to be as popular as ever (Eisenberg et al., 1993). This survey found that in 1990 an estimated 61 million Americans used an alternative therapy and 22 million saw a provider of alternative therapies for a principal medical condition.

More intriguing, Americans appear to have made more total visits to practitioners of alternative medicine than to conventional primary care physicians—425 million visits versus 388 million—even though most of these visits to alternative practitioners were paid out of pocket (i.e., were not covered by medical insurance). Americans spent an estimated $13.7 billion on alternative therapies in 1990, of which $10.3 billion was paid out of pocket. This is almost as much as the out-of-pocket expenditure for all hospital care in the United States that year ($12.8 billion), and it is nearly half the amount spent out of pocket for all physicians' services in the United States ($23.5 billion). Thus, alternative medicine appears to represent a significant portion of Americans' health care expenditures. Furthermore, as the Eisenberg and Kessler survey showed, the majority of people seeking alternative medical therapies are those with chronic illnesses who believe that conventional medicine has few, if any, effective treatments for their conditions.

Distinction Between Alternative and Conventional Medicine

In a narrow sense, alternative medical practices today are often defined as those that are not widely practiced in hospitals or taught in conventional U.S. medical school curriculums (Eisenberg et al., 1993). However, "alternative" medicine can refer to any one of a number of practices, techniques, and systems that may challenge the commonly assumed viewpoints or bureaucratic priorities of our dominant professionalized system of health care.

Besides wide differences in the philosophical underpinnings and the types of therapies offered by mainstream and alternative medicine, there are also major differences in how therapies are administered and how the practitioners and patients interact. For example, conventional medicine practitioners tend to give their patients standardized treatments (typically drugs or surgery or both) and medical advice on the basis of whether the patient fits into one of a number of broadly defined symptomatic categories. Furthermore, the educational theory most familiar to conventional physicians and the one they most frequently use when interacting with their patients is "physician centered." In this model, the physician is the authoritative expert and the patient is a receptive participant (Brunton, 1984). This type of communication has been found to be lacking in addressing patient needs; it encourages passivity in patients, which may undermine the patient's commitment and determination to carry out the recommended treatment regimen (McCann and Blossom, 1990).

In comparison, because alternative medical practitioners often see each patient as unique, they tend to individualize treatment to the extreme and to create elaborate procedures for identifying individual suitability and sensitivity to the interventions. They also frequently use multiple treatment modalities and judge effectiveness by using multiple or unusual outcomes, many of them subjective and patient de-rived (Jonas, 1993). Furthermore, many alternative systems of medicine are converging toward a client-centered relationship, where emphasis is placed on the patient's responsibility in the healing process. Patient-centered exchanges have been found to maximize the collaboration be-tween the physician and patient, thus enhancing the benefits of a therapy. Indeed, Rosenberg (1971) showed that patients who feel they have some control over their treatment have better outcomes.

Unifying Threads among the Alternative Medical Systems

Because the term *alternative medicine* is used to describe such a wide variety of medical systems and therapies, they cannot easily be categorized. Despite this diversity, most alternative systems of medi-cine do hold some common beliefs. First, there is the overarching be-lief that humans have built-in recuperative powers, such as when a cut heals into a scar. Most alternative medicine adherents believe that this phenomenon, referred to as *vis medicatrix naturae* (the healing power of nature), can be speeded up, sometimes to an astonishing degree, by the proper stimuli (Inglis, 1965). Thus, alternative medi-cal practitioners typically focus on therapies designed to stimulate the patient's constitution to fight on its own behalf, on the assumption that this emphasis on enhancing the natural healing process is the most appropriate foundation of any medical therapy.

In addition, several other unifying threads are common to most alternative medical systems. These include emphasis on the

- *Integration of individuals in the "stream of life,"* that is, one's relationships and place in society, one's sense of value and self-esteem, and the various meanings and values one perceives in life (Dossey, 1991).

- *Importance of religious and spiritual values to health.* These factors are largely ignored or considered of secondary impor-tance in contemporary medical science (Larson and Larson, 1991; Larson et al., 1992; Levin and Schiller, 1987).

- *Attribution of a causal, independent role to the various "mani-festations of consciousness."* One's thoughts, attitudes, feelings, emotions, values, and perceived meanings are capable of directly affecting one's physical function. This causal view of the mind has been called "downward causation" by Nobel laureate Roger Sperry; it contrasts with the idea of "upward causation," which is currently favored in medical science. Upward causation views all mental activity as a derivative of the biochemical and physiological processes of the brain; essentially, the mind is equated with the brain, and thus the mind is regarded as a "brain in disguise." Almost all alternative medical systems maintain that consciousness may manifest itself "through" or "via" the brain, but they do not equate the two (Sperry, 1987, 1991).

- *Maintaining the Hippocratic injunction: first do no harm.* In general, many alternative practitioners use the least harmful therapies first. In addition, most alternative therapies tend to avoid suppressing symptoms because the symptoms are understood to be a manifestation of a more profound underlying imbalance—in physiology, attitude, and lifestyle—that must be addressed. Therefore, most alternative medical practitioners tend to rely primarily on diet, exercise, relaxation techniques, and lifestyle and changes in attitude to bring about changes in health.

- *Use of whole substances.* Alternative practitioners understand that pharmacological agents, which may be extracted or synthesized from plants, may be more potent and fast acting. However, whole foods and herbs are believed to produce fewer adverse side effects.

In addition, the following concepts often are used by alternative systems of medicine and their practitioners and are important in understanding the rationale for such treatments:

- *Holism.* Holism is the principle that all aspects of the person—physical, emotional, mental, and psychosocial health; diet; lifestyle; and so on—are interrelated and must be considered in treatment, not just the specific disease or specific body part that is affected. The holistic practitioner looks equally at the relationship among these aspects of the total person and at the presenting disorder. Closely associated with the principle of holism is the principle of balance.

- *Balance and imbalance.* Balance refers to harmony among organs in the body and among body systems, in a person's diet, and in relationships to other individuals, society, and the environment.

Balance or imbalance in any of these systems is understood to holistically affect other systems as well. Thus people who are out of balance with society find their organs affected because of the societal imbalance. The quality of imbalance is expressed in similar but slightly different ways in different alternative medical systems—too hot or too cold, too *yin* (weak, quiet) or too *yang* (strong, loud), too high or too low, too wet or too dry, too sweet or too salty. To achieve balance, energy must be equalized between the imbalanced portions. People who use this term often do not use the concept of "disease"[2] or use it in a much modified form.

- *Energy* refers to the force necessary to achieve balance; the part of the system that is deficient needs to acquire energy while the part that has excess needs to release energy. Thus (in traditional Chinese medicine, for example) when an organ is imbalanced, it is either too yang or too yin. Therefore, *qi* (the Chinese term for energy) must be transferred from the yang organ to the yin organ to restore balance and reestablish harmony among the organs; the harmony achieved extends holistically into all aspects (mental, physical, and psychosocial) of the person with beneficial effect. In practice, the holistic practitioner is likely to boost the vis medicatrix naturae by, for example, stimulating the immune system, balancing organ function by moving energy from the excessive organ to the deficient organ, altering diet to include more (or less) hot (or cold) foods, and prescribing more (or less) specific exercise or other lifestyle changes.

- *Healing and curing.* Because of the focus on the total person, many alternative practitioners often measure their treatment success, or lack of it, on healing the total person—bringing all aspects of the person into better balance, rather than just focusing on curing a given disease or disorder. In this view, where total outcome is more important than specific result, it is possible for the person to be *healed* without the disease being *cured*, although the intent is always to do both.

Interface Between Alternative and Conventional Medicine

In some areas, the distinction between what is alternative and what is conventional is not always so clear-cut, because there is a constant progression of therapies from the "fringe" into the mainstream. For example, manipulative therapies such as chiropractic were considered fringe therapies 20 years ago but now are gaining increasing acceptance in mainstream medicine in the United States (Cherkin et al., 1989). In a recent survey of conventional physicians in Britain, 75 percent said that some alternative practices had become conventional between 1982 and 1987. Fifty-four percent said that musculoskeletal manipulation had become conventional, 47 percent reported the same for hypnosis, and 45 percent said that acupuncture had become conventional for certain problems (Reilly and Taylor, 1991).

This increasing acceptance of some forms of alternative medicine is demonstrated by the fact that in the past few decades, a small but growing number of M.D.s in America have organized and taken courses in manipulative medicine to better serve their patients (Gevitz, 1993). In addition, an estimated 3,000 conventionally trained physicians—M.D.s and D.O.s (doctors of osteopathy)—have been trained to incorporate acupuncture as a treatment modality in their medical practices through courses such as those affiliated with the University of California, Los Angeles, School of Medicine; the New York University School of Medicine and Dentistry; and St. Louis University Medical School (Lytle, 1993).

Furthermore, a number of tenets of naturopathy, especially those linking particular foods to the incidence of certain diseases such as cancer, are beginning to gain more credence in mainstream science. Many recent case control and cohort studies indicate associations between high intake of red meat and increased risk of some forms of cancer (Willett, 1990); other studies have focused on the anticancer protective effects of a vegetarian diet (Rao and Janezic, 1992). Such associations have led to increased interest among researchers worldwide in investigating the role that micronutrients and other substances in fruits and vegetables may play in preventing or inhibiting serious disease (Lee, 1993).

Given that what is considered alternative today may be the accepted treatment for a particular condition in a decade or two, the following question arises: Could any of today's fringe therapies have a significant, immediate impact on the pressing and costly medical problems facing the Nation if they were more widely available?

Barriers to Progress on Alternative Medicine Research

Barriers to a fair, unbiased, scientific evaluation of alternative therapies can be categorized as structural barriers (problems caused by classification, definition, cultural, or language barriers), regulatory and economic barriers (the legal and cost implications of compliance or noncompliance with Federal and State regulations), and belief barriers (obstacles caused by ideology, misconceptions, myths, etc.).

Structural Barriers

As mentioned previously, a basic problem in investigating alternative therapies is that a clear definition of alternative medicine is almost impossible to devise. Alternative therapies are often referred to by a diverse group of sometimes derogatory pseudonyms, including "unconventional," "unorthodox," "integrated," "non-mainstream," "traditional," "nontraditional," "natural," "unscientific," "holistic," "wholistic," and many others, making classification difficult (Jonas, 1993). Other questions arise: Is the use of megavitamins, food supplements, or nutritional regimens to treat disease considered medicine, or is it a lifestyle change, or both? Can having one's aching back massaged be considered a medical therapy? How should spiritual healing and prayer—some of the oldest, most widely applied, and least studied unconventional approaches—be classified?

Because the line between conventional and alternative is imprecise and frequently changing, an approach to evaluation must be devised that is useful for comparing all types of therapy. The unfamiliar diagnostic outcome categories in many alternative approaches may require two sets of classification criteria (Wiegart et al., 1991). Traditional acupuncture, for example, classifies patients according to excesses or deficiencies in vital energy, or *chi*, in contrast to Western diagnostic classifications that are based on pathological or symptom complexes (coronary artery disease, depression, etc.). Scientists rarely understand and may oversimplify these alternative medicine concepts and thus may design methodologically correct research on the basis of incorrect classifications, resulting in unusable data (Bensoussan, 1991; Patel, 1991).

In addition, reprints of original research in alternative medicine are difficult to locate. Many alternative medicine research studies, especially those conducted in other countries, are not published in scientifically reviewed literature, and much of what does exist is not in English. For example, more than 600 research articles or abstracts have been published on the medical effects of *qigong* (a Chinese term for a form of energy), but few have been translated from Chinese (Sancier et al., 1993). The retrieval of information on alternative medicine from online databases is often inadequate, because these databases do not routinely collect articles from alternative medicine journals (Bareta et al., 1990; Dickerson, 1990; Easterbrook et al., 1991) or because the ones they do collect are not accessible by standard search languages.

Many alternative medicine practitioners are primarily clinicians rather than researchers, and medical practice is their primary priority. Therefore, case series and anecdotal reports are often their only evidence that a practice is effective. Even so, the quality of the research presented by alternative medical practitioners is not always poor, and the fact that an article is published in an alternative medical journal does not mean the study is inferior. For example, a meta-analysis of 107 published controlled trials of homeopathic treatments to assess their methodological quality found that while many of the trials were of "low" methodological quality, there appeared to be an overall positive effect from the homeopathic treatment regardless of the quality of the trial. The authors of the study noted that while no definitive conclusions about the effectiveness of homeopathic treatments could be drawn, the meta-analysis supported a legitimate case for the further evaluation of homeopathy (Kleijnen et al., 1991).

Therefore, one cannot assume that practices unfamiliar to conventional physicians and researchers are necessarily backed by poor-quality research. Surprisingly, adequate methods for judging the quality of research in individual alternative medicine studies, both published and unpublished, still remain an underdeveloped research area. Scientists who conduct reviews of the literature on alternative medicine must be comprehensive, systematic, and explicit (Fuchs and Garber, 1990; Larson et al., 1986; Sachett et al., 1991).

Finally, many conventional physicians remain virtually unaware that alternative approaches exist, even though their patients are seeing them and alternative medical practitioners simultaneously for the same condition. The Eisenberg-Kessler survey (Eisenberg et al., 1993) found that 70 percent of patients seeking alternative practices did not reveal to their conventional physicians that they had done so. Patients' unwillingness to reveal this information to their conventional physicians may be largely due to the physician-centered model discussed above. Recently, an increasing number of members of the conventional medical community have called for physicians to move toward a patient-centered model for educating and interacting with patients. The impetus for this is a realization that the majority of patients want to participate in their clinical decision-making and are more likely to adhere to a prescribed therapy using this approach (Brody and Larson, 1992; Brunton, 1984; Titus et al. 1980).

Regulatory and Economic Barriers

Today there are literally hundreds of treatments that are considered alternative, or outside the range of conventional medical treatment modalities. These treatments include various forms of behavioral, psychological, and spiritual interventions, as well as a host of herbal, pharmacological, nutritional, and mechanical therapies. Promoters of these therapies include trained physicians and other allied health care practitioners as well as laypersons.

The U.S. Food and Drug Administration (FDA) is the Federal agency most responsible for protecting consumers against unsafe and ineffective medicines and health products in the marketplace. Armed with broad regulatory powers delegated to the agency by the Food, Drug, and Cosmetic Act (FDCA), FDA oversees distribution of the Nation's food supply, oversees development and marketing of new drugs and medical devices, and generally supervises the promotion of these items to ensure that consumers are not harmed or defrauded.

Under the FDCA, new drugs require extensive laboratory and animal testing before their sponsors can petition FDA for an investigational new drug (IND) application for limited testing in humans. IND applications must state in detail how the clinical trials will be conducted (e.g., how subjects will be selected and how many will be involved with the studies), where the studies will be done and by whom, and how the product's safety and effectiveness will be evaluated.

Clinical trials are generally done in three phases. Phase I studies are designed to determine the safety of the product using small numbers of healthy subjects. Phase II studies are concerned more with the effectiveness of the product, usually employ up to several hundred volunteers diagnosed with the particular disease or condition under investigation, and may take two years or more to complete. Phase III studies, which may require several hundred to several thousand subjects and take four years or more to complete, are then designed to elaborate the correct dosage and frequency of administration of the product (Evers, 1988).

The entire drug approval process is time-consuming and extremely expensive, forcing treatment sponsors to spend millions of dollars each year to comply with FDA's safety and efficacy regulations. For example, a manufacturer must submit more than 100,000 pages of supporting documentation in connection with a single new drug application (Hect, 1983). It can take up to 10 years and cost hundreds of millions of dollars to obtain FDA approval of a new drug (Evers, 1988). These astronomical costs are beyond the reach of all but a few

17

corporations and can be recouped only by exercising the legal 17-year monopolies conferred by the U.S. patent laws. With a patent, drug companies can and do charge whatever the market will bear.

Thus, the current Federal mechanisms of regulating medical research do not favor the evaluation of many forms of alternative treatment. Because the costs of developing, evaluating, and marketing new drugs are so prohibitive, pharmaceutical companies are not likely to invest time and effort in therapies, such as nutritional or behavioral approaches, that cannot be patented and are therefore unlikely to offer the opportunity to recover their investment and provide a return to stockholders. This means that many alternative therapies are likely to be casualties of the formal research process.

Although foods are exempt from such extensive premarketing clearance, the FDA often regulates foods as if they were drugs whenever any health claims are associated with a product, even though the same product may also qualify as a food or as a cosmetic. A recent controversy surrounding the advertising campaign of a popular breakfast cereal demonstrates how overzealous FDA can be at times. FDA disapproved of the manufacturer's claims that its cereal would help prevent colon cancer, even though the company had prepared the advertisement in cooperation with the National Cancer Institute. FDA launched a probe into the matter, which it later had to abandon (Evers, 1988).

FDA has long attempted to regulate vitamins and minerals as drugs. The AMA supports this view and has urged Congress to grant FDA such authority (U.S. Congress, 1984). To date, Congress has not chosen to extend FDA's drug jurisdiction to encompass vitamins and minerals, except in cases where therapeutic claims are made for products.

Although the FDCA is the most comprehensive law designed to prevent interstate marketing of unapproved drugs, several other Federal statutes also are applicable to promotion or sale. The Federal Trade Commission (FTC) often uses the term false advertisement under the Federal Trade Commission Act to prevent the manufacturers of alternative therapies from promoting their products or services. Courts have generally held that the FTC does not have to show that an advertiser lacked good faith or intended to deceive, nor must it show that actual deception occurred. Rather, it has to show only that the potential to deceive might be there.

The FTC frequently seeks to hinder what it considers false advertising dealing with disease prevention or cure. For example, in 1983 the FTC sought to prohibit the manufacturer of a dietary supplement—which contained vitamins A, C, and E; selenium; beta-carotene;

and dehydrated vegetables—from advertising its product as reducing the risk of certain cancers. The manufacturer's claims were based on the findings of a report entitled *Diet, Nutrition, and Cancer*, published by the National Research Council (1982). The FTC successfully argued that the manufacturer's representations went well beyond the report's conclusions and thus were false, misleading, and deceptive because they conveyed the impression that simply consuming daily portions of the product would prevent cancer. Accordingly, an injunction was issued prohibiting such advertisements (Evers, 1988).

In addition to FDA and FTC restrictions and regulations, the Federal Government routinely uses numerous other statutes to curtail the promotion of alternative treatments and practices. Statutes such as the mail fraud and wire fraud statutes and the "smuggling statute" are among the many laws that provide criminal penalties for those who promote unapproved products through the mail or on the radio or attempt to import them from overseas. Penalties can be fines of up to $10,000 or five years' imprisonment or both.

Another major barrier to the investigation and acceptance of alternative medicine is the existence in all States of medical practice acts that limit the practice of healing arts to holders of medical licenses. The history of medical licensure illustrates not only the enormous power bestowed on professional groups by regulation, but also the ways licensing has been used to eliminate or curtail the activities of alternative medical practitioners, regardless of whether their methods have been proved harmful. For example, throughout this century the medical professional organizations have used a variety of weapons to harass osteopathic and chiropractic physicians. Indeed, conventional medical organizations have historically prohibited their members from even consulting with "sectarian" practitioners such as homeopaths and chiropractors (see below). Medical organizations establish such prohibitions for reasons that have to do as much with ideology as with economics. The ideological reasons are discussed below.

Belief Barriers

Conventional physicians in general adhere to a number of beliefs and misconceptions about themselves and the type of medicine they practice that prevent them from viewing anything labeled "alternative" in a positive light or taking it seriously. The following are some of the ideological grounds for conventional physicians' skepticism of alternative systems of medicine and their therapies.

- **Confidence in high technology.** High-tech diagnostic and therapeutic procedures in modern medicine are often enormously attractive to the physician. However, confidence in these instruments and procedures often exceeds the evidence for their effectiveness (Grimes, 1993). As a result, many alternative therapies, which are often relatively "low tech," may be considered ineffective.

- **Safety in the status quo.** Once in place, established therapies often tend to prevail over new or alternative treatments. How much and what kind of evidence is necessary for implementing an alternative therapy? This question has not been fully answered even for conventional therapies. For example, acceptance of a new drug therapy usually requires repeated, double-blind, placebo-controlled, randomized clinical trials, whereas implementation of new surgical techniques may at times be done without any controlled trials at all (Eddy, 1990).

- **The "one true" medical profession.** A longstanding belief held by many conventional medical practitioners is that there should be only one representative voice for the whole of medicine (Gevitz, 1989). That is, only the members of their profession, holders of a certain degree from approved institutions, are the bona fide, rightful, and exclusive representatives of medicine, and they should be allowed to control all aspects of medical practice (Inglis, 1965). For example, in the 1960s the AMA decided to contain and eliminate chiropractic as a profession. To do so, in 1963 the AMA formed its Committee on Quackery, which worked aggressively—both overtly and covertly—to find ways to cut off chiropractors from their base of patients. One of the AMA's principal means of achieving this goal was to make it unethical for a medical physician to associate with an "unscientific practitioner." Then, in 1966, the AMA's House of Delegates passed a resolution calling chiropractic an "unscientific cult." To complete the circle, the AMA's Judicial Council issued an opinion holding that it was unethical for a physician to associate professionally with chiropractors (Gevitz, 1989).

Although the AMA gradually relaxed some of its taboos regarding chiropractors, these relaxed positions were generally not communicated to AMA members (Gevitz, 1989). However, in the August 1987 *Wilk et al. V. the American Medical Association* decision, a Federal judge found that the AMA, the American College

of Radiology, and the American College of Surgeons had con-
spired to intentionally harm the chiropractic profession and
were thus guilty of violating the Sherman Antitrust Act (Special
Communication, 1988). Under the court's ruling, the AMA was
ordered to cease and desist its hampering of chiropractors and
to send a copy of the injunction to each of its members.

- *Stereotypes.* One stereotype of alternative medicine that is
widely propagated is that it attracts people with "weak" minds
(i.e., the uneducated and the poor) who easily succumb to the
"sideshow" lures of "snake oil" salespeople, who are not qualified to give medical advice or to practice medicine. However, recent studies of cancer patients indicate that, much to the
contrary, well-educated persons with higher incomes are more
likely to use alternative treatments, primarily because they
want to take charge of their health (Lerner and Kennedy, 1992;
McGinnis, 1991). Furthermore, more than 60 percent of practitioners of alternative treatments for cancer hold an M.D., a
Ph.D., or both from an accredited medical school or graduate
school (Cassileth et al., 1984). In addition, the term *quack*, as a
blanket indictment of all those who practice alternative forms of
medicine, is often used more as an insult than as an objective
assessment of someone's skills and intentions. According to Dr.
David J. Hufford, professor of behavioral science at the Pennsylvania State College of Medicine, the term *quack* generally
means "one who pretends to have medical knowledge but does
not; that is, it implies the element of fraud." Hufford contends
that most alternative healers do not pretend to have medical
knowledge but possess some other sort of knowledge that they
and their clients believe is relevant to health. "Certainly the use
of caution to protect oneself and one's family from unscrupulous
and incompetent health care pretenders should be part of
everyone's concern. But this is not limited to alternative medicine," he maintains (Hufford, 1990).

The barriers facing many aspects of alternative medicine today are
typical of the barriers that have faced novel scientific ideas throughout the centuries. At the root of this conflict is the fact that alternative and mainstream medical scientists often have two diametrically
opposed views, not just on which drugs and vaccines are appropriate
or most effective for a particular condition, but on the nature of life
itself.

The 20th-century scientific philosopher Thomas Kuhn put this age-old conflict into perspective by saying that scientific doctrines rest not just on facts, but more fundamentally on paradigms (i.e., broad views of how those facts should be organized).[3] Differences in views among groups of people are a reflection of the different scientific paradigms they adhere to. According to Kuhn, because unusual scientific discoveries often require more than incremental adjustments to the dominant scientific paradigm, the hapless innovator who stumbles upon some new set of facts that run counter to the dominant paradigm often finds it necessary to elaborate a whole new paradigm to accommodate them. When this happens, the innovator often becomes a scientific outcast, for, as Kuhn wrote, "to desert the paradigm is to cease practicing the science it defines" (Kuhn, 1970). For example, Louis Pasteur, the father of microbiology, was thrown out of the Academy of Medicine for suggesting that microbes that could not be seen by the naked eye were responsible for causing food to spoil and that spontaneous generation (life arising from nonliving matter) was an impossibility (Kostychev, 1978). Thus, bridging the gap between the different paradigms of the conventional medical and alternative medical communities is and always has been a formidable challenge. However, as the public turns increasingly to alternative medical practitioners for treatment, pressure is mounting on the mainstream scientific and medical communities as well as on Federal and State scientific and regulatory bodies to speed up the investigation and evaluation of "novel" approaches. The public is demanding a streamlined evaluation process not only to provide it with more health care options, but also to provide definitive answers about the safety and efficacy of alternative therapies that are being offered. Claire Cassidy, Ph.D., James S. Gordon, M.D., Ralph W. Moss, Ph.D., and Richard Pavek contributed to this section.

Footnotes

1. *This is the more accurate technical term for the style of medical practice in which practitioners hold either an M.D. (medical doctor) or D.O. (doctor of osteopathy) degree. Other terms for this system include allopathy, Western medicine, regular medicine, conventional medicine, mainstream medicine, and cosmopolitan medicine. All these terms have some applicability, but none is as accurate as biomedicine. Allopathy, the most specific of these terms, denotes a tendency to choose therapies that oppose symptoms (allo = opposite) and enables parallels with terms such as osteopathy, homeopathy, and naturopathy.*

The other terms (mainstream, conventional, etc.) are less accurate but are better known and thus will be used throughout this text interchangeably with biomedicine.

2. Disease is a technical concept, especially developed in biomedicine, that refers to a limited, well-defined condition such as a specific infection (measles) or deficiency (beri-beri). It has expanded to take in many less well-defined conditions for which the "cause" is complex, such as duodenal ulcer, stroke, or breast cancer. Some conditions, especially psychosocial conditions such as alcoholism and depression, which straddle the line between moral failing and disease, are becoming "medicalized," or pushed away from the moral fading category and into the disease category. In contrast, illness and sickness are social terms that emphasize sensations of unwellness and discomfort and imply a change in relationship toward family and work. Sociologically speaking, people take on the "sick role" at the time when they claim sickness and those around them accept the claim. People can have a disease and not know it, in which case they are not ill or sick because they have not recognized their condition of frailty and have not sought the sick role. Or a person can feel ill or sick and seek the sick role but be denied it, at least by medical specialists, if they "can find no wrong." When both sickness and disease overlap, everyone involved in the communication agrees that "something is wrong with this person."

3. A paradigm is an overarching cosmological conceptual scheme; an explanatory model explains a limited set of events or observations from within a paradigm and using the guidance of a paradigm. Alternative words for paradigm include world-view, framework, and weltanschauung, all of which suggest the largeness of the concept. A paradigm tells whole societies in whole historical periods how to think about such "big issues" as goodness, success, holiness, love, and evil. Much of a paradigm is out of awareness—that is, people act on it without realizing that they have other choices. In contrast, an explanatory model is the way one discipline, denomination, or health care system explains itself—the details of its assumptions, logic, and rationale—and much of this is within the awareness of its practitioners, and is therefore open to argument, criticism, and change.

—by Larry Dossey, M.D. and James P. Swyers, M.A.

23

Chapter 3

Cultural Diversity, Folk Medicine, and Alternative Medicine

"Alternative medicine," a relatively recent term, has important connections with "folk medicine." For example, botanical or phytomedicine has developed from the folk herbalist traditions of many cultures; modern midwifery has recent historical roots in the folk health practices of women; and spiritual approaches to alternative medicine, even when described in the language of quantum mechanics, have developed from and remain parallel with folk religious healing traditions. Such connections have important ethical, legal, and clinical implications that grow out of cultural diversity issues in healthcare.

The ethnic and cultural diversity of the US population has grown constantly throughout history. During much of that time, established American groups assumed that newcomers would be assimilated into existing cultural patterns (the "melting pot" model). Now, late in the 20th century, this assimilation model has been recognized as neither a good description of what has happened nor a plausible prediction of what can happen as our population continues to diversify. The linguistic, religious, and other cultural patterns of American society are now more varied than ever, and medicine, like other institutions, works to develop appropriate methods for a pluralistic society.

In an essay titled "Culture and Clinical Care," pediatrician Lee Pachter[1] discusses the clinical importance of cultural differences in beliefs about health and disease, using the folk medical beliefs of Latinos to illustrate the point. More recently, the third edition of

Mosby's Guide to Physical Examination devotes an entire chapter[2] to cultural awareness, emphasizing cultural values and beliefs and their impact on health behavior and, by extension, on care. This chapter provides a chart of cultural characteristics including a column of health and diet practices for Americans from 10 different ethnic groups including Chinese Americans, African-Americans, Mexican Americans, and Native Americans. The health practices listed range from the use of herbs and dietary manipulations to acupuncture or acupressure to spiritual practices invoking supernatural intervention.

The importance of such information, as Pachter points out, is that people with medically unconventional beliefs may still present in medical clinics for care. In fact, not only is it the case that in "culturally pluralistic settings, people go to 'doctors for 'medical' illness and to 'folk healers' for folk illnesses," but also patients sometimes use medical doctors and folk practitioners simultaneously.

Because these cultural differences are medically significant, there have been efforts to identity those patients most likely to have strong convictions about "ethnocultural health beliefs and behaviors." Pachter[1(p130)] characterizes those patients in six categories; they are those who:

1. are recent immigrants to the mainland United States,
2. who live in ethnic enclaves,
3. who prefer to use their native tongue,
4. who are educated in their country of origin,
5. who migrate back and forth to the country of origin, and
6. who are in constant contact with older individuals who maintain a high degree of ethnic identity.

Pachter says that these people may be considered less acculturated.

Although recent writing on this subject has been done in a sensitive and sophisticated fashion, it consistently omits what is probably the largest group of American patients possessing cultural health beliefs and practices that are medically unconventional. These are American-born, English-speaking, middle-class people with college educations. Every good study of medically unconventional health beliefs and practices in the past 25 years has shown that this group possesses and acts on a great variety of health beliefs and practices—including many borrowed from the cultural groups cited in Mosby, Pachter, and other publications on cultural diversity.

The best quantitative study[3] to date was published in 1993 in *The New England Journal of Medicine* by David Eisenberg, MD, and colleagues at Harvard. Their large national survey found that 34 percent of those surveyed used alternative medicine, and that those with more education and higher income were most likely to use it.

The Harvard study simply confirmed earlier work, including a 1986 Harris poll done for the US Department of Health and Human Services. My own studies in central Pennsylvania have shown the same phenomena.

It is true that middle-class American English speakers fit rather well with Pachter's criteria. They do tend to live in "ethnic enclaves," they "prefer their native tongue," they were "educated in their country of origin," and they do have contact with "older individuals who maintain a high degree of ethnic identity." But this is clearly not what Pachter had in mind. These patients are not recent immigrants and they do not have to "migrate frequently to their country of origin." They are most definitely not "less acculturated." And yet they share with "recently arrived groups" the simultaneous use of conventional medicine and a host of other treatments ranging from self-care to healers operating outside medicine. And now, evidence suggests that newly immigrated groups share the tendency for the more acculturated members to be the most likely to use their culture's "folk medicines."

For example, a study[4] published in 1990 found that those most likely to use traditional Korean health practitioners such as acupuncturists and herbalists were "the most educated and assimilated Korean immigrants."

How can we account for this apparent paradox? Perhaps the first step is to account for the very fact that it seems paradoxical. One hundred years ago healthcare in America was provided by a welter of competing "medical sects." It would not have been news to anyone that patients in the American "mainstream" frequently used a great variety of "alternative practitioners." In 1910, when Abraham Flexner published his famous report revolutionizing medical education, part of his purpose was to bring an end to the popularity of folk and alternative health practices in favor of scientifically grounded medicine. By establishing consistent standards for the scientific and clinical education of physicians, Flexner expected that homeopathy, chiropractic, osteopathy, Christian Science—in short, systems competing with regular or "allopathic" medicine—would disappear. With good education and science, medicine would come to include everything that research showed to be effective. What was not shown to be effective would wither and die. There would not be different kinds of medicine (apart from legitimate medical specialties). There would just be good, rationally founded medicine.

27

The regulatory developments that followed did have substantial success in suppressing competition to regular medicine, but although the competing practices were rendered considerably less visible for several decades, they did not disappear. In fact, they now flourish. They are represented by the Office of Alternative Medicine at the National Institutes of Health. They are increasingly being covered by insurers. And studies such as those by Eisenberg show that they command a substantial share of the healthcare market.

For 60 or 70 years following the Flexner Report, alternative medicine, generally called "folk medicine" or "unorthodox medicine"—or sometimes "marginal medicine"—was studied by several disciplines, and the particular interests and approaches of each have had an impact on current images. Anthropologists have traditionally studied non-Western cultures, including their medical systems. In recent years they have increasingly turned their attention to the United States, but their selection of populations for study continues to be influenced by their discipline's history. They have therefore tended to focus on new immigrant groups, Native Americans, and others isolated from the cultural mainstream by political, ethnic, linguistic, or geographical barriers; that is, those who—as Pachter suggested—are relatively unacculturated to modern, North American culture.

Sociology has generally given less attention to folk medicine. However, medical sociologists have shown an increasing awareness that "self-treatment, folk medicine, and home remedies . . . [are] far and away the major source of healthcare in the United States.

Within sociology the interest in class differences and the importance of the concept of "deviance" has resulted in an image of alternative health practices similar to that produced in anthropology; that is, an image that emphasizes its difference and the distance from scientific medicine. Finally, the success with which historians of medicine have traced elements of folk medicine back through the millennia has combined with other trends in health systems research to depict folk or alternative medicine as vestigial. Even Erwin Ackerknecht,[6(p7,8)] a medical historian who cautioned against "medical historians [being] obsessed with the evolutionary idea," characterized folk medicine as "10 percent primitive medicine, 50 percent Galenism and 40 percent misunderstood modern technology."

These academic ideas have created an impression that North American mainstream culture is monolithic and relatively homogeneous, and that education has directly led to a consensus that the biomedical healthcare system is the only proper authority on health. At the same time, North American ethnic subcultures have come to be viewed as archaic and deviant, at least to the extent that their health beliefs do not reflect and accept modern medical views. But not only do well-educated, native English-speaking Americans—those assumed to be most "acculturated"—have their own array of alternative health practices, they also make use of the practices of other cultures around the world and of immigrant groups! Acupuncture and moxibustion from China, Ayurveda from India, shamanism from South America, and herbs from all over the world are as influential with middle-class Americans today as the classic Western European alternative systems such as homeopathy, chiropractic, and the health food movement.

What does all this mean? First of all, we should not be too surprised that a cultural circumstance that is ancient and ubiquitous has not changed in just 70 or 80 years. All cultures have diverse health resources ranging from self-care and home first aid through a variety of kinds of healer specialists. And those societies that have had substantial cross-cultural contact have always borrowed and assimilated the health beliefs and practices of those with whom they came in contact. American society is no different in this regard.

But the history of folk and alternative medicine does not bear out that idea. The high-fiber diet and reduced animal fat intake were urged by people whom regular medicine called charlatans and quacks, from the mid-19th century until they became conventional health recommendations less than 20 years ago. Acupuncture was used as an illustration of medical irrationality before Nixon's China trip and James Reston's fortuitous appendicitis brought it to the United States. From the impact of the LaLeche League on the advisability of breast-feeding to current studies of botanical medicines such as ginger, echinacea, and ginkgo biloba, folk and alternative medicines have continuously influenced medical research and practice. And these influences have originated outside conventional medicine. Western neurology would not have created acupuncture. The number of plants in the world and their possible health applications make it very unlikely that even a prodigious effort such as the National Cancer Institute's plant screening program would eventually find all useful botanicals for a single disease. Therefore, the experience of millions of individuals in hundreds of different herbal traditions offers a wealth of leads toward plant medicines. From religious healing traditions and the research they have inspired on the health effects of meditation (such as Herbert Benson, MD'S research at Harvard) to the growing number of studies comparing the spinal manipulation of chiropractors with other interventions for back pain, ideas from outside conventional medicine continue to suggest new investigations and applications. The greater the diversity of theories and observations, the greater the variety of ideas available for empirical testing.

Cultural diversity—including diverse health beliefs and practices—characterizes the entire patient population. It is something that new immigrants have in common with those already here—and something to which they add. It is something that does not fade away in the process of assimilation; rather it becomes more complex. Chinese immigrants have given acupuncture to thousands of Americans just as Indians have been giving yoga to Americans for generations. At the same time that the United States exports modern biomedicine around the world, as well as chiropractic and other distinctively American alternatives, it imports and reconfigures the health practices of cultures all over the globe. This growing cultural complexity is a good thing, and it holds the potential for great benefits. Both alternative and conventional practitioners must keep folk medicine in view as they seek new routes to health— and recall that many of those new routes are in fact ancient.

References

1. Pachter LM. culture and clinical care. *JAMA*. 1994; 271(9):127-131.

2. Sediel HM, Ball JW, Dains JE, Benedict GW. cultural awareness. In: *Mosby's Guide to Physical Examination*. 3rd ed. St. Louis, Mo: Mushy; 1995.

3. Eisenberg DM. Kessler RC, Foster C, Norlock FE, Calkins DR. Delbanco TL.. unconventional medicine in the United States. *N Engli Med*. 1993; 328(4):246-252.

4. Miller JK. Use of traditional Korean health care by Korean immigrants to the United States. *Sociol Soc Rec* 1990:75(1):38.

5. Wolinsky FD. Alternative healers and popular medicine. In: *The Sociology of Health*. Boston. Mass: Little, Brown and Ca: 1980:291-302.

6. Ackerknecht EH. *Medicine and Ethnology: Selected Essays*. Baltimore, Md: Johns Hopkins Press; 1971.

—by David J Hufford, PhD

David J Hufford is director of The Doctors Kienle Center for Humanistic Medicine and a professor of medical humanities. He holds a joint appointment in behavioral science and is an adjunct professor at the University of Pennsylvania.

Chapter 4

A Food and Drug Administration Guide to Choosing Alternative Medical Treatments

Medical treatments come in many shapes and sizes. There are "home remedies" shared between families and friends. There are prescription medicines, available only from a pharmacist, and only when ordered by a physician. There are over-the-counter drugs that you can buy—almost anywhere—without a doctor's order. Of growing interest and attention in recent years are so-called alternative treatments, not yet approved for sale because they are still undergoing scientific research to see if they really are safe and effective. Of course, there are those "miracle" products sold through "back-of-the-magazine" advertisements and TV infomercials.

How can you tell which of these may really help treat your medical condition, and which will only make you worse off—financially, physically, or both?

Many advocates of unproven treatments and cures contend that people have the right to try whatever may offer them hope, even if others believe the remedy is worthless. This argument is especially compelling for people with AIDS or other life-threatening diseases with no known cure.

Clinical Trials

Before gaining Food and Drug Administration marketing approval, new drugs, biologics, and medical devices must be proven safe and effective by controlled clinical trials.

FDA Consumer, June 1995.

31

In a clinical trial, results observed in patients getting the treatment are compared with the results in similar patients receiving a different treatment or placebo (inactive) treatment. Preferably, neither patients nor researchers know who is receiving the therapy under study.

To the FDA, it does not matter whether the product or treatment is labeled alternative or falls under the auspices of mainstream American medical practice. (Mainstream American medicine essentially includes the practices and products the majority of medical doctors in this country follow and use.) It must meet the agency's safety and effectiveness criteria before being allowed on the market.

In addition, just because something is undergoing a clinical trial doesn't mean it works or the FDA considers it to be a proven therapy, says Donald Pohl, of the FDA's Office of AIDS and Special Health Issues. "You can't jump to that conclusion," he says. A trial can fail to prove that the product is effective, he explains. And that's not just true for alternative products. Even when the major drug companies sponsor clinical trials for mainstream products, only a small fraction are proven safe and effective.

Many people with serious illnesses are unable to find a cure, or even temporary relief, from the available mainstream treatments that have been rigorously studied and proven safe and effective. For many conditions, such as arthritis or even cancer, what is effective for one patient may not help another.

Real Alternatives

"It is best not to abandon conventional therapy when there is a known response [in the effectiveness or that therapy]," says Joseph Jacobs, M.D., former director of the National Institutes of Health's Office of Alternative Medicine, which was established in October 1992. As an example he cites childhood leukemia, which has an 80 percent cure rate with conventional therapy.

But what if conventional therapy holds little promise?

Many physicians believe it is not unreasonable for someone in the last stages of an incurable cancer to try something unproven. But, for example, if a woman with an early stage of breast cancer wanted to try shark cartilage (an unproven treatment that may inhibit the growth of cancer tumors, currently undergoing clinical trials), those same doctors would probably say, "Don't do it," because there are so many effective conventional treatments.

Jacobs warns that, "If an alternative practitioner does not want to work with a regular doctor, then he's suspect."

Alternative medicine is often described as any medical practice or intervention that:

- lacks sufficient documentation of its safety and effectiveness against specific diseases and conditions.
- is not generally taught in U.S. medical schools.
- is not generally reimbursable by health insurance providers.

According to a study in the Jan. 28, 1993, *New England Journal of Medicine*, one in three patients used alternative therapy in 1990. More than 80 percent of those who use alternative therapies used conventional medicine at the same time, but did not tell their doctors about the alternative treatments. The study's authors concluded this lack of communication between doctors and patients "is not in the best interest of the patients, since the use of unconventional therapy, especially if it is totally unsupervised, may be harmful." The study concluded that medical doctors should ask their patients about any use of unconventional treatment as part of a medical history.

Many doctors are interested in learning more about alternative therapies, according to Brian Berman, M.D., a family practitioner with the University of Maryland School of Medicine in Baltimore. Berman says his own interest began when "I found that I wasn't getting all the results that I would have liked with conventional medicine, especially in patients with chronic diseases."

"What I've found at the University of Maryland is a healthy skepticism among my colleagues, but a real willingness to collaborate. We have many people from different departments who are saying, let's see how we can develop scientifically rigorous studies that are also sensitive to the particular therapies that we're working with."

Anyone who wants to be treated with an alternative therapy should try to do so through participation in a clinical trial. Clinical trials are regulated by the FDA and provide safeguards to protect patients, such as monitoring of adverse reactions. In fact, the FDA is interested in assisting investigators who want to study alternative therapies under carefully controlled clinical trials.

Some of the alternative therapies currently under study with grants from NIH include:

- acupuncture to treat depression, attention-deficit hyperactivity disorder, osteoarthritis, and postoperative dental pain.
- hypnosis for chronic low back pain and accelerated fracture healing.

- Ayurvedic herbals for Parkinson's disease. (Ayurvedic medicine is a holistic system based on the belief that herbals, massage, and other stress relievers help the body make its own natural drugs.)

- biofeedback for diabetes, low back pain, and face and mouth pain caused by jaw disorders. (Biofeedback is the conscious control of biological functions, such as those of the heart and blood vessels, normally controlled involuntarily.)

- electric currents to treat tumors.

- imagery for asthma and breast cancer. (With imagery, patients are guided to see themselves in a different physical, emotional or spiritual state. For example, patients might be guided to imagine themselves in a state of vibrant health and the disease organisms as weak and destructible.)

While these alternative therapies are the subject of scientifically valid research, it's important to remember that at this time their safety and effectiveness are still unproven.

Avoiding Fraud

The FDA defines health fraud as the promotion, advertisement, distribution, or sale of articles, intended for human or animal use, that are represented as being effective to diagnose, prevent, cure, treat, or mitigate disease (or other conditions), or provide a beneficial effect on health, but which have not been scientifically proven safe and effective for such purposes. Such practices may be deliberately deceptive, or done without adequate knowledge or understanding of the article.

Health fraud costs Americans an estimated $30 billion a year. However, the costs are not just economic, according to John Renner, M.D., a Kansas City-based champion of quality health care for the elderly. "The hidden costs—death, disability—are unbelievable," he says.

To combat health fraud, the FDA established its National Health Fraud Unit in 1988. The unit works with the National Association of Attorneys General and the Association of Food and Drug Officials to coordinate federal, state and local regulatory actions against specific health frauds.

Regulatory actions may be necessary in many cases because products that have not been shown to be safe and effective pose potential hazards for consumers both directly and indirectly. The agency's priorities for regulatory action depend on the situation; direct risks to health come first.

Unproven products cause direct health hazards when their use results in injuries or adverse reactions. For example, a medical device called the InnerQuest Brain Wave Synchronizer was promoted to alter brain waves and relieve stress. It consisted of an audio cassette and eyeglasses that emitted sounds and flashing lights. It caused epileptic seizures in some users. As a result of a court order requested by the FDA, seventy-eight cartons of the devices, valued at $200,000, were seized by U.S. marshals and destroyed in June 1993.

Indirectly harmful products are those that do not themselves cause injury, but may lead people to delay or reject proven remedies, possibly worsening their condition. For example, if cancer patients reject proven drug therapies in favor of unproven ones and the unproven ones turn out not to work, their disease may advance beyond the point where proven therapies can help.

"What you see out there is the promotion of products claiming to cure or prevent AIDS, multiple sclerosis, cancer, and a list of other diseases that goes on and on," says Joel Aronson, director of FDA's Health Fraud Staff, in the agency's Center for Drug Evaluation and Research. For example, he says, several skin cream products promise to prevent transmission of HIV (the virus that causes AIDS) and herpes viruses. They are promoted especially to healthcare workers. Many of the creams contain antibacterial ingredients but, "there is no substantiation at all on whether or not [the skin creams] work" against HIV, says Aronson. The FDA has warned the manufacturers of these creams to stop the misleading promotions.

People at Risk

Teenagers and the elderly are two prime targets for health fraud promoters.

Teenagers concerned about their appearance and susceptible to peer pressure may fall for such products as fraudulent diet pills, breast developers, and muscle-building pills.

Older Americans may be especially vulnerable to health fraud because approximately 80 percent of them have at least one chronic health problem, according to Renner. Many of these problems, such as arthritis, have no cure and, for some people, no effective treatment. He says their pain and disability lead to despair, making them excellent targets for deception.

Arthritis

Although there is no cure for arthritis, the symptoms may come and go with no explanation. According to the Arthritis Foundation, "You may think a new remedy worked because you took it when your symptoms were going away."

Some commonly touted unproven treatments for arthritis are harmful, according to the foundation, including snake venom and DMSO (dimethyl sulfoxide), an industrial solvent similar to turpentine. The FDA has approved a sterile form of DMSO called Rimso-50, which is administered directly into the bladder for treatment of a rare bladder condition called interstitial cystitis. However, the DMSO sold to arthritis sufferers may contain bacterial toxins. DMSO is readily absorbed through the skin into the bloodstream, and these toxins enter the bloodstream along with it. It can be especially dangerous if used as an enema, as some of its promoters recommend.

Treatments the foundation considers harmless but ineffective include copper bracelets, mineral springs, and spas.

Cancer and Aids

Cancer treatment is complicated because in some types of cancer there are no symptoms, and in other types symptoms may disappear by themselves, at least temporarily. Use of an unconventional treatment coinciding with remission (lessening of symptoms) could be simply coincidental. There is no way of knowing, without a controlled clinical trial, what effect the treatment had on the outcome. The danger comes when this false security causes patients to forgo approved treatment that has shown real benefit.

Some unapproved cancer treatments not only have no proven benefits, they have actually been proven dangerous. These include Laetrile, which may cause cyanide poisoning and has been found ineffective in clinical trials, and coffee enemas, which, when used excessively, have killed patients.

Ozone generators, which produce a toxic form of oxygen gas, have been touted as being able to cure AIDS. To date this is still unproven, and the FDA considers ozone an unapproved drug and these generators to be unapproved medical devices. At least three deaths have been connected to the use of these generators. Four British citizens were indicted in 1991 for selling fraudulent ozone generators in the United States. Two of the defendants fled to Great Britain, but the other two pleaded guilty and served time in U.S. federal prisons.

The bottom line in deciding whether a certain treatment you have read or heard about might be right for you: Talk to your doctor. And keep in mind the old adage: If it sounds too good to be true, it probably is.

Tip-offs to Rip-offs

New health frauds pop up all the time, but the promoters usually fall back on the same old cliches and tricks to gain your trust and get your money. According to the FDA, some red flags to watch out for include:

- claims the product works by a secret formula. (Legitimate scientists share their knowledge so their peers can review their data.)

- publicity only in the back pages of magazines, over the phone, by direct mail, in newspaper advertisements in the format of news stories, or 30-minute commercials in talk show format. (Results of studies on bona fide treatments are generally reported first in medical journals.)

- claims the product is an amazing or miraculous breakthrough. (Real medical breakthroughs are rare, and when they happen, they're not touted as "amazing" or "miraculous" by any responsible scientist or journalist.)

- promises of easy weight loss. (For most people, the only way to lose weight is to eat less and exercise more.)

- promises of a quick, painless, guaranteed cure.

- testimonials from satisfied customers. (These people may never have had the disease the product is supposed to cure, may be paid representatives, or may simply not exist. Often they're identified only by initials or first names.)

Approaching Alternative Therapies

The NIH Office of Alternative Medicine recommends the following before getting involved in any alternative therapy:

- Obtain objective information about the therapy. Besides talking with the person promoting the approach, speak with people who have gone through the treatment—preferably both those who were treated recently and those treated in the past. Ask about the advantages and disadvantages, risks, side effects, costs, results, and over what time span results can be expected.

- Inquire about the training and expertise of the person administering the treatment (for example, certification).

- Consider the costs. Alternative treatments may not be reimbursable by health insurance.

- Discuss all treatments with your primary care provider, who needs this information to have a complete picture of your treatment plan.

For everyone—consumers, physicians and other health-care providers, and government regulators—the FDA has the same advice when it comes to weeding out the hopeless from the hopeful: Be open-minded, but don't fall into the abyss of accepting anything at all. For there are—as there have been for centuries—countless products that are nothing more than fraud.

—by Isadora B. Stehlin

Isadora B. Stehlin is a staff writer for FDA Consumer.

Part Two

Alternative Systems of Medical Practice

Chapter 5

Families of Alternative and Complementary Medicine

Background

In the United States many people think of mainstream biomedicine as the world's standard health care system, assuming it is used by most people most of the time.[1] Actually, careful estimates reveal that worldwide only 10 to 30 percent of human health care is delivered by the conventional, biomedically oriented health care system. The remaining 70 to 90 percent of health care sought out by people includes everything from self-care according to folk principles to care rendered in an organized health care system based on an alternative tradition of practice (Dean, 1981; Hufford, 1992).

Such strikingly high usage of alternative health care systems also is reflected in a number of recent surveys. For example, a nationwide telephone survey of 1,539 people, conducted in 1990, indicated that up to one in three Americans used alternative therapies (Eisenberg et al., 1993). Another telephone survey conducted in 1992 in the States of Maryland and Pennsylvania reported that someone in 33 percent of 1,165 households consulted chiropractors, 25 percent, massage therapists; and 16 percent, spiritual healers (Kirby, 1992). One biomedical clinic survey of 660 cancer patients showed that 54 percent

Extracted from NIH Publication No. 94-066 from the Office of Alternative Medicine. December 1994. Due to space considerations, bibliographic data have not been reprinted in this chapter. However, to aid readers who wish to consult the original document or do further research, the in-text references have been retained.

41

used alternative medical care along with conventional care, and 8 percent used strictly alternative care (Cassileth et al., 1984). In addition, a survey of 628 cancer patients found the utilization rate of folk treatments for cancer to be 70 percent (Hufford, 1992). Finally, an acupuncture clinic survey of 180 general-care patients showed that 70 percent sought other alternative professional or community-based health care in addition to biomedical and acupuncture care (Cassidy, 1994).

Given the immense political and economic investment this country has made in its "mainstream" medicine, these statistics are quite surprising. However, to better understand why alternative systems of medicine not only survive but thrive, it is worthwhile to first examine how people typically go about choosing their health care.

Studies show that most people go through a "hierarchy of resort" when seeking health care assistance (Romanuicci-Ross, 1969). That is, when ill, they usually begin by trying simple home remedies, often consulting friends and family about what to do. Only if the condition persists and worsens do people typically seek help from health care specialists.

The hierarchy of health care specialists includes the *popular, community-based, and professionalized* (Hufford, 1988; Kleinman, 1980). All are similar in that they aim to help people stay or get well and use manipulation (from laying on of hands to surgery), chemical substances (foods and drugs), or psychospiritual approaches (e.g., talking, suggesting, praying, drumming) as therapeutic techniques. They differ, however, in factors such as how much training they require of practitioners, how intensely they scrutinize and theorize about their own methods, how widely their practice is spread, and to whom they primarily aim their care.

Popular health care is what most people practice and receive at home, such as drinking hot honey and lemonade to relieve a sore throat. People get information about popular health care primarily from family or friends; it can be centuries old or relatively new to that family or social circle. People also learn about popular medicine from magazines, television, and other informal sources. In the United States, popular medicine often uses the words but not necessarily the underlying thinking of biomedicine.

Community-based health care refers to the nonprofessionalized yet specialized health care practices of both rural and urban people. The term community-based is used to avoid the stereotypes associated with the terms *folk* and *tribal*. Information in such systems is commonly passed on orally (through workshops, apprenticeships, and so on) and through informal and popular media sources. Some community-based practices have ancient roots (such as rootwork among African-Americans, pow-wowing among European-Americans, *curanderismo* among Hispanic-Americans, and religious pilgrimage and psychic healing traditions), while others have developed relatively recently, such as the various 12-step programs (e.g., Alcoholics Anonymous), popular weight loss programs, and various health and natural foods dietary practices. In contrast to popular and professionalized systems, these community-based systems characteristically focus on community health care or on the individual as part of the community. They also usually fuse concepts of medicine and religion or spirituality in such a way that all care is explained as being influenced by a "higher power."

Professionalized health care is characteristically urban and com-plexly organized. It is the most intellectualized and formalized type of health care. Certain of these have been called the "Great Tradition" medical care systems. Examples of such professionalized health care systems include conventional Western biomedicine, Asian-Indian Ayurveda, traditional oriental medicine, and traditional Persian medi-cine (Unani), all of which have evolved over time within major urban cultures. Other systems such as chiropractic medicine, osteopathic medicine, anthroposophically extended medicine, environmental medicine, and homeopathic medicine have been the result of the for-malization and expansion of the teachings of a specific creative founder within the Western rational and intellectual culture. Each of these major formal systems of medical practice has the following general characteristics:

1. A theory of health and disease;

2. An educational scheme to teach its concepts;

3. A delivery system involving practitioners who usually practice in offices, clinics, or hospitals;

4. A material support system to produce its medicines and thera-peutic devices;

5. A legal and economic mandate to regulate its practice;

6. A set of cultural expectations on the role of the medical sys-tem; and

7. A means to confer "professional" status on the approved pro-viders.

Two major types of illnesses are recognized in most of these sys-tems, though one or the other is usually emphasized: the *naturalistic* illness (which results from an accident, infection, intoxication, malformation, aging, environmental stress, etc.) and the *personalistic* illness (which is the result of malfunction in relationships between people). A third category of illness is increasingly proposed: the *energetic* illness, which is the result of abnormalities in the flow of subtle energies.

Studies show that people are quite astute at knowing what sorts of conditions to take to what sorts of practitioners. The practitioners at the top of the hierarchy, those that are the most "socially foreign" (i.e., hard to reach from the point of view of the patient), are consulted last and usually only when the condition is unresponsive, very serious, or chronically debilitating. For example, rural Mexicans go to the *curandero* or *curandera* for "folk" illnesses, to the nun or nurse for mild biomedical conditions, and to the biomedical physician for the most serious conditions (Young, 1981). Likewise, in urban America many people consult a registered nurse, pharmacist, or health food salesperson before taking their concerns to the medical doctor. One-third of the users of unconventional therapy are estimated to use it for "nonserious" conditions, health promotion, or disease prevention. However, in the case of more serious health problems, the medical doctor is not the most socially foreign type of practitioner in the United States, because M.D.s and D.O.s (doctors of osteopathy) are abundant. People consulting alternative practitioners for an identified health problem are much more likely to have first consulted a medical doctor (Eisenberg et al., 1993). This point suggests that many of the alternative practitioners are rendering care to people with conditions either unresponsive to or unsatisfactorily treated by standard biomedical care.

Of the types of health care listed above, only the professionalized practitioners have received much, if any, scientific study regarding the causes of illness and the explanations and results of treatment. Indeed, community-based practices have been virtually ignored by conventional medicine on the assumption that these superstitious ways are dying out. On the other hand, popular and community-based systems have been studied primarily by social scientists, historians, and folklorists. These researchers, though not primarily concerned with clinical results or health outcomes, have provided most of the clinical material currently available. Health educators have made use of such studies in designing culturally sensitive outreach programs (see the "Diet and Nutrition" chapter.)

In recent years, the professionalized biomedical health care system has initiated a number of programs in an attempt to influence popular health practices on the basis of sound epidemiological concerns, addressing such issues as smoking and health, diet and cardiovascular disease, sexual behavior and human immunodeficiency virus (HIV), and healthy childbirth practices. The comparative clinical effectiveness of indigenous community-based health care practices remains, however, a fruitful field for further research.

Professionalized Health Systems

This section includes discussions of representative health systems whose practitioner base and standards of practice are such that outcomes research may lead to generalizable conclusions applicable to the improvement of the Nation's health care delivery system. These systems are:

- traditional oriental medicine,
- acupuncture,
- Ayurvedic medicine,
- homeopathic medicine,
- anthroposophically extended medicine,
- naturopathic medicine, and
- environmental medicine.

Traditional oriental medicine and Ayurvedic medicine are professionalized health systems that are enjoying popularity beyond the ethnic Asian community and are building practitioner bases, educational systems, and popular awareness in North America. Likewise, acupuncture, both as a treatment method and as a formal professional medical system, has an established formal educational base, extensive legal sanction for a variety of practitioners, and a broad base of public support and acceptance in the United States.

Homeopathic medicine has maintained a sound educational base for both professional practitioner training and popular self-help support and has the only officially established "alternative" drug production system regulated by the Food and Drug Administration (FDA). Naturopathy has a base in two formally accredited naturopathic medical schools in the United States and legal recognition of practitioners in a number of States. Anthroposophically extended medicine, while limited in availability in the United States, has a track record of thoughtful research and drug development in Europe that exemplifies the possibilities for "scientific alternatives" in our own health care system. Environmental medicine is a modern specialty area within biomedicine that has developed in ecological theory of health and disease.

Discussion of these professionalized systems is intended as an overview only. The serious student or researcher will find an extensive global database for future research. Each of the following subsections ends with a discussion of current research issues and recommendations for future research.

Chapter 6

Traditional Oriental Medicine and Acupuncture

Overview. Traditional oriental medicine is a sophisticated set of many systematic techniques and methods. Many of these methods are widely known in the United States, including acupuncture, herbal medicines, acupressure, qigong, and oriental massage techniques. Traditional oriental medicine is rooted in Chinese culture and has spread, with variations, throughout other Asian countries, particularly Japan, Korea, and Vietnam. As a professionalized health system, it has a range of applications from health promotion to the treatment of illness.

The fundamental concepts of oriental medicine are embedded in the philosophical and metaphysical worldviews of Taoism, Confucianism, and Buddhism, which began evolving and spreading throughout East Asia 2,500 years ago. Whereas the religions and philosophies of the Western world developed around the theme of separation of mind, body, and spirit, the Eastern philosophies undergirding oriental medicine consider the whole person and nature to be systematically interrelated.

Chinese medicine developed concurrently with Chinese culture out of its shamanic, tribal origins in the pre-Christian era. By the beginning of the Han Dynasty (200 B.C.E.) the Chinese had acquired and documented formidable medical experience. The first mention of the

Extracted from NIH Publication No. 94-066 from the Office of Alternative Medicine. December 1994. Due to space considerations, bibliographic data have not been reprinted in this chapter. However, to aid readers who wish to consult the original document or do further research, the in-text references have been retained.

Shen Nung pharmacopoeia dates from the first century A.D. (Unschuld, 1986). Anatomic dissections and surgeries were practiced during the earlier eras, although in later centuries the Confucian belief in the sacredness of the human body prevented further developments in surgery and anatomic research. The early Chinese State distinguished various sorts of doctors, including medical physicians, surgeons, dietitians, veterinary surgeons, and community-based health officers. By the close of the Han era (220 A.D.), the Chinese had a clear idea of preventive medicine and first aid, knew pathology and dietetics, and had devised breathing practices to promote longevity. After Buddhist influences were assimilated, particularly a tolerance for judging medical practices by their results and not by their theories, the characteristic qualities and components of Chinese medicine had developed by 500 A.D. These qualities and components were expanded during periods of cultural intellectual growth that paralleled the Middle Ages and the Renaissance in Western Europe (Unschuld, 1985).

During the colonial periods of encounter with Western culture, the systems of oriental medicine became fragmented. As Western medical science followed the spread of Western social and political power throughout East Asia, some traditional methods were relegated to folk and quasi-religious practitioners. However, since 1949, traditional Chinese medicine has enjoyed a Government-sponsored renaissance in the People's Republic of China (PRC) (Hiller and Jewel, 1983; Unschuld, 1992). Today, both traditional- and Western-oriented medical training, research, and institutional practice are available throughout mainland China (Quinn, 1972). In addition, traditional practices survive in various degrees in other East Asian countries (Sonoda, 1988).

The most striking characteristic of oriental medicine is its emphasis on diagnosing disturbances of qi (pronounced "chee"), or vital energy, in health and disease (Unschuld, 1985; Wiseman et al., 1985). There are many aspects of healthy balance and function in oriental medicine, and these aspects are described qualitatively or metaphorically as "disharmonies" among forms of vital energy. The concept of yin and yang harmony is a basic description of the interaction between the active and passive, stimulating and nurturing, masculine and feminine, and "heavenly" and "earthly" qualities that characterize living things. Imbalances of yin and yang can manifest within the functions of internal organs in their generation of metabolic energy, can propagate along energetically active channels represented on the body as the acupuncture meridians, and can undergo transformations of expression according to the system of "five phases." Each phase of energy has a characteristic quality of material expression represented by the elemental natures of fire, earth, metal, water, and wood. The Chinese systematically incorporated into their theories new discoveries of environmental and infectious influences on healthy qi and incorporated the emotional, psychological, and personality aspects of illness into the five-phase system.

Diagnosis in oriental medicine involves the classical procedures of observation, listening, questioning, and palpation, including feeling the quality of the pulses and the sensitivity of various body parts. The well-trained physician is taught to use all procedures together in evaluating the patient and to search for details of habit, lifestyle, nutritional indulgence, and specific mediating circumstances. Physical and emotional aspects of health are assumed to be interrelated; for example, fullness of the lungs is said to produce dreams of sorrow and weeping. A range of traditional therapies is prescribed to correct physical symptoms, restore energetic balance, and redirect and normalize the patient's qi.

The professionalization of oriental medicine has taken diverse paths in both East Asia and the United States. Currently, the model in the PRC, which was established after the 1949 revolution, involves the organized training of practitioners in schools of traditional Chinese medicine. The curriculum of these schools includes acupuncture, oriental massage, herbal medicine, and pharmacology, though the theoretical style of making a diagnosis and designing a treatment plan is the one traditionally associated with herbal medicine (Flaws, 1993). The graduates of these colleges are generally certified in one of the four specialty areas at a training level roughly equivalent to that of the Western bachelor's degree (Flaws, 1993). In contrast, in Japan there is a distinct profession of acupuncture, and the herbs used in traditional herbal medicine products (*kampo*) are prescribed by medically trained physicians or pharmacists (Birch, 1993).

In the United States the professional practitioner base for oriental medicine is organized around acupuncture and oriental massage. There are about 6,500 acupuncturist practitioners in the United States. The American Oriental Bodywork Therapy Association has approximately 1,600 members representing practitioners of tuina, shiatsu, and related techniques (Flaws, 1993). Many American schools of acupuncture are evolving into "colleges of oriental medicine" by adding courses in oriental massage, herbal medicine, and dietary interventions. They are also offering diplomas and master's or doctor's degrees in oriental medicine. Although graduates of these programs are exposed to herbal medicine pharmacology, only the States of California and Nevada include a specific section evaluating knowledge of herbal medicine in the state acupuncturist licensing examination. The legal sanctioning of oriental medical practice is most extensive in New Mexico, where the acupuncturists have established an exclusive profession of oriental medicine. Their legal scope of practice is currently similar to that of primary care M.D.s and D.O.s, and their State statute restricts other licensed New Mexico health professionals' ability to advertise or bill for oriental medicine or acupuncture services (New Mexico Association of Acupuncture and Oriental Medicine, 1993).

As with any new profession in the United States, the issues of appropriate formal training, State-by-State legal scope of practice, official title and privileges of practitioners, and professional monopoly on health practices are currently controversial, even among the community of oriental medicine advocates. Furthermore, the position of oriental medicine practices and practitioners within the broader U.S. health care system continues to be a subject of heated political, economic, and intellectual debate (Birch, 1993; Flaws, 1993; National Council Against Health Fraud, 1991; New Mexico Association of Acupuncture and Oriental Medicine, 1993).

The treatment modalities most associated with traditional oriental medicine and used regularly by practitioners include acupuncture, moxibustion, acupressure, remedial massage, cupping, qigong, herbal medicine, and nutritional and dietary interventions. These are discussed below. Acupressure, massage, and qigong are also discussed in the "Manual Healing Methods" chapter.

Acupuncture. It is important to remember that acupuncture was but one branch among several therapies. It involves the direct manipulation of the network of energetic meridians, which are believed to connect not only with the surface or structural body parts but also to influence the deeper internal organs. The needle is inserted at appropriately chosen energetic points to disperse or activate the qi by a variety of technical manipulations. Western-style research showing that acupuncture could relieve pain and cause surgical analgesia through the release of pain-inhibiting chemicals (endorphins) in the nervous system led to the first theories of how acupuncture might work in terms of a biomedical science model (Han, 1987). This model does not, however, account for the many different ways acupuncture is used clinically to improve or correct ailing body functions. Because acupuncture has attracted major interest in the United States, an expanded section on acupuncture is included in this chapter.

Moxibustion. Moxibustion using *Artemisia vulgaris* (a plant of the composite, or daisy, family) evolved in early times in northern China. In this cold, mountainous region, the effect of heating the body on the energetically active points was a logical development. Moxibustion is thought to have preceded the use of needles. The crushed leaves, or moxa, of vulgaris may be used in loose or cigar form. In theory, the burning from the moxa releases a radiant heat that penetrates deeply and is used to affect the balance and flow of qi.

Acupressure. The energy points and channels can be treated with direct physical pressure by the fingertips or hands of the therapist. Simple points may be used for first aid or symptomatic relief or entire systems of manual therapy (e.g., shiatsu, jin shin jyutsu) may be used to effect the overall well-being of the body.

Remedial massage. The techniques of remedial massage (an-mo and tuina) are described in medical texts of the Han period. Later, in the Tang dynasty, massage was taught in special institutes. An-mo tonifies the system using pressing and rubbing hand motions, while tuina soothes and sedates using thrusting and rolling hand motions. Both systems employ a complex series of hand movements called the eight *kua* on specific body areas to produce the desired effects.

Cupping. Cupping is a technique of applying suction over selected points or zones in the body. A vacuum is created by warming the air in a jar of bamboo or glass and overturning it onto the body to disperse areas of local congestion. This therapy is used in the treatment of arthritis, bronchitis, and sprains, among other ailments.

Qigong. Qigong is the art and science of using breath, movement, and meditation to cleanse, strengthen, and circulate the vital life energy and blood.[2] Three basic principles are observed in the performance of the exercises: relaxation and repose; association of breathing with attention; and the interaction of movement and rest. Tai chi and other practices of oriental physical culture emphasize maintaining internal and external balance while encountering one's environment. Certain of the qigong exercises, particularly the *gou lin* form, have been used for immune stimulation and selfhelp in cancer patients (Sancier, 1991, 1993). These personal practices are the "internal" qigong type. Certain qigong "masters" are considered to be "energetic healers," who via "external" qigong use some of their own energy to strengthen the vitality of others who have ailments.

51

Herbal medicine. There is a complex series of practices regarding the preparation and administering of herbs in Chinese medicine (Unschuld, 1986). The traditional *materia medica* in China included approximately 3,200 herbs and 300 mineral and animal extracts (Bensky and Gamble, 1986). Herbal prescriptions cover the entire range of medical ailments, including pain, hormone disturbances, breathing disorders, infections, and chronic debilitating illnesses. Medications are classified according to their energetic qualities (e.g., heating, cooling, moisturizing, drying) and prescribed for their action on corresponding organ dysfunction, energy disorders, disturbed internal energy, blockage of the meridians, or seasonal physical demands. One unique aspect of traditional prescribing is the use of complex mixtures containing many ingredients. Such prescriptions are systemically compounded to have several effects: to principally affect the disease or disharmony, to balance out any potential side effects of the principal therapy, and to direct the therapy to a specific area or a physical process in the body. (See the "Herbal Medicine" chapter for details on specific Chinese herbs and how they are used).

Nutrition and dietetics. Dietary interventions are also individualized on the basis of the physical characteristics of both the patient's constitution and the patient's illness disturbance. Foods are characterized according to their energetic qualities (e.g., tonifying, dispersing, heating, cooling, moistening, drying). Emphasis is given to eating in harmony with seasonal shifts and life activities.

Research base. Although extensive research has been done in China through the institutions of traditional Chinese medicine, much of this clinical research has been empirical, that is, reports of observed results of various treatments. Many of these reports have been difficult to translate into Western languages and into the standard formulas or analysis typical for Western biomedical research. Because of the interest in applying acupuncture for pain and for chronic conditions, much research has focused on these two areas. However, clinical practice experience in the Asian countries suggests there is a role for complementary use of traditional therapies with a myriad of modern Western "scientific" medical interventions (Sun, 1988; Unschuld, 1992; Wong et al., 1991).

Only in the past quarter-century have biomedical scientists in China been characterizing and identifying the active agents in much of the traditional medical formulary (Hsu et al., 1982, 1985). However, extensive research has been published detailing the pharmacology and toxicity of many traditional oriental herbs (Bensky and Gamble, 1986; Hsu et al., 1982, 1985; Ng et al., 1991). How many clinical trials of traditional oriental herbal medicine have been conducted and what extent and validity the findings have are unclear. Few references to published studies appear in the databases available in the West. Although some individual studies appear quite promising, only preliminary conclusions can be drawn about the field until more complete literature searches are conducted. (See the "Herbal Medicine" chapter for a more complete discussion of the status of herbal medicine research in China.)

Tsutani conducted an extensive search to find the number of clinical trials of herbal medicine in China (Tsutani, 1993). Of 148 studies retrieved from computerized databases, 39 were double blind, used random allocation, or were randomized controlled clinical trials. He conducted a combined computerized and manual search of the Japanese literature and retrieved references to 59 controlled studies on the use of kampo (Japanese traditional herbal medicine). An additional unpublished search by Birch of computer indexed herbal medicine studies published in the period 1978-92 located 23 studies in English and 44 in other languages (Chinese 37, Japanese 5, German 1, French 1). In general, the methodological quality of these studies was poor, and they had multiple study design problems, including poor experimental design, lack of randomization, unclear entry criteria and end points, and lack of consideration of the traditional uses of the herbs (Birch, 1993).

Research in the medical effects of qigong has been a subject of interest in the PRC in recent years and was the topic of six international conferences between 1986 and 1991. Patients who practice internal qigong exercises combining meditation and gentle body movement were shown to have better results in therapy for hypertension, cancer, and coronary artery disease (Sancier, 1991, 1993). Qigong exercise also was shown to affect the blood chemistry of individuals practicing it. In addition, studies on external qigong have included measurements of the effect of qi emitted by master practitioners on cell cultures, germination rate of seeds, and electroencephalographic measurements of human recipients (Sancier and Hu, 1991).

Measurements of emissions from external qigong practitioners suggested that infrasonic energy was present in frequency ranges from 8 to 12.5 hertz (lower than the human ear can hear) and in intensities measurably different than background-noise level (Sancier and Hu, 1991). These suggestive findings parallel certain studies done in the West on mind-body interactions and nonlocal or "energetic" healing. (See the "Manual Healing Methods" and "Mind-Body Interventions" chapters.) Unfortunately, these Chinese studies are available only in abstract or conference proceedings formats in English. It is not known whether the complete papers are published in the Chinese literature with supporting data that would allow a methodological evaluation of the quality of the studies.

Future research opportunities. Although many diseases may be helped by the modalities of traditional oriental medicine, documenting its benefit in conditions of greatest concern to the United States should have research priority: cancer, acquired immune deficiency syndrome (AIDS), cardiovascular diseases, neuromuscular disabilities, chronic fatigue syndrome, psychosomatic problems, alcohol and drug addictions, and chronic pain.

Clinical research into the nondrug modalities of traditional oriental medicine includes opportunities for investigating manual healing therapies, bioelectricity and magnetic physical interventions, and the use of body-mind interactions for health purposes. Issues and criteria for such future research are discussed in other chapters of this report.

The use of traditional oriental herbal medicines and formulas in China and Japan has been studied for therapeutic value in the following areas: chronic hepatitis; rheumatoid arthritis; hypertension; atopic eczema; various immunologic disorders, including AIDS; and certain cancers (Hirayama et al., 1989; Sheehan and Atherton, 1992; Smith, 1987; Sun, 1988; Tao et al., 1989; Wong et al., 1991; Xu et al., 1989; Zhao et al., 1993). It would be useful to repeat these studies in the United States using high-quality research criteria. Research into the application of traditional oriental products could be roughly organized in three levels: first, publication of appropriate safety studies; second, pharmacological studies characterizing the contents, action, and components of single herbs and herbal formulas; and third, controlled clinical trials for specified conditions. The expense of this research endeavor can be lessened if World Health Organization proposals (see the "Herbal Medicine" chapter) allowing the documentation of traditional use are adopted by U.S. regulatory authorities (McCaleb, 1993). Given the large-scale use of over-the-counter herbal products as "food supplements" in the U.S. market, studies involving postmarketing surveillance of the use, clinical results, and complications of currently available products also would be appropriate (Ng et al., 1991).

Examples of creative basic research would include viewing the pH balance of body fluids as a representation of yin-yang balance, noting changes in organ and tissue receptor sites following treatment with herbal preparations, and investigating various neurological responses to massage and acupressure interventions. There is a major opportunity for cataloging and translating research done in China, Japan, and Korea in order to stimulate further development of the field in the United States.

Outcomes research can also address the application of traditional oriental medicine as a system. Such research would involve comparing (a) the overall health improvement and cost of care of a population working with a program of mixed interventions prescribed by practitioners of traditional oriental medicines with (b) the health indices of a control group using conventional care.

Acupuncture

Overview. Acupuncture involves stimulating specific anatomic points in the body for therapeutic purposes. Puncturing the skin with a needle is the usual method of application, but practitioners may also use heat, pressure, friction, suction, or impulses of electromagnetic energy to stimulate the points. Acupuncture was an evolving part of the medical practices of the Chinese people and is described in two surviving historical texts: the well-known medical treatise *Huang Ti Nei Ching Su Wen (The Yellow Emperor's Classic of Internal Medicine)*, and *Shi Ji (Book of History)*, both dating to the period 200-100 B.C.E.

Over the centuries, acupuncture spread throughout the medical practices of the Asiatic peoples around the Pacific Rim. However, it has been practiced as a medical art in Western Europe for several hundred years, having been brought home by the traders, diplomats, and missionary priests who encountered it during their travels in the Orient. By the late 19th century, acupuncture was known and used on the east coast of the United States. Sir William Osler's American medical textbook, which was first published in 1892 and was updated periodically through 1947, recommended acupuncture for treating lumbago or lower back pain (Lytle, 1993). Acupuncture also reached the United States on the west coast as an ethnic practice among Asian immigrants in the 19th and 20th centuries.

George Soulie de Morant, a French diplomat in China at the turn of the century, became an accomplished acupuncturist. On his return to France he began systematically introducing the full range of acupuncture to the French and European medical community. He published significant texts in 1934, 1939, 1941, and 1955 that represent a landmark effort to expand Western biomedical explanations of the physiology of health and disease to include the classical and empirical observations of Chinese acupuncture. His influence did much to establish acupuncture as an accepted clinical art in Europe (Zmiewski, 1994).

In the past 40 years acupuncture has become a well-known and reasonably available treatment in both developed and developing countries. Since the reopening of relations between the United States and the PRC, acupuncture has attracted increased attention from the American public and governmental agencies (Chen, 1973). With the emergence of traditional Chinese medicine as an organized system of practice in the PRC, formal training programs in acupuncture and oriental medicine have expanded throughout the world. Schools and training programs of acupuncture in the United States incorporate varying degrees of traditional Chinese medicine as well as European acupuncture approaches and elements of the traditional and modern practice traditions from Japan, Korea, and Vietnam.

Because the traditional view of health and illness in oriental medicine is related to a proper balance of qi, or energy, in the body, acupuncture is used to regulate or correct the flow of qi to restore health. Acupuncture treatment points are chosen on the basis of diagnosis of a medical problem by history and physical exam using one or more models of how the body operates in health and disease. The model, or "tradition," that is used to guide treatment may vary according to the cultural background and education of the practitioner as well as the nature of the patient's problem. Acupuncture prescriptions can be simple or sophisticated. A series of 10 or more treatments is usually prescribed for a chronic illness or physical rehabilitation. On the other hand, one to four treatments may suffice for minor injuries, a self-limited illness, or a seasonal "tune up." Modern theories of acupuncture are based on laboratory research conducted in the past 40 years. Acupuncture points have been found to have certain electrical properties, and stimulation of these points has been shown to alter the chemical neurotransmitters in the body. Many of the therapeutic effects of acupuncture can be clearly related to the mechanism of neurotransmitter release via peripheral nerve stimulation. This mechanism is associated with changes in the balance of the natural physiological chemicals in the body, which can be used for a therapeutic effect (Pomeranz, 1986). Other therapeutic effects may be related to mechanical stimulation or alteration of the natural electrical currents or electromagnetic fields in the body.

Although the physiological effects of acupuncture stimulation in experimental animals have been well documented, the use of acupuncture treatments for clinical illness in humans has remained controversial within much of the mainstream medical community in the United States. Some controversy comes from the "foreignness" of traditional Chinese interpretations of medical illness, and some may be due to an unfamiliarity with the existing global research base. In 1973 the commissioner of the FDA announced that devices used in acupuncture, including the specialized needles, electrical stimulators, and associated paraphernalia, would be considered investigational on the basis of the perception at that time that "the safety and effectiveness of acupuncture devices [had] not yet been established by adequate scientific studies to support the many and varied uses for which such devices are being promoted including uses for analgesia and anesthesia" (Lytle, 1993). This designation is still official FDA policy.

In the subsequent 20 years, however, acupuncture has become an increasingly established health care practice in the United States. Furthermore, there are currently more than 40 schools and colleges of acupuncture and oriental medicine in the United States, 20 of which are either approved or in candidacy status with the National Accreditation Commission for Schools and Colleges of Acupuncture and Oriental Medicine. There are licensure or registration statutes in 28 States for the practitioner graduates of these programs. There are an estimated 6,500 acupuncturist practitioners in the United States, of whom 3,300 have taken the examination of the National Commission for the Certification of Acupuncturists. In addition to these practitioners, naturopathic and chiropractic physicians also can legally incorporate acupuncture in their practice in a limited number of States.

Besides the "alternative" medical practitioners who are trained in acupuncture, an estimated 3,000 conventionally trained physicians (M.D.s and D.O.s) have taken courses to incorporate acupuncture as a treatment modality in their medical practices. Such courses have been affiliated with the UCLA School of Medicine, the New York University School of Medicine and Dentistry, and St. Louis University Medical School (Helms, 1993). Proficiency certification examination for physician acupuncturists has been offered for a number of years in Canada by the Acupuncture Foundation of Canada, and similar examinations are currently in development in the United States, Australia, and New Zealand (Williams, 1994). The gradual acceptance of acupuncture therapeutics based on clinical practice experience in American medicine is reflected by the incorporation of descriptions of this discipline into most current textbooks of physical medicine and pain management (Chapman and Gunn, 1990; Lee and Liao, 1990). Moreover, a recent review estimated that patient visits for acupuncture to physician and nonphysician practitioners are occurring at a rate of 9 to 12 million per year in the United States (Lytle, 1993). Thus, the continued FDA "experimental" designation, which is echoed by the reference committee of the American Medical Association (AMA), is considered by many to be obsolete in the face of the large-scale use of acupuncture by legally sanctioned practitioners in the United States as well as in many other countries' health care systems.

Research base. Acupuncture is one of the most thoroughly researched and documented of the so-called alternative medical practices. A series of controlled studies on the treatment of a variety of conditions has shown compelling, though not statistically conclusive, evidence for the efficacy of acupuncture. These conditions are osteoarthritis (Dickens and Lewith, 1989), chemotherapy-induced nausea (J. Dundee et al., 1989), asthma (Fung and Chow, 1986), back pain (Gunn and Milbrandt, 1980), painful menstrual cycles (Helms, 1987), bladder instability (Phillip et al., 1988), and migraine headaches (Vincent, 1990). Moreover, in spite of the unenviable challenge of serving as the "alternative" therapy of "last resort," acupuncture studies have shown positive results in managing chronic pain (Patel et al., 1989) and drug addiction (Bullock et al., 1989; Smith, 1988), two areas where conventional Western medicine has generally failed. Indeed, the criminal justice systems in New York City and Portland, OR, have mandated acupuncture as part of their detoxification and probation programs for drug abusers.

In addition, basic science research in animal models suggests that neurological pathways are the mechanism by which acupuncture relieves pain (Pomeranz, 1986). There also is work showing acupuncture effects in treating veterinary medical problems, such as bacteria-induced diarrhea in pigs (Hwang and Jenkins, 1988). A broad range of applications in human medicine also has been explored.

The risk and safety issues in acupuncture also have been thoroughly investigated (Lytle, 1993). In a recent review of 3,255 acupuncture citations in the world scientific literature, the conditions of study in 365 Western and 344 Chinese clinical research papers were tabulated (American Foundation of Medical Acupuncture,1993). See Table 6.1 for the number of studies per topic.

The diversity of clinical applications and supporting basic physiology studies points to acupuncture having a therapeutic effect that exceeds a purely placebo or culturally dependent action.

Acupuncture research involves tailoring the study design and question to one of several levels of clinical investigation. At the most basic

Table 6.1.

surgical applications	77
pain (chronic and acute pain of all types)	222
neurological disorders	62
organic illness (e.g., heart, lungs)	200
women's reproductive disorders	43
mental illness	29
addiction therapy	54
acupuncture treatment complications	11

level, one can study the effect of stimulating a specific acupuncture point on a specific physiological response. For example, Dundee and colleagues conducted a series of investigations involving more than 500 patients for a 5-year period, evaluating the effect on nausea of stimulating the acupuncture point PC-6 (*neiguan*). These studies involved manual needling, electrical stimulation on the needle, acupressure, and noninvasive electrical stimulation. Control groups included patients with no treatment as well as patients who were needled at a sham point (a point unrelated to the accepted treatment meridian). The patients being investigated were undergoing minor gynecologic operations under general anesthesia. Results of the active acupuncture treatments showed better response than was shown by controls or by those who received sham acupuncture treatments. Indeed, needle acupuncture gave slightly better results than the then-standard antinausea drugs (R. Dundee et al., 1989).

Moreover, the effect of acupuncture in the treatment of specific clinical conditions has been measured. For example, Helms (1987) studied 43 women suffering from dysmenorrhea (painful menstrual periods); the patients were divided into four groups: real acupuncture, sham acupuncture, standard controls (no intervention), and visitation controls (visits to the treating physician). The patients were free to take their previously used pain medications during the 3-month treatment period and a followup period. Ninety-one percent of the real acupuncture treatment group showed improvement, whereas only 36 percent of the sham acupuncture group showed improvement. Only 18 percent of the standard control group and 10 percent of the visitation control group showed improvement. In addition, there was a 41-percent decrease in use of pain medication in the real acupuncture group, versus no change in the others (Helms, 1987). Furthermore, the improvement noted in the real acupuncture treatment group persisted beyond the end of the active treatment period.

Although acupuncture effects on pain problems can be considered purely subjective phenomena, acupuncture treatments also can be studied in terms of their effect on altering patient behavior and use of medical care. Bullock et al. (1989) studied 80 severe alcoholics through the Hennipen County, MN, alcohol detoxification program. These patients all had a history of repeated hospital admissions for alcoholism, or were severe recidivists. They were divided into two groups, a treatment group receiving acupuncture at specific ear acupuncture points and a control group treated with sham acupuncture points on the ear. The patients were treated for 45 days from the date of their last acute alcoholism hospital admission.

Six months after the treatment program the control (sham) group had nearly twice as many drinking episodes and admissions to detox centers as the treatment groups (Bullock et al., 1989). These types of results have caught the attention of public agencies and criminal justice systems across the country who are concerned with the cost of managing the social impact of people with severe drug abuse behavior.

Promising early evidence suggests that acupuncture can be cost-effective in conventional medical practice settings as well. In France, for example, statistics from the insurance syndicate show that physicians whose practice is at least 50 percent acupuncture cost the system considerably less for laboratory examinations, hospitalizations, and medication prescriptions than their non-acupuncture-practicing colleagues (Helms, 1993). In the United States, a pilot study on followup of chronic pain patients receiving acupuncture in a managed-care setting demonstrated a reduction of clinic visits, physical therapy visits, telephone consultations, and prescription costs in the 6 months following a short course of acupuncture therapy (Erickson, 1992).

In Denmark a study was made involving the 58 patients on a county health system's waiting list for elective knee replacement surgery. Forty-eight of these patients were considered candidates for a controlled trial of acupuncture therapy, and two-thirds (32) participated in the study. The subgroup treated with acupuncture initially showed improvement in both objective and subjective measures of knee function and a 50-percent reduction in nonsteroidal anti-inflammatory drug (NSAID) use after six treatments when this group was compared with its own baseline findings and with the untreated subgroup. The untreated patients were then treated with acupuncture and also showed improvement. Five of these were called for their elective surgery, and the remaining 17 continued in long-term followup for 49 weeks with monthly acupuncture treatments for maintenance. At the 1-year followup point, NSAID use in the group as a whole was still 20 percent less than the baseline measurements, and 22 percent (seven) of the study group had responded so well that they no longer desired knee replacement surgery. These seven patients constituted 12 percent of the original elective surgery waiting list (Christensen et al., 1992). Taken as a whole, these results suggest that wider use of acupuncture in the United States might reduce health care costs significantly as well as improve outcomes of selected conditions.

Future research opportunities. Basic research is needed to examine the effects of acupuncture beyond the pain management field. This extended basic research in acupuncture should address the broad range of clinically observed effects of acupuncture treatments, including improved physical health, improved emotional stability and cognitive functioning, and overall improvement in quality of life. State-of-the-art techniques for monitoring and detecting changes in body physiology (e.g., electroencephalography, brain mapping, single-photon emission tomography scans, positron emission tomography scans, and electromyographic mapping) could be used. Such techniques are useful in evaluating medical conditions in which patients do not show gross changes in standard biochemical measures.

Basic research in the bioelectromagnetic effect of acupuncture on the physical and energetic phenomena of the human body might present another modern correlation to the traditional concept of qi. (See the "Bioelectromagnetics Applications in Medicine" and "Manual Healing Methods" chapters.) The alterations by acupuncture of the neuropeptide chemicals involved in the digestive and immune responses also could be studied. This biochemical research would parallel the existing studies on pain relief with acupuncture. Another promising area is research into disorders of the autonomic nervous system and their alteration or correction by acupuncture.

Acupuncture's traditionally reported effects on improving the well-being of the whole person should be investigated using established psychological and behavioral health measures as well as standardized measurements of health status and quality of life. Since acupuncture is a procedural therapy involving an intentional interaction between the practitioner and the patient, acupuncture research is an appropriate area in which to investigate the interpersonal and transpersonal aspects of mind-body healing. (See the "Mind-Body Interventions" chapter.)

Acupuncture research in clinical medicine is entering a challenging period. With a broad base of research and practice supporting the safety and promising results of acupuncture in many clinical conditions, studies now need to be done to firmly establish the efficacy of acupuncture in comparison with other medical interventions for relevant health problems. There are three appropriate questions for clinical studies of acupuncture:

1. Is acupuncture efficacious for the condition under study in comparison with conventional or other alternative treatments?

2. Is acupuncture more than a placebo intervention for the specific conditions being studied?

3. Is the mechanism of acupuncture more than that of a nonspecific irritant stimulation? That is, does it matter where you stick the needle?

These levels of research, done as controlled clinical trials, are necessary to answer treatment efficacy questions that are equivalent to those being studied in Phase III drug treatment trials. These initial studies should assist in correcting the "experimental" designations imposed by the FDA and the AMA on the practice of acupuncture.

Key issues. Because of the entrenched skepticism in American medicine regarding acupuncture, an extremely high standard of biostatistical and clinical expertise will be required for these acupuncture clinical trials. Unfortunately, as an operator-dependent procedure— a type of procedure that has individualized treatment protocols—acupuncture can be studied in a full-scale, blinded, randomized, placebo-controlled fashion in only a limited number of clinical conditions. Suggested areas for such placebo controlled acupuncture research studies include treatment of acute low back pain, chronic osteoarthritis of the knee, cancer chemotherapy-induced nausea and vomiting, and pain related to dental procedures. Issues for which existing studies have been criticized, such as sample bias, inadequate statistical power, lack of appropriate controls, practitioner incompetence, and inappropriate treatment design, must be addressed to ensure that the data generated in new clinical trials are of the highest possible quality (ter Riet et al., 1990).

Furthermore, the drug model of biomedical research is appropriate for only a limited range of acupuncture investigations. For most clinical applications, acupuncture research trials will have to compare clinical effectiveness, that is, compare the outcome of courses of acupuncture treatment with clinical outcomes in non-acupuncture-treated or conventionally treated patients. The priority areas for these acupuncture research studies should be based on considerations of public health importance, the inadequacy of current treatment methods owing to excessive side effects or cost, and the existing promising data in the global acupuncture research base. Attention to specificity of the diagnostic, therapeutic, and outcome criteria is necessary to allow compelling conclusions to be drawn about the effectiveness of acupuncture in disorders such as chronic headaches, urinary system dysfunction, respiratory disorders, allergies, neurological and orthopedic problems, and substance abuse problems.

Since acupuncture treatments for many of these health problems are individually designed and directed at improving the function of the whole person, specific research methods must be involved that will not only document alterations in a specific disease process but also validate the improved quality-of-life outcomes reported by patients who have been treated by experienced acupuncture practitioners.

Chapter 7

Ayurvedic Medicine

Overview

Ayurveda is the traditional, natural system of medicine of India, which has been practiced for more than 5,000 years. Ayurveda provides an integrated approach to the prevention and treatment of illness through lifestyle interventions and a wide range of natural therapies. The term *Ayurveda* has its origins in the Sanskrit roots *ayus*, which means "life," and *veda*, which means "knowledge."

Ayurvedic theory states that all imbalance and disease in the body begin with imbalance or stress in the awareness, or consciousness, of the individual. This mental stress leads to unhealthy lifestyles, which further promote ill health. Therefore, mental techniques such as meditation are considered essential to the promotion of healing and to prevention.

Ayurveda describes all physical manifestations of disease as due to the imbalance of three basic physiological principles in the body, called *doshas*, which are believed to govern all bodily functions. Evaluation of these three doshas—*vata, pitta*, and *kapha*—is accomplished primarily by feeling the patient's pulse at the radial artery, which is a detailed and systematic technique called *nadi vigyan*. This evaluation

Extracted from NIH Publication No. 94-066 from the Office of Alternative Medicine. December 1994. Due to space considerations, bibliographic data have not been reprinted in this chapter. However, to aid readers who wish to consult the original document or do further research, the in-text references have been retained.

determines the types of herbs prescribed, and it guides the physician in the application of all other ayurvedic therapies.

Specific lifestyle interventions are a major preventive and therapeutic approach in Ayurveda as well. Each patient is prescribed an individualized dietary, eating, sleeping, and exercise program depending on his or her constitutional type and the nature of the underlying dosha imbalance at the source of the illness. The Ayurvedic practitioner uses a variety of precise body postures, all derived from the age-old discipline of yoga; breathing exercises; and meditative techniques. These postures are used to create an individualized self-care program to improve both physical health and personal consciousness. In addition, herbal preparations are added to the patient's diet for preventive and rejuvenative purposes as well as for the treatment of specific disorders.

In addition to mental factors, lifestyle, and dosha imbalance, Ayurveda identifies a fourth major factor in disease: the accumulation of metabolic byproducts and toxins in the body tissues. Ayurvedic physical therapy, called *panchakarma*, consists of physical applications, including herbalized oil massage, herbalized heat treatments, and elimination therapies (e.g., therapies to improve bowel movements), which promote internal cleansing and removal of such toxic metabolic wastes. Certain of the agents used in panchakarma therapy are proposed to have free-radical scavenging, or antioxidant, effects (Fields et al., 1990). Free radicals are naturally occurring atoms or molecules that are highly reactive with anything they come into contact with. A recently developed theory suggests that free radicals play important roles in causing a wide range of degenerative and chronic disorders, including cancer and aging. Thus, substances with antioxidant properties may be effective in preventing, or even treating, myriad conditions. (See the "Diet and Nutrition" chapter for more information on free radicals and antioxidants.)

Ayurveda emphasizes the interdependence of the health of the individual and the quality of societal life. Therefore, measures to ensure the collective health of society, such as pollution control, community hygiene, the collective practice of meditation programs, and appropriate living conditions, are supported.

There are currently approximately 10 Ayurveda clinics in North America, including one hospital-based clinic, which together have served an estimated 25,000 patients since 1985 (Lonsdorf, 1993). More than 200 physicians have received training as Ayurvedic practitioners through the American Association of Ayurvedic Medicine, have received continuing medical education credit for Ayurvedic training programs, and have incorporated Ayurveda into their clinical practices as an adjunct to modern medicine (Lonsdorf, 1993). A modern revitalization of Ayurveda now being practiced in the United States and internationally is known as Maharishi Ayurveda. This approach utilizes a full range of physical and mental therapies from the Ayurvedic tradition.

In India, Ayurvedic practitioners receive State-recognized and -institutionalized training along with their physician counterparts in the Indian state-supported systems for conventional Western biomedicine and homeopathic medicine. A number of these Indian-trained Ayurvedic physicians practice or teach Ayurveda in the United States.

Research base. There have been extensive studies of the physiological effects of meditative techniques and yoga postures in both the Indian medical literature and the Western psychological literature (Funderburk, 1977; Murphy, 1992a; Murphy and Donovan, 1988). For example, students in hatha yoga classes showed improvement in fitness measures, including flexibility, strength, equilibrium, and stamina (Jharote, 1973).

In addition, effects of yogic postures and breathing on finger blood flow showed consistent changes with various breathing practices, changes that were more pronounced in trained yogic practitioners (Gopal et al., 1973). Changes in endocrine hormone measurements also have been associated with certain Ayurvedic practices (Glaser et al., 1992; Udupa et al., 1971). Measurement of metabolic rate, oxygen exchange, lung capacity, and red and white blood cell counts have been found to be associated with general yogic training and in some cases with specific *asanas* (posture) (Gopal et al., 1974). Similar basic research on meditative practices has led to the development in Western medicine of biofeed-back and relaxation training (see the "Mind-Body Interventions" chapter).

Yogic and meditative practices also have been studied as specific interventions for disease states such as asthma and hypertension (Bhole, 1967; Patel, 1973). A recent pilot study performed in Holland followed a group of patients who used a combination of Ayurvedic therapies. The study documented improvements with Ayurvedic therapies in 79 percent of patients who were studied for a 3-month treatment period with a number of chronic disease conditions, including rheumatoid arthritis, asthma, chronic bronchitis, eczema, psoriasis, hypertension, constipation, headaches, chronic sinusitis, and noninsulin-dependent diabetes mellitus (Janssen, 1989).

In addition, published studies have documented reductions in cardiovascular disease risk factors, including blood pressure, cholesterol, and reaction to stress, in individuals practicing Ayurvedic methods (Schneider et al., 1992) and have shown improvement in overall health care utilization measures among meditators (Orme-Johnson, 1988).

The "technology" of meditative practices has been subjected to studies showing physiological changes of heart rate, blood pressure, brain cortex activity, metabolism, respiration, muscle tension, lactate level, skin resistance, salivation, and pain and stress responses (improvement), and both negative and positive behavioral effects (Murphy, 1992a).

Further laboratory and clinical studies on Ayurvedic herbal preparations and other therapies have shown them to have a wide range of potentially beneficial effects for the prevention and treatment of certain cancers, including breast, lung, and colon cancers (Sharma et al., 1990). They have also been shown effective in the treatment of mental health (Alexander et al., 1989b) and infectious disease (Thyagarajan et al., 1988), in health promotion (Schneider et al., 1990), and in treatment of aging (Alexander et al., 1989a; Glaser et al., 1992). Mechanisms underlying these effects are believed to include free-radical scavenging effects (Fields et al., 1990), immune system modulation, brain neurotransmitter modulation, and hormonal effects (Glaser et al., 1992). The National Cancer Institute (NCI) has included Ayurvedic compounds on its list of potential chemopreventive agents and has recently funded a series of in vitro studies on the cancer-preventive properties of two Ayurvedic herbal compounds, *maharadis amrit kalash* 4 and 5 (MAK-4 and MAK-5). In preliminary studies, NCI researchers have demonstrated that MAK-4 and MAK-5 significantly inhibited cancer cell growth in both human tumor and rat tracheal epithelial cell systems (Arnold et al., 1991).

Future research opportunities and priorities. Because of the potential of ayurvedic therapies for treating conditions for which modern medicine has few, if any, effective treatments, this area is a fertile one for research opportunities. For example, when NCI researchers began testing MAK-4 and MAK-5 for effects against tumor cell growth, they also found that similar compounds such as ferulic acid, catechin, bioflavonoids, retinoic acid (vitamin A), ascorbyl palmitate, and glycyrrhetinic acid also showed chemopreventive activity (Arnold et al., 1991).

Known scientific data on the intrinsic rhythms and laterality (right side vs. left side) patterns in the autonomic nervous system can provide a model for understanding how stress disrupts healthy physical function. Certain meditative and yogic practices have been proposed as noninvasive "technologies" to self-regulate the neural matrices that couple mind and metabolism in the body (Shannahoff-Khalsa, 1991). Translation of the traditional concepts of yogic medicine into the language of modern medicine could stimulate creative research in the neurophysiology of stress and adaptation.

The following are the research opportunities as well as the priorities for investigations in this area of alternative medicine:

1. Performing a critical review of world literature to identify potentially useful Ayurvedic therapies for various conditions.

2. Conducting long-term health care utilization and cost effectiveness studies on individuals who use Ayurvedic therapies, lifestyle programs, and meditation regularly for prevention.

3. Studying the effectiveness of Ayurvedic therapies and lifestyle for the prevention and treatment of diseases such as cardiovascular disease, cancer, AIDS, osteoporosis, autoimmune disorders, Alzheimer's, and aging.

4. Assessing the cost and treatment effectiveness of Ayurvedic therapies in the treatment of specific functional or chronic disorders such as chronic fatigue syndrome, premenstrual syndrome, chronic pain, functional bowel and digestive problems, insomnia, allergies, and neuromuscular disorders.

5. Identifying the mechanisms underlying therapeutic effects of herbal therapies, diet, Ayurvedic physical therapies such as panchakarma, meditation, yogic practices, and other treatment modalities.

6. Studying the effects of the collective practice of meditation on community health indices and health care costs in cities, the Nation, and other social groups.

Chapter 8

Homeopathic Medicine

Overview

The term homeopathy is derived from the Greek words *homeo* (similar) and *pathos* (suffering from disease). The first basic principles of homeopathy were formulated by the German physician Samuel Hahnemann in the late 1700s. Curious about why quinine could cure malaria, Hahnemann ingested quinine bark and experienced alternating bouts of chills, fever, and weakness, the classic symptoms of malaria. From this experience he derived the principle of similars, or "like cures like": that is, a substance that can cause certain symptoms when given to a healthy person can cure those same symptoms in someone who is sick.

Hahnemann spent the rest of his life extensively testing, or "proving," many common herbal and medicinal substances to find out what symptoms they could cause. He also began treating sick people, prescribing the medicine that most closely matched the symptoms of their illness. The information from this experimentation has been carefully recorded and makes up the homeopathic materia medica, a listing of

---

This chapter contains information from two documents: NIH 94-066 and *FDA Consumer*, December 1996. The first section is extracted from NIH Publication No. 94-066 from the Office of Alternative Medicine. December 1994. Due to space considerations, bibliographic data have not been reprinted in this chapter. However, to aid readers who wish to consult the original document or do further research, the in-text references have been retained. The second part reprints an article from the *FDA Consumer*, December 1996 titled "Homeopathy: Real Medicine or Empty Promises?"

medicines and their indications for use. According to the *Homeopathic Pharmacopoeia of the United States*, homeopathic medicines, or remedies, are made from naturally occurring plant, animal, and mineral substances.

By the end of the 19th century, homeopathy was widely practiced in the United States, when there were 22 homeopathic medical schools, more than 100 homeopathic hospitals, and an estimated 15 percent of physicians practicing homeopathy. The practice of homeopathy (along with other types of alternative medicine) declined dramatically in the United States following the publication of the Flexner Report in 1910, which established guidelines for the funding of medical schools. These guidelines favored AMA-approved institutions and virtually crippled competing schools of medicine. In the past 15 years, however, there has been a resurgence of interest in homeopathy in this country. It is estimated that approximately 3,000 physicians and other health care practitioners currently use homeopathy, and a recent survey showed that 1 percent of the general population, or approximately 2.5 million people, had sought help from a homeopathic doctor in 1990 (Eisenberg et al., 1993).

Those who are licensed to practice homeopathy in the United States vary according to state-by-state "scope of practice" guidelines, but they include M.D.s, D.O.s, dentists, naturopaths (N.D.s), chiropractors, veterinarians, acupuncturists, nurse practitioners, and physician assistants. Three states now have specific licensing boards for homeopathic physicians: Arizona, Connecticut, and Nevada. Specialty certification diplomas for those prescribing homeopathic drugs are established through national boards of examination for M.D.s/D.O.s and N.D.s. Selfhelp as well as professional training courses in homeopathy are offered through the National Center for Homeopathy (NCH) in Alexandria, Virginia. NCH serves as an umbrella organization for consumer support of homeopathy as well as a focus for coordination among an increasing number of organizations and specialty societies offering lay and professional training programs in homeopathy.

Homeopathic medicine also is currently widely practiced worldwide, especially in Europe, Latin America, and Asia. In France, 32 percent of family physicians use homeopathy, while 42 percent of British physicians refer patients to homeopaths (Bouchayer, 1990; Wharton and Lewith, 1986). In India, homeopathy is practiced in the national health service, and there are more than 100 homeopathic medical colleges and more than 100,000 homeopathic physicians (Kishore, 1983).

In the United States today, the homeopathic drug market has grown to become a multimillion-dollar industry; a significant increase has occurred in the importation and domestic marketing of homeopathic drugs. Homeopathic remedies are recognized and regulated by the FDA and are manufactured by established pharmaceutical companies under strict guidelines established by the *Homeopathic Pharmacopoeia of the United States*. Products that are offered for the treatment of serious conditions must be dispensed under the care of a licensed practitioner. Other products offered for the use of self-limiting conditions such as colds and allergies may be marketed as over-the-counter drugs.

Homeopathy is used to treat both acute and chronic health problems as well as for health prevention and promotion in healthy people. Homeopathic medicines are prescribed on the basis of a wide constellation of physical, emotional, and mental symptoms. The one remedy that most closely fits all of the symptoms of a given individual is called the *similimum* for that person. Thus, homeopathic treatment is individualized, and two or more people with the same diagnosis may be given different medicines, depending on the specific symptoms of illness in each person. A person with a sore throat, for instance, may need one of six or seven common remedies for sore throats, depending on whether the pain is worse on the right or left side, what time of day it is worse, what the person's mood is, and his or her body temperature, thirst, and appetite (Jouanny, 1980).

Hahnemann also discovered that if the homeopathic remedies were "potentized" by diluting them in a water-alcohol solution and then shaking, side effects could be diminished. He found that after the medicines were potentized to high dilutions, there was still a medicinal effect, and side effects were minimal. Some homeopathic medicines are diluted to concentrations as low as 10^{-30} to $10^{-20,000}$. This particular aspect of homeopathic theory and practice has caused many modern scientists to reject homeopathic medicine outright. Critics of homeopathy contend that such extreme dilutions of the medicines are beyond the point at which any molecules of the medicine can theoretically still be found in the solution (When to believe . . . , 1988).

On the other hand, scientists who accept the validity of homeopathic theory suggest several theories to explain how highly diluted homeopathic medicines may act. Using recent developments in quantum physics, they have proposed that electromagnetic energy may exist in the medicines and interact with the body on some level (Delinick, 1991). Researchers in physical chemistry have proposed the "memory of water" theory, whereby the structure of the water-alcohol solution is altered by the medicine during the process of dilution and retains this structure even after none of the actual substance remains (Davenas et al., 1988).

Recent research accomplishments. Basic science research in homeopathy has primarily involved investigations into the chemical and biological activity of highly diluted substances. The most thought-provoking research has involved observation of the physiological responses of living systems to homeopathically potentized solutions. For example, in the 1920s a German researcher conducted a series of studies spanning 12 years in which he showed periodic variations in the growth patterns of plants that had been exposed to a series of homeopathic dilutions of metallic salts (Kolisko, 1932). With the focus of modern biological laboratory research on cellular and organ function, homeopathic studies have more recently been conducted in this area. Such laboratory studies have shown positive effects of homeopathically prepared microdoses on mouse white blood cells (Davenas et al.,1987), arsenic excretion in the rat (Cazin et al., 1987), bleeding time with aspirin (Doutremepuich et al., 1987), and degranulation of human basophils—blood cells that mediate allergic reactions—(Davenas et al., 1988; Poitevin et al., 1988).

Furthermore, recent clinical trials in Europe have suggested a positive effect of homeopathic medicines on such conditions as allergic rhinitis (Reilly et al., 1986), fibrositis (Fisher et al., 1989), and influenza (Ferley et al., 1989), while an earlier study showed no apparent effect in the treatment of osteoarthritis by a homeopathic medicine (Shipley et al., 1983). The *British Medical Journal* published a meta-analysis in 1992 of homeopathic clinical trials, which found that 15 of 22 well-designed studies showed positive results. This study concluded that more methodologically rigorous trials should be done to address the question of efficacy of homeopathic treatment (Kleijnen et al., 1991). A recent double-blind study comparing homeopathic treatment with placebo in the treatment of acute childhood diarrhea found a statistically significant improvement in the group receiving the homeopathic treatment (Jacobs et al., 1993).

Homeopathic research study design has used different methodologies depending on the question being asked. One of the earliest studies of homeopathy in a peer-reviewed conventional medical journal asked the question, "Is the homeopathic medical system taken *as a whole* more effective or less detrimental than another treatment or placebo in the condition studied?" In this study, which focused on rheumatoid arthritis, 195 patients who had previously been treated with nonsteroidal anti-inflammatory drugs were allocated to placebo treatment or active treatment. The active-treatment population then was divided between aspirin and a homeopathic medication. The homeopathic doctors were allowed to prescribe any medication at whatever interval, frequency, or potency they considered appropriate.

The trial was conducted for a year, and by the end of the year almost 43 percent of the homeopathic treatment group had stopped other treatments and were judged to have improved since the beginning of the study. Another 24 percent of the homeopathic group improved, but they continued their conventional medications. In contrast, only 15 percent of the aspirin group were maintained and improved on the treatment. The entire placebo group had dropped out within six weeks.

This study, however, was criticized on some methodological grounds—principally that the homeopathic prescribers were more committed to the treatment and the patients were easily able to determine who was in the placebo group (Gibson et al., 1978). Subsequently, the same researchers conducted another trial of this type, in which a specific disease was subjected to homeopathic treatment by any one of a number of clinically indicated homeopathic medications. This time, a placebo-controlled, double-blind study showed that the improvements among the homeopathically treated patients were statistically more significant than those of the placebo group (Gibson et al., 1980).

A second type of homeopathic study has been used to ask a more specific question, namely, is a particular homeopathic medication more effective than another treatment or placebo for a particular disease? Fisher and colleagues (1989) asked this question in a study of primary fibromyalgia, a type of inflammation; patients who met recognized diagnostic criteria for fibromyalgia were further stratified as patients for whom a particular homeopathic medicine, rhus toxicodendron 6C, was homeopathically indicated. Patients with the active treatment were better on all variables, and a number of their tender points were reduced by 25 percent at the end of four weeks of active treatment in comparison with controls.

In a similar study, Reilly and colleagues (1986) used homeopathic medications with hay fever patients to address the issue of whether homeopathic medications are in fact placebos. The researchers directly treated matched groups of approximately 70 patients with a homeopathic medication made from mixed grass pollens at the dilution of one part in 10^{60}. This was done to address the assertion that a potency lacking in any of the original substances could act as more than a placebo. Patients took one tablet twice daily of either placebo or the test drug and were free to use a standard antihistamine at any time during the 5-week study. Only the homeopathically treated group showed a clear reduction in symptoms, and in comparison with the placebo-treated group, twice as many of the homeopathically treated patients had discontinued their antihistamines. This study also demonstrated that even a simple study design requires careful analysis of potential confounding variables, including the clinical observations that some homeopathically treated patients experience temporary aggravation of their symptoms before achieving a sustained improvement.

A third type of study simply looks at comparative utilization figures for homeopathic practitioners in a health care system with or without attention to the comparative clinical outcomes. For example, in France, research on cost-effectiveness has shown that the annual cost to the social security system for a homeopathic physician is 54 percent lower than the cost for a conventional physician. Moreover, the same study found that the price of the average homeopathic medicine is one-third that of standard drugs (CNAM, 1991).

Research opportunities. Research into the basic science areas of quantum physics, physical chemistry, and biochemistry may determine whether a homeopathic medicine's mechanism of action can be elucidated. Existing studies of the effects of the succussion process on the physical-energetic nature of medicinal dilutions should be repeated and extended (Smith and Boericke, 1967). Moreover, modern-day herbal, biological, or pharmaceutically synthesized agents should be subjected to homeopathic "provings." This scientific documentation of effects and side effects in healthy people would enable new homeopathic drug development.

Evaluating the clinical efficacy of homeopathy using randomized, double-blind clinical trials for the treatment of acute problems such as diarrhea, otitis media, and postoperative pain as well as for chronic illnesses is a fertile area for research. Existing studies should be repeated with different investigators, giving attention to rigorous methodology. Special emphasis should be given to research in areas where modern medicine does not have an established, satisfactory solution, such as arthritis, AIDS, asthma, headaches, and inflammatory bowel disease.

More clinical research also needs to be directed toward analyzing and improving the accuracy of the clinical data in the homeopathic literature, much of which is currently at least a century old. Indeed, homeopaths in Great Britain are currently establishing a system using a modern, computerized medical database and standardized subjective and objective outcome measures to analyze the outcomes of patients treated with various homeopathic medications (van Haseln and Fisher, 1990). This sort of study will help homeopathic clinicians to investigate the differential efficacy of various homeopathic medications and allow for an updating of the prescribing criteria for various medications in the homeopathic materia medica.

In addition to clinical trials on conditions with specific diagnoses, studies also need to be done to evaluate the possible benefits of long-term treatment with the system of homeopathic medicine. Since proponents of this discipline claim that homeopathy improves overall physical and mental health, health status indicators should be used to evaluate changes in health in patients treated this way for several months or years.

Recent surveys in the United States found that most homeopathic patients seek care for chronic illnesses (Jacobs and Crothers, 1991) and that homeopathic physicians spend twice as much time with their patients, order half as many laboratory tests and procedures, and prescribe fewer drugs (Jacobs, 1992). Since treatment of chronic illness accounts for a large proportion of health care expenditures in the United States, the cost effectiveness of homeopathic medicine should be investigated by comparing homeopathy with conventional treatments for specific chronic illnesses such as recurrent childhood ear infections, allergies, arthritis, headaches, depression, and asthma. Clinical outcomes should be measured as well as such factors as utilization of health services, number of missed days of work or school, patient satisfaction, and overall cost of health care. This research will help determine whether incorporating homeopathy into the national health care scheme would significantly reduce health care costs.

Homeopathy: Real Medicine or Empty Promises?

Some of the medicines of homeopathy evoke positive images—chamomile, marigold, daisy, onion. But even some of Mother Nature's cruelest creations—poison ivy, mercury, arsenic, pit viper venom, hemlock—are part of homeopathic care. Homeopathy is a medical theory and practice that developed in reaction to the bloodletting, blistering, purging, and other harsh procedures of conventional medicine as it was practiced more than 200 years ago. Remedies made from many sources—including plants, minerals or animals—are prescribed based on both a person's symptoms and personality. Patients receiving homeopathic care frequently feel worse before they get better because homeopathic medicines often stimulate, rather than suppress, symptoms. This seeming reversal of logic is a relevant part of homeopathy because symptoms are viewed as the body's effort to restore health.

The Food and Drug Administration regulates homeopathic remedies under provisions of the Food, Drug, and Cosmetic Act.

Kinder, Gentler Medicine

In the late 1700s, the most popular therapy for most ailments was bloodletting. Some doctors had so much faith in bleeding that they were willing to remove up to four-fifths of the patient's blood. Other therapies of choice included blistering—placing caustic or hot substances on the skin to draw out infections—and administering dangerous chemicals to induce vomiting or purge the bowels. Massive doses of a mercury-containing drug called calomel cleansed the bowels, but at the same time caused teeth to loosen, hair to fall out, and other symptoms of acute mercury poisoning.

Samuel Hahnemann, a German physician disenchanted with these methods, began to develop a theory based on three principles: the law of similars, the minimum dose, and the single remedy.

The word homeopathy is derived from the Greek words for like (*homoios*) and suffering (*pathos*). With the law of similars, Hahnemann theorized that if a large amount of a substance causes certain symptoms in a healthy person, smaller amounts of the same substance can treat those symptoms in someone who is ill. The basis of his theory took shape after a strong dose of the malaria treatment quinine caused his healthy body to develop symptoms similar to ones caused by the disease. He continued to test his theory on himself as well as family and friends with different herbs, minerals and other substances. He called these experiments "provings."

But, as might be expected, the intensity of the symptoms caused by the original proving was harrowing. So Hahnemann began decreasing the doses to see how little of a substance could still produce signs of healing.

With the minimum dose, or law of infinitesimals, Hahnemann believed that a substance's strength and effectiveness increased the more it was diluted. Minuscule doses were prepared by repeatedly diluting the active ingredient by factors of 10. A "6X" preparation (the X is the Roman numeral for 10) is a 1-to-10 dilution repeated six times, leaving the active ingredient as one part per million. Essential to the process of increasing potency while decreasing the actual amount of the active ingredient is vigorous shaking after each dilution.

Some homeopathic remedies are so dilute, no molecules of the healing substance remain. Even with sophisticated technology now available, analytical chemists may find it difficult or impossible to identify any active ingredient. But the homeopathic belief is that the substance has left its imprint or a spirit-like essence that stimulates the body to heal itself.

Finally, a homeopathic physician generally prescribes only a single remedy to cover all symptoms—mental as well as physical—the patient is experiencing. However, the use of multi-ingredient remedies is recognized as part of homeopathic practice.

FDA Regulation

In 1938, Sen. Royal Copeland of New York, the chief sponsor of the Food, Drug, and Cosmetic Act and a homeopathic physician, wrote into the law a recognition of any product listed in the *Homeopathic Pharmacopeia* of the United States. The *Homeopathic Pharmencopeia* includes a compilation of standards for source, composition and preparation of homeopathic drugs.

FDA regulates homeopathic drugs in several significantly different ways from other drugs. Manufacturers of homeopathic drugs are deferred from submitting new drug applications to FDA. Their products are exempt from good manufacturing practice requirements related to expiration dating and from finished product testing for identity and strength. Homeopathic drugs in solid oral dosage form must have an imprint that identifies the manufacturer and indicates that the drug is homeopathic. The imprint on conventional products, unless specifically exempt, must identify the active ingredient and dosage strength as well as the manufacturer.

"The reasoning behind [the difference] is that homeopathic products contain little or no active ingredients," explains Edward Miracco, a consumer safety officer with FDA's Center for Drug Evaluation and Research. "From a toxicity, poison-control standpoint, [the active ingredient and strength] was deemed to be unnecessary."

Another difference involves alcohol. Conventional drugs for adults can contain no more than 10 percent alcohol, and the amount is even less for children's medications. But some homeopathic products contain much higher amounts because the agency has temporarily exempted these products from the alcohol limit rules.

"Alcohol is an integral part of many homeopathic products," says Miracco. For this reason, the agency has decided to delay its decision concerning alcohol in homeopathic products while it reviews the necessity of high levels of alcohol.

"Overall, the disparate treatment has been primarily based on the uniqueness of homeopathic products, the lack of any real concern over their safety because they have little or no pharmacologically active ingredients, and because of agency resources and priorities," explains Miracco.

However, homeopathic products are not exempt from all FDA regulations. If a homeopathic drug claims to treat a serious disease such as cancer it can be sold by prescription only. Only products sold for so-called self-limiting conditions—colds, headaches, and other minor health problems that eventually go away on their own—can be sold without a prescription (over-the-counter).

Requirements for nonprescription labeling include:

• an ingredients list
• instructions for safe use
• at least one major indication
• dilution (for example 2X for one part per hundred, 3X for one part per thousand).

Over the past several years, the agency has issued about 12 warning letters to homeopathic marketers. The most common infraction was the sale of prescription homeopathic drugs over-the-counter. "It's illegal, it's in violation, and we're going to focus on it," says Miracco.

Other problems include:

• products promoted as homeopathic that contain non-homeopathic active ingredients, such as vitamins or plants not listed in homeopathic references

• lack of tamper-resistant packaging

• lack of proper labeling

• vague indications for use that could encompass serious disease conditions. For example, a phrase like "treats gastrointestinal disorders" is too general, explains Miracco. "This phrase can encompass a wide variety of conditions, from stomachache or simple diarrhea to colon cancer," he says. "Claims need to be specific so the consumer knows what the product is intended to treat and the indication does not encompass serious disease conditions that would require prescription dispensing and labeling."

In addition to enforcement, the agency is also focusing on preventing problems by educating the homeopathic industry about FDA regulations. "Agency representatives continue to meet with homeopathic trade groups to tell them about problems we've had, difficulties we've seen, and trends we've noticed," says Miracco.

FDA is aware of a few reports of illness associated with the use of homeopathic products. However, agency review of those reported to FDA discounted the homeopathic product involved as the cause of the adverse reaction. In one instance, arsenic, which is a recognized homeopathic ingredient, was implicated. But, as would be expected, FDA analysis revealed the concentration of arsenic was so minute there wasn't enough to cause concern, explains Miracco. "It's been diluted out."

Homeopathic Treatment

Homeopathy consists of highly individualized treatments based on a person's genetic history, personal health history, body type, and present status of all physical, emotional and mental symptoms.

Jennifer Jacobs, M.D., who has a family practice and is licensed to practice homeopathy in Washington state, spends at least an hour and a half with each new patient. "What I do is review the lifetime history of the patient's health," she explains. "Also I ask a lot of questions about certain general symptoms such as food preferences and sleep patterns that usually aren't seen as important in conventional medicine. In looking to make the match between the person and the remedy, I need to have all of this sort of information."

Why does someone trained in conventional medicine turn to homeopathy? "With chronic illnesses such as arthritis and allergies, conventional medicine has solutions that help control the symptoms but you don't really see the patients getting better," says Jacobs. "What I have seen in my homeopathic work is that it really does seem to help people get better. I'm not saying I can cure everyone but I do see where people's overall health is improved over the course of treatment."

Jacobs hasn't abandoned conventional medicine completely. "My daughter is 17 and she's never taken antibiotics, but I would have no hesitation to use antibiotics if she had pneumonia, or meningitis, or a kidney infection," says Jacobs.

About a third of Jacobs' practice is children, and ear infections are one of the most common problems she treats. "Ear infections are something that seems to respond well to homeopathy," she says. "Of course, if a child is not better within two or three days, or if the child develops a high fever, or if I feel that there's a serious complication setting in, then of course I will use antibiotics. But I find that in the majority of cases, ear infections do resolve without antibiotics."

In addition to treating patients, Jacobs has conducted a clinical trial the results of which suggest that homeopathic treatment might be useful in the treatment of acute childhood diarrhea. The results were published in the May 1994 issue of *Pediatrics*. In the article, Jacobs concluded that further studies should be conducted to determine whether her findings were accurate. A subsequent article appearing the November 1995 issue of *Pediatrics* indicated that Jacobs' study was flawed in several ways.

Although *Pediatrics* is published by the American Academy of Pediatrics, Jacobs' study and several others published in such journals as *The Lancet* and the *British Medical Journal* are considered "scanty at best" by the academy. "Given the plethora of studies that are published [on other topics] in scientific journals, I wouldn't say there are a lot of articles coming out," says Joe M. Sanders Jr., M.D., the executive director of the academy. "Just because an article appears in a scientific journal does not mean that it's absolute fact and should be immediately incorporated into therapeutic regimens. It just means that the study is [published] for critique and review and hopefully people will use that as a stepping stone for further research."

More studies are under way. For example, the Office of Alternative Medicine at the National Institutes of Health has awarded a grant for a clinical trial of the effects of homeopathic treatment on mild traumatic brain injury

Even with the dearth of clinical research, homeopathy's popularity in the United States is growing. The 1995 retail sales of homeopathic medicines in the United States were estimated at $201 million and growing at a rate of 20 percent a year, according to the American Homeopathic Pharmaceutical Association. The number of homeopathic practitioners in the United States has increased from fewer than 200 in the 1970s to approximately 3,000 in 1996.

When looking for a homeopathic practitioner, it's important to, find someone who is licensed, according to the National Center for Homeopathy. Each state has its own licensing requirements. "Whether that person is a medical doctor or a physician's assistant or a naturopathic physician, I feel that anyone who's treating people who are sick needs to have medical training," says Jacobs.

Real Medicine or Wishful Thinking?

Many who don't believe in homeopathy's effectiveness say any successful treatments are due to the placebo effect, or, in other words, positive thinking.

But homeopathy's supporters counter that their medicine works in groups like infants and even animals that can't be influenced by a pep talk. Jacobs adds that sometimes she mistakenly gives a patient the wrong remedy and he or she doesn't get better. "Then I give the right remedy, and the person does get better," she says. "So it's not like everybody gets better because it's all in their head. I think it's only because we don't understand the mechanism of action of homeopathy that so many people have trouble accepting it."

The American Medical Association does not accept homeopathy, but it doesn't reject it either. "The AMA encourages doctors to become aware of alternative therapies and use them when and where appropriate," says AMA spokesman Jim Fox.

Similarly, the American Academy of Pediatrics has no specific policy on homeopathy. If an adult asked the academy's Sanders about homeopathy, he would tell that person to "do your own investigation. I don't personally prescribe homeopathic remedies, but I would be open-minded."

That open-mindedness applies only to adults, however. "I would have problems with somebody imposing other than conventional medicine onto a child who's incapable of making that decision," he says.

Even professionals who practice homeopathy warn that nothing in medicine—either conventional or alternative—is absolute. "I'm not saying we can cure everyone [with homeopathy]," says Jacobs.

—by Isadora Stehlin

Isadora Stehlin is a member of FDA's public affairs staff.

Chapter 9

Anthroposophically Extended Medicine

Overview

The foundations of anthroposophically extended medicine were laid down by the Austrian philosopher and spiritual scientist Rudolf Steiner, Ph.D. (1861-1925). Steiner's "anthroposophy" (*anthropos* [human]; *sophia* [wisdom]) proposed a philosophical or spiritual-scientific model of human individuality. He took rigorous precision and methodologies of scientific empiricism and extended them into the spiritual domain, into what he called the "supersensible world," the domain underlying all human life, thought, and physical well-being. Steiner's theories were applied to agriculture (biodynamics), education (Waldorf Schools), and social theories (threefold social order) as well as art, painting, sculpture, dance (eurythmy), architecture, music, and speech (e.g., for performance, education, and therapeutics).

In the 1920s Ita Wegman, M.D. (a Dutch physician, 1876-1943), and Steiner coauthored a foundational work for physicians seeking to broaden their medical practice according to these anthroposophical principles (Steiner and Wegman, 1925). Steiner's intention was to outline a "rationally exact medical mode of thinking" as part of his larger, lifelong program of approaching issues of spiritual knowledge

Extracted from NIH Publication No. 94-066 from the Office of Alternative Medicine. December 1994. Due to space considerations, bibliographic data have not been reprinted in this chapter. However, to aid readers who wish to consult the original document or do further research, the in-text references have been retained.

as a scientist. He gave an extended series of lectures and training courses for physicians, nurses, social workers, and pastoral counselors. This effort to extend therapeutics through the anthroposophical paradigm was based on Steiner's 34 years of work with the scientific method and encompassed therapeutic efforts based on botany, anatomy, natural sciences, and the dynamics of healing. Steiner and his physician followers attempted to reorient medical therapeutics so that they would encompass the spiritual depths of human existence. "Medicine will be broadened by a spiritual conception of man to an art of healing or else it will remain a souless technology that removes only symptoms. Through the concrete inclusion of the spirit and soul of man, a humanization of medicine is possible" (Wolff, undated).

As an extension of Western medicine, anthroposophical medicine builds on three preexisting movements and therapeutics. The first is natural medicine or naturopathy, which involves the use of material substances in nondegraded, nonchemically separated forms. Naturopathy, established in Europe in the early 19th century, is now practiced in an increasing number of States in the United States. The second foundation is homeopathy, introduced by the German physician Samuel Hahnemann in the 18th century (see the "Homeopathic Medicine" section). The third foundation for anthroposophical medicine is modern scientific medicine itself. Steiner insisted that anthroposophically extended medicine be practiced only on the foundation of a Western medical training and credentials, and thus only M.D.s could become anthroposophical physicians.

Estimates of the number of M.D.s who mainly or exclusively practice anthroposophical medicine range from 1,000 to 6,000 worldwide with between 30 and 100 such physicians in the United States (Ministry of Science and Technology, Federal Republic of Germany, 1992; Scharff, 1993). Most practitioners are concentrated in Switzerland, Germany, Sweden, and Holland, and there are more than a dozen hospitals and clinics in Europe specializing in anthroposophically extended medicine. The Witten-Herdecke Medical School, established in 1983 near Dortmund, Germany, teaches anthroposophical medicine and grants M.D. degrees. Efforts are under way to formally certify physicians with anthroposophical training, and the Board of the American College of Anthroposophically Extended Medicine has been established in the United States (Scharff, 1993).

Hundreds of uniquely formulated medications are used in anthroposophical practice. Some are prepared by a multiple dilution and succussion (potentization) process, which is similar to that used in standard homeopathic pharmaceuticals. About 85 percent of the remedies are such potentized preparations, and the remaining 15 percent are similar to other botanical or traditional herbal medicines. All the basic substances go through a standardized pharmaceutical process and are made into remedies according to the official pharmacopoeia of the country of manufacture. The preparation of medications seeks to match the "archetypal forces" in plants, animals, and minerals with disease processes in humans and, through this correspondence, to stimulate healing.

Two major pharmaceutical firms prepare anthroposophical medications for physicians around the world: Waleda and Wala, which are both located in Europe with subsidiaries in many countries, including the United States. Use of these products is not limited exclusively to anthroposophical medicine specialists. In the United States approximately 300 physicians regularly order anthroposophical pharmaceuticals, while in Germany up to 15,000 physicians prescribe these products, mainly preparations of the mistletoe plant for treatment of cancers (Ministry of Science and Technology, Federal Republic of Germany, 1992).

Today, anthroposophical physicians augment conventional science by including new scientific approaches to the living processes of nature, the soul, and the human spirit. One model for approaching this task is to identify three different interdependent aspects of a human's body-mind processes. First, the "sense-nerve" system, which includes the nervous system and the brain organization that support the mind and the thinking process. Second, there is the "rhythmic" system, which includes physical processes of a rhythmic or periodic nature (e.g., the pulse, breathing, intestinal rhythms) and supports the emotional or feeling processes. Third is the "metabolic-limb" system, which includes digestion, elimination, energetic metabolism, and the voluntary movement processes. This third system supports the aspects of human behavior that express the will.

This threefold model gives the physician a diagnostic scheme for understanding an illness as a deviation from the harmonious internal balance of the functions of the bodily self and the spiritual self. In this approach, a person's physical, human makeup is seen as continually interacting with the soul or spiritual nature of that person. This anthroposophical model is used by practitioners as a creative entry for therapeutic insight into what are now recognized as the processes of mind-body interactions in health and disease.

Research base. Much of the research in the field of anthroposophically extended medicine has been connected with attempts to understand the nature of disease, assess it qualitatively, and understand how the essential properties of the objects under investigation could be applied in therapy. For instance, Steiner suggested that mistletoe might have a role in cancer therapy. It was observed that mistletoe had unusual biological properties as a relatively undifferentiated plant as well as a tendency to show regular rhythmic changes in both a seasonal and a lunar cycle. From this observation came an extensive series of studies in Europe on iscador, iscucin, abnoba, vysorel, and helixor, cancer remedies made from mistletoe. This work suggests that these mistletoe remedies can stimulate the body's immunological defense systems and act as chemostatic agents to prevent further growth of tumors. Mistletoe extracts have been analyzed for their chemical fractions, which include lectins, polysaccharides, and proteins. A review of 36 controlled clinical trials using mistletoe in cancer therapy showed six as statistically significant, having results pointing to a life-extending effect (Keine, 1989). (See the "Pharmacological and Biological Treatments" chapter and the "Research Methodologies" chapter for further information on mistletoe research.)

In recent years, collaboration between anthroposophical scientists and established university-based researchers has led to improvement in the quality and mutual acceptability of "unconventional" anthroposophical research in Germany. Of particular note is the work done by Professor G. Hildebrandt and his colleagues at the University of Marburg. In the past 30 years they have contributed more than 500 papers to the world's scientific literature, placing particular emphasis on the chronobiology (biorhythms) of body physiology in stress, disease, and therapy (Hildebrandt and Hensel, 1982; Hildebrandt, 1986). An example of the application of this line of research is shown by the work of von Laue and Henn, who reported studies of the time rhythms of cancer patients and tumor growths and how these abnormal rhythmic functions in cancer could be altered with mistletoe therapy (von Laue and Henn, 1991).

The qualitative and analytical aspects of anthroposophical research are further illustrated in the psychosomatic field by the work of Fischer and Grosshans with colitis patients at Herdecke Hospital. They conducted a structured interview with 60 patients admitted with ulcerative colitis or Crohn's disease (inflammations of the bowel) for a 2-year period and found that in addition to the well-known physical characteristics of these two diseases, the patients displayed other characteristic behaviors, including distinct underlying mood tendencies, communication styles, self-perceptions, and typical attitudinal relationships to past and future events. These psychological responses differentiated the Crohn's disease and ulcerative colitis patients along a pattern that could be interpreted as a parallel to the clinical symptoms (Fischer and Grosshans, 1992).

Cost and effectiveness issues in health care delivery are important in European countries as well as the United States. In Germany, von Hauff and Praetorius, an economist and a political scientist, conducted a pilot study (1990) on the performance structure of alternative medical practices. They used a nonrandom poll of established practitioners of conventional, homeopathic, or anthroposophical practices and were able to qualitatively analyze the practices under consideration as well as show quantitative differences in health care utilization. They found that the patients being treated by homeopathic and anthroposophical practitioners claimed 30 percent to 50 percent fewer illness days, respectively, than patients being treated by conventional practitioners. Furthermore, the homeopathic and anthroposophical practices had fewer referrals for hospitalization, fewer referrals to specialists, and fewer laboratory tests.

Research opportunities. Anthroposophical physicians approach issues of medical research by stressing basic methodological issues. For instance, the current dominant model of medical practice based on classical physics is seen as inadequate for understanding the laws of living organisms. This criticism extends to clinical research, where anthroposophical principles emphasize the overall therapeutic strategies being studied and not the isolated effect of specific chemical medicines. A truly scientific research agenda, according to the anthroposophical approach, must match the study methods and questions posed with the subject under investigation. In other words, inorganic systems require one type of science, living organic systems require another, psychological processes another, and intellectual-spiritual activities yet another. Although a single rational scientific method may be valid throughout these various domains of human endeavor, the specific nature of the scientific approach must be different and appropriate to the context of each domain. A recent poll in Germany of anthroposophical physicians identified this methodological issue as the major problem for future medical research (Ministry of Science and Technology, Federal Republic of Germany, 1992).

Particular areas of recommended research for anthroposophical medicine include the following:

- Establishing comprehensive valid criteria for assessing quality-of-life outcomes in therapy trials.

- Conducting comparison trials of isolated active ingredients versus extracts from the whole plant.

- Comparing a single-therapy approach to a combination-therapy approach (e.g., medical treatment, diet, and curative eurythmy artistic therapies for groups of patients with given clinical conditions).

- Documenting the effect of the use of anthroposophical remedies from a chronobiological perspective.

- Prospectively evaluating the effect of using anthroposophical methods for early detection and correction of tendencies toward illness before they manifest as serious pathology requiring expensive medical interventions.

Chapter 10

Naturopathic Medicine

Overview

As a distinct American health care profession, naturopathic medicine is almost 100 years old. It was founded as a formal health care system at the turn of the century by a variety of medical practitioners from various natural therapeutic disciplines. By the early 1900s there were more than 20 naturopathic medical schools, and naturopathic physicians, called "eclectic" physicians at the time, were licensed in most of the States. After the Flexner Report in 1910 and the rise in belief that pharmaceutical drugs could eliminate all disease, the practice of naturopathic medicine experienced a dramatic decline. It has experienced a resurgence in the past two decades, however, as a health-conscious public began to seek natural therapies delivered by professionals skilled in these modalities.

Today, there are more than 1,000 licensed naturopathic doctors (N.D.s) in the United States. Currently, there are two accredited U.S. naturopathic medical schools: the National College of Naturopathic Medicine (NCNM) in Portland, OR, and Bastyr College of Natural Sciences in Seattle, WA, which graduate approximately 50 physicians each per year. A third naturopathic medical school, Southwest Col-

---

Extracted from NIH Publication No. 94-066 from the Office of Alternative Medicine. December 1994. Due to space considerations, bibliographic data have not been reprinted in this chapter. However, to aid readers who wish to consult the original document or do further research, the in-text references have been retained.

lege of Naturopathic Medicine in Scottsdale, AZ, began classes in September 1993. Seven U.S. States and four Canadian provinces grant licenses to practice naturopathic medicine. In addition, a number of other States have legal statutes that allow the practice of naturopathic medicine within a specific context. The American Association of Naturopathic Physicians publishes the *Journal of Naturopathic Medicine*, which includes articles on original research, research reviews, and news and review articles relating to naturopathic medicine.

As it is practiced today, naturopathic medicine integrates traditional natural therapeutics—including botanical medicine, clinical nutrition, homeopathy, acupuncture, traditional oriental medicine, hydrotherapy, and naturopathic manipulative therapy—with modern scientific medical diagnostic science and standards of care. Naturopathic physicians are trained in anatomy, cell biology, nutrition, physiology, pathology, neurosciences, histology, pharmacology, biostatistics, epidemiology, public health, and other conventional medical disciplines, and they receive specialized training in the alternative medicine disciplines. They integrate this knowledge into a cohesive medical practice and tailor their approaches to the needs of an individual patient according to these eight primary principles:

1. Recognition of the inherent healing ability of the body.

2. Identification and treatment of the cause of diseases rather than mere elimination or suppression of symptoms.

3. Use of therapies that do no harm.

4. The doctor's primary role as teacher.

5. Establishment and maintenance of optimal health and balance.

6. Treatment of the whole person.

7. Prevention of disease through a healthy lifestyle and control of risk factors.

8. Therapeutic use of nutrition to promote health and to combat chronic and degenerative diseases.

Research base. Medical research on naturopathic practice is based on the empirical documentation of treatments with case history observations, medical records, and summaries of practitioners' clinical experiences. Naturopathic physicians have conducted scientific research in natural medicines in China, Germany, India, France, and England as well as U.S. research in clinical nutrition.

The two current accredited naturopathic medical schools have active research departments. For example, NCNM participated in a 10-year nationwide study of the cervical cap as a method of birth control. Study conclusions were submitted to the FDA (National College of Naturopathic Medicine Clinical Faculty, 1991). Naturopathic researchers also have investigated the pharmacology and physiological effects of nutritional and natural therapeutic agents (Barrie et al., 1987a, 1987b; Mittman, 1990). Digestive tract stresses and their treatment with natural methods also have been a focus of study (Blair et al., 1991; Collins and Mittman, 1990; Thom, 1992), and naturopathic physicians have been active in the investigation of new homeopathic remedies (Brown and Lange, 1992).

Naturopathic medical researchers have shown a particular interest in the natural treatment of women's health problems. One series of clinical research studies evaluated a naturopathic treatment protocol for women with cervical dysplasia (abnormal Pap smears). All subjects received oral nutritional and botanical supplementation, local topical cleansings, and suppositories made from herbal and nutritional agents (Hudson, 1991). Eight distinct naturopathic protocols were used depending on the severity of the abnormal Pap smears. Treatment included topical applications of *Bromelia, Calendula*, zinc chloride, and *Sanguinaria*. Additional home treatments included vaginal suppositories with myrrh, *Echinacea, Usnea, Hydrastis, Althaea*, geranium, and yarrow. The patients also used vitamin A suppositories, vitamin C, beta-carotene, folic acid, selenium, and *Lomatium* systemically as well as a botanical formula including (a) *Trifolium*, (b) *Taraxacum*, (c) *Glycyrrhiza* and *Hydrastis*, or (d) *Thuja* plus *Echinacea* and *Ligustrum* (Hudson, 1993b).

Of the 43 women in the study, 38 returned to normal Pap smears and normal tissue biopsy. Three had partial improvement, two showed no change, and none progressed toward more advanced disease states during treatment (Hudson, 1993a). It was suggested that partial use of these protocols might also benefit the long-term outcome in patients undergoing conventional treatment of cervical dysplasia including cryosurgery, conization, or loop electrosurgical excision procedures.

The most recently completed naturopathic study in women's health tested the clinical and endocrine effects of a botanical formula as an alternative to estrogen replacement therapy. Results of this study suggest a clinically significant benefit (measured as reduction in the total number of menopausal symptoms) in 100 percent of the women versus 17 percent in the placebo group (Hudson and Standish, 1993).

Future research opportunities. The following areas in the field of naturopathy offer the best opportunities for yielding significant research results:

Clinical trials on naturopathic botanical formulas as an alternative to hormone replacement therapy.

Effects of individual herbs on specific disease, for example, *Glycyrrhiza* for peptic ulcer disease, *Crataegus* for hypertension, *Echinacea* as an antiviral, *Ulmus fulva* for irritable bowel, and *Taraxacum* as a diuretic.

- Evaluations of the postsurgical outcomes of patients who have used naturopathic medicine to accelerate healing and improve their recovery.

- Evaluations of naturopathic protocols for treatment of hyperlipidemia, cervical dysplasia, otitis media, diabetes, and hypertension.

- Clinical trials on the outcome of breast cancer patients who use naturopathic medicine with their conventional therapy versus patients who use only conventional treatment.

- Facilitation of research into ethnomedicines by documenting oral traditions and studying them in the context of their cultures—for example, hydrotherapy and European traditions, native plants of developing countries and their local use by native healers, and traditional diets of native peoples.

- Clinical trials to evaluate the effectiveness of combination naturopathic medical protocols and rigorous evaluation of single-agent botanical medicines and naturopathic modalities in the treatment of HIV and AIDS.

Chapter 11

Environmental Medicine

Overview

Environmental medicine is an alternative system of medical practice based on the science of assessing the impact of environmental factors on health. It is the result of continuing study of the interfaces among chemicals, foods, and inhalants in the environment and the biological function of the individual.

Environmental medicine traces its roots to the practice of allergy treatment. In the 1940s Theron Randolph, the founding father of environmental medicine, identified a wide range of medical problems he believed were caused by food allergies. Working with the techniques developed by Herbert Rinkel, Randolph identified multiple symptoms due to a variety of common foods such as corn, wheat, milk, and eggs—symptoms previously unrecognized as caused by food exposure. Using Rinkel's method of unmasking food allergies by avoiding the suspect food for at least four days before challenging, Randolph was able to identify food-related triggers for symptoms such as arthritis, asthma, depression and anxiety, enuresis, colitis, fatigue, hyperactivity, and others (Randolph, 1962).

In the 1950s Randolph noted that in small amounts, chemicals such as natural gas, industrial solvents, pesticides, car exhaust, and

Extracted from NIH Publication No. 94-066 from the Office of Alternative Medicine. December 1994. Due to space considerations, bibliographic data have not been reprinted in this chapter. However, to aid readers who wish to consult the original document or do further research, the in-text references have been retained.

formaldehyde were also responsible for significant and previously un-recognized health problems (Randolph, 1962). It was noted that certain individuals were more sensitive to these minute exposures and that illness could be triggered in such hypersensitive individuals by amounts of chemicals that most people could tolerate without apparent symptoms.

Many of the findings of Randolph and others were originally identified through the use of environmental control units (strictly controlled environments in hospitals). In these settings, patients' allergies and sensitivities were unmasked through fasting and complete avoidance of incitant chemicals. When foods or chemicals were introduced in a systematic fashion, cause and effect could be identified. Today there are several environmental control units in the United States and a Canadian Government-sponsored unit in Nova Scotia, Canada.

Through careful and detailed environmentally focused clinical observations of thousands of patients, Randolph and others developed a new model and associated clinical principles that helped explain and treat many of the complex problems seen in medical practice today. By assessing the interaction between the individual's internal state and exposure to external factors, the physician may understand the cause of an illness. This type of medical practice goes beyond traditional medical concepts because it emphasizes the effects of food and chemicals in health.

The problems treated by environmental medicine include both diagnosis of problems that are traditionally considered allergic problems—asthma, hay fever, allergic rhinoconjunctivitis, eczema, and anaphylactic food allergies mediated by immunoglobulin E (IgE) antibody as well as other factors—and other diagnoses for which the underlying immunological aspects are not yet understood: arthritis, colitis, depression, fatigue, attention deficit disorder, cardiovascular disease, migraine and other headaches, urinary tract disorders, and other functional illnesses.

Of particular importance is the recognition of the effects of chemicals in the home and workplace, such as in the "sick building syndrome." With the changing environment found in workplaces and homes as well as outdoors, the incidence of environmentally triggered illness has increased. Chemically induced environmental illness is already affecting four million to five million Americans, and it is estimated that no more than 5 percent have been identified and treated. If patients with problems stemming from environmental exposure are not seen by a physician knowledgeable in environmental illness, they are often misdiagnosed or told they have psychiatric problems or hypochondriases (Randolph and Moss, 1980; Rea and Mitchell, 1982).

In 1965, Randolph and his colleagues founded the Society for Clinical Ecology to further explore the connection between the environment and illness. Today, courses organized by the American Academy of Environmental Medicine are available for training in the techniques and principles of this field. This organization, the successor to the Society for Clinical Ecology, has annual scientific meetings to further research and education. It publishes the peer-reviewed journal *Environmental Medicine* (formerly *Clinical Ecology*).

Today, environmental medicine is a medical specialty practiced by more than 3,000 physicians worldwide, most of them in the United States, Canada, and Great Britain. Many of these clinicians and researchers are members of one of the following professional medical organizations: the American Academy of Environmental Medicine, the Pan American Allergy Society, or the American Academy of Otolaryngologic Allergy. More than 50 percent of the members in the American Academy of Environmental Medicine are board certified in one or more of 19 medical specialties. The binding factor in these diverse physicians' backgrounds is an expanded view of health and illness, including an emphasis on the role the environment plays in a wide variety of medical disorders. This view of health and illness allows environmental medicine to be considered as an "alternative system" of medical practices developed from within the Western heritage of biomedical science.

Principles of environmental medicine. Many complex problems in medicine are called *idiopathic*: there is no readily apparent cause for the illness. The conventional medical model holds that similar illnesses have the same cause in all patients and should be treated similarly. This is not the case in the paradigm of environmental medicine.

Environmental medicine recognizes that illness in the individual can be caused by a broad range of inciting substances, including foods; chemicals found in the home and workplace; chemicals in air, water, and food; and inhalant materials, including pollens, molds, dust, dust mites, and danders. Individual susceptibility to these exposures can vary widely. The response to these exposures over time is specific to each person's own level of susceptibility and can manifest differently from person to person. Therefore, the specific symptoms and illnesses developed depend on all these factors, and environmental medicine attempts to answer the question why a particular patient has a particular symptom at a particular time.

One key to understanding the diagnosis in environmental medicine is a detailed chronological history. The emphasis of this history is on environmentally focused events and stressors over time. A thorough medical history and a physical examination are also needed. The detail of the home and work environment is explored to identify possible incitants.

The factors contributing to the sensitivity of the patient are related to genetics, nutritional status, effectiveness of detoxification pathways, and total allergic and chemical load at the time. Biochemical individuality determines the adequacy of nutritional stores and influences the ability to operate the detoxification pathways effectively and thus contributes to the individual's degree of sensitivity. Other factors that can induce immune system dysfunction, such as emotional stress, may have a major impact on the outcome of an exposure to a chemical toxin, a food exposure, or an inhalant contact.

The onset of illness coincides with the person's inability to continue coping with the *total allergic load*. This onset can occur either with a large acute exposure or with low-level, gradual exposures. The total allergic load is defined as the total level of exposure to substances that the person can be sensitive to, and it varies significantly over time. The total allergic load is often the determining factor in maintaining health (homeostasis) versus falling ill.

Environmental medicine practitioners believe that large amounts of toxic substances affect all those exposed, but minute amounts affect only those who are susceptible to the material. This fact explains the varied response to a material such as formaldehyde; 10 percent of the population is highly sensitive to small amounts of this poison and 90 percent is not. Thus, a susceptible person may get sick from a small workplace exposure, while others who are not susceptible suffer no ill effects. This situation often leads to missing a diagnosis while ignoring the patient's individual susceptibility. Indeed, many patients and physicians are unaware of the effects of chemical exposures as a contributing factor in illnesses. As a result, patients are often labeled "hypochondriacs" or told their illness is psychosomatic ("all in their mind") (Choffres, 1987; Davis, 1985; Saifer and Saifer, 1987).

Another concept that can help to explain the course of events in environmental illnesses is adaptation. Adaptation is the process by which the body attempts to maintain homeostasis. There are four distinct phases of adaptation: *preadapted-nonadapted* (alarm), *adapted* (masked), *maladapted*, and *exhausted-nonadapted*. The first three stages occur sequentially and if left uninterrupted can lead to the *exhausted* stage, or the onset of disease.

An example of adaptation phenomena is a sensitivity to wheat. At first exposure, wheat might cause symptoms such as fatigue (preadapted phase). After further exposure, the homeostatic mechanism creates an adapted state with no reactions. On further and frequent exposure, however, overt symptoms can occur (maladapted phase); for example, headaches to wheat may be labeled migraine and treated with medication. Eventually, with continued exposure, more serious symptoms can occur (exhausted phase). If the person stops being exposed to the food for at least four days and challenging (deadaptation) then causes the symptoms to reappear, cause and effect have been observed clearly. This sequence can also be seen with low-level chemical exposures.

Another observed phenomenon in environmental medicine is the *spreading phenomenon*. There are two aspects:

1. New onset of acute or chronic susceptibility to previously tolerated substances, and.

2. Spreading of susceptibility to new target organs. These events can occur with a single large exposure to a chemical that damages particular biological mechanisms and causes sensitivity to occur to other chemicals in addition to the primary incitant substance. This phenomenon is frequently seen with solvent or pesticide exposure causing a person to become a "universal reactor" to many other chemicals.

The type of symptoms experienced in the reaction to an offending substance (food, chemical, or inhalant) is not specific to the substance but is determined by a combination of factors specific to the person. In contrast, all individuals exposed to a highly toxic chemical have similar symptoms (e.g., respiratory symptoms from exposure to formaldehyde). Symptoms of sensitivity to small levels of exposure can affect many target organs; widespread central nervous system effects such as fatigue, depression, anxiety, or poor memory and concentration may occur and can differ from person to person. This observation often makes the cause of these problems extremely difficult to identify and underlines the need for the multifactorial approach, which is the basis of environmental medicine.

The final pattern described in environmental medicine is labeled the *switch phenomenon*. In this situation, symptoms change and can affect different organ systems; symptoms may range from psychological (e.g., anxiety) to asthma, fatigue, and hyperactivity. This movement of symptoms was described by Randolph as bipolar and biphasic responses of the biological mechanism ranging from stimulatory phases (+1 to +4) to withdrawal phases (-1 to - 4). It is possible to range from stimulation to withdrawal in the course of the illness (Randolph, 1976).

Diagnostic and treatment techniques. Several aspects of the assessment and treatment approaches employed in environmental medicine are unique to this specialty. The key to proper treatment is an accurate environmental history. With a broader view of the connection between environment and illness, many illnesses that are attributed to other causes by traditional medicine are assessed in terms of environmental aspects.

The environmental history details the chronology of the symptoms as well as the current form of the illness. Using the chronological history and the assessment of the detailed circumstances of the symptoms can lead to a greater understanding of the etiology. There is a search for a history of adverse reactions to specific environmental substances, including biological inhalants, foods, and chemicals. A detailed description of the home, the workplace, and the effects of season, activity, and other environmental factors is necessary. A thorough understanding of the pathophysiology of the dysfunctioning systems is also required. The effects of total allergic load, the spreading phenomenon, the switch phenomenon, and biochemical individuality need to be recognized so that the etiology of the illness can be assessed.

The physical examination and laboratory assessment look for evidence of nutritional deficiencies, organ system dysfunction, and disorders of detoxification systems. Blood tests might include standard assessments such as chemistry panels, blood counts, and hormonal function tests. In addition, tests that further assess immune function are required, such as lymphocyte subset panels, immunoglobulin levels, autoantibody screens, viral and chemical antibody panels, and in vitro assessment of allergy to foods, inhalants, and chemicals. Furthermore, assessment of nutritional status is often included, involving in vitro analysis of minerals and vitamins through enzyme system activation, as well as serum, plasma, leukocyte, or erythrocyte levels. Levels of toxic chemicals and minerals may be measured in serum or other biological markers.

In-office testing for allergies and hypersensitivity is often the most important aspect of assessing a patient with environmental illness. The techniques employed include serial end-point titration, provocative neutralization, and bronchoprovocation. These techniques test a wide range of antigens including bacteria, foods, chemicals, and inhalants such as dust, mites, pollens, and molds. The antigen sources are the same ones used in traditional allergy testing, but these techniques can more effectively assess the non-IgE sensitivity reaction (King, 1989; McGovern, 1981; Miller, 1972; Morris, 1981; Rinkel, 1963). Although the validity of these techniques is controversial, a significant number of studies support these approaches (Brostoff, 1988; Gerdes, 1993; King, 1981).

Provocative testing is in essence a quantitative bioassay. Individual skin tests with progressively weaker blinded dilutions of extract can reproduce many of the patient's symptoms. Subjective and objective monitoring can show changes in heart rate, blood pressure, nasal patency, respiratory function, cognitive function, and handwriting during and after single allergy tests.

When complex patients cannot be evaluated as outpatients, inpatient environmental control units are available in several locations in the United States and Canada. In these settings, the patients are in hospital rooms that are environmentally controlled and are free of all common chemical exposures. They are fasted on water until all symptoms disappear. At this point, they are challenged with foods by mouth and with chemicals in inhalant booths. The symptomatic response to these substances can help clarify the cause of the illness.

Treatment approaches to these complex problems require a full understanding of the nature of environmentally induced illness. Immunotherapy based on the results of the in vivo allergy testing techniques can be used to reduce the sensitivity to these antigens through a variety of mechanisms, including modulation by T-suppressor cells and altering the ratio of antibody to antigen, which affects the formation of immune complexes and histamine release (Rapp, 1986).

Educating the patient is critical in environmental medicine. A thorough understanding of the factors contributing to illness must be emphasized for long-term improvement to occur. Emphasis is placed on environmental controls in the home and workplace to reduce exposure to inhalants as well as chemicals. Where possible, the patient is informed about alternatives to using chemicals such as pesticides in the home and the workplace.

Dietary management is based on avoidance of food antigens and on the four day rotary diversified diet. With the rotary diet and avoidance of repetitive food exposures, it is possible to reduce sensitivity to foods and hasten recovery from food allergies. Nutritional supplements are prescribed as indicated by both objective nutritional testing and symptomatology. Improving the xenobiotic detoxification pathways through therapeutic nutrition is often required. In this respect the practice of environmental medicine overlaps "orthomolecular" nutrition practices. (See the "Diet and Nutrition" chapter.)

Research accomplishments. Research in the field has been directed at both clinical treatment of ill patients and evaluation of the diagnostic and treatment techniques used by practitioners. Studies have been done that support the approach of environmental medicine in arthritis (Panush, 1986), asthma (Gerrard, 1989), chemical sensitivity (Rea, 1991), colitis (Lake, 1982), depression (Randolph, 1959), eczema (Atherton, 1988), eye allergy (Shirakawa and Rea, 1990), fatigue (Rowe, 1950), food allergy (Rapp, 1947), hyperactivity (Rapp, 1979), migraine (Munro et al., 1980), psychological complaints (Campbell, 1973), urticaria (August, 1989), and vascular disease (Rea, 1991). Published bibliographies on environmental medicine discuss other studies and background in this area (Oberg, 1990; Randolph, 1987; Rapp, 1981).

Rea et al. (1984) studied twenty patients with known food sensitivity. Using neutralization therapy in a double-blind study they found significant improvement ($p < 0.001$) in signs and symptoms of allergy reactions to those foods. Mabry (1982), treating women with premenstrual tension syndrome, used progesterone neutralization and found that 65 percent of them preferred the active treatment to placebo.

Gerdes (1993) performed critical reviews of thirty-one studies of the provocation-neutralization technique done between 1969 and 1988. Twenty-one studies showed evidence for the effectiveness of the technique, and ten had negative results. Only ten of the thirty-one studies reviewed were methodologically sound, however. Among these potentially replicable studies, eight were supportive of the technique, one was not, and one could be cited by either side in the controversy. (See the "Diet and Nutrition" chapter for data on food allergy studies.)

Future directions for research. Despite its designation as an "alternative" professional specialty within the biomedical community, environmental medicine remains a controversial field. Practitioners of environmental medicine have been criticized for "nonstandard" diagnostic techniques and "unorthodox" treatment methods, as have other practitioners of alternative forms of medicine. The principal detractors have been the American Academy of Allergy and Immunology and the American College of Allergy and Immunology (Gerdes, 1993). Proponents claim, however, that the basic principles of environmental medicine are critical to designing the types of studies that could further validate the field. Research has also been hampered by application of the "unconventional" label to practices that attract patients who have failed to be helped by conventional internal medicine, allergy, and psychological approaches. The problem of chemical hypersensitivity and chemically induced illness and worker's disability led to a report by the New Jersey State Department of Health in 1989, which summarizes much of the controversy in this area (Ashford and Miller, 1989). Another major review of the complex medico-legal and social problems encountered with workers with multiple chemical sensitivities was published by Rosenstock and Cullen in 1994.

Although the belief that humans may get sick from accumulated low-level environmental stress is not well accepted in the conventional community, sick building syndrome and other diseases of the 20th century are being seen with greater frequency. Indeed, according to The National Research Council of the National Academy of Sciences, the U.S. population is exposed to at least 50,000 chemicals, most of which have not been studied sufficiently in relation to their effects on human health (National Research Council, 1975). Those that have been studied are assessed only in terms of their carcinogenicity in animal models and not in terms of a myriad of other aspects affecting human health. In addition, no work has been done on the additive effects of repeated low-level exposures to pesticides, solvents, formaldehyde, and the other common substances found in the immediate environment (Elkington, 1986).

Future occupational toxicology studies should include clinicians trained in environmental medicine. Peer review committees in allergy and toxicology grant review processes should not be dominated by persons whose belief system is threatened by the environmental medicine philosophy.

The testing techniques of environmental medicine need further validating studies, as do the various immunological and nutritional treatment methods. The research protocols must, however, actually test the paradigm. For example, food or chemical challenges in the exhausted stage of illness might yield different results if the study subjects were first deadapted (allowed to recover) before being challenged. Careful qualitative research might be needed to validate variable biological responses such as those described in the switch phenomenon.

Since quality-of-life issues surround many of the complex illnesses treated by environmental medicine, qualitative outcomes research comparing patients treated by these principles versus "orthodox medicine" could give insight into the best use of this approach in the U.S. health care system.

Summary. Environmental medicine offers an alternative view of the causation, prevention, and treatment of many common illnesses. It emphasizes self-care and the use of nonpharmaceutical approaches. Environmental medicine presents a dynamic and potentially cost-effective paradigm to deal with the many common illnesses seen in today's increasingly complex environment. It has been estimated by the U.S. Public Health Service (1990) that diet and environment play a role in 90 percent of cancers and cardiovascular disease. Environmental medicine is in a position to be a leading force in the investigation of ways to reduce the incidence of these and other disorders.

Chapter 12

Community-Based Health Care Practices

Overview

All of the systems discussed in this section are community based in several ways. Most important, an individual's sickness is viewed as a sickness of the entire community. That is, when one person becomes sick, the whole community is believed to be in danger. Therefore, the treatment must address the whole community rather than just the patient.

Because the concepts of "medicine" and "religion" in these systems often are fused, no sickness can affect only one part of the body. Rather, it affects the whole network of existence, the natural world, and the spiritual world. Accordingly, in addition to their expertise in naturalistic healing (i.e., the use of herbs), community-based health care practitioners are expected to have expertise in dealing with relationships (between partners, between parents and children, etc.), mediating disputes and communicating with the spirit world. Also, health care is delivered in public, with members of the family and community present.

Community-based health care practices are varied and found throughout the United States, although many people would not consider that they were participating in such a system when they attend

Extracted from NIH Publication No. 94-066 from the Office of Alternative Medicine. December 1994. Due to space considerations, bibliographic data have not been reprinted in this chapter. However, to aid readers who wish to consult the original document or do further research, the in-text references have been retained.

a healing service at a local church or go to a meeting of Weight Watchers. Like other health care specialists, community-based healers may emphasize naturalistic, personalistic, or energetic explanatory models or a combination. Traditional midwives and herbalists—and nowadays, pragmatic weight loss specialists—are probably the best known of community-based practitioners who follow the naturalistic model[3].

Though most traditional healers will accept gifts, many refuse pay for their healing work. They believe they are the agents of God or the spirit world and that their power and skill should be used to help the needy. Most community-based healers do not advertise their skills, which are therefore mainly known locally. There are two types of personalistic healers: the shaman, and others who do not quite fit this model and whose practice can be called "shamanistic."

A *shaman* is a type of spiritual healer distinguished by the practice of journeying to nonordinary reality to make contact with the world of spirits, to ask their direction in bringing healing back to people and the community (Atkinson, 1987, 1992; Brown, 1988; Eliade, 1964; Halifax, 1979; Harner, 1990; Ingerman, 1991; Laderman, 1988; McClenon, 1993; Myerhoff, 1976). The journey is a controlled trance state that practitioners induce by using repetitive sound (drums, rattles) or movement (dancing) and occasionally by consuming plant substances (e.g., peyote or certain mushrooms). Characteristically experiential and cooperative, shamanic healing is found worldwide. It is fundamental to much traditional European, African, Asian, and Native American Indian folk practice and is rapidly gaining popularity among nonnative urban Americans, in which setting it is sometimes called neo-shamanism (Hufford, 1990).

Shamanic practices define healing broadly: not only are people to be healed of their spiritual and psychic wounds, but shamans also attempt to heal communities, modify the weather, and find lost objects. Many traditional shamans are also skilled in manipulative or herbal practices (Atkinson, 1987; Brown, 1988).

Clinical evidence of results is anecdotal, consisting of the stories successful shamans tell of their curing and healing activities (Black Elk and Lyon, 1990; Harner, 1990; Ingerman, 1991; Yellowtail and Fitzgerald, 1991; Young, 1989). Some interpretations of shamanism have tended to categorize its effectiveness in the same range as psychotherapy, but wider interpretations may be more accurate (Atkinson, 1992; Brown, 1988; Laderman, 1988; McClenon, 1993).

Shamans are concerned with helping patients discover "meaning," but such meaning is not limited to the interior dialog. It expands to include the entire natural and spiritual community. For example, shamanic journeying and the precision with which shamans can "tell" a patient's life and concerns to a patient convince many that the spirit world is real and supportive. Also, shamans commonly help individual patients see their illness not as a personal failure but as a concern of the larger sociopolitical unit, thus drawing community support toward the sick. Shamanic care can also result in physical "curing." In summary, the shamanic approach is complex and paradigmatically quite different from mainstream Western explanatory models.

Personalistic specialists who do not practice journeying are not shamans. Nor can practices that depend on fixed rituals or charms, and thus are not experiential, be considered shamanic practices. However, to the extent that mediums, channelers, prayer healers, and others call on the unseen or on the spirit world to intervene for the benefit of people in the material world, they are "shamanistic."

In contrast to professionalized practitioners, community-based healers often do not have set locations—such as offices or clinics—for delivering care but do so in homes, at ceremonial sites, or even right where they stand. Community-based healing of the personalistic variety can also be "distant," that is, it does not require that practitioner and patient be in each other's presence. Prayers or shamanic journeys, for example, can be requested and "administered" at any time, and charm cures are sometimes delivered by telephone.

An example of rural community-based practitioners is the "powwowers." These are "wise women" or elders who by reason of birth or calling have been recognized as having the requisite "power" to say the verbal charms or prayers to cure trauma and disease in powwowing (Hostetler, 1976; Yoder, 1976). The term is borrowed from the Algonquin Indians, although the practices did not originate with the Native American Indian. Instead they date back many centuries in Europe. The original German dialect words, *brauche* or *braucherei*, are still sometimes used.

Powwowing closely resembles traditional European practices found elsewhere in the United States (Hufford, 1988, 1992; Kirkland, 1992; Reimansnyder, 1989; Wigginton, 1972; Wilkinson, 1987). "Granny women" deliver care in the Appalachians, *traiteurs* in Louisiana, and "power doctors" in the Ozarks, and similar ideas may be found in almost any State. A similar niche in African-American communities is filled by "rootwork." This community-based system is found throughout the Southern United States and in African-American communities elsewhere, sometimes under alternate names such as "conjure" and "hoo-doo" (Lichstein, 1992; Mathews, 1987, 1992; Snow, 1993; Terrell, 1990; Weidmann, 1978). Although not familiar to most urban peoples, these systems serve considerable numbers of rural Americans.

Meanwhile, community-based systems also thrive in urban areas. These systems include the popular weight loss programs and other 12-step programs. Often the practitioners rent office space and emphasize contact between client and practitioner, and they may charge considerable fees. Since these practitioners depend on their healing practice for their livelihood, they advertise and so may be easier to identify and contact for study purposes.

The following discusses the community-based health care practices of certain Native American Indian tribes, rural Latin American communities, and urban self-help systems.

Native American Indian Health Care Practices

Although each Native American Indian community-based medical system has its distinct characteristics, all share the following rituals and practices.

Sweating and purging. Both techniques are intended to purify the body as well as the spirit. Herbal preparations, such as the famous "black drink" of the southeastern tribes, were formerly used to induce vomiting (Hudson, 1979). The goal was to strengthen the body and prepare it for challenges—a form of preventive medicine. Sweating continues to be widely practiced, often in special "sweat lodges" (McGaa, 1990). Typically, these are small conical structures where hot rocks are doused with water to create steam. Participants pray, sing, and drum to purify their spirits while sweating to cleanse their bodies. This practice is also considered a means of preventing imbalance and illness; in some cases it is also used to heal. In the Lakota community, a complete lodge ceremony lasts several hours and is recommended both for general purification (e.g., monthly for men, a kind of parallel to women's monthly menses) and for help in reaching major life decisions or dealing with major life challenges. In addition, praying in the sweat lodge commonly precedes and follows vision questing and sun dancing.

Herbal remedies. All indigenous Americans depended on a variety of herbal remedies gathered from the surrounding environment and sometimes traded over long distances. The "Herbal Medicine" chapter gives more details on the types and applications of herbal remedies used by certain tribes.

108

Shamanic healing. Shamanic healing is also an important part of virtually all Native American Indian health care. Most tribal people have one or more types of health care specialists in naturalistic or personalistic healing. Frequently, the two overlap—thus a midwife or a medicine man or woman might focus primarily on naturalistic explanations and healing but sometimes also uses prayer, suggestion, or other techniques characteristic of a personalistic framework. "Holy people" or shamans (each tribe has its own name for this specialist type) emphasize personalistic healing but often are also knowledgeable about herbs, massage, and other naturalistic techniques.

Shamanic practice is relatively well maintained in a number of tribes today and in several cases is expanding into the larger society. On the other hand, herbal and other practices have largely disappeared in many localities. There are some current efforts to save vanishing knowledge, and the next few years may see more young people apprentice themselves to elders and become naturalistic or personalistic healing specialists.

Below, major practices in two Native American Indian tribal communities are briefly outlined: the Lakota Sioux and the Dineh (Navajo).

These two were selected because traditional healing practices have been relatively well maintained and well studied in these communities, and because they help to show the wide variety of practices used by Native American Indian peoples. There is a large literature on different groups, however, and the reader is also referred to sources such as Johnston, 1982; Morse et al., 1991; Naranjo and Swentzell, 1989; and Young, 1989.

Lakota practices. The Lakota—one of several branches of a tribe often called Sioux, who live primarily in North and South Dakota, Minnesota, and Manitoba—are perhaps unique in their recent efforts to inform the wider society of their psychosocial healing techniques (Black Elk and Lyon, 1990; McGaa, 1990; Neihardt, 1932; Powers, 1977, 1982). Though the Lakota have their own distinctive ways of practice, in broad outline their techniques are shared with other Plains tribes as well as with other groups from Wisconsin to Washington (Farrer, 1991; Harrod, 1992; Storm, 1972; Yellowtail and Fitzgerald, 1991).

Lakota techniques are based on the assumption of the absolute continuity of body and spirit; for the Lakota, "medicine" and "religion" are not separate. The two most famous Lakota religiomedical practices are the sweat lodge and the medicine wheel (sacred hoop.) Other techniques, such as the vision quest and sun dance, are familiar to many non-Native American Indians. Other practices, such as the *yuwipi* ceremony (Powers, 1982), are little known to outsiders.

All these healing ceremonials are led by specialists, usually called medicine women or men or holy men or women, who are essentially shamanic in their approach to healing (Hultkrantz, 1985). Some also have knowledge of herbal remedies or manipulative techniques. One usually discovers that one's path is to become a medicine person through a dream or vision, sometimes sought (as in the vision quest), sometimes unsought (appearing during the course of serious illness or in lucid dreaming). Shamanic skills also tend to run in families. Once called, one seeks training, usually by apprenticing oneself to a successful medicine man or woman, often for several years. Training is complete when the teacher says it is complete and when the candidate has practiced his or her skills publicly and with success.

The medicine wheel or sacred hoop is both a conceptual scheme and a major ceremonial. The wheel or hoop represents all of cosmology and life in a circle of four quarters, plus the directions of up, down, and center. Each of the four quarters has a character or power, which can be expressed in many ways; as an aspect of some form of wisdom, as an animal, as a color, as an energy, or as a season. The four quarters are separated by two "roads," one red for happiness, one black for sorrow. Everyone is born with the gift of one of the powers, and the thoughtful person will "journey" his or her life to develop the other forms of wisdom, know that happiness and sorrow come to everyone, and recognize the relatedness of the whole. This deeply ecological cosmology is expressed in virtually all Lakota prayer, and with the phrase *"Mitakuye oyasin"* ("Thanks to all our relatives"). The wheel or hoop is represented on much Lakota artwork; periodically it is represented as a stone circle on the ground, around which a ceremonial is held. Participation in the ceremonial is considered generally healing, and in addition, individuals can seek specific healing through prayer.

Dineh or Navajo practices. The Dineh are a herding people who have lived in the southwestern United States for some centuries; they are the largest tribe in North America today. Like the Lakota, in their traditional practice the Dineh make essentially no distinction between religious and medical practices. Here, discussion is limited to the famous Navajo healing "sings" or "chants" and the specialists who make them possible (Luckert and Cooke, 1979; Morgan, 1931/1977; Reichard, 1939, 1950; Sandner, 1979, 1991; Topper, 1987; Wyman and Haile, 1970).

110

A sing is a healing ceremonial that lasts from two to nine days and nights. It is guided by a highly skilled specialist called a "singer." Although focused on helping an individual, sings are commonly attended by as many in the community as can come, for just being present is considered healing. Navajo cosmology teaches that health is present when all things are in harmony. The full concept is impossible to translate into English, so it is often rendered as the Navajo word *hozro*, which summarizes many things such as happiness, connection, and balance. Its opposite is something like "evil"; indeed, where there is disharmony, there is sickness and disease, and vice versa. A long-time student of Navajo singers notes:

> *This "evil" must be controlled or banished and goodness restored. To implement this desired state of affairs, the Navajos have created a great body of symbolic rituals [that] attempt to placate or expel the destructive powers and attract the good, helpful ones. By doing this they reestablish the basic harmony, cure individual illness, and bring general blessing to the tribe (Sandner, 1979, p. 118).*

There are three basic categories of chants: "holyway," "ghostway," and "lifeway." Holyway chants—including the most famous, called "blessingway"—are used to attract good, to cure, and to repair. Ghostway chants are used to remove evil and are often performed to heal Dineh who have had too much contact with strangers (non-Navajo), as in the armed forces or at college, or who have had contact with dead bodies. Lifeway chants are used to treat what westerners would call "physical" injuries and accidents; such treatment includes both restoring cosmological harmony and repairing trauma—by setting broken bones, for example.

The two kinds of healing specialists among the Dineh are the "diagnosticians" and the aforementioned singers. Diagnosticians are usually "called" to their profession by nonordinary experiences and receive little formal training in their skill. They diagnose deep cause by going into trance. While in trance, "hand tremblers" pass their shaking hands over the body of the patient; when the hands stop trembling, the locale of the illness is shown and the cause is usually nameable. "Star gazers" also enter trance to read cause in the stars. "Listeners" do not go into trance but listen to the patient's story and on that basis diagnose deep cause. Once cause is known—and it is always phrased in terms of harmony and disharmony—patients seek a singer who can provide the indicated treatment.

111

Singers are specialists of symbology who have a good deal in common both with priests and with psychotherapists; in addition, their moral probity and high intellectual powers mean that they usually perform as community leaders as well. They are not shamans and are not "called" by supernatural powers to their profession. Instead, interest and patience are the prerequisites, as well as demonstrated dependability and economic success. To learn a single chant can take up to several years, for the performance of each chant involves memorizing what amounts to a long epic poem (one that takes two to nine nights to repeat) along with the recipes for the accompanying herbal preparations and sand paintings. The singer must also know where to find the herbs, how to prepare them, and how to use them. He must know where to find the colored sands necessary for the sand paintings, and he must learn to make—without error—the intricate sand paintings specific to the chant he is learning. Because the training is so arduous, most singers learn only a few chants in a lifetime.

The Dineh have depended on singers and chants for many centuries; today they are used in combination with conventional medicine. It remains common for Dineh both on and off the reservation to seek sings to treat conditions that conventional medicine does not recognize and to use sings for healing along with conventional medicine used curatively.

Numerous observers have asked why the sings "work." Topper (1987, p. 248) remarks that sings are restorative: "They restore an individual's ego functions and integrate the patient back into the social setting from which he or she has become estranged." Sandner (1979, 1991) analyzes the process further: First, the herbal remedies often have requisite physiological effects. Second, the patient's expectation is encouraged time and again during the chant by its intricate psychological structure. Third, the patient is socially supported by the entire community, who are centrally concerned since, by Navajo cosmology, the well-being of all is threatened by disharmony in one. Fourth, the chant wordings guide the sick person to finding culturally appropriate answers to difficult cosmological problems, such as the management of evil and the inevitability of death.

Formal research into the healing ceremonies and herbal medicines conducted and used by bona fide Native American Indian healers or holy people is almost nonexistent, even though Native American Indians believe they positively cure both the mind and body. Ailments and diseases such as heart disease, diabetes, thyroid conditions, cancer, skin rashes, and asthma reportedly have been cured by Native

American Indian doctors who are knowledgeable about the complex ceremonies. Among Native American Indians living today there are many stories about seemingly impossible cures that have been wrought by holy people. However, the information on what was done is closely guarded and not readily rendered to non-Native American Indian investigators. It has been suggested that if Congress restored religious freedom to Native American Indians, then collaborative research into Native American Indian healing and healing practices could be possible (Locke, 1993).

Latin American Rural Practices

Curanderismo is a folk system used in Latin America and among many Hispanic-Americans in the United States. Hispanic-American refers to Americans of Spanish or Spanish-American descent; in the United States most trace their roots to Mexico (63 percent), Puerto Rico (12 percent), and Cuba, but increasing numbers of immigrants are arriving from Central America (Wright, 1990). The population of Hispanics is rapidly growing in the United States, and today about 22 million people call themselves Hispanic. More than half of this population lives in Texas and California, and large populations are also in Colorado, Arizona, Florida, Illinois, New Jersey, New Mexico, and New York.

Curanderismo typically includes two distinct components, a humoral model for classifying activity, food, drugs, and illness; and a series of folk illnesses such as "evil eye," "fright," "blockage," and "fallen fontanelle." Curanderismo as described herein is most characteristic of Mexican-Americans, especially those who are little assimilated; variants on the humoral component typify most of Latin America, while the folk diseases and the treatment modalities reflect national background. Thus the Cuban-American folk system is not curanderismo, but *santeria*, and it is African influenced.

Although no formal effectiveness studies seem to have been done on this system, its wide popularity and the research suggesting the relevance of the folk diagnoses for biomedical practice indicate the need for further demographic and effectiveness studies.

In the humoral component of curanderismo things could be classified as having qualitative (not literal) characteristics of hot or cold, dry or moist. (Harwood, 1971; Messer, 1981; Weller, 1983). According to this theory, good health is maintained by maintaining a balance of hot and cold. Thus, a good meal will contain both hot and cold foods, and a person with a hot disease must be given cold remedies and vice versa. Again, a person who is exposed to cold when excessively hot may "take cold" and become ill.

While this model is simple in theory, how people perceive in practice the hotness or coldness of substances varies greatly by region. Thus, while most can be expected to classify chili peppers as "hot" and milk as "cold," the classification of pork or penicillin is not so predictable.

The second component, the folk illnesses, is actively in use in much of Mexico and among less educated Hispanic U.S. citizens (Rubel, 1960, 1964; Rubel et al., 1984; Young, 1981). Trotter (1985) did more than 2,000 clinic interviews in Texas, Arizona, and New Mexico and found that 32 percent to 96 percent of Mexican-American households (more frequent in the less Americanized communities) treated members for Hispanic folk illnesses. Baer and colleagues found similarly high use patterns among Mexican migrant workers in Florida and Mexico (Baer and Penzell, 1993: Baer and Bustillo, 1993).

Four important Mexican-American folk illnesses are *mal de ojo*, *susto*, *empacho*, and *caida de mollera*. Mal de ojo, or evil eye, is a worldwide disease concept in which a person can make another sick by looking at him or her. The one who gets sick, typically an infant, is usually "weak." The one who causes the illness is usually thought not to do it on purpose—the person just has the misfortune to have a "piercing" glance. Typical symptoms of mal de ojo include fussiness, refusal to eat, and refusal to sleep. Infants are protected from evil eye with amulets or by having their faces covered in the presence of strangers. Treatment is primarily symbolic.

Caida de mollera, or fallen fontanelle, is an illness of infants before the anterior fontanelle (crown of the head) closes. Common symptoms include diarrhea, excessive crying, fever, loss of appetite, and irritability. Usual folk treatments focus on raising the fontanelle by, for example, pushing up on the palate.

Empacho is thought to be caused by something getting stuck in the intestines, causing blockage. Common symptoms are diarrhea, constipation, indigestion, vomiting, and bloating. The commonest treatment is massage along with herbal teas; the former is for dislodging the blockage, and the latter is for washing it out.

Susto, or fright (sometimes called magical fright), develops when a person has had a sudden shock—a mother may develop fright if she sees her child nearly drown, or someone may experience fright after participating in an unusually intense argument. The sick person experiences such symptoms as daytime sleepiness combined with nighttime insomnia, irritability and easy startling, palpitations, inability to stop thinking about the shocking event, anxiety that it will be repeated, and sometimes a sense of loss or a sadness that will not leave. The mild form is treated with herb tea; more severe cases are treated with ritual cleansings (barridas) to restore the harmony of body and soul.

When mild, these folk illnesses are commonly treated at home, but if they persist, the help of specialists—curanderos (men) or curanderas (women)—is sought. The training of curanderos and curanderas varies widely. Most practice a combination of shamanic healing and herbal or practical first aid healing. Most are also astute at manipulating symbols and "reading" the prevailing psychological and social indicators. Some curanderas specialize in midwifery and infant care. In some areas, becoming a healer is a matter of inheritance; the skills are passed from mother to daughter or perhaps aunt to niece. In some areas it is a matter of being called. Typically, curanderos and curanderas spend several years in apprenticeship; their subsequent reputation depends on the number of their patients and how successful their patients judge them.

Treatment techniques, usually a combination of the shamanic and the naturalistic, vary widely; interested readers should consult specialist texts. An issue of concern is that some curanderismo treatments, particularly for empacho, involve feeding lead- or mercury-based remedies. Investigators' efforts to test whether the amounts ingested were causing medical complications were inconclusive. Although curanderas were found to be largely aware of the danger of the remedies and used them sparingly, intervention programs to limit use of these remedies were begun (Baer ot al., 1989: Trotter, 1985).

Trotter (1985) collected symptomatology lists from more than 2,000 interviews and submitted symptom clusters to medical doctors for "blind" diagnoses. He found, for example, that caida de mollera appears to be symptomatic of serious dehydration secondary to gastroenteritis or respiratory infection. Trotter also found that people who are sicker than average are more likely to be diagnosed with susto. Baer and Penzell (1993) similarly report that migrant workers most affected in a pesticide poisoning incident were also those most likely to report suffering from susto. Susto fits the pattern of "soul loss" (Ingerman, 1991), a shamanically recognized disorder known worldwide that resembles several serious psychotherapeutically recognized conditions, including depression and posttraumatic stress syndrome. Therefore, people being treated for folk diseases could be considered to have conventional illnesses that are being treated outside the conventional biomedical health care system.

115

Community-Based Systems

Alcoholics Anonymous (AA) is a community-based healing system for helping people whose lives are damaged by the consumption of alcohol to stop drinking (Encyclopaedia Britannica, 1990; Scott, 1993; Trice and Staudenmeier, 1989). Founded in 1935 by Bob Smith, M.D., and Bill Wilson, two alcoholics, it is a patient-centered self-help fellowship of men and women. AA has burgeoned and today is widely considered the most successful existing method for supporting sobriety.

Habitual excessive drinking or craving for alcohol was first proposed as constituting a disease by Magnus Huss in 1849. Currently many definitions of the condition exist, but most emphasize that the drinker has "lost control" (is addicted or dependent) and that alcohol use is causing physical, social, mental, or economic harm to the drinker. The concept of loss of control is especially important to AA, which requires its members, as the first step toward sobriety, to comprehend the extent to which they have lost control of their lives. Only then—when they have understood that "playing God" has led them to their sickness, that in fact they are limited human beings in need of salvation—can they begin the breakthroughs that support sobriety (Scott, 1993).

In contrast to most community-based systems, a very large literature exists analyzing AA. Several models attempt to explain its success. One popular psychometric model interprets AA as a "cult" and the achievement of sobriety as a "conversion experience" (Galanter, 1990; Greil and Rudy, 1983; Rudy, 1987). Another model accepts AA's interpretation of itself (Hufford, 1988; Kurtz, 1982; Scott, 1993): members recover by integrating their own experiences with alcohol with those of others in the group and by learning and practicing some new ways to behave. Through these new ways, AA members feel as if they are living apart from the urban materialist norm; that the cause of alcoholism is not at issue; that people should share, not compete; and that the individual need not rise above the rest (spiritual anonymity). In contrast to the "conversion" theory of AA membership, learning to live in the "new way" is not achieved through catharsis but is an intellectual and educational process requiring considerable work and perseverance. As Kurtz comments, "AA addresses itself not to alcoholism, but to the alcoholic" (Kurtz 1982).

AA, by most accounts, is more successful than any other system aimed at helping individuals to achieve sobriety. Estimates put membership at about a half-million members worldwide, and although it was originally an American urban phenomenon, AA has found its way into isolated and rural communities of completely different cultural backgrounds (Slagle and Weibel-Orlando, 1986; Sutro, 1989). Recently, AA has seen a rise in membership proportions of women, people younger than 30, and people dually addicted to alcohol and drugs (Emrick, 1987). Studies have concluded that active AA membership allows 60 percent to 68 percent of alcoholics to drink less or not at all for up to a year, and 40 percent to 50 percent to achieve sobriety for many years (Emrick, 1987). More active or dedicated members (those who attend meetings more often) remain sober longer. However, because AA defines alcoholism as a disease controllable only by the cessation of drinking, it is a less appropriate choice for those who simply want to cut down on their drinking (Ogborne, 1989).

Despite these interesting effectiveness data, some authors argue that no appropriate controlled studies of AA effectiveness have been done (Peele, 1990); others hold that difficult research design issues have not been sufficiently addressed, such as how to measure psychosocial functioning before and after AA, or the effects of AA plus some other intervention (Glaser and Ogborne, 1982). Given the popularity and the apparent success rates of AA, further careful research on AA seems highly appropriate. The research design issues applicable to studying AA's effectiveness would be relevant to other alternative practices that include an individual's commitment to a shared belief system and a social behavior pattern.

Research Opportunities

Community-based health practices are specific to many subcultural groups in the United States, including immigrant, rural, and Native American communities. The first step in research would be to categorize and characterize these forms of ethnomedicine practices using qualitative research methods developed in the field of anthropology. Clinical research could begin promptly on those systems that have already been well described and are used widely and in which practitioners of the systems are open to dialog.

A study of various symbolic or nonmaterial concepts of healing such as shamanic healing might identify effective principles of body-mind intervention that would be useful to integrate in the training of future primary care practitioners in the general community. Herbal agents and ethnic herbal practitioners deserve study to identify fruitful clinical areas for research in phytopharmaceutics (pharmacology of plants). Practices and techniques that are rapidly spreading beyond their original cultural confines, such as AA and the sweat lodge, would be candidates for outcomes research. Careful investigation of tribal and folk practices may illuminate larger issues of health care and provide guidelines for low-cost alternatives to existing conventional biomedical interventions. Utilization studies of tribal and folk health care practices could develop a realistic sense of the self-care patterns used by the Nation's ethnic and cultural minorities and inform national public health policies about these minority communities.

Research Barriers

To effectively research and study the alternative health practices people are using, it is necessary to recognize that the operating assumptions of the conventional biomedical way of thinking have led to these alternative systems being ignored or suppressed. Historically the practices of these systems have been scorned as cultic, superstitious, or sectarian, and these systems have been suppressed economically, politically, and scientifically.

From an economic standpoint it is not surprising that the institutions and agents charged with maintaining the exclusive professional mandates of the biomedical system have sought to eliminate competition from alternative professionalized systems as well as folk and tribal practitioners. This anticompetitive tendency is also extended to popular health practices. Popular self-help health books now routinely have a "consult your professional" disclaimer to protect the authors from law suits for practicing "unscientific" medicine in the media without a license.

In the political arena, current concerns about FDA regulation of the health food industry have resulted from an attempt to extend a level of governmental control mandated for a professionalized drug-dispensing health care system into a whole system of self-help and demand-driven popular health care. In addition, the suppression of the tribal health care practices of Native American Indian groups has been primarily due to the dominant political and cultural view that it is in the best interest of these peoples to be forcibly assimilated into the mainstream.

Community-based practitioners themselves may present barriers to research: some may not want to share their knowledge. In some cases the explanatory model of the folk system states that to share the knowledge, except under particular circumstances, is to lose one's power, even to call down punishment on one's head. In other cases, especially among Native American Indians, it is felt that the sharing of traditional secular and sacred knowledge has resulted in the misuse of that knowledge, especially when it has been applied without sufficient awareness of the social and environmental context.

Key Research Issues

In the current climate of concern about the adequacy of the U.S. health care delivery system, a culturally sensitive and scientifically grounded dialog about alternative systems of health care is required. Therefore, cross-cultural researchers must heed the insights of professionals who do health care outreach.

The concept of cultural sensitivity means that issues of conflicts between basic paradigms, worldviews, or belief systems are recognized and openly dealt with when a dominant culture tries to study, influence, or assist a different culture or subculture. The goal of cultural sensitivity—to find common ground among different cultures—has been widely understood among outreach specialists for perhaps twenty years. Cultural sensitivity is a worthy and necessary goal, but it is not easy to achieve. Hufford (1992) notes that understanding the other's position does not imply acceptance or agreement. Nor does it imply that bridging models to accomplish good research is easy. These studies require patience and often extensive negotiation. In addition, the tendency to see differences can sometimes overwhelm the ability to see similarities, thereby unnecessarily focusing people on conflict and negotiation.

Most published studies in these areas have been done by social scientists, folklorists, and historians. Literature on the topic is extensive, including books (e.g., Harwood, 1981; Pedersen et al., 1989) and many articles. From this database one can begin exploring the role of nonprofessionalized health care in the human community.

The first job is, of course, to establish that significant differences exist, and then to detail them. For example, Aitken (1990), speaking as an insider, claims that Native American Indians have distinctive values, and researchers such as Dubray (1985) and Fox (1992) find ways to measure the differences. Often, researchers do their best to identify the differences, and outreach proceeds with certain assumed values, for example, that clients should be asked to help in designing programs intended to benefit them (e.g., Broken Nose, 1992).

Subsequently, evaluations can show which research or outreach models were most successful in given locales. For example, May (1986) and May and Smith (1988) report that alcoholism is better controlled on reservations when indigenous concepts are included in treatment plans; Guilmet and Whited (1987), Marburg (1983), and Manson and colleagues (1987) compare mental health outreach programs among Native American Indians and conclude that the most effective ones reflect indigenous value systems, such as team-based approaches in using group and family therapy rather than individual one-on-one counseling. Beauvais and LaBoueff (1985) state that the control of drug and alcohol abuse will come about through "bolstering the spirit of the community."

Thus, doing clinical research in community-based health care requires questioning certain common assumptions of researchers who are schooled in the biomedical model. These assumptions include:

1. That community-based systems are disappearing and are not delivering health care to many people;

2. That the care they deliver is psychosomatic or not really significant, an idea made more sensible by the segregation of body and mind that is characteristic of mainstream medicine; and

3. That existing clinical research methods are sufficient to analyze community-based practices.

A careful, culturally sensitive analysis of the function and intent of various community-based practices will help sort out the psychic from the somatic aspects of health care. While similarities between systems may allow researchers to pose interesting questions, the research must take into account the particularities of the folk or tribal system being studied. For example, Navajo singers share some characteristics with psychotherapists, but they are not psychotherapists. Likewise, members of AA share their experiences and thus "counsel" other members, but they are not alcohol counselors. Researchers must resist trying to fit these systems into their existing categories.

Research Priorities

The following are general recommendations and priorities for research in the area of alternative professionalized medical systems and community-based practices:

1. Establish a database with descriptive information about traditional medical practice from medical and nonmedical sources. Included should be a review of existing scientific data, including a meta-analysis of studies in selected disciplines.

2. Promote and publish consumer-based surveys describing which alternative systems and traditional ethnic medical practices are being used and for what illnesses.

3. Explore alternative and ethnic medical systems, including historical traditions that may not be replicable in the biomedical model, and recognizing the role of body, mind, spirit, and environmental factors in health and disease.

4. Conduct basic science research to investigate the existence, nature, and role of "energy" (chi, vital force) as a phenomenon active in health and disease.

5. Develop cross-agency guidelines to facilitate research on alternative systems and traditional practices by reducing legal barriers for research that may already exist in other Federal agencies; encourage best case series research, as has been done by NCI in other Federal research agencies; and create an ongoing database of activities in alternative systems and traditional medical practices.

6. Initiate an evaluation program for traditional remedies and herbal medicines, including a global ethnobotany inventory, investigation into issues of toxicity and safety, and creation of an appropriate regulatory category for herbal therapeutic agents.

7. Establish collaboration standards for alternative medical practice research to ensure that the research team respects the paradigm under study; that there is joint involvement of representatives of alternative and traditional practitioners along with existing biomedical research institutions; and that joint involvement occurs at all stages of the research project: conception, method design, funding, data collection, evaluation, and publication.

8. Support the legislative intent of Congress in creating the Office of Alternative Medicine by focusing on socially and economically critical health conditions through cost-effectiveness research.

9. Encourage the addition of alternative systems or ethnomedicine research components to current clinical studies sponsored by the National Institutes of Health; for example, adding traditional Asian therapy, naturopathic, or homeopathic interventions to current studies in the Women's Health Initiative.

10. Expand studies such as the International Cooperative Biodiversity Group so that whole plant material is used rather
than isolating an active ingredient for pharmaceutical usage.

Footnotes

1. The term health care system is used two ways. In one sense, a
health care system encompasses all the health care available
to a nation of people. According to this meaning, in the United
States all people are immersed in the health care system to
the extent that they are connected to the health-protective infrastructure (e.g., clean water, sewer systems, vaccinations)
and use any form of specialist health care, including both
community-based and professionalized health care practitioners. In the second sense, a health care system is all the components that together make up the practice of any particular
form of medical care, such as osteopathy, acupuncture, psychotherapy, biomedicine, or hands-on healing. Each such system provides explanations for the cause and cure of illness;
identifies and trains specialists; provides locales, equipment,
and materia medica for practice; and arranges for social and
legal mandates for practice. All health care provided by specialists (that is, apart from household and popular remedies)
is delivered from within a health care system. However, the
complexity and extension of health care systems vary widely,
from the relatively experiential and localized practices of community-based traditional healers to the extensive, complex,
and intensely professionalized practices of cosmopolitan doctors.

2. The word qi is principally used in relation to the biofield flux,
the material of the biofield. The former phonetic spelling is
ch'i; both are pronounced "chee"; originally also used as a root
word similar to the use of the word energy. It was used with
modifiers to describe hormones, nutrition factors, etc., such as
the following. Ching qi: (merudian qi)—the qi that flows
through the twelve meridians. Fa qi—external qi (wei qi) used
in healing. Jing qi—essence (sexual essence—ancient usage,
hormones in current usage). Ku qi—caloric energy from plants.
Qi density—relative quantity of qi. Ren qi—internal qi that
fills the spaces between the meridians in the body. Wei qi—external portion of the body's qi (aura). Receiving hand-hand

with a polarity that receives the flow (qi). Sending hand—
hand with a polarity that sends the flow (qi). Flows—movement of qi through the body or movement of qi from one of the
practitioner's hands to the other through the patient's body.

3. The Native American "medicine man" or "medicine woman" is
    a traditional healer with primarily naturalistic skills, that is,
    the skills of a herbalist in particular (Hulfkrantz, 1985). Some
    medicine people are also shamans, in which case they are of-
    ten distinguished as "holy" men and women. This distinction
    is usually not made in popular writing, though it is under-
    standably important to the Native American Indian users.

Chapter 13

Healing and the Mind/Body Arts: Massage, Acupuncture, Yoga, T'ai Chi, and Feldenkrais

The great victories of modern medicine have been won on two fronts: surgery, and the control of infectious diseases. No one can dispute the value of these victories, nor the extraordinary virtuosity they display. Nevertheless, the health practitioner is still faced with a vast array of problems that are no less deadly for being ill defined. From minor aches and pains and the various levels of depression and anxiety, to the multitude of degenerative diseases, stress related disorders, alcoholism, drug addiction, and suicide, modern medicine appears unable to deal with many systemic complaints.

Western culture has long been dominated by an analytic tradition that seeks to take things apart to understand them, to reduce complex phenomena to their constitutive elements. In particular, Western tradition has been dominated by the notion that a chasm exists between the body and the mind. When confronted with a disease, medicine tends to look for a single, malfunctioning entity or disease-causing agent and to develop a specialty to deal with it. This approach, for certain problems, is extremely powerful. But for others, it does not work.

When confronted with problems that are resistant to habitual modes of attack, it is useful to approach them from a different perspective; for example, by consulting the health traditions of other cultures.

©1993 American Association of Occupational Health Nurses. *AAOHN Journal*. July 1993, vol 41, No. 7. Reprinted with permission.

In most non-Western cultures to be ill is to be out of balance. Instead of looking for a single disease causing entity, it is assumed that what is damaged is a set of relationships. Instead of setting the body and the mind apart from each other, these traditions see the body as an outgrowth of the mind, just as a cell is the outgrowth of the intelligence coded into DNA. Given this perspective, when confronted by disease, one seeks to strengthen the whole, instead of isolating and treating the diseased part.

Movement and Touch

Living in a highly verbal culture, one can easily forget the rich language of movement and touch. Movement and touch are prior to all speech. Feeling is the foundation upon which culture is built. In his classic work, *Touching: The Human Significance of the Skin*, Ashley Montagu calls the skin, "the mother of the senses" (Montagu, 1986). All human senses are a specialization of the sense of touch; touch remains the deepest, the most intimate, the most primal means of knowing, the most elemental form of communication. Infants, when they see an object, are impelled to touch it or to mouth it, to know it fully. Even adults often feel that they truly know a person when they have touched them.

When people feel something deeply they say that they are touched or moved. Movement and sensation are interdependent functions. The quality of the one depends on the quality of the other, and the quality of both is determined by the attention given to the self in movement.

Good health requires that humans attend both internally to the myriad sensations and feelings that guide choices and decisions and, externally, to our relationship with the environment and, especially, relationships with other human beings. At every level the quality of life depends on the quality of the attention bestowed on it.

Even in the case of accidents in which one has no prior participation, the quality of recovery largely depends on the quality of one's attention. Is treatment sought immediately? How does one care for one's self during convalescence? Does one focus on feelings of frustration, anger, or self pity? Does one attend to the circumstances that allowed the accident to happen, or blithely proceed, all but asking the accident to happen again?

All of the mind/body arts reviewed below can help a client focus attention inwardly in new ways. The number of such arts is very nearly limitless. The choice of which to present is based on the popularity of the art and the author's interest and expertise.

126

Mind/Body Arts

Massage

Massage is the most widely known and practiced mind/body healing art. It may be the oldest healing art of all. Hippocrates, in the early fifth century BC, wrote, "the physician must be experienced in many things, but assuredly in rubbing" (White, 1988).

Massage is instinctive. All humans rub their own aches and pains, and comfort others by holding or stroking them. Classical therapeutic massage is an elaboration of this response. Frequently cited benefits of massage include relaxation; improved breathing, circulation, and oxygen carrying capacity of the blood; improved lymph flow and decreased edema; strengthening of the immune system; reduction of fatigue, pain, and anxiety; diminished feelings of isolation; improved sleep; healthier skin; and a generalized sense of well being.

Studies have suggested that massage may facilitate learning and development in both healthy and premature infants, as well as help develop feelings of closeness between parents and infants. Mothers who learn to massage their infants report that the infants seem to enjoy it and are calmer afterward. Parents who massage their infants appear afterwards to handle them with more confidence (White, 1988).

Acupressure/Acupuncture

Shiatsu, or acupressure, is a specialized form of massage that developed in China and Japan. Along with acupuncture, these forms are based on the theory that the body contains subtle energy pathways that correspond to no known physical structure, but that may be traced along points of decreased electrical resistance on the skin. Stimulating these points by deep pressure, as in shiatsu, or by needles as in acupuncture, is said to improve this energy flow and beneficially affect organs distant from the point stimulated.

Western scientists initially met acupuncture with much skepticism about the notion of subtle energy pathways following no observable anatomical structure. However, clinical success with a variety of conditions has led to increasing respect.

Acupuncture is most widely used in the West as a method of pain relief. The stimulation of specific points releases endorphins. In addition, there is growing interest in using acupuncture as a method of treating drug, alcohol, and food addictions (George, 1992). The World Health Organization has declared that acupuncture is suitable for treating ear, nose, and throat; respiratory; gastrointestinal; eye; neurological; and muscular disorders.

Yoga

Hatha Yoga is an ancient Hindu discipline that combines stretching and breathing exercises, deep relaxation, and meditation. Its practitioners claim a wide variety of physical, mental, and emotional benefits. A recent controlled study described in *Lancet* concluded that yogic breathing exercises "may result in improved control of asthma in mild cases" (Singh, 1990).

T'ai Chi

T'ai chi ch'uan is a slow motion, dance like, Chinese martial art. Practitioners move with great concentration, flowing smoothly from one graceful pose to another. T'ai chi has been likened to swimming in air.

A National Institute on Aging three-year study on ways to enhance fitness among older Americans includes T'ai chi. Although results will not be released until next spring, preliminary reports suggest that it is extremely effective in helping seniors improve their coordination and balance (Down, 1992).

Feldenkrais

The Feldenkrais method was developed in this century by Dr. Moshe Feldenkrais, a physicist and electronics engineer, and recipient of the first European black belt in Judo. In 1942, while still in his thirties, an old knee injury threatened to cripple him. Suspecting that the problem was not in his knee but in the way he was using it, Feldenkrais began an intensive study of anatomy, physiology, and movement. Applying his discoveries, he recovered the full use of his knee without surgery.

The Feldenkrais method teaches that many pains and movement restrictions are not the result of actual physical defect or the inevitable deteriorations of age, but of habitual poor use. This results, over time, in fatigue, disability, and pain. The antidote is to experience again the profound pleasure and deep satisfaction that comes from learning how to move organically.

To this end Feldenkrais developed two modes of instruction. The first consists of gentle, exploratory, Yoga like movements that are performed in response to verbal instruction. Feldenkrais movements are designed to break up habitual patterns—for example, moving one's head in one direction and shoulders and eyes in the other (Feldenkrais, 1972).

In the second mode of instruction, functional integration, the client lies on a low, padded table and is guided into non-habitual movements by the hands of a trained practitioner. While both modes are relaxing, more than mere relaxation is achieved. The central nervous system learns how to coordinate movement more efficiently. One learns how to consciously imitate the strategy of learning spontaneously adopted as infants—experimenting and playing with movement. Feldenkrais creates a learning environment in which there is no right or wrong, in which every action is evaluated solely in terms of how it feels.

Clients report profound relaxation, feelings of lightness, groundedness, and even the urge to dance (Stern, J. Breaking free: Feldenkrais method seeks to eliminate areas of tension. The *Huguenot Herald*, July 16, 1992). One of the author's recent clients, whose cerebral palsy was sufficiently severe to have occasioned two hip surgeries in an only partially successful attempt to correct extreme inward rotation of the feet, laughed like a little girl when, sitting on one side of the table after her first lesson, she looked down and saw her feet resting easily on the floor, "like two perfectly normal feet!" The method that Feldenkrais developed to teach himself to overcome the effects of internalized social fears is exactly applicable to those whose learning disabilities are the result not of socialization but of accident or birth defect.

As yet no published studies document the effectiveness of this method, although some are in progress.

In summary, a number of nontraditional therapies rely on touch and movement. Practitioners seek to help clients integrate the mind and body to achieve health or a sense of balance.

References

Down, L. (1992). T'ai Chi. *Modern Maturity* June-July.

Feldenkrais, M. (1972) *Awareness Through Movement: Health Exercises for Personal Growth*. San Francisco: Harper & Row. George, L. (1992). Alternative medicine. American Health: Fitness of Body and Mind, 45.

Montagu, A. (1986). *Touching: The Human Significance of the Skin*. New York, NY: Harper & Row.

Singh, V., Wisniewski, A, Britton, J., & Tattersfield, A. (1990). Effect of yoga breathing exercises (pranayama) on airway reactivity in subjects with asthma. *Lancet*, 335, 1381-1383. White, J. (1988). *Touching with intent: Therapeutic massage.* Holistic Nursing Practice.

— by Thomas Wanning, BA

Mr Wanning is a Guild Certified Feldenkrais Practitioner, Saugerties, NY

Part Three

Bioelectromagnetics

Chapter 14

Bioelectromagnetics: Applications in Medicine

Overview

Bioelectromagnetics (BEM) is the emerging science that studies how living organisms interact with electromagnetic (EM) fields. Electrical phenomena are found in all living organisms. Moreover, electrical currents exist in the body that are capable of producing magnetic fields that extend outside the body. Consequently, they can be influenced by external magnetic and EM fields as well. Changes in the body's natural fields may produce physical and behavioral changes. To understand how these field effects may occur, it is first useful to discuss some basic phenomena associated with EM fields.

In its simplest form, a magnetic field is a field of magnetic force extending out from a permanent magnet. Magnetic fields are produced by moving electrical currents. For example, when an electrical current flows in a wire, the movement of the electrons through the wire produces a magnetic field in the space around the wire (fig. 14.1). If the current is a direct current (DC), it flows in one direction and the magnetic field is steady. If the electrical current in the wire is pulsing, or fluctuating—such as in alternating current (AC), which means the current flow is switching directions—the magnetic field also fluctuates. The strength of the magnetic field depends on the amount of

Extracted from NIH Publication No. 94-066 from the Office of Alternative Medicine. December 1994. Due to space considerations, bibliographic data have not been reprinted in this chapter. However, to aid readers who wish to consult the original document or do further research, the in-text references have been retained.

133

current flowing in the wire; the more current, the stronger the magnetic field. An EM field contains both an electrical field and a magnetic field. In the case of a fluctuating magnetic or EM field, the field is characterized by its rate, or frequency, of fluctuation (e.g., one fluctuation per second is equal to 1 hertz [Hz], the unit of frequency).

A field fluctuating in this fashion theoretically extends out in space to infinity, decreasing in strength with distance and ultimately becoming lost in the jumble of other EM and magnetic fields that fill space. Since it is fluctuating at a certain frequency, it also has a wave motion (fig. 14.2). The wave moves outward at the speed of light (roughly 186,000 miles per second). As a result, it has a wavelength (i.e., the distance between crests of the wave) that is inversely related to its frequency. For example, a 1-Hz frequency has a wavelength of millions of miles, whereas a 1-million-Hz, or 1-megahertz (MHz), frequency has a wavelength of several hundred feet, and a 100-MHz frequency has a wavelength of about 6 feet.

All of the known frequencies of EM waves or fields are represented in the EM spectrum, ranging from DC (zero frequency) to the highest frequencies, such as gamma and cosmic rays. The EM spectrum includes x rays, visible light, microwaves, and television and radio frequencies, among many others. Moreover, all EM fields are force fields that carry energy through space and are capable of producing an effect at a distance. These fields have characteristics of both waves and particles. Depending on what types of experiments one does to investigate light, radio waves, or any other part of the EM spectrum, one will find either waves or particles called photons.

A photon is a tiny packet of energy that has no measurable mass. The greater the energy of the photon, the greater the frequency associated with its waveform. The human eye detects only a narrow

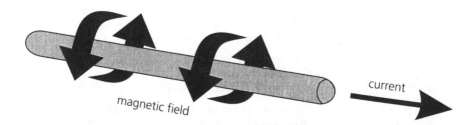

Figure 14.1. *An electrical current in a wire produces a magnetic field in the space around the wire.*

band of frequencies within the EM spectrum, that of light. One photon gives up its energy to the retina in the back of the eye, which converts it into an electrical signal in the nervous system that produces the sensation of light.

Table 14.1 shows the usual classification of EM fields in terms of their frequency of oscillation, ranging from DC through extremely low frequency (ELF), low frequency, radio frequency (RF), microwave and radar, infrared, visible light, ultraviolet, x rays, and gamma rays. For oscillating fields, the higher the frequency, the greater the energy.

Endogenous fields (those produced within the body) are to be distinguished from exogenous fields (those produced by sources outside the body). Exogenous EM fields can be classified as either natural, such as the earth's geomagnetic field, or artificial (e.g., power lines, transformers, appliances, radio transmitters, and medical devices). The term electropollution refers to artificial EM fields that may be associated with health risks.

In radiation biophysics, an EM field is classified as ionizing if its energy is high enough to dislodge electrons from an atom or molecule. High-energy, high-frequency forms of EM radiation, such as gamma rays and x rays, are strongly ionizing in biological matter. For this reason, prolonged exposure to such rays is harmful. Radiation in the middle portion of the frequency and energy spectrum—such as visible, especially ultraviolet, light—is weakly ionizing (i.e., it can be ionizing or not, depending on the target molecules).

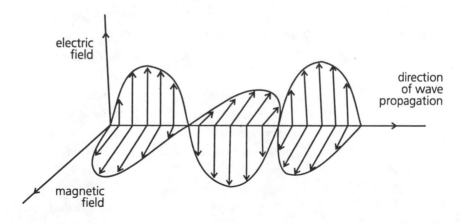

Figure 14.2. *Electromagnetic theory showing a wave in which the electric field is perpendicular to the magnetic field and also to the direction of propagation.*

Although it has long been known that exposure to strongly ionizing EM radiation can cause extreme damage in biological tissues, only recently have epidemiological studies and other evidence implicated long-term exposure to nonionizing, exogenous EM fields, such as those emitted by power lines, in increased health hazards. These hazards may include an increased risk in children of developing leukemia (Bierbaum and Peters, 1991; Nair et al. 1989; Wilson et al., 1990a).

However, it also has been discovered that oscillating nonionizing EM fields in the ELF range can have vigorous biological effects that may be beneficial and thus nonharmful (Becker and Marino, 1982; Brighton and Pollack, 1991). This discovery is a cornerstone in the foundation of BEM research and application.

Specific changes in the field configuration and exposure pattern of low-level EM fields can produce highly specific biological responses. More intriguing, some specific frequencies have highly specific effects on tissues in the body, just as drugs have their specific effects on target tissues. The actual mechanism by which EM fields produce biological effects is under intense study. Evidence suggests that the cell membrane may be one of the primary locations where applied EM fields act on the cell. EM forces at the membrane's outer surface could modify ligand-receptor interactions (e.g., the binding of messenger chemicals such as hormones and growth factors to specialized cell membrane molecules called receptors), which in turn would alter the state of large membrane molecules that play a role in controlling the

Table 14.1. Electromagnetic Spectrum

Frequency range (Hz)*	Classification	Biological effect
0	Direct current	Nonionizing
0 – 300	Extremely low frequency	Nonionizing
$300 – 10^4$	Low frequency	Nonionizing
$10^4 – 10^9$	Radio frequency	Nonionizing
$10^9 – 10^{12}$	Microwave and radar bands	Nonionizing
$10^{12} – 4 \times 10^{14}$	Infrared band	Nonionizing
$4 \times 10^{14} – 7 \times 10^{14}$	Visible light	Weakly ionizing
$7 \times 10^{14} – 10^{18}$	Ultraviolet band	Weakly ionizing
$10^{18} – 10^{20}$	X rays	Strongly ionizing
Over 10^{20}	Gamma rays	Strongly ionizing

* Division of the EM spectrum into frequency bands is based on conventional but arbitrary usage in various disciplines.

cell's internal processes (Tenforde and Kaune, 1987). Experiments to establish the full details of a mechanistic chain of events such as this, however, are just beginning.

Another line of study focuses on the endogenous EM fields. At the level of body tissues and organs, electrical activity is known to exhibit macroscopic patterns that contain medically useful information. For example, the diagnostic procedures of electroencephalography (EEG) and electrocardiography are based on detection of endogenous EM fields produced in the central nervous system and heart muscle, respectively. Taking the observations in these two systems a step further, current BEM research is exploring the possibility that weak EM fields associated with nerve activity in other tissues and organs might also carry information of diagnostic value. New technologies for constructing extremely sensitive EM transducers (e.g., magnetometers and electrometers) and for signal processing recently have made this line of research feasible.

Recent BEM research has uncovered a form of endogenous EM radiation in the visible region of the spectrum that is emitted by most living organisms, ranging from plant seeds to humans (Chwirot et al., 1987, Mathew and Rumar, in press, Popp et al., 1984, 1988, 1992). Some evidence indicates that this extremely low-level light, known as biophoton emission, may be important in bioregulation, membrane transport, and gene expression. It is possible that the effects (both beneficial and harmful) of exogenous fields maybe mediated by alterations in endogenous fields. Thus, externally applied EM fields from medical devices may act to correct abnormalities in endogenous EM fields characteristic of disease states. Furthermore, the energy of the biophotons and processes involving their emission as well as other endogenous fields of the body may prove to be involved in energetic therapies, such as healer interactions.

At the cutting edge of BEM research lies the question of how endogenous body EM fields may change as a result of changes in consciousness. The recent formation and rapid growth of a new society, the International Society for the Study of Subtle Energies and Energy Medicine, is indicative of the growing interest in this field.[1]

Figure 14.3 illustrates several types of EM fields of interest in BEM research.

Medical Applications of Bioelectromagnetics

Medical research applications of BEM began almost simultaneously with Michael Faraday's discovery of electromagnetic induction in the late 1700s. Immediately thereafter came the famous experiments of the 18th-century physician and physicist Luigi Galvani, who showed with frog legs that there was a connection between electricity and muscle contraction. This was followed by the work of Alessandro Volta, the Italian physicist whose investigation into electricity led him to correctly interpret Galvani's experiments with muscle, showing that

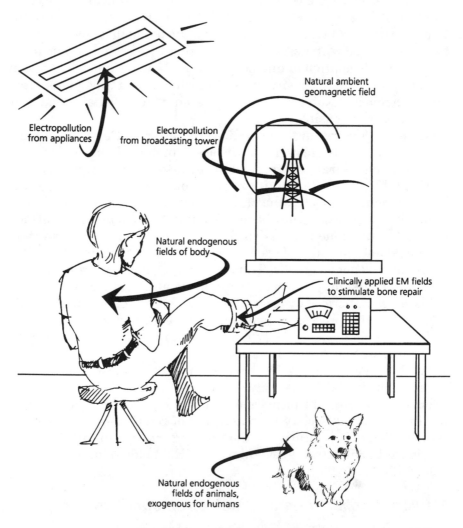

Natural ambient geomagnetic field

Electropollution from appliances

Electropollution from broadcasting tower

Natural endogenous fields of body

Clinically applied EM fields to stimulate bone repair

Natural endogenous fields of animals, exogenous for humans

Figure 14.3. Examples of natural and created EM fields, exogenous and endogenous.

the metal electrodes and not the tissue generated the current. From this early work came a plethora of devices for the diagnosis and treatment of disease, using first static electricity, then electrical currents, and, later, frequencies from different regions of the EM spectrum. Like other treatment methods, certain devices were seen as unconventional at first, only to become widely accepted later. For example, many of the medical devices that make up the core of modern, scientifically based medicine, such as x-ray devices, at one time were considered highly experimental.

Most of today's medical EM devices use relatively large levels of electrical, magnetic, or EM energy. The main topic of this chapter, however, is the use of the nonionizing portion of the EM spectrum, particularly at low levels, which is the focus of BEM research.

Nonionizing BEM medical applications may be classified according to whether they are thermal (heat producing in biologic tissue) or nonthermal. Thermal applications of nonionizing radiation (i.e., application of heat) include RF hyperthermia, laser and RF surgery, and RF diathermy.

The most important BEM modalities in alternative medicine are the nonthermal applications of nonionizing radiation. The term nonthermal is used with two different meanings in the medical and scientific literature. Biologically (or medically) nonthermal means that it "causes no significant gross tissue heating"; this is the most common usage. Physically (or scientifically) nonthermal means "below the thermal noise limit at physiological temperatures." The energy level of thermal noise is much lower than that required to cause heating of tissue; thus, any physically nonthermal application is automatically biologically nonthermal.

All of the nonthermal applications of nonionizing radiation are nonthermal in the biological sense. That is, they cause no significant heating of tissue. Some of the newer, unconventional BEM applications are also physically nonthermal. A variety of alternative medical practices developed outside the United States employ nonionizing EM fields at nonthermal intensities. For instance, microwave resonance therapy, which is used primarily in Russia, employs low-intensity (either continuous or pulse modulated), sinusoidal microwave radiation to treat a variety of conditions, including arthritis, ulcers, esophagitis, hypertension, chronic pain, cerebral palsy, neurological disorders, and side effects of cancer chemotherapy (Devyatkov et al., 1991). Thousands of people in Russia also have been treated by specific frequencies of extremely low-level microwaves applied at certain acupuncture points.

The mechanism of action of microwave resonance therapy is thought to involve modifications in cell membrane transport or production of chemical mediators or both. Although a sizable body of Russian-language literature on this technique already exists, no independent validation studies have been conducted in the West. However, if such treatments prove to be effective, current views on the role of information and thermal noise (i.e., order and disorder) in living systems, which hold that biological information is stored in molecular structures, may need revision. It may be that such information is stored at the level of the whole organism in the endogenous EM field, which may be used informationally in biological regulation and cellular communication (i.e., not due to energy content or power intensity). If exogenous, extremely low-level nonionizing fields with energy contents well below the thermal noise limit produce biological effects, they may be acting on the body in such a way that they alter the body's own field. That is to say, biological information would be altered by the exogenous EM fields.

The eight major new (or "unconventional") applications of nonthermal, nonionizing EM fields are as follows:

1. Bone repair.
2. Nerve stimulation.
3. Wound healing.
4. Treatment of osteoarthritis.
5. Electroacupuncture.
6. Tissue regeneration.
7. Immune system stimulation.
8. Neuroendocrine modulations.

These applications of BEM and the evidence for their efficacy are discussed in the following section

Research Base

Applications 1 through 5 above have been clinically tested and are in limited clinical use. On the basis of existing animal and cellular studies, applications 6 through 8 offer the potential for developing new clinical treatments, but clinical trials have not yet been conducted.

Bone Repair

Three types of applied EM fields are known to promote healing of nonunion bone fractures (i.e., those that fail to heal spontaneously):

140

- Pulsed EM fields (PEMFs) and sinusoidal EM fields (AC fields).
- DC fields.
- Combined AC-DC magnetic fields tuned to ion-resonant frequencies (these are extremely low-intensity, physically nonthermal fields) (Weinstein et al., 1990).

Approval of the U.S. Food and Drug Administration (FDA) has been obtained on PEMF and DC applications and is pending for the AC-DC application. In PEMF and AC applications, the repetition frequencies used are in the ELF range (Bassett, 1989). In DC applications, magnetic field intensities range from 100 microgauss to 100 gauss (G), and electric currents range from less than 0.1 microampere to milliamperes (Baranowski and Black, 1987).2 FDA approval of these therapies covers only their use to promote healing of nonunion bone fractures, not to accelerate routine healing of uncomplicated fractures.

Efficacy of EM bone repair treatment has been confirmed in double-blind clinical trials (Barker et al., 1984; Sharrard, 1990). A conservative estimate is that as of 1985 more than 100,000 people had been treated with such devices (Bassett et al., 1974, 1982; Brighton et al., 1979, 1981; Goldenberg and Hansen, 1972; Hinsenkamp et al., 1985).

Stimulation and Measurement of Nerve Activity

These applications fall into the following seven categories:

1. **Transcutaneous electrical nerve stimulation (TENS).** In this medical application, two electrodes are applied to the skin via wires attached to a portable electrical generating device, which may be clipped to the patient's belt (Hagfors and Hyme, 1975). Perhaps more than 100 types of FDA-approved devices in this category are currently available and used in physical therapy for pain relief. All of them operate on the same basis.

2. **Transcranial electrostimulation (TCES).** These devices are similar to the TENS units. They apply extremely low currents (below the nerve excitation threshold) to the brain via two electrodes applied to the head and are used for behavioral/psychological modification (e.g., to reduce symptoms of depression, anxiety, and insomnia) (Shealy et al., 1992). A recent meta-analysis covering at least 12 clinical trials selected from more than 100 published reports found that TCES can alleviate anxiety disorders (Klawansky et al., 1992). With support

141

from the National Institutes of Health (NIH), TCES is under evaluation for alleviation of drug dependence.

3. **Neuromagnetic stimulation.** In this application, which has both diagnostic and therapeutic uses, a magnetic pulse is applied noninvasively to a part of the patient's body to stimulate nerve activity. In diagnostic use, a pulse is applied to the cerebral cortex, and the patient's physiological responses are monitored to obtain a dynamic picture of the brain-body interface (Hallett and Cohen, 1989). As a treatment modality, it is being used in lieu of electroshock therapy to treat certain types of affective disorder (e.g., major depression) and seizures (Anninos and Tsagas, 1991). Neuromagnetic stimulation also is used in nerve conduction studies for conditions such as carpal tunnel syndrome.

4. **Electromyography.** This diagnostic application detects electrical potentials associated with muscle contraction. Specific electrical patterns have been associated with certain abnormal states (e.g., denervated muscle). This method, along with electromyographic biofeedback, is being used to treat carpal tunnel syndrome and other movement disorders.

5. **Electroencephalography.** This neurodiagnostic application detects brainwaves. Coupled with EEG biofeedback it is used to treat a variety of conditions, such as learning disabilities, attention deficit and hyperactivity disorders, chronic alcoholism, and stroke.

6. **Electroretinography.** This diagnostic application monitors electrical potentials across the retina to assess eye movements. This is one of the few methods available for noninvasive monitoring of rapid eye movement sleep.

7. **Low-energy emission therapy.** This application uses an antenna positioned in the patient's mouth to administer amplitude-modulated EM fields. It has been shown to affect the central nervous system, and pilot clinical studies show efficacy in treating insomnia (Hajdukovic et al., 1992) and hypertension (Pasche et al.,1989).

Soft-tissue Wound Healing

The following studies have demonstrated accelerated healing of soft-tissue wounds using DC, PEMF. and electrochemical modalities

- When wound healing is abnormal (retarded or arrested), electric or magnetic field applications may trigger healing to occur. A review of several reports indicates that fields may be useful in this regard (Lee et al., 1993; Vodovnik and Karba, 1992).

- PEMFs have been used clinically to treat venous skin ulcers. Results of several double-blind studies showed that PEMF stimulation promotes cell activation and cell proliferation through an effect on the cell membrane, particularly on endothelial cells (Ieran et al., 1990; Stiller et al., 1992).

- ELF and RF fields are applied to accelerate wound healing. Since skin wounds have unique electrical potentials and currents, stimulation of these electrical factors by a variety of exogenous EM fields can aid in the healing process by causing dedifferentiation (i.e., conversion to a more primitive form) of the nearby cells followed by accelerated cell proliferation (O'Connor et al., 1990).

- An electrochemical treatment that provides scarless regenerative wound healing uses electricity solely to introduce active metallic ions, such as silver, into the tissue. The electric field plays no role itself (Becker, 1987, 1990, 1992).

- PEMF increases the rate of formation of epithelial (skin) cells in partially healed wounds (Mertz et al., 1988).

- EM fields promote the repair of injured vascular networks (Herbst et al., 1988).

- EM devices have been patented for treating atherosclerotic lesions (i.e., small blood clots that build up on the walls of arteries and cause cardiovascular disease) and to control tissue growth (Gordon, 1986; Liboff et al., 1992b).

Osteoarthritis

In a recent clinical trial using a double-blind, randomized protocol with placebo control, osteoarthritis (primarily of the knee) treated noninvasively by pulsed 30-Hz, 60-G PEMFs showed the treatment group improved substantially more than the placebo group (Trock et al., 1993). It is believed that applied magnetic fields act to suppress inflammatory responses at the cell membrane level (O'Connor et al 1990).

Electroacupuncture

Electrical stimulation via acupuncture needles is often used as an enhancement or replacement for manual needling. Clinical benefits have been demonstrated for the use of electrical stimulation (electrostimulation) in combination with acupuncture as well as for electrostimulation applied directly to acupuncture points.

As an enhancement of acupuncture, a small-scale study showed electrostimulation with acupuncture to be beneficial in the treatment of post-operative pain (Christensen and Noreng, 1989). Other controlled studies have shown good success in using electrostimulation with acupuncture in the treatment of chemotherapy-induced sickness in cancer patients (Dundee and Ghaly, 1989). In addition, electrical stimulation with acupuncture was recently shown to be beneficial in the treatment of renal colic (Lee et al., 1992).

As a replacement for acupuncture, electrostimulation applied in a controlled study to acupuncture points by a TENS unit was effective in inducing uterine contractions in post-term pregnant women (Dunn and Rogers, 1989). Further, research with rats has shown that electrostimulation at such points can enhance peripheral motor nerve regeneration (McDevitt et al., 1987) and sensory nerve sprouting (Pomeranz et al., 1984).

Regeneration

Animal research in this area indicates that the body's endogenous EM fields are involved in growth processes and that modifications of these fields can lead to modest regeneration of severed limbs (Becker, 1987; Becker and Spadero, 1972; Smith, 1967). Russian research and clinical applications, along with studies now under way in the United States, indicate that low-intensity microwaves apparently stimulate bone marrow stem cell division and may be useful in enhancing the effects of chemotherapy by maintaining the formation and development, or hematopoiesis, of various types of blood cells (Devyatkov et al., 1991).

The following studies are also relevant to the use of BEM for regeneration:

- PEMF applications to promote peripheral nerve regeneration (Orgel et al., 1992; Sisken, 1992).

- The "diapulse" method of using pulsed, high-frequency EM fields for human wrist nerve regeneration (Wilson et al., 1974).

- DC applications to promote rat spinal cord regeneration (Fehlings et al., 1992; Hurlbert and Tator, 1992).

144

- Swedish work showing that BEM promotes rat sciatic nerve regeneration (Kanje and Rusovan, 1992; Rusovan and Kanje, 1991, 1992; Rusovan et al., 1992).

Immune System

During the past two decades, the effects of EM exposure on the immune system and its components have been extensively studied. While early studies indicated that long-term exposure to EM fields might negatively affect the immune system, there is promising new research showing that applied EM fields may be able to beneficially modulate immune responses. For example, studies with human lymphocytes show that exogenous EM or magnetic fields can produce changes in calcium transport (Walleczek, 1992) and cause mediation of the mitogenic response (i.e., the stimulation of the division of cellular nuclei; certain types of immune cells begin to divide and reproduce rapidly in response to certain stimuli, or mitogens). This finding has led to research investigating the possible augmentation by applied EM fields of a type of immune cell population called natural killer cells, which are important in helping the body fight against cancer and viruses (Cadossi et al., 1988a, 1988b; Cossarizza et al., 1989a, 1989b, 1989c).

Potential Neuroendocrine Modulations

Low-level PEMFs have typically been shown to suppress levels of melatonin, which is secreted by the pineal gland and is believed to regulate the body's inner clock (Lerchl et al., 1990; Wilson et al., 1990b). Melatonin, as a hormone, is oncostatic (i.e., it stops cancer growth). Thus, if melatonin can be suppressed by certain magnetic fields, it also may be possible to employ magnetic fields with different characteristics to stimulate melatonin secretion for the treatment of cancer. Other applications may include use of EM fields to affect melatonin secretion to normalize circadian rhythms in people with jet lag and sleep cycle disturbances

Table 14.2 provides an overview of selected citations to the refereed literature for these application.

Future Research Opportunities

Although to date there is an extensive base of literature on the use of BEM for medical applications, the overall research strategy into this phenomenon has been quite fragmented. Because of BEM's potential

Table 14.2. Selected Literature Citations on Biomedical Effects of Nonthermal EM Fields *(continued on next page)*

Location or type of bioeffect	DC	Frequency range of EM fields			Review articles and monographs
		ELF, including sinusoidal, pulsed, and mixed	RF and microwave	IR, visible, and UV light	
Bone and cartilage, including treatments for bone repair and osteoporosis	Brighton et al., 1981; Baranowsi & Black, 1987; Papatheofanis, 1989	Bassett et al., 1982; Barker et al., 1984; Brighton et al., 1985; Hinsenkamp et al., 1985; Huraki et al., 1987; Bassett, 1989, Madroñero, 1990; Sharrard, 1990; Grande et al., 1991; Magee et al., 1991; Pollack et al., 1991; Skerry et al., 1991; Ryaby et al., 1992			Brighton et al., 1979
Soft tissue, including wound healing, regeneratrion, and vascular-tissue effects	Becker, 1987; Becker, 1990; Becker, 1992; Vodovnik & Karba, 1992	Gordon, 1986; Herbst et al., 1988; Mertz et al., 1988; Yen-Patton et al., 1988; Albertini et al., 1990; Ieran et al., 1990; Im & Hoopes, 1991; Kraus, 1992; Liboff et al., 1992b; Stiller et al., 1992; Vodovnik & Karba, 1992	Devyatkov et al., 1991		Vodovnik & Karba, 1992
Neural tissue, including nerve growth and regeneration		Wilson et al., 1974; Rusovan & Kanje, 1991; Subramanian et al., 1991; Horton et al., 1992; Rusovan & Kanje, 1992; Rusovan et al., 1992			

Table 14.2. Selected Literature Citations on Biomedical Effects of Nonthermal EM Fields *(continued from previous page; continued on next page)*

Location or type of bioeffect	DC	Frequency range of EM fields			Review articles and monographs
		ELF, including sinusoidal, pulsed, and mixed	RF and microwave	IR, visible, and UV light	
Neural stimulation effects, including TENS and TCES		Hagfors & Hyme, 1975; Hallett & Cohen, 1989; Anninos & Tsagas, 1991; Klawansky et al., 1992			
Psychophysiological and behavioral effects			Pasche et al., 1989; Devyatkov et al., 1991; Hajdukovic et al., 1992	Thomas et al., 1986	O'Connor & Lovely, 1988
Electroacupuncture	McDevitt et al., 1987	Pomeranz et al., 1984; Christensen & Noreng, 1989; Dundee & Ghaly, 1989; Lee et al., 1992			
Neuroendocrine effects, including melatonin modifications	Feinendegen & Muhlensiepen, 1987	Lerchl et al., 1990; Wilson et al., 1990a, 1990b			O'Connor & Lovely, 1988
Immune system effects		Cadossi et al., 1988a; Cadossi et al., 1988b; Cossarizza et al., 1989a; Cossarizza et al., 1989b; Rosenthal & Obe, 1989; Phillips & McChesney, 1991; Walleczek, 1992			
Arthritis treatments		Grande et al., 1991; Trock et al., 1993	Devyatkov et al., 1991		

147

Table 14.2. Selected Literature Citations on Biomedical Effects of Nonthermal EM Fields *(continued from previous page)*

Location or type of bioeffect	DC	Frequency range of EM fields			Review articles and monographs
		ELF, including sinusoidal, pulsed, and mixed	**RF and microwave**	**IR, visible, and UV light**	
Cellular and subcellular effects, including effects on cell membrane, genetic system, and tumors	Easterly, 1982; Liburdy & Tenforde, 1986; Foxall et al., 1991; Miklavčič et al., 1991; Short et al., 1992	Cohen et al., 1986; Takahashi et al., 1987; Adey, 1992; Marron et al., 1988; Onuma & Hui, 1988; Brayman & Miller, 1989; Cossarizza et al., 1989a, 1989b; De Loecker et al., 1989; Goodmann et al., 1989; Rodemann et al., 1989; Brayman & Miller, 1990; Lerchl et al., 1990; Omote et al., 1990; Greene et al., 1991; Liboff et al., 1991	Guy, 1987; Chen & Ghandi, 1989; Brown & Chattpadhyay, 1991; Devyatkov et al., 1991		Adey & Lawrence, 1984; Marino, 1988; Blank & Findl, 1987; Ramel & Norden, 1991; Grundler et al., in press
Endogenous EM fields, including biophotons		Mathew & Rumar, in press	Mathew & Rumar, in press	Popp et al., 1984; Chwirot et al., 1987; Chwirot, 1988; Popp et al., 1988	Wijk & Schamhart, 1988; Popp et al., 1992

Note: Reports listed in table 2 are selected from refereed medical and scientific journals, multiauthor monographs, conference proceedings, and patents. See References for identification of sources. This is a representative selection from a large body of relevant sources and is not meant to be exhaustive or definitive.

for the treatment of a wide range of conditions, an integrated research program is needed that includes both basic and clinical research in BEM. These two approaches should be pursued vigorously and simultaneously along parallel tracks.

Basic research is needed to refine or develop new BEM technologies with the aim of establishing the fundamental knowledge about the body's endogenous EM fields and how they interact with clinically applied EM fields. A basic understanding of the BEM of the human body might provide insight into the scientific bioenergetic or bioinformational principles by which other areas of alternative medicine, such as homeopathy, acupuncture, and energetic therapies, may function. Furthermore, fundamental knowledge of BEM principles in the human body, in conjunction with psychophysiological states, might help facilitate understanding of mind-body regulation.

Clinical research, including preclinical assessments, is also essential, with the aim of bringing the most promising BEM treatments and diagnostics from limited use into widespread use as quickly as possible. Although a number of BEM devices show promise as new diagnostics or therapeutics, they must be tested on humans to show exactly when they are effective and when they are not. Moreover, measures of clinical effectiveness and safety are required for FDA approval of BEM medical devices. Ultimately, knowledge about the safety of new BEM medical devices can be ascertained only from the appropriate clinical trials.

Basic

The current status of basic research in BEM may be summarized as follows:

- Nonionizing, nonthermal exogenous EM fields exert measurable bioeffects in living organisms. In general, the organism's response to applied EM fields is highly frequency specific and the dose-response curve is nonlinear (i.e., application of an additional amount of the EM field does not elicit a response of equal magnitude; the response eventually diminishes no matter how additional EM stimuli are applied). Extremely weak EM fields may, at the proper frequency and site of application, produce large effects that are either clinically beneficial are harmful.

- The cell membrane has been proposed as the primary site of transduction of EM field bioeffects. Relevant mechanisms may include changes in cell-membrane binding and transport processes, displacement or deformation of polarized molecules, modifications in the conformation of biological water (i.e., water that comprises organisms), and others.

- The physical mechanisms by which EM fields may act on biomolecules are far too complex to discuss here. However, the following references propose such physical mechanisms: Grundler et al., in press; Liboff, 1985, 1991; and Liboff et al., 1991.

- Endogenous nonthermal EM fields ranging from DC to the visible spectral region may be intimately involved in regulating physiological and biochemical processes.

Consequently, the following pressing needs should be addressed in developing a basic BEM research program:

- Standardized protocols for measuring dosages for therapeutically applied EM fields should be established and followed uniformly in BEM research. Protocols are needed for characterizing (i.e., defining and measuring) EM field sources (both exogenous and endogenous) and EM parameters of biological subjects. Such variables must be characterized in greater detail than is commonly practiced in clinical research. Artifacts caused by ambient EM fields in the laboratory environment (e.g., from power lines and laboratory equipment) must be avoided.

- In general, a balanced, strategic approach to basic research—including studies in humans, animals, and cells along with theoretical modeling and close collaboration with other investigators in alternative medicine—will produce the most valuable results in the long run.

- Many independent parameters characterize nonthermal nonionizing EM fields, including pulsed vs. nonpulsed and sinusoidal vs. other waveforms; frequency; phase; intensity (as a function of spatial position); voltage; and current. If multiple fields are combined, these parameters must be specified for each component. Additional parameters necessary for characterizing the medical application of EM fields include the site of application and the time course of exposure. All of these can be experimentally varied, producing an enormous range of possibilities. To date, there has been little systematic research to explore the potential biological effects of this vast array of applied field parameter characteristics.

Clinical

Clinical trials of BEM-based treatments for the following conditions may yield useful results relatively soon: arthritis, psychophysiological states (including drug dependence and epilepsy), wound healing and regeneration, intractable pain, Parkinson's disease, spinal cord injury, closed head injury, cerebral palsy (spasticity reduction), learning disabilities, headache, degenerative conditions associated with aging, cancer, and acquired immunodeficiency syndrome (AIDS).

EM fields may be applied clinically as the primary therapy or as adjuvant therapy along with other treatments in the conditions listed above. Effectiveness can be measured via the following clinical markers:

- In arthritis, the usual clinical criteria, including decrease of pain, less swelling, and thus a greater potential for mobility.

- In psychophysiological problems, relief from symptoms of drug withdrawal and alleviation of depressive anxiety and its symptoms.

- In epilepsy, return to greater normality in EEG, more normal sleep patterns, and reduction in required drug dosages.

- In wound healing and regeneration, repair of soft tissue and reduction of collagenous tissue in scar formation; regrowth via blastemal (primitive cell) formation and increase in tensile strength of surgical wounds; alleviation of decubitus chronic ulcers (bedsores); increased angiogenesis (regrowth of vascular tissue such as blood vessels); and healing of recalcitrant (i.e., unresponsive to treatment) chronic venous ulcers.

For instance, a short-term, double-blind clinical trial of magnetic field therapy could be based on the protocol of Trock et al. (1993) for osteoarthritis of the knee or elbow. This protocol is as follows:

- A suitable patient population is divided into treatment and control groups. Individual assignments are coded and remain unknown to patients, clinicians, and operators until treatment and assessment are complete.

- Pretreatment clinical markers are assessed by clinicians or by patients themselves or both.

- Treatments consist of 3 to 5 half-hour sessions each week for a total of 18 treatments over 5-6 weeks.

- During treatment, each patient inserts the affected limb into the opening of a Helmholtz coil (a solenoid about 12 inches in diameter and 6 inches long) and rests while appropriate currents are applied to the coil via a preset program.

- The treatment is noninvasive and painless; the patient feels nothing; there is no measurable transfer of heat to the patient.

- The control group follows the same procedure except that, unknown to operator and patient, a "dummy" apparatus (altered internally so that no current flows in the coil) is used.

- Patients' posttreatment clinical markers are assessed.

- Appropriate data reduction (scoring of assessments, decoding of the treatment and control groups, and statistical analysis) is performed.

Clinical trials of BEM-based treatments for a variety of other conditions could follow a similar general outline.

Key Issues

Certain key issues or controversies surrounding BEM have inhibited progress in this field. These issues fall into several distinct areas: medical controversy, scientific controversy, barriers, and other issues.

Medical Controversy

A number of uncharacterized "black box" medical treatment and diagnostic devices—some legal and some illegal—have been associated with EM medical treatment. Whether they operate on the basis of BEM principles is unknown. Among these devices are the following: radionics devices, Lakhovsky multiple-wave oscillator, Priore's machine, Rife's inert gas discharge tubes, violet ray tubes, Reich's orgone energy devices, EAV machines, and biocircuit devices. There are at least six alternative explanations for how these and other such devices operate:

1. They are ineffectual and are based on erroneous application of physical principles.

2. They may be operating on BEM principles, but they are uncharacterized.

3. They may operate on acoustic principles (sound or ultrasound waves) rather than BEM.

4. In the case of diagnostic devices, they may work by focusing the intuitive capacity of the practitioner.

5. In the case of long-distance applications, they may operate by means of nonlocal properties of consciousness of patient and practitioner.

6. They may be operating on the energy of some domain that is uncharacterized at present.

A recent survey (Eisenberg et al., 1993) showed that about 1 percent of the U.S. population used energy healing techniques that included a variety of EM devices. Indeed, more of the respondents in this 1990 survey used energy healing techniques than used homeopathy and acupuncture in the treatment of either serious or chronic disease. In addition to the use of devices by practitioners, a plethora of consumer medical products that use magnetic energy are purported to promote relaxation or to treat a variety of illnesses. For example, for the bed there are mattress pads impregnated with magnets; there are magnets to attach to the site of an athletic injury; and there are small pelletlike magnets to place over specific points on the body. Most of these so-called therapeutic magnets, also called biomagnets, come from Japan. However, no known published journal articles demonstrating effectiveness via clinical trials exist.

Some of the medical modalities discussed in this report, although presently accepted medically or legally in the United States, have not necessarily passed the most recent requirements of safety or effectiveness. FDA approval of a significant number of BEM-based devices, primarily those used in bone repair and neurostimulation, was "grandfathered." That is, medical devices sold in the United States prior to the Medical Device Law of the late 1970s automatically received FDA approval for use in the same manner and for the same medical conditions for which they were used prior to the law's enactment. Grandfathering by the FDA applies not only to BEM devices but to all devices covered by the Medical Device Law. However, neither the safety nor the effectiveness of grandfathered devices is established (i.e., they are approved on the basis of a "presumption" by the FDA, but they usually remain incompletely studied). Reexamination of devices in use, whether grandfathered or not, may be warranted.

There are three possible ways of resolving controversies associated with BEM and its application:

1. elucidating the fundamental principles underlying the device, or at least the historical basis for the development of the device;

2. conducting properly designed case control studies and clinical trials to validate effects that have been reported or claimed for BEM-based treatments; and

3. increasing the medical community's awareness of well-documented, controlled clinical trials that indicate the effectiveness of specific BEM applications (see table 14.2).

Scientific Controversy

Some physicists claim that low-intensity, nonionizing EM fields have no bioeffects other than resistive (joule) heating of tissue. One such argument is based on a physical model in which the only EM field parameter considered relevant to biological systems is power density (Adair, 1991). The argument asserts that measurable nonthermal bioeffects of EM fields are "impossible" because they contradict known physical laws or would require a "new physics" to explain them.

However, numerous independent experiments reported in the refereed journal research literature conclusively establish that nonthermal bioeffects of low-intensity EM fields do indeed exist. Moreover, the experimental results lend support to certain new approaches in theoretical modeling of the interactions between EM fields and biological matter. Most researchers now feel that BEM bioeffects will become comprehensible not by forsaking physics but rather by developing more sophisticated, detailed models based on known physical laws, in which additional parameters (e.g., frequency, intensity, waveform and field directionality) are taken into account.

Barriers

The following barriers to BEM research exist:

• Members of NIH review panels in medical applications might not be adequately knowledgeable about alternative medical practices or BEM. This is the most serious barrier.

• Funding in BEM research is weighted heavily toward the study of hazards of EM fields; there is little funding for potential beneficial

medical applications or the study of basic mechanisms of EM interactions with life processes. Also, the bulk of EM field research is
administered by the Department of Defense and the Department
of Energy, agencies with missions unrelated to medical research.
The small amount of BEM work funded by NIH thus far has addressed mostly the hazards of EM fields. In late 1993 the National Institute of Environmental Health Sciences issued requests
for grant application in the areas of (1) cellular effects of low-
frequency EM fields and (2) effects of 60-Hz EM fields in vivo. The
latter project is concerned solely with safety in power line and ap-
pliance exposures. However, the former apparently does not rule
out the investigation of possible beneficial effects from low-fre-
quency fields, although the focus is clearly on assessing previously
reported effects of 60-Hz EM fields on cellular processes.

- Regulatory barriers to making new BEM devices available to
  practitioners are formidable. The approval process is slow and
  exorbitantly expensive even for conventional medical devices.

- Barriers in education include the following: (1) basic education in
  biological science is weak in physics, (2) undergraduate- and
  graduate-level programs in BEM are virtually nonexistent, and (3)
  multidisciplinary training is lacking in medicine and biology.

- The mainstream scientific and medical communities are basically conservative and respond to emerging disciplines, such as
  BEM, with reactions ranging from ignorance and apathy to
  open hostility. Consequently, accomplished senior researchers
  may not be aware of the opportunities for fruitful work in (or in
  collaboration with others in) BEM, while junior researchers
  may be reluctant to enter a field perceived by some as detrimental to career advancement.

Other Issues

Other key issues that need to be considered in developing a comprehensive research and development agenda for BEM include the following:

- Separate studies prepared for the Office of Technology Assessment, the National Institute of Occupational Safety and Health,
  and the Environmental Protection Agency have recommended
  independently that research on fundamental mechanisms of EM
  field interactions in humans receive high priority (Bierbaum and

Peters, 1991; Nair et al., 1989; U.S. EPA, 1991). Moreover, a 1985 report prepared by scientists at the Centers for Devices and Radiological Health recommended that future research on EM field interactions with living systems "be directed at exploring beneficial medical applications of EMR (electromagnetic radiation) modulation of immune responses" (Budd and Czerski, 1985).

- Elucidation of the physical mechanisms of BEM medical modalities is the single most powerful key to developing efficient and optimal clinical intervention. Even a relatively small advance beyond present knowledge of fundamental mechanisms would be of considerable practical value. In addition, progress in the development of a mechanistic explanation of the effects of alterative medicine could increase its acceptability in the eyes of mainstream medicine and science.

- BEM potentially offers a powerful new approach to understanding the neuroendocrine and immunological bases of certain major medical problems (e.g., wound healing, cancer, and AIDS). However, substantial funding and time are required to perform the basic research needed in developing this approach.

- BEM may provide a comprehensive biophysical framework grounded in fundamental science, through which many alternative medical practices can be studied. BEM offers a promising starting point for scientifically exploring various traditional alternative medical systems (Becker and Marino, 1982).

Basic Research Priorities

The most fruitful topics for future basic research investigations of BEM may include the following:

- Developing assay methods based on EM field interactions in cells (e.g., for potassium transport, calcium transport, and cytotoxicity). These assays could then be applied to existing studies of such phenomena in cellular systems.

- Developing BEM-based treatments for osteoporosis, on basis of the large body of existing work on EM bone repair and other research (e.g., Brighton et al., 1985; Cruess and Bassett, 1983; Liboff et al., 1992a; Madronero, 1990; Magee et al., 1991; Skerry et al., 1991). NASA researchers have already expressed interest in collaborative work to develop BEM treatments for weightlessness-induced osteoporosis.

- Measuring neurobiochemical changes in the blood in response to microcurrent skin stimulation in animals or humans with different frequencies, waveforms, and carrier waves. Such measurements should be made for preclinical evaluation of neurostimulation devices.

- Furthering studies of mechanisms of EM field interactions in cells and tissues with emphasis on coherent or cooperative states and resonant phenomena in biomolecules; and on coherent brainwave states and other long-range interactions in biological systems.

- Studying the role of water as a mediator in biological interactions with emphasis on the quantum EM aspects of its conformation (i.e., "structure," as implied in some forms of homeopathy). The response of biologic water to EM fields should be studied experimentally. A novel informational capacity of water in relation to EM bioeffects may provide insights into homeopathy and healer interactions (i.e., "laying on of hands").

- Studying in detail the role of the body's internally generated (endogenous) EM fields and the body's other natural electromagnetic parameters (see the "Manual Healing Methods" chapter). Knowledge of such processes should be applied to develop novel diagnostic methods and to understand alternative medical treatments such as acupuncture, electroacupuncture, and biofield therapies. Furthermore, exploratory research on the role of the body's energy fields in relation to the role of states of consciousness in health and healing should be launched.

- Establishing a knowledge base (an intelligent database) to provide convenient access to all significant BEM work in both basic and clinical research.

- Performing systematic reviews as well as meta-analytic reviews of existing BEM studies to identify the frequency and quality of research concerning BEM as well as most promising clinical end points for BEM treatments in humans.

Summary

Just as exposure to high-energy radiation has unquestioned hazards, radiation has long been a key weapon in the fight against many types of cancers. Likewise, although there are indications that some

157

EM fields may be hazardous, there is now increasing evidence that there are beneficial bioeffects of certain low-intensity nonthermal EM fields.

In clinical practice, BEM applications offer the possibility of more economical and more effective diagnostics and new noninvasive therapies for medical problems, including those considered intractable or recalcitrant to conventional treatments. The sizable body of recent work cited in this chapter has established the feasibility of treatments based on BEM, although the mainstream medical community is largely unaware of this work.

In biomedical research, BEM can provide a better understanding of fundamental mechanisms of communication and regulation at levels ranging from intracellular to organismic. Improved knowledge of fundamental mechanisms of EM field interactions could lead directly to major advances in diagnostic and treatment methods.

In the study of other alternative medical modalities, BEM offers a unified conceptual framework that may help explain how certain diagnostic and therapeutic techniques (e.g., acupuncture, homeopathy, certain types of ethnomedicine, and healer effects) may produce results that are difficult to understand from a more conventional viewpoint. These areas of alternative medicine are currently based entirely on empirical (i.e., experimentation and observation rather than theory) and phenomenological (i.e., the classification and description of any fact, circumstance, or experience without any attempt at explanation) approaches. Thus, their future development could be accelerated as a scientific understanding if their mechanisms of action are ascertained.

Footnotes

1. A more detailed introduction to the field of BEM and an overview of research progress is available in the following monographs and conference proceedings: Adey, 1992; Adey and Lawrence, 1984; Becker and Marino, 1982; Blank, 1993; Blank and Findl, 1987; Brighton and Pollack, 1991; Brighton et al., 1979; Liboffand Rinaldi, 1974; Marino, 1988; O'Connor et al., 1990; O'Connor and Lovely, 1988; Popp et al., 1992; and Ramel and Norden, 1991.

2. Gauss is a unit of magnetic flux density. For comparison, a typical magnet used to hold papers vertically on a refrigerator is 200 G.

Chapter 15

Electroacupuncture

Conditioned Healing with Electroacupuncture

Abstract

Increasing interest in mind-body medicine has spawned numerous methods that demonstrate the power of imagery and belief to favorably influence the course of disease. Few methods, however link the occurrence of a healing response with a demonstrated, specific, targeted body chemical. Even hypnosis and biofeedback, which direct their effects at targeted body systems, have been hypothesized to work by means of general relaxation. Research from China has demonstrated that neuroelectric acupuncture with stimulation at specific frequencies releases neuropeptides in human cerebrospinal fluid. Combining such stimulation with imagery as the conditional stimulus opens up the possibility for a conditioning paradigm of mind-body, patient-participant healing using specific healing neurohormones. This chapter discusses developments leading to the scientization of traditional acupuncture and its possible mechanism as a means for such conditioned healing. The demonstrated usefulness of this technique is based on patients' reports of symptom relief. Many variables should he considered, though ultimate verification will depend on serial sampling of cerebrospinal fluid. (*Alternative Therapies in Health and Medicine.* 1996, 2(5). 56-60)

An old Chinese proverb states that one generation travels the road built by a previous generation. This is particularly true in the case of contemporary acupuncture. Most civilizations have healing practices based on areas of the skin that have an unusual sensitivity. Three thousand years ago ancient Chinese physicians vigorously stimulated such spots with fragments of bone and bamboo. Through the ages these instruments were replaced by heavy metal needles of iron and, later, gold and silver. Steel needles were developed with special handles to aid with twisting and insertion. Finally, with concern about the transmission of bloodborne diseases such as AIDS, fine steel disposable needles became the standard.

Acupuncture was incorporated early into traditional Chinese medicine. Ideally holistic, traditional Chinese medicine involved careful examination of the whole person including the tongue, eyes, skin, pulse, diet, habits, emotions, and behavior. Treatment included advice, special diets, exercises, and two major interventions: herbs and acupuncture.

The practice of acupuncture spread to Korea by the year 300, and from there on to Japan. By 1800 there was considerable interest in Europe, where acupuncture has continued to experience a substantial growth. The World Health Organization estimates that acupuncture is now a major mode of therapy for one third of the world's population.

Acupuncture was late in coming to the United States. The story is an interesting one, mentioned in a surgical treatise by Billroth in 1863 and again by Sir William Osler in 1912. In his book, *Principles and Practice of Medicine*, Osler wrote, "For lumbago, acupuncture is, in acute cases, the most efficient treatment"—a statement that was deleted from subsequent editions. There was then a hiatus of some 60 years before this advice was again taken seriously in the United States.

Increased attention to acupuncture began with the visit of President Nixon to China in 1971. At that time a member of the press corps, James Reston, had an emergency appendectomy performed in China; relief from his post-appendectomy gas pain was produced by acupuncture needling. On his return to the United States, Reston presented to American readers a glowing picture of acupuncture treatment. With the parting of the "bamboo curtain," there was considerable interest in things Chinese; the idea that tiny needles could relieve pain fascinated the American public. Its use as an "anesthetic" in surgical procedures prompted curiosity among members of the medical profession. Reports in the popular press presented acupuncture as a cure-all, which created an instant demand for such treatments by patients with chronic pain and other complaints.

Explanation of the acupuncture phenomenon in terms of yin and yang, meridians, and other Oriental metaphysical and cosmological ideas was unacceptable to American doctors who described its action as hypnosis, placebo, or simply Oriental stoicism. In 1974 the American Medical Association (AMA) cautioned against "acupuncture quackery" (St Louis Post Dispatch. August 4, 1974). Since then, despite a growing body of literature supporting its widely demonstrated effectiveness, acupuncture has been labeled by the AMA as an "experimental procedure." As a result of this stance, acupuncture has become an enigma and has been shunned by most MDs; thus, the bulk of acupuncture in the US is performed by practitioners without medical degrees.

My coworkers and I received the first NIH grant for the study of acupuncture. Our investigation compared acupuncture with hypnosis for the control of experimental pain. We found that acupuncture successfully modulated experimental pain and was not hypnosis. Despite claims that acupuncture was "merely a placebo," we remained convinced that its healing was more than a mind-body effect. Particularly intriguing was our observation that, while needles alone could decrease experimental pain, when electrical stimulation was added to the needles the relief from pain became statistically significant and as strong as a 10 mg intramuscular injection of morphine.

Electroacupuncture

It is commonly accepted that mechanical stimulation of fibrous tissue in the human body can produce a piezoelectric effect. Undoubtedly those early Chinese acupuncturists who inserted and vigorously manipulated heavy slivers of bone and bamboo may well have "pried loose" a few electrons. It was not until 1764, however, that Gennai Hiraga of Envo, Japan, gave the first report of electrical stimulation of acupuncture needles.

In 1825 Chevalier Sarlandiere of France described the application of an electric current from Leyden jars applied to inserted acupuncture needles for the treatment of rheumatic conditions. The Chinese reported the use of electrical acupuncture as an anesthetic for surgery in the 1950s.

In 1973 Wen of Hong Kong reported that electrical stimulation of needles in the concha of the ear could be useful in detoxifying drug addicted patients, presumably through vagus innervation. In subsequent years, Wen's advocacy of electrical stimulation somehow was ignored and "needles only" auriculotherapy without electrical stimulation became the standard US treatment for drug addiction. Using a hypothesized map of the body in the ear, specific points have been recommended for addiction. A paper by Wells et al, however, reported no significant treatment differences between such specific and placebo points. Following the advice of Wen and a reported study on heroin addiction from Han's group in China, the authors successfully have used electrical stimulation—not of the ear, but of the Hoku point on the hand—in the treatment of drug addiction.

Papers by Laitinen and Fox and Melzack have compared acupuncture (needles twirled) without electrical stimulation and stimulation done with electrically stimulated conductive polymer electrodes for the treatment of low-back pain. They found that in general electroacupuncture and transdermal electrical nerve stimulation (TENS) treatments were equally effective. Later work from Han's laboratory (on animals) supported the view that as long as the proper parameters of electrical stimulation are used, needles and polymer conducting pads are equally effective for acupuncture treatments. Of special significance is the work of Han and Sun, demonstrating that different frequencies of electrical stimulation release different neuropeptides in the central nervous system. Two-hertz stimulation is specific for ß-endorphin. (For additional milestones, see Table 15.1 below)

Conditioned Reflexes

Ivan Pavlov (1849-1936) was the father of conditioned reflex theory. His scientific life and effort can be divided into four periods: (1) early research on circulation and the heart, (2) investigation of the physiology of digestion, (3) the bulk of work on conditioned reflexes, and (4) the period from age 80 until his death at age 86, during which he ventured into the field of psychiatry. Acupuncture is used widely in Russia, and Russian electrosleep treatment parallels work with neuroelectric acupuncture. (Had Pavlov continued his work in psychiatry and lived a few decades longer to witness the discovery of endorphins, he might well have written this very paper.)

Influenced by the teachings of Sherrington, Pavlov envisioned the nervous system functioning as an integrated whole. He believed strongly that it retained the characteristic of plasticity and hence could be trained. From his assumptions, Pavlov proceeded to develop his theory and ultimate demonstration of conditioned reflexes. He showed how the combination of an indifferent conditional stimulus

(CS) with an unconditioned stimulus (UCS) will lead to the formation of a conditioned reflex (CR). With repetition this conditioned reflex becomes stronger; if not repeated over time, it leads to extinction. However, if repeated frequently it can become increasingly stronger and, with training over a long period of time, it undergoes almost no regression at all.

The CS is always a certain complex situation activating a number of receptors. The stronger the UCS, the stronger the CR and the larger the neuron field involved. The more elements in common processed by the neural centers, the stronger the generalization. These laws developed by Pavlov apply to the technique of conditioned healing.

The possibility of using conditioning clinically with patients suffering from chronic pain and various psychiatric complaints was suggested by the work of Robert Ader. Ader and Cohen showed that the immune response in experimental animals could be classically conditioned. Watkins et al induced analgesia in rats by neuroelectrical stimulation of the front paws. When the electrical stimulation was paired with a tone in repeated experiments, it later became possible to produce analgesia by presenting the tone alone; this has been termed "auto-analgesia." The same thing happened when animals merely were put into the cage where the conditioning had occurred. This response could be blocked by nalorphine, demonstrating that opioids were involved in what could be termed a conditioned analgesic phenomenon. Conditioned reflexes are readily established in humans.

It appeared to us possible to set up a classical conditioning paradigm in human subjects to teach them to self-release heating neuropeptides including enkephalins, endorphins, and adrenocorticotropic hormone (ACTH). The secretion of these neuropeptides, demonstrated by Han and others, is a phenomenon produced regularly in the treatment of our patients by the use of neuroelectric acupuncture as the treatment modality.

The use of a tone or bell as the CS seemed neither reasonable nor convenient; rather, in humans it was preferable to use a mental image that would always be readily available. Unlike a tone (an external conditional signal), images are electrochemical events that already are intricately woven into the fabric of the brain.

Pavlov's concept of an integrated nervous system functioning as a whole is consistent with current ideas about memory, in which a nerve net links various parts of the sensory nervous system (Pavlov's "analysers"). These analysers are concerned with hearing, sight, smell, and so on, and—colored by a link to encode emotions—they give rise to the imagery "engram," which is the conditional signal.

163

Imagery

Imagery always has played a key role in medicine and is assuming an increasingly important place in holistic healing. Coupled with relaxation, imagery could have considerable therapeutic significance in strengthening the effect of electroacupuncture stimulation. Clinically, imagery has been used to stimulate the body so as to strengthen the immune system.

Enkephalins and endorphins are important in imagery. The placebo effect is a dramatic example of belief and imagination in action, a mechanism mediated by endorphins. Endorphins are formed in the anterior pituitary gland and in opioid neurons in the brain as part of a precursor, proopiomelanocortin. On activation this precursor releases endogenous opioids and ACTH. Enkephalins are endogenous immunomodulators. This relationship of endorphins to the immune system and of ß-endorphin to the imagination suggests that these compounds can play a role in conditioned healing. Accessing this system by a combined imagery conditioning electrostimulation approach should provide a particularly strong signal for neuropeptide release, and thus be of considerable significance in healing.

Training patients to use this technique at home produces a strong means for involving them in their own treatment. It provides a means for the self-release of healing neuropeptides.

Conditioned Healing (Electroacupuncture, Imagery, and Conditioning)

Even if the image is only a small part of the total experience, it can, according to Pribram's holographic model of brain functioning, create much of the positive experience and affect of the original situation. With this in mind, the authors ask patients to self-select a relaxing scene from their past experiences. A relaxation tape is used to induce a state of relaxation or self-hypnosis, during which the patient recalls to mind the scene that will become the CS. This pairing occurs during a 30-minute session of electroacupuncture in which the stimulus frequency of a HAN ACU-TENS unit is varied between 2 and 15 Hz in 3-second stimulation periods. This "dense/disperse" stimulation setting alternates the two frequencies at 3-second intervals, thus releasing endorphins, enkephalins, and possibly other healing neuropeptides. The polymer-pad electrodes are placed bilaterally on the Hoku points located on the web between the thumb and first finger. This location is the motor point of the dorsal interosseus muscle and is one of the most widely used points in traditional Chinese acupuncture. It is of interest that the dorsal interosseus muscle permits opposition of the thumb to the fingers, which is the basis of the prehensile hand of humans and thus an essential element in the development of civilization. Accordingly the thumb area has one of the largest representations on the surface of the cortex, graphically illustrated in "homunculus" diagrams. If one wishes to stimulate as many neurons as possible with a single body stimulus point, this is the one to use.

The conditioning procedure—repairing imagery with the release of neuropeptides in the cerebrospinal fluid—is repeated over a period of 10 to 12 weeks. Between weekly office treatment sessions the patient is directed to practice at home three or more times daily, sitting quietly while visualizing the conditional scene. In this manner the patient learns to self-release neuropeptides that can be helpful in regulating the body's homeostatic mechanisms.

The Hoku points are used as standard procedure with all patients. In those who have chronic pain, this strong point is useful to induce a centrally controlled modulation of pain. In addition, in patients with chronic pain we often use body points in the neurotome of the affected area with a frequency of stimulation set at 100 Hz to release dynorphins. When we treat psychiatric patients who are experiencing anxiety or patients with psychosomatic illnesses with symptoms resulting from sympathetic hyperactivity, we stimulate the concha of the ear. This produces a homeostatic response of the parasympathetic nervous system, which also may become part of the conditioning effect.

That the imagery occurs during a condition of relaxation may also play a significant role in pain modulation. Dahlgren et al noted that hypnotic suggestions of relaxation significantly reduce reports of pain and unpleasantness. Similar effects of relaxation on pain control were reported at the recent NIH consensus meeting on this subject. Relaxation may be a common thread in many holistic healing treatments.

In our technique, conditioned reflexes are formed by pairing imagery, the CS, with the electrically stimulated UCS of neuropeptide release and autonomic regulation. These procedures now have been used on several hundred patients, who have reported gratifying clinical results. Following are some clinical illustrations:

- RR, a 49-year-old female computer analyst, was diagnosed with schizoaffective disorder and migraine. The referring psychiatrist had her on Dexadrine, Zoloft, lithium, Wellbutrin, Depakote, Xanax, and Tylenol 3 and Caffergot taken as needed for headaches. She is receiving monthly neuroelectric acupuncture sessions with imagery conditioning. After four sessions she was able to reduce her medications and now is on only Risperdal and lithium, with headaches mostly controlled by her conditioned imagery.

- JW, a 62-year-old minister, developed severe and incapacitating situational panic reactions when required to speak before groups. Heavy doses of benzodiazepines had been only partly helpful and caused drowsiness. A series of six neuroelectric acupuncture sessions with imagery conditioning were sufficient to give him a tool to conquer his anxiety reactions. He now can successfully control his symptoms by using imagery for 5 minutes before his public appearances. He returns yearly for a single session to help maintain his conditioned ability.

- NJ, a 49-year-old Vietnam War veteran with posttraumatic stress disorder, had symptoms of insomnia, recurrent nightmares, panic attacks, and vasomotor instability. He was greatly improved and able to reduce his dependencies on benzodiazepines following a series of 12 weekly treatments.

Conclusion

The imagery and relaxation that occur with this procedure lie within the paradigm of mind-body medicine. The release of neuropeptides in the cerebrospinal fluid by neuroelectrical stimulation is a demonstrated physiological action. Combining the two for the development of a conditioned reflex uses a widely accepted psychoneurophysiological phenomenon. This method of conditioned healing is thus a psychosomatic technique used to enhance patients' ability for self-healing.

To date we have developed and tested this procedure, demonstrating its usefulness through enthusiastic patient response and symptom relief. Further development and validation of the technique will depend on planned research.

—by George A Ulett, MD, PhD

George A Ulett is clinical professor of psychiatry at the Missouri Institute of Mental Health, St Louis of the University of Missouri-Columbia School of Medicine and clinical professor in the department of community and family medicine in the St Louis University School of Medicine. He is in the private practice of psychosomatic medicine and psychiatry.

Table 15.1. Historical Developments in Understanding New Scientific Chinese Acupuncture (NSCA)

1965	Melzack and Wall formulated the "gate theory" of pain.
1973	Pert and Snyder demonstrated opiate receptors on nerve cells.
1975 and 1977	Liu et al. and Gunn recognized the correspondence between some important acupuncture points and motor points.
1975	Kosterlitz and Hughes described the significance of endorphins, the body's own pain killers.
1977	Sjolund et al demonstrated that electroacupuncture increased endorphins in cerebrospinal fluid.
1977	Mayer et al. showed that naloxone could halt the action of opiate compounds.
1978	Peets and Pomeranz reported that a strain of mice deficient in opiate receptors responded poorly to acupuncture.
1987	Professor Ji Sheng Han (a member of China's National Academy of Sciences) of Beijing Medical University published The Neurochemical Basis of Pain Relief by Acupuncture.
1990	Han and Sun demonstrated that specific frequencies of electrical stimulation induce endorphin gene expression, thus releasing specific neuropeptides in both animal and human cerebrospinal fluid.
1990	Lou et al demonstrated that neuroelectric acupuncture is as effective as amitriptyline for the treatment of serious depression.
1992	Li et al showed electroacupuncture to be effective for gastrointestinal disorders.
1993	Johansson et al reported the effectiveness of electroacupuncture for the rehabilitation of stroke patients.
1994	Jin et al demonstrated that the electroacupuncture inhibition of gastric acid secretion is mediated by endorphins.
1994	Han et al. demonstrated a specific frequency of electroacupuncture for treating spinal spasticity.
1996	Ulett and Nichols reported that neuroelectrical stimulation of the Hoku point with pad electrodes was a successful treatment for addiction.

167

Part Four

Diet, Nutrition, and Lifestyle Changes

Chapter 16

Diet and Nutrition as Medicine

Introduction:
The Prevention and Treatment of Chronic Disease

Status of Diet and Nutrition Research in the United States

Diet and nutrition research goes on in almost every medical school, university, and pharmaceutical laboratory throughout the world. Thus, the knowledge of how to prevent illness and maintain health through nutrition grows every year. However, for such areas as reversing the effects of chronic disease through dietary or nutritional intervention or determining levels of nutrients required to achieve optimal metabolic or immune system functioning, there often is no critical mass of researchers or funds to follow up promising initial experimental results.

In fact, the history of nutrition research is marked by examples where, for one reason or another, preliminary reports of a positive therapeutic effect of a certain vitamin, mineral, or nutritional manipulation appear but are often not followed up by the overwhelming majority of the medical community. In cases where such therapies eventually are proven to be safe and effective, it is sometimes not until

Extracted from NIH Publication No. 94-066 from the Office of Alternative Medicine. December 1994. Due to space considerations, bibliographic data have not been reprinted in this chapter. However, to aid readers who wish to consult the original document or do further research, the in-text references have been retained.

years or even decades after the initial reports. The result is that many individuals may die or suffer needlessly, while effective interventions are available but not yet validated.

For example, in the 1930s, Australian psychiatrist John Cade began a series of crude experiments on guinea pigs in which he injected them with the urine of psychiatric patients to test his hypothesis that mania—a mood disorder characterized by, among other things, periods of euphoria—might represent a state of intoxication resulting from an excess of some commonly occurring metabolite. Depression, on the other hand, might represent the effects of abnormally low levels of the same metabolite (Johnson, 1984). Although all the urine samples proved toxic to the guinea pigs—Cade traced the toxicity to the urea component of the urine—the urine from the manic patients was far more toxic than urine from the schizophrenic or depressive patients.

In his attempts to find out what was increasing the toxicity of the urea in the manic patients' urine, Cade happened upon the compound lithium citrate, which he eventually began injecting by itself into the guinea pigs to judge its effect. To his amazement, the guinea pigs became lethargic and unresponsive for several hours after receiving lithium, before fully recovering. In 1949, Cade published the results of a crude clinical trial, stating that lithium salts given to 10 manic patients resulted in a dramatic improvement in each one's condition (Cade, 1949). Unfortunately for Cade, just as his results were reaching the United States, a number of table salt substitutes containing lithium chloride had just been recalled by the Food and Drug Administration (FDA) due to toxic side effects and, in some cases, death with heavy use. So much publicity was given to the toxicity associated with these salt substitutes—which were marketed for use by people on salt-restricted diets—that for five years after Cade's original report, relatively little work with lithium was undertaken (Georgotas and Gershon, 1981).

According to medical historian Frederick Johnson (1984), "Cade's report of lithium treatment of mania might well have succumbed to the same fate as that suffered by many proposed therapeutic techniques before and after that time . . . had lithium salts been at all expensive or hard to come by . . . " Instead, because canisters of lithium salts were to be found in most hospitals and pharmacies at the time, many psychiatrists in the mid-1950s, for lack of adequate treatments for manic disorders, simply started experimenting with lithium on their own. By the mid-1960s, a spate of reports appeared in the medical literature reporting on the effectiveness of lithium in the treatment of manic and other psychiatric disorders (Gershon-and Yuwiler,

1960; Schlagenhauf et al., 1966). Today lithium, in some patients with bipolar disorders (i.e., mood swings), is the most successful therapeutic drug of the five major types of drugs currently used in psychiatry (Horrobin, 1990), often producing normalization in acute mania patients in one to three weeks.

A situation analogous to the lithium story occurred in the late 1980s in the United States. Just as reports were emerging that suggested the effectiveness of the amino acid L-tryptophan in treating mild depression (Boman, 1988), chronic insomnia (Demisch et al., 1987), and mood disorders (Maurizi, 1988), there was a severe outbreak of a sometimes deadly inflammatory disorder called eosinophilia myalgia syndrome (EMS). The cause of the EMS outbreak was linked by epidemiologists to the over-the-counter use of tryptophan (Varga et al., 1993). Although all cases of this disorder were eventually found to be caused by contaminants in batches of tryptophan produced by a single manufacturer in Japan (Barnhart et al., 1990) and not by the effects of tryptophan itself, this nutritional supplement was taken off the market by the FDA and is no longer available over the counter. Just as with lithium, the publicity about toxicities associated with tryptophan may have hindered rational scientific discourse about the effectiveness of this nutritional therapy for some time to come. In fact, FDA uses the tryptophan example to justify its efforts to regulate as drugs most dietary and nutritional supplements whose manufacturers make any health claims (U.S. Food and Drug Administration, 1992).

There have been numerous other instances in recent decades when individuals or groups of individuals have advocated nutritional interventions or alternative dietary lifestyles as a means of preventing or even treating disease and have met not only indifference but often hostility. This was especially true for those advocating vegetarianism or an extremely low-fat diet as a means of preventing or treating illnesses such as heart disease (see below). As was the case with John Cade and lithium, it took many decades for the facts to win out over misconceptions and biases.

The rest of this chapter discusses a number of areas of diet and nutrition research in which there is at least preliminary scientific evidence indicating the need for more in-depth studies, but for which there often is no critical mass of researchers or funds to follow up promising initial experimental results. However, it should be noted that only an overview of the field is presented, and it is by no means comprehensive. This field of research is so complex and diverse that no more than a few examples can be offered for each subsection.

First, however, it is instructive to discuss briefly the evolution of the modern affluent diet and evidence relating chronic disease with its excesses and micronutrient deficiencies. Also presented is a discussion of the evolution of present dietary guidelines and why some consider them inadequate

Evolution of the Modern "Affluent" Diet

Over the course of evolution, human beings (and their primate predecessors) adapted gradually to a wide range of naturally occurring foods, but the types of food and mix of nutrients (in terms of carbohydrates, fats, and proteins) remained relatively constant. Food supplies were often precarious, and the threat of death from starvation was a constant preoccupation for most of the Earth's inhabitants.

About 12,000 years ago, an agricultural revolution brought profound dietary changes to many human populations. The ability to produce and store foods became widespread, and some foods, such as grains, were preferentially cultivated. These new techniques and the overabundance of some foods they produced presented novel challenges to the human digestive system.

The Industrial Revolution, which began about 200 years ago in Europe and soon spread to North America, introduced more radical changes in the human diet due to advances in food production, processing, storage, and distribution. Recent technological innovations, along with increased material well-being, or affluence, and lifestyles that have allowed people more freedom in deciding what and when they wish to eat (amplified by modern marketing techniques), have led to even further major dietary changes in developed countries. Indeed, such innovations as sugared breakfast cereals and a variety of snack items were unheard of before World War II; Hampe and Wittenberg (1964) estimated that 60 percent of the items on supermarket shelves in 1960 came into existence in the 15 years following World War II.

Health Consequences of the Modern Affluent Diet

Because changes in the dietary patterns of the more technologically developed countries, such as the United States, have been so dramatic and rapid, the people consuming these affluent diets have had little time to adapt biologically to the types and quantities of food available to them today. The longer term adverse health effects of the affluent diets prevailing in these countries—characterized by an excess of energy-dense foods rich in animal fat, partially hydrogenated vegetable oils, and refined carbohydrates but lacking in whole grains, fruits, and vegetables—have become apparent only in recent decades.

Comparisons of population groups have demonstrated a close and consistent relationship between the adoption of this affluent diet and the emergence of a range of chronic, noninfectious diseases, such as coronary heart disease, cerebrovascular disease, various cancers, diabetes mellitus, gallstones, dental caries (cavities), gastrointestinal disorders, and various bone and joint diseases (World Health Organization, 1990). Some nutrition and health experts believe that the relationship between rapid changes in a population's diet and rapidly changing disease and mortality profiles is reflected in many recently acculturated (i.e., adapted to the dominant culture) groups in the United States who are now eating a diet more akin to that of the northern European and U.S. general populations.

For example, increasing rates of diabetes mellitus have been reported in Native American and other populations that suddenly switch from a traditional to a more modern lifestyle (West, 1974). This disease has only recently become a major health problem for Native Americans, who now often have rates much higher than those found in either U.S. Caucasian or African-American populations. Indeed, although the overall rate of diabetes in the general U.S. population is between 1 and 3 percent, and 5 to 6 percent for those over age 35, it ranges from 10 to 50 percent among Pima Indians 35 years of age and older (Bennett et al., 1979; Neel, 1976). Furthermore, in Hawaii, the incidence of breast cancer for Caucasians is similar to U.S. mainland rates, but the incidence among Hawaii's Japanese population is more than twice the rate in Japan and approaches the rate for Caucasians (Muir et al., 1987).

The reasons for these abnormally high disease rates in American Indian and other non-Caucasian populations are complex; however, they include obesity related to changes in activity patterns and, probably, the increased consumption of refined carbohydrates and sugar. Also, intake of dietary fiber has decreased dramatically. Excessive caloric consumption in some of these populations also may be a major contributor; one study found that obese American Indians consumed 250 to 1,600 more calories than were recommended for persons of their height, gender, age, and level of activity (Joos, 1984).

In one of the few studies of its kind, a group of Native Hawaiians with multiple risk factors for cardiovascular disease believed to be related to consuming a nontraditional diet were placed on a "pre-Western contact," or traditional, Hawaiian diet to assess its effect on obesity and cardiovascular risk factors. Twenty individuals were placed on a diet low in fat (7 percent), high in complex carbohydrates (78 percent), and moderate in protein (15 percent) for 21 days. The subjects were encouraged to eat as much as they wanted. At the end of the diet modification period, the average weight loss was 7.8 kilograms (approximately 17 lbs.), and the average serum cholesterol dropped by about 14 percent. Blood pressure decreased an average of 11.5 mm Hg systolic and 8.9 mm Hg diastolic (Shintani et al., 1991).

Evolution of Federal Dietary Guidelines

Due to the rapid rise in chronic illness related to diet in recent decades, the focus of nutrition research has shifted from eliminating nutritional deficiency resulting from undernutrition to dealing with chronic diseases caused by nutritional excess, or "overnutrition." Since the 1950s, researchers have identified a number of types of dietary excess that appear to influence the incidence and course of specific chronic diseases.

Another growing concern among nutrition researchers is the accumulation of evidence indicating that inadequate intakes of some micronutrients over a long time may increase the risk of developing a variety of disease conditions, including coronary heart disease, many cancers, cataracts, and birth defects. Earlier, many of these conditions were not even considered diet-related. Furthermore, many other components of foods, in addition to those traditionally considered nutrients, may be important in achieving optimal health. Unfortunately, the "standard" American diet, while rich in calories, contains processed foods deficient in many important micronutrients and other components of the original unrefined foods.

The Federal Government has been involved in developing nutrition guidelines for the American public since the mid-1800s, when the U.S. Department of Agriculture (USDA) was established. However, such guidelines traditionally had dealt with how to prevent nutritional deficiencies, as well as how to promote the consumption of U.S. agricultural products. Only in the past several decades, as the focus of public health policy has shifted from preventing disease caused by nutritional deficiencies to preventing disease caused by overnutrition or nutritional imbalances, have Federal dietary guidelines attempted to address the latter. Today, such guidelines are becoming more difficult to develop and often meet fierce resistance from various lobbying groups when they are disseminated (Nestle, 1993).

Nevertheless, since the early 1970s, USDA and other Federal agencies and advisory groups have periodically released diet and nutrition

Table 16.1. Food and Nutrition Board, National Academy of Sciences—National Research Council Recommended Dietary Allowances[a], Revised 1989

Designed for the maintenance of good nutrition of practically all healthy people in the United States

Category	Age (years) or Condition	Weight[b] (kg)	Weight[b] (lb)	Height[b] (cm)	Height[b] (in)	Protein (g)	Fat-Soluble Vitamins — Vitamin A (µg RE)[c]	Vitamin D (µg)[d]	Vitamin E (mg α-TE)[e]	Vitamin K (µg)	Water-Soluble Vitamins — Vitamin C (mg)	Thiamin (mg)	Riboflavin (mg)	Niacin (mg NE)[f]	Vitamin B6 (mg)	Folate (µg)	Vitamin B12 (µg)	Minerals — Calcium (mg)	Phosphorus (mg)	Magnesium (mg)	Iron (mg)	Zinc (mg)	Iodine (µg)	Selenium (µg)
Infants	0.0–0.5	6	13	60	24	13	375	7.5	3	5	30	0.3	0.4	5	0.3	25	0.3	400	300	40	6	5	40	10
	0.5–1.0	9	20	71	28	14	375	10	4	10	35	0.4	0.5	6	0.6	35	0.5	600	500	60	10	5	50	15
Children	1–3	13	29	90	35	16	400	10	6	15	40	0.7	0.8	9	1.0	50	0.7	800	800	80	10	10	70	20
	4–6	20	44	112	44	24	500	10	7	20	45	0.9	1.1	12	1.1	75	1.0	800	800	120	10	10	90	20
	7–10	28	62	132	52	28	700	10	7	30	45	1.0	1.2	13	1.4	100	1.4	800	800	170	10	10	120	30
Males	11–14	45	99	157	62	45	1,000	10	10	45	50	1.3	1.5	17	1.7	150	2.0	1,200	1,200	270	12	15	150	40
	15–18	66	145	176	69	59	1,000	10	10	65	60	1.5	1.8	20	2.0	200	2.0	1,200	1,200	400	12	15	150	50
	19–24	72	160	177	70	58	1,000	10	10	70	60	1.5	1.7	19	2.0	200	2.0	1,200	1,200	350	10	15	150	70
	25–50	79	174	176	70	63	1,000	5	10	80	60	1.5	1.7	19	2.0	200	2.0	800	800	350	10	15	150	70
	51+	77	170	173	68	63	1,000	5	10	80	60	1.2	1.4	15	2.0	200	2.0	800	800	350	10	15	150	70
Females	11–14	46	101	157	62	46	800	10	8	45	50	1.1	1.3	15	1.4	150	2.0	1,200	1,200	280	15	12	150	45
	15–18	55	120	163	64	44	800	10	8	55	60	1.1	1.3	15	1.5	180	2.0	1,200	1,200	300	15	12	150	50
	19–24	58	128	164	65	46	800	10	8	60	60	1.1	1.3	15	1.6	180	2.0	1,200	1,200	280	15	12	150	55
	25–50	63	138	163	64	50	800	5	8	65	60	1.1	1.3	15	1.6	180	2.0	800	800	280	15	12	150	55
	51+	65	143	160	63	50	800	5	8	65	60	1.0	1.2	13	1.6	180	2.0	800	800	280	10	12	150	55
Pregnant						60	800	10	10	65	70	1.5	1.6	17	2.2	400	2.2	1,200	1,200	320	30	15	175	65
Lactating	1st 6 months					65	1,300	10	12	65	95	1.6	1.8	20	2.1	280	2.6	1,200	1,200	355	15	19	200	75
	2nd 6 months					62	1,200	10	11	65	90	1.6	1.7	20	2.1	260	2.6	1,200	1,200	340	15	16	200	75

[a] The allowances, expressed as average daily intakes over time, are intended to provide for individual variations among most normal persons as they live in the United States under usual environmental stresses. Diets should be based on a variety of common foods in order to provide other nutrients for which human requirements have been less well defined. See text for detailed discussion of allowances and of nutrients not tabulated.

[b] Weights and heights of Reference Adults are actual medians for the U.S. population of the designated age, as reported by NHANES II. The median weights and heights of those under 19 years of age were taken from Hamill et al. (1979) (see pages 16–17). The use of these figures does not imply that the height-to-weight ratios are ideal.

[c] Retinol equivalents. 1 retinol equivalent = 1 µg retinol or 6 µg β-carotene. See text for calculation of vitamin A activity of diets as retinol equivalents.

[d] As cholecalciferol. 10 µg cholecalciferol = 400 IU of vitamin D.

[e] α-Tocopherol equivalents. 1 mg d-α tocopherol = 1 α-TE. See text for variation in allowances and calculation of vitamin E activity of the diet as α-tocopherol equivalents.

[f] 1 NE (niacin equivalent) is equal to 1 mg of niacin or 60 mg of dietary tryptophan.

177

guidelines dealing with preventing chronic illness related to nutrition. This material typically targets public health policy makers, medical doctors, or the general public. Two of the better known current Federal dietary and nutritional guidelines, from which public health policy is made, are the recommended daily allowances (RDAs) and the Food Guide Pyramid.

RDAs are defined as the average daily amounts of essential nutrients estimated, on the basis of available scientific knowledge, as adequate to meet the physiological needs of practically all healthy persons (Monsen, 1990). (See Table 16.1.) To establish the standards for RDAs, which are updated periodically (most recently with the 10th edition in 1989; see Monsen, 1990), the Food and Nutrition Board of the National Academy of Sciences critically evaluates the literature on human requirements for each nutrient, examines the individual variability of requirements, and tries to estimate the efficiency with which the nutrients are biologically available and used from foods consumed. The RDAs are levels that should be reached as averages in a period of several days, not necessarily daily.

RDAs are not meant to be guidelines for consumers; they were initially designed to serve as standards for planning food supplies for population groups (National Research Council, 1989). However, they are used as a partial basis for the development of other guidelines that are intended for consumers, such as the Food Guide Pyramid, which was released by USDA in 1992 to replace the old "basic four" food groups. The Food Guide Pyramid is designed to give consumers information on how to eat a "balanced" diet that will provide them with the RDAs for essential nutrients while lowering their risks of chronic illness due to nutritional excesses (Journal of the American Dietetic Association, 1992). Sweets, fats, and oily foods are at the top of the pyramid, indicating that they should be consumed in small amounts. Dairy products such as milk, yogurt, and cheese, and meats, poultry, fish, dried beans, eggs, and nuts are just below, indicating they should be consumed in moderation. Fruits and vegetables follow; bread, cereal, rice, and Pasta are at the bottom of the pyramid, indicating that they should be consumed in rather large amounts in comparison with the foods at the top of the pyramid (see figure 16.2).

Guidelines such as the Food Guide Pyramid are intended to inform consumers, as well as public health policy makers, about what kinds and amounts of certain foods are best suited for maintaining health and lowering the risks of nutrition-related illnesses. Generally, this approach to affecting health through diet and nutrition interventions involves manipulating the "typical," or mainstream, diet so that foods with less nutritional value are eaten less and foods with more nutritional value are eaten more.

The Federal Government's approach to dietary intervention, which has been formulated over the years by boards composed of nutrition scientists, generally does not recommend supplementing this "typical" diet with vitamins or nutritional supplements (National Research Council, 1989). It also does not take a "good food" or "bad food" approach (Herron, 1991) or suggest that certain foods are "off limits" because of their propensity to cause chronic disease (Nestle, 1993).

However, this is only one approach to promoting health and preventing illness through dietary intervention. There are many "alternative" dietary approaches that contend that no matter how much one manipulates the typical American diet, it is not enough to promote optimal health or stave off eventual chronic illness. Alternative approaches represent a continuum of philosophies, from the idea that diet supplementation somewhat beyond RDAs is necessary to promote optimal health to the idea that supplementation well above RDAs is

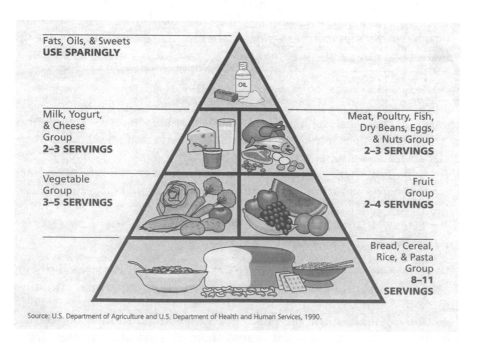

Source: U.S. Department of Agriculture and U.S. Department of Health and Human Services, 1990.

Figure 16.1. The Food Guide Pyramid.

often required to treat some chronic disorders. Further along this continuum is the approach advocating drastic modification of patients' diets either completely eliminating or adding certain types of foods—to treat specific types of conditions, such as cancer and cardiovascular disease. Finally, there is the approach that promotes eating a less refined, more "naturalistic" diet as the only way to promote optimal health and prevent illness. This last approach holds that staples of the typical American diet (e.g., meat and dairy products) are basically unhealthful and should be avoided altogether. The remainder of this chapter describes representative alternative therapies along this continuum.

Alternative Approaches to Diet and Nutrition That May Prevent or Control Chronic Illness as Well as Promote Health

The Standard American Diet

The mainstream, or "standard," American diet, which is one of the world's most affluent diets, is derived primarily from the traditions of the British and German cultures. The British tradition emphasizes meat and bread. These staples traditionally form the core of the meal, with vegetables serving as side dishes and fruits either eaten as snacks between meals or mixed with wheat, milk, and eggs to form a sweet pudding, pie, or cake, which is called a "dessert" (Kittler and Sucher, 1989).

The German tradition emphasizes dairy foods, especially; milk and cheese (Kittler and Sucher, 1989). Pork is a staple for Germans and is the second most important red meat for Americans, who like it in every form from roast to "lunch meat" (cold cuts) to sausages and bacon. Two core American meat-and-grain foods are actually of German origin: hamburgers and frankfurters (or wieners) (Yoder, 1981).

The Use of Vitamins and Other Nutritional Supplements in the Prevention of Chronic Disease

Vitamins are organic substances required by all living organisms for healthy life and growth. Among their many properties, vitamins function as coenzymes (helpers to the primary enzyme) in metabolic reactions. Higher animals, particularly humans, cannot synthesize vitamins and therefore must ingest them as part of their diet. Deficiency in a particular vitamin results in a specific vitamin deficiency disease, such as rickets (a bone deformity from lack of vitamin D) and scurvy (the infamous sailors' deficiency disease of old, caused by lack of vitamin C-containing fruits and vegetables on sailing ships). Each type of deficiency disease is typically characterized by a "classic" set of symptoms.

Vitamins of the B complex and vitamin C are water soluble (i.e., they dissolve readily in water). The B complex vitamins are found in food sources such as whole wheat bread, fruits, green and yellow leafy plants, and animal sources such as eggs, dairy products, and liver. They include B1 (thiamine), B2 (riboflavin), B3 (nicotinic acid, or niacin), pantothenic acid, B6 (pyridoxine), biotin, folic acid, and B12. Certain other substances, such as choline, also may be considered as belonging to the B complex. Vitamin C (ascorbic acid) is present in certain fruits and green vegetables.

All the remaining vitamins (A, D, E, and K) are fat, or lipid, soluble (i.e., they dissolve more readily in oil than in water). Vitamin A (in the form of carotenoids) occurs naturally in green leafy and yellow vegetables; spinach, collards, kale, chard, carrots, and sweet potatoes are particularly good sources. Vitamin E (tocopherol) is found in many plant oils, such as corn oil. In adults vitamin K is supplied by intestinal bacteria.

A number of other minerals and nutrients, such as iron, calcium, magnesium, selenium, and zinc, have been found essential for preventing deficiency diseases. For example, magnesium, which is required for the activation of more than 300 enzymes in the body and for the use of some vitamins and minerals, is required for normal function and structure of the arteries, heart, kidneys, and bone (Seelig, 1980), and for the neuromuscular system (Durlach, 1988; Galland, 1991). There also are a number of "essential" amino acids and fats (that is, humans cannot synthesize them). Some other amino acids are considered "semi-essential" because humans cannot synthesize them fast enough to meet metabolic needs.

Research base. The relatively few studies that have explicitly investigated the role of vitamin and mineral supplements in promoting health and preventing disease have generally found benefits from the supplements. In fact, evidence is increasing rapidly for a beneficial role of supplementation with a number of nutrients, including vitamins B6, C, and E; beta-carotene and other carotenes; folic acid; calcium; magnesium; and other factors. Although there is little dispute about the importance and functions of many vitamins and nutrients, questions arise regarding the levels necessary to produce optimum health. Many contend that the optimal levels of these compounds can be obtained in a normal diet and that the effect of additional amounts is negligible (National Research Council, 1989). To answer such questions, it is first necessary to compare some nutrient levels in the typical American diet with current RDAs as well as with what some now consider to be optimal levels based on the most recent research. The following includes data from recent studies on the minerals calcium, iron, and magnesium as well as the vitamins C, D, E, beta-carotene, and folic acid.

Calcium. Some authorities have recommended that women (including young women) consume 1,000 to 1,500 milligrams (mg) of calcium per day to develop and maintain bone health and prevent osteoporosis (Office of Medical Applications of Research, 1984). Although it is technically feasible to achieve this level by diet alone, most people in the United States do not get that much calcium in their diet. In fact, the median intake among American women is only 600 mg per day, or around half the optimal level. Furthermore, 25 percent of women consume less than 400 mg per day (based on an average of four nonconsecutive days over one year) (U.S. Department of Agriculture, 1988).

Iron. Approximately 8 percent of low-income women and 10 to 20 percent of low-income children are believed to be iron deficient (Public Health Service, 1989). While the RDA for women is 15 mg per day, only slightly more than 10 percent of women achieve this goal from diet alone; less than 10 percent of low-income women achieve this level (Block and Abrams, 1993; U.S. Department of Agriculture, 1988). Iron deficiency is not an important public health problem among men; indeed, some evidence suggests that iron overload in men may be a source of illness, such as heart disease (Sullivan, 1992). Absorption of iron from supplements and plant sources is quite low if body stores of iron are adequate; however, iron from red meat continues to be absorbed even if body stores of iron are plentiful (Ascherio and Willett, 1994). Therefore, until this hypothesis can be more fully studied, it may be prudent for men to avoid daily consumption of red meat.

Magnesium. Extensive metabolic balance studies done by the USDA Research Service showed that the ratio of dietary calcium to magnesium that best maintained equilibrium (i.e., output equaling intake) was 2:1 (Hathaway, 1962). This ratio is achieved at the median magnesium intake of approximately 600 mg per day. However, dietary surveys taken in the last decade have found that most Americans' diets provide less than 300 mg/day (Lakshmanan et al., 1984; Morgan and Stampley, 1988; Spillman, 1987). Thus, like that of calcium, the median daily intake of magnesium in the United States appears to be inadequate.

Long-term magnesium deficiency causes damage to arteries and the heart in all species of animals tested—rodents, cats, dogs, cattle, and monkeys (Seelig, 1980; Seelig and Heggtveit, 1974). It also adversely affects fat metabolism, increasing the "bad" lipids—low-density lipoprotein (LDL) cholesterol and triglycerides, which are associated with atheromas (fat deposits in arteries)—and decreasing the levels of "good" lipids—high-density lipoprotein (HDL) cholesterol, which remove fat deposits from the arterial wall (Altura et al., 1990; Rayssiguier, 1981, 1984, 1986; Rayssiguier et al., 1993).

On the other hand, magnesium supplementation appears to be effective in reversing this process. For example in a double-blind, placebo-controlled study, 47 patients with coronary artery disease and heart attacks were treated with oral magnesium or placebo for three months. Those who received the magnesium experienced a 27-percent decrease in the "bad" lipids in contrast to a slight increase in the placebo group. There was also a tendency toward increased HDL in the magnesium group (Rasmussen et al., 1989a). The investigators observed that these findings support the assumption that magnesium deficiency might be involved in the causation of coronary artery disease. Oral magnesium preparations have also favorably influenced blood lipids in diabetes mellitus, lowering high levels of LDL and raising low levels of HDL (Corica et al., 1994)

In another study in which about half of 374 men at high risk for serious cardiovascular disease were put on a diet high in magnesium (a predominantly vegetarian diet containing 900 to more than 1,200 mg of magnesium daily) and half were put on a regular diet (containing about 300 to 500 mg of magnesium daily), sudden cardiac deaths were 1.5 times more common in the low-magnesium group. Total complications occurred in 60 percent of the low-magnesium group versus 28.6 percent of the high-magnesium group (Singh, 1990). Total mortality was 18 percent and 10.7 percent in the low- and high-magnesium groups, respectively. Furthermore, in a 6-week study of 206 non-insulin-dependent diabetic patients there was significant lowering of LDL levels and slight raising of HDL levels on a high-magnesium diet versus no change in 194 comparable patients on their usual diets (Singh et al., 1991).

Epidemiological evidence also supports the premise that magnesium protects against cardiovascular disease in humans. Areas of the world where the intake of magnesium is high from either drinking water or diet have low prevalence of cardiovascular disease (Anderson et al., 1980; Durlach et al., 1989; Eisenberg, 1992; Hopps, 1981; Leary, 1986; Marier, 1978). In the United States, the Southeast (where water is soft and is low in magnesium) is known as the heart attack—kidney stone belt, whereas the northern Midwest Plains states (where water is hard and is high in magnesium) have lower cardiovascular disease rates and longer life expectancies (Hopps, 1981; Hopps and Feder, 1986).

In Germany, large-scale retrospective studies of nearly 5,000 patients indicate that magnesium supplements added to drugs used to prevent pre-term delivery resulted in improved weights of infants, reducing incidence of low birth weights (whether due to prematurity or intrauterine growth retardation), and decreased the incidence of toxemias of pregnancy, including pregnancy-induced hypertension, preeclampsia, and eclampsia (Conradt, 1984; Conradt and Weidinger, 1982; Conradt et al., 1984). Two randomized double-blind studies of a total of 1,500 pregnant women, half of whom received placebo and the other half a magnesium salt supplement, showed that significantly fewer of the magnesium group developed eclampsia; in addition, there were significantly fewer low birth weights among the infants of the magnesium group. The conclusion was that magnesium supplements during pregnancy improved the outcome (Civics et al., 1988; Spaetling and Spaetling, 1987). It has been suggested that magnesium deficiency is a contributory factor in these conditions (Conradt et al., 1984; Kontopoulos et al., 1980; Seelig, 1980; Waiver), a concept that has been proved in magnesium deficiency-induced hypertension of pregnancy and in low birth weight of lambs born to ewes fed low-magnesium diets (Weaver, 1986, 1988). That preeclamptic women retain more magnesium after a loading test (injection of magnesium salt solution) than normal women do is direct evidence of the magnesium deficit in toxemia of pregnancy (Kontopoulos et al., 1980; Valenzuela and Munson, 1987).

Vitamin C. Vitamin C is an important antioxidant nutrient that is synthesized by most animal species but not by humans. The current RDA is 60 mg, an amount easily obtainable in diet. Nevertheless, 25 percent of women consume less than 40 mg per day in their 4-day average (U.S. Department of Agriculture, 1988). The optimal level of vitamin C intake is unknown, but a diet rich in fruits and vegetables can provide 250 to 500 mg per day (Becker, 1993). Interestingly, estimates of nutrition during the Paleolithic Age (the Old Stone Age, roughly 1,000,000 to 9,000 BC) suggest that early humans

184

may have consumed as much as 390 mg per day of vitamin C (Eaton and Konner, 1985). As with vitamin E (see below), there is evidence that intakes well above 60 mg per day may reduce the risks of cataracts. The potential therapeutic attributes of vitamin C are discussed in detail in the next section, Orthomolecular Medicine.

Vitamin D. The current RDA for adults is 200 international units (IUs). However, there are few studies in adults to verify that this is the optimal level (Gloth et al., 1991). Although this vitamin can be synthesized by humans by exposure to the sun, many elderly persons, for example, who are often inside much of the day get little or no sun. Since fortified milk is the principal dietary source of vitamin D, persons who obtain little calcium from milk or who have inadequate sun exposure may have inadequate vitamin D intake (Gloth et al., 1991).

Vitamin E. Vitamin E, or alpha-tocopherol, is another important antioxidant nutrient. The current RDA for vitamin E is 8 IU for women and 10 for men. This is a reduction from an earlier RDA of 30 IU for both men and women. A well-selected diet containing numerous servings of fruits and vegetables, nuts, whole-grain breads, and vegetable oils can achieve a diet containing 30 IU (Becker, 1993). However, few Americans consume such a diet. Current median intake in the U.S. population is approximately 5 IU, with 10 percent of the population consuming little more than 3 IU. Levels of 100 IU or higher have been associated with significantly reduced risk of coronary heart disease in both men and women (Rimm et al., 1993; Stampfer et al., 1993). However, this effect has been seen at levels obtainable only from supplements. Indeed, the use of vitamin E supplements for two or more years was associated with a 41-percent decrease in risk of coronary disease among women (Stampfer et al., 1992) and a 37-percent decrease in men (Rimm et al., 1993). In addition, consumption of supplements containing vitamin E has been associated with significant reduction in risk of oral cancer (Gridley et al., 1992). This effect was seen even after controlling for factors such as smoking and alcohol consumption. Moreover, although persons with a high intake of fruits and vegetables had a 40-percent reduction in risk of oral cancer, those who used a vitamin E supplement in addition to high fruit and vegetable intake had an 80-percent reduction in risk.

Cataracts are a major cause of blindness worldwide and represent a significant fraction of health care costs in the United States. A number of studies have found that ingesting antioxidants, such as vitamin E, significantly reduced the risk of cataracts (Taylor, 1992). In one study, daily supplementation with 400 IU of vitamin E was associated with a 60-percent reduction in risk of cataracts, whereas daily use of 300 mg or more of vitamin C resulted in a 75-percent reduction in cataract risk (Robertson et al., 1989). Others have also found a high intake of dietary carotenoids associated with reduced cataract risk (Hankinson et al., 1992; Jacques et al., 1988).

Beta-carotene. This antioxidant is found in orange fruits and vegetables such as carrots, sweet potatoes, and squash, and in dark green leafy vegetables. As much as 20 to 30 mg can be obtained from just a few fresh carrots. This also is the level currently being used as the test dose in a number of intervention studies to determine whether it can reduce cancer risk (see below). However, current median intake is less than 2 mg per day, and approximately 25 percent of Americans consume 1 mg per day or less (U.S. Department of Agriculture, 1988). There also is evidence that other naturally occurring carotenoids, in addition to beta-carotene, may be important as antioxidants in reducing the risk of disease.

A number of recent studies have suggested that beta-carotene, among other antioxidants, may have a protective effect against certain cancers. For example, low blood levels of beta-carotene are consistently associated with the subsequent development of lung cancer (Ziegler, 1991).

Furthermore, in a recent prospective trial in China funded by the National Cancer Institute (NCI) and the Cancer Institute of the Chinese Academy of Medical Sciences, 29,584 adults were given several combinations of vitamin and mineral supplements. Linxian, a rural county in Henan province, northern China, has one of the highest rates of esophageal cancer in the world. Death rates for this cancer in Linxian are 10 times higher than the Chinese average and 100 times greater than for American whites.

During the period of the study, there were 2,127 deaths among study participants, with 32 percent of all deaths resulting from esophageal or stomach cancer. Only the combination of beta-carotene, vitamin E, and selenium significantly reduced death rates in the study population, and most of the reduction was due to lower cancer rates. This included not only a reduction in esophageal cancer and stomach cancer but also a 45-percent reduction in fatal lung cancer that did not reach statistical significance (Blot et al., 1994). The doses in the study were typically two to three times the U.S. RDA, and the risk reduction appeared to begin one to two years after vitamin and mineral supplementation began.

However, two other recent trials to assess the ability of beta-carotene to prevent cancer have not shown such positive results. A Finnish study in which almost 30,000 male smokers aged 50 to 59 were given daily supplements of vitamin E (alpha-tocopherol), beta-carotene, or both found no reduction in the incidence of lung cancer (Heinonen and Albanes, 1994). In fact, the study observed a higher incidence of lung cancer among men who received the beta-carotene than among those who did not. Nor was there any reduction in the formation of colon polyps—a precursor of colon cancer—in a study in which 864 individuals received placebo or beta-carotene (25 mg daily), vitamin C (1 g daily), and vitamin E (400 mg daily) for four years (Greenberg et al., 1994).

There are several problems with trying to compare these studies. Most important is whether a period of four to six years is sufficient to detect a beneficial effect of an agent that acts early in the development of cancer—which could be decades before the cancer is diagnosed. Also, it is possible that only persons with low levels of beta-carotene may benefit from supplementation. The New England Journal of Medicine managing editors warned in a recent editorial that consumers should not overinterpret the latest negative findings, just as they should not overinterpret the earlier positive findings (Angell and Kassirer, 1994).

Folic acid (folate). The current RDA for folate is 180 micrograms (ug) per day for women, but recent studies have shown that intake of 400 ug by pregnant women can greatly reduce the risk of neural tube defects (i.e., defects of the spinal cord tube) (Willett, 1992). Intake must be at this level in the earliest weeks after conception to be effective. Unfortunately, most women are not yet aware that they are pregnant then.

Researchers examining the role of folate in preventing cancer and cardiovascular disease have found that less than optional levels of folate may be linked to these diseases. For example, a recent study of almost 1,500 male physicians revealed that the risk of suffering a heart attack was elevated more than threefold by a common metabolic abnormality called homocysteinemia, which is correctable by consuming more folate. None of the study participants who suffered heart attacks would be considered folate deficient by current nutritional standards. However, the results of this study indicate that their intake of folate was clearly less than optimal for preventing cardiovascular disease (Stampfer et al., 1992). In addition, folic acid supplementation was associated with reduced risk of colorectal cancer

(Giovannucci et al., 1993). In contrast, folate from food alone was not significantly related to reduced risk of colon cancer.

In another double-blind, placebo-controlled trial of 96 healthy persons over age 65, the consumption of vitamin and mineral supplements was associated with a significant reduction in illness from infections and improved immune function (Chandra, 1992). The vitamin used was a therapeutic-level, multiple vitamin containing, among other nutrients, 400 ug of folate and 16 mg of beta-carotene. Participants receiving the vitamin formulation experienced half as many days of infection-related illness over the treatment year as did persons receiving the placebo (i.e., 23 days for the treatment group compared with 48 days for the untreated group).

Thus, it may be that approximately 400, ug per day of folic acid is necessary for men and women of all ages. Although this level can be obtained from a well-chosen diet containing, for example, six servings of fruit or vegetables and fortified cereal per day (Block and Abrams, 1993), few in the United States consume such a diet. In fact, a recent study found that 25 percent of pregnant women who were surveyed consumed only 128 ug or less of folate and 10 percent consumed only 90 ug per day in their 4-day average (Johnson et al., 1994).

Risks Associated with Vitamin and Mineral Supplementation.

All vitamins, as well as other substances, including water, can be toxic at some upper level. Under certain conditions or for particular subgroups, dangers may arise in taking large doses of some vitamins and minerals. For example, persons on anticoagulant (blood-thinning) therapy should avoid high doses of vitamin E, because prolonged bleeding can occur. Accidental poisonings of children have occurred with a number of vitamins, most notably with large doses of iron and vitamins A and D. Indeed, the accidental fatal poisoning of children by ingestion of their mothers' high-dose iron tablets is a health problem that deserves wider recognition. Childproof caps have been required on iron tablets for several years, but greater awareness among parents is needed to prevent children from removing such protective devices.

Nevertheless, evidence suggests that most vitamins are safe for long-term use at levels well above the RDAs for most adults. For example, Hathcock (1991) found a "possible adverse effect level" for vitamins C, E, B6, and folate only with long-term ingestion at 10 times the RDA or greater and at 5 times the RDA for vitamin A. Minerals such as iron, zinc, and selenium, however, may be associated with greater risk of toxicity at levels of less than 10 times the RDA for long-term use.

The use of pharmacological doses (i.e., levels of intake substantially above those traditionally assumed necessary to prevent deficiency) of some vitamins and magnesium salts is an accepted practice in mainstream medicine for treatment of a few established conditions. However, such cases are relatively isolated, and the use of pharmacological doses of vitamins for many diseases remains controversial. This subject is discussed next.

Orthomolecular Medicine: Therapeutic Use of High-dose Nutrient Therapy in Treatment of Chronic Disease

Varying the concentrations of substances normally present in the body may control mental disease.

—Linus Pauling

In theory, the concept behind orthomolecular medicine is quite simple. Orthomolecular medicine is the pursuit of good health and the treatment of disease with the optimal concentration of substances normally present in the body. Nobel laureate Linus Pauling first used the term orthomolecular in his 1968 article, "Orthomolecular Psychiatry," in the journal *Science* (Pauling, 1968). The prefix ortho implies correct or proper; in using the term orthomolecular, Pauling was calling for the "right molecules in the right amounts" (Huemer, 1986).

Pauling's *Science* article concentrated on the psychiatric implications of the concept. It referred to the work of two Canadian psychiatrists, Abram Hoffer and Humphrey Osmond, who had for several years been treating acute schizophrenia with large doses of nicotinic acid (vitamin B3) and vitamin C as enhancements to or replacements for the then state-of-the-art therapies, electroconvulsive therapy (ECT) and major tranquilizer therapy. Hoffer and Osmond first became interested in vitamin B3 as a therapeutic biochemical agent because of reports in the literature that patients with pellagra, a disease caused by a vitamin B3 deficiency, displayed many of the same psychiatric symptoms as did patients with schizophrenia.

In a series of double-blind, placebo-controlled clinical trials in the 1950s and early 1960s, Hoffer and Osmond began giving patients with schizophrenia up to six grams a day of vitamin B3, as well as large doses of vitamin C and other vitamins, in addition to the normal treatment regimen. They reportedly doubled the recovery rate, halved the

189

rehospitalization rate, and practically eliminated the suicide rate among this patient group in comparison with the patients receiving only ECT or tranquilizers. These positive results were reported in 5-, 10-, and 15-year follow ups (Hoffer and Osmond, 1960, 1964; Osmond, 1969).

In his *Science* article, Pauling indicated some of the ways orthomolecular concepts could be usefully applied to many other areas of medicine. He then suggested that increasing the intake of such nutrients to levels well above those usually associated with prevention of overt deficiency disease could have previously unrecognized health benefits for some, but not all, people (Pauling, 1968).

One outcome of the increased attention focused on the megavitamin issue by Pauling's *Science* article was the publication of a report by the American Psychiatric Association's Task Force on Megavitamin Therapy in Psychiatry (Lipton et al., 1973), which roundly criticized the work of Hoffer and Osmond and declared megavitamin therapy to be of no value. Proponents of this new form of medical intervention criticized these reports as having numerous misstatements and inaccuracies. In particular, orthomolecular psychiatry proponents argued that the two reports had based their conclusions on flawed studies that attempted to replicate the use of niacin for the treatment of schizophrenia in chronically hospitalized psychotic patients. The treatment, according to proponents, had been shown effective only in acute schizophrenia of relatively recent onset (i.e., within a few months to a year or two), which meant that trials in chronically ill patients were doomed to failure (Hoffer, 1974; Pauling, 1974).

Concurrent with the studies of niacin in psychiatry in the early 1970s, Pauling began collaborating with Scottish surgeon Evan Cameron on a series of retrospective studies to determine whether vitamin C was effective in the treatment of cancer. In the late 1970s, Pauling and Cameron reported a significant prolongation of lifespan of vitamin C-treated patients over that of cancer patients who did not receive vitamin C therapy (Cameron and Pauling, 1976). These studies were undertaken as follow ups to a clinical trial conducted by Cameron with Alan Campbell, which reported complete cessation of tumor progression in 3 patients and complete tumor regression in 5 patients of 50 advanced-cancer patients treated intravenously for long periods with high doses of vitamin C (Cameron and Campbell, 1974).

The results of Pauling and Cameron's retrospective studies were published in the *Proceedings of the National Academy of Sciences* (PNAS), which took the unusual step of running an accompanying editorial along with the second PNAS paper criticizing its methodology and calling for better designed double-blind prospective studies to confirm or refute vitamin C's anticancer activity. Following this, the NCI funded two highly publicized clinical trials of vitamin C at the Mayo Clinic in Rochester, MN, both of which reported negative results for the use of vitamin C in the treatment of cancer (Creagan et al., 1979; Moertel et al., 1985). However, Pauling argued that the first Mayo Clinic study was flawed because almost all the patients had previously received chemotherapy, which may have affected their response to vitamin C. He contended that the second study was flawed as well, in part, because it did not use Cameron's protocol and vitamin C therapy was not carried out for long enough (Richards, 1986).

Despite the negative results of the Mayo Clinic studies, Pauling and others continued to promote vitamin C and other immune-modulating substances as important adjuvants to the treatment of cancer. They believed that neither surgery, radiation, nor chemotherapy could ever be completely effective in eliminating all the cancer cells from a patient's body. Thus it is necessary, they argued, to enhance the patient's immune defenses against cancer with large doses of vitamin C (Cameron and Pauling, 1976). The rationale for this is based on earlier observations that cancer patients tended to be significantly depleted of vitamin C (Baird and Cameron, 1973; Bodansky et al., 1951) and that those animals that have the ability to produce their own vitamin C significantly increased their own production of vitamin C-to an equivalent of 16 grams per day for the average human—when challenged with a potent carcinogen or when experimentally burdened with cancer (Burns et al., 1960; Schmidt et al., 1963). However, Cameron and Pauling never suggested that vitamin C (or other nutrients) should be used instead of conventional cancer therapy but rather as an adjunct to therapy (Cameron and Pauling, 1976). Pauling and others also have advocated high doses of vitamin C as a means of treating or preventing other diseases, including the common cold and influenza (Pauling, 1976).

Although the negative results from the Mayo Clinic studies as well as results from the American Psychiatric Association study managed to put a damper on claims made by the proponents of orthomolecular medicine for more than a decade, interest in this subject has been renewed recently. One reason is that in isolated instances, orthomolecular treatments have indeed proved effective in treating certain chronic illnesses. For example, megadose niacin is now routinely prescribed to treat hypercholesterolemia (i.e., abnormally high levels of LDL cholesterol in the blood) and has been shown to reduce cardiac mortality in large-scale trials (Vega and Grundy, 1994; Zhao et al.,

191

1993). Likewise, vitamin A in dosages substantially higher than the RDA is a highly effective treatment for an uncommon form of leukemia (Bunce et al., 1994; Skrede et al., 1994), and the effectiveness of high-dose vitamin E in surgical wound healing and burn therapy has been recognized for years (Haberal et al., 1987; Zhang et al., 1992).

Finally, as the data have mounted on the role such antioxidants as vitamin C may play in preventing disease and maintaining health, younger investigators are increasingly being attracted to this field. These investigators are now equipped with more accurate and sensitive methods for exploring the validity of theories that were previously rejected outright but were never adequately tested (Barinaga, 1991).

Research base. The following are examples of orthomolecular treatments for which there is at least preliminary evidence suggesting their effectiveness in treating various chronic, debilitating illnesses but for which larger, more detailed studies are needed. This is by no means a comprehensive list. For the reader's convenience, these therapies are presented by type of conditions for which they are applied. These conditions include AIDS, cancer, a variety of heart and vascular conditions, lymphedema, and mental and neurological disorders.

Acquired Immunodeficiency Syndrome (AIDS).

AIDS is a clinical disorder caused by a retrovirus infection (i.e., human immunodeficiency virus, or HIV), which is the end stage of a progressive sequence of immunosuppressive changes. The drawbacks of current pharmacological therapy for HIV infection, such as zidovudine (AZT), include deleterious toxic side effects, inability to improve the immune dysfunctions and undernutrition initiated by the retrovirus infection, and the occurrence of AZT-resistant HIV strains. These drawbacks necessitate new strategies for developing novel therapies to treat AIDS. Low toxicity nutritional agents with immuno-enhancing and antioxidant activities may help normalize retrovirus-induced immune dysfunctions, undernutrition, and other pathological symptoms, thereby retarding the progression of the disease to AIDS. Data on the immune-stimulating effects of vitamin A and beta-carotene in HIV-infected individuals are presented below.

Vitamin A. In the early 1980s, Seifter and colleagues showed through a series of experiments that vitamin A or beta-carotene (its precursor) decreases the immune deficiency that results when animals are exposed to a wide variety of immuno-compromising conditions such as trauma, infection, irradiation, and treatment with cytotoxic agents (Seifter et al., 1982, 1983a, 1983b, 1984). Seifter and others also studied the effects of vitamin A supplementation in animals infected with the Moloney murine sarcoma virus, a retrovirus having many features in common with human immunodeficiency virus (HIV), the virus that causes AIDS (Kanofsky et al., 1987, 1990; Seifter et al., 1982, 1985, 1991). The vitamin A supplementation Seifter and his colleagues used in those experiments was approximately 10 to 15 times the recommended dietary allowance.

There is evidence suggesting that vitamin A supplementation in immune-compromised individuals may be necessary to correct a vitamin A deficiency caused by HIV infection. For example, Lack and colleagues (1993) found that approximately 50 percent of 120 HIV-positive patients, who were both symptomatic and asymptomatic, had a low serum vitamin A level. In another study, Semba and colleagues (1993) measured serum vitamin A levels in HIV-positive drug abusers and concluded that vitamin A deficiency may be common during HIV infection. Low vitamin A status was independently associated with decreased CD4 cells and a much greater mortality rate.

Beta-carotene. Alexander and colleagues (1985) reported that extremely large oral doses of beta-carotene (180 mg per day) can increase the number of CD4 cells in the blood of healthy humans, with no observable toxicity. The CD4 cell is the white blood cell that becomes markedly depressed in AIDS patients. According to these researchers, "Our data suggest that beta-carotene administration might be considered for patients with AIDS."

Coodley and colleagues (1993), in an 8-week, double-blind crossover study of 21 HIV-positive patients, compared 180 mg per day of beta-carotene with placebo. The results showed a statistically significant increase in total white blood cell count, percent change in CD4 count, and percent change in CD4:CD8 ratios. The CD4:CD8 ratio is often used as an indicator of whether a patient's status is getting worse, holding steady, or improving.

Watson and colleagues gave a much smaller dose of beta-carotene (60 mg per day) to 11 HIV-infected patients over four months. The authors saw no change in T-helper lymphocytes (CD4), T-suppressor lymphocytes (CD8), or total T-cell lymphocytes. However, they did see an increase in the number of cells with natural killer markers and markers of activation (IL-2R, transferrin receptors) (Garewal et al., 1992). This indicates that beta-carotene may be enhancing certain aspects of the immune response.

Furthermore, Fryburg and colleagues (1992) gave 120 mg per day of beta-carotene and one multivitamin tablet a day to seven AIDS patients for four weeks. The mean CD4 count at baseline (i.e., before treatment) was approximately 53 cells/mm^3. After 4 weeks of beta-carotene therapy, it rose to 76 cells/mm^3. However, it returned to approximately 53 cells/mm^3 6 weeks after treatment was stopped. A recommendation was made for beta-carotene to be tried in larger groups of patients.

Bianchi-Santamaria and colleagues (1993) gave 60 mg per day of beta-carotene 20 days of each month for 21 months to 64 patients with AIDS-related complex, which is the stage of HIV infection that occurs just before full-blown AIDS. This is the study with by far the longest duration and also is the largest and most recent. Mean CD4 count at baseline was approximately 451 cells/mm^3. After 21 months of beta-carotene treatment, the mean CD4 count rose to approximately 519 cells/mm^3, an increase of 15 percent. Normally, the mean CD4 count in these patients would be expected to drop. Furthermore, the authors suggested that the beta-carotene accounted for the apparent recovery of patients from asthenia, fever, nocturnal sweating, diarrhea, and weight loss. Unfortunately, this study did not have a control group.

Bronchial Asthma.

Asthma, better termed hyperactive airway disease, is an autoimmune disease characterized by increased responsiveness of the tracheobronchial tree to exogenous and endogenous stimuli. The hallmark of this illness is widespread inflammation and narrowing of the tracheobronchial tree. This is manifested clinically by dyspnea (shortness of breath), wheezing, and cough, which generally occur simultaneously.

Asthma is typically managed with bronchodilator therapy and/or anti-inflammatory drugs. However, currently used pharmaceutical formulations for bronchodilation, such as theophylline, have a narrow therapeutic margin because adverse effects often occur at concentrations high enough to be effective (Taburet and Schmit, 1994). In addition, prednisone, the most common anti-inflammatory drug used to treat asthma, is also associated with a variety of adverse side effects. Such limited effectiveness of presently available treatments has recently sparked research into less toxic, immune-enhancing nutritional approaches to treating asthma. Data on the efficacy of vitamin C and magnesium in the treatment of this condition are presented below.

194

Vitamin C. Bielory and Gandhi (1994) conducted a comprehensive literature search of relevant English-language papers pertaining to the use of vitamin C in the treatment of asthma and allergy and analyzed the studies according to their design, inclusion and exclusion criteria, population studied, variables or factors tested, method of intervention or treatment with vitamin C, and results and conclusions. They found a number of studies that support the use of vitamin C in asthma and allergy. Significant results included positive effects of vitamin C on pulmonary function tests; bronchoprovocation challenges with methacholine, histamine, or allergens; improvement in white blood cell function and motility; and a decrease in respiratory infections. On the other hand, their review also revealed several studies that did not support a beneficial role for vitamin C in asthma and allergy. These studies did not report improvements in pulmonary function tests or bronchoprovocation challenges or on other reactivity or specific immunologic factors and levels.

From their review, the researchers concluded that the majority of the studies were too short term and assessed immediate effects of vitamin C supplementation. Rather, long-term supplementation with vitamin C or delayed effects need to be examined for the studies to be valid. The researchers went on to note that although the current literature does not support a definite indication for the use of vitamin C in asthma and allergy, the promising and positive studies were worth following up. Furthermore, the researchers suggested, with a large portion of health care dollars being spent on alternative medicine and vitamin C in particular, further studies are needed to define its role, if any, in the treatment of this condition.

Magnesium. First reported almost 50 years ago (Haury, 1938), the efficacy of magnesium in the treatment of bronchial asthma has received considerably more attention in the past few years. Its bronchodilating effect was reported in patients with mild asthmatic attacks, and when that was found effective, applied to those with severe attacks (Okayama et al., 1988). Intravenous magnesium sulfate was found to relieve respiratory failure in asthmatic patients not responsive to standard drug therapy (Hauser and Braun, 1991; McNamara et al., 1989; Neves et al., 1991; Noppen et al., 1990; Okayama et al., 1991; Skobeloff et al., 1989) and has been considered lifesaving (Dellinger, 1991; Kuitert and Kletchko, 1991).

Not all published trials of magnesium treatment of bronchial asthma, however, have been successful (Green and Rothrock, 1992; Kufs, 1990). However, the protocols of those studies reporting no therapeutic benefit of magnesium in asthma patients have been criticized on the grounds that insufficient dosages were used, with the result that the serum levels found effective in the treatment of preeclampsia and eclampsia (see below) were not achieved (Fesmire, 1993). Another criticism leveled at the negative efficacy reports was that the study group was too small for significance; this was countered by pointing out that analysis of results from the first 40 patients indicated withholding magnesium from comparably compromised patients would be unethical, so the study was ended and the results were reported (Skobeloff and McNamara, 1993).

Cancer

The rationale for the use of high dosages of vitamins, particularly vitamin C, to treat cancer was discussed in the beginning of this section. The following is a review of more recent data that have emerged since the negative results of the Mayo Clinic studies for vitamin C, as well as quite intriguing data on the use of high dosages of coenzyme Q10 in the treatment of certain cancers.

Vitamin C. The possible value of vitamin C as an adjuvant in cancer therapy is supported in animal and human studies. Indeed, vitamin C, used in conjunction with other treatment modalities, has been shown to improve the effectiveness of those treatments (Meadows et al., 1991; Poydock, 1991; Tsao, 1991). Of equal interest, vitamin C supplementation has been shown to reduce the toxicity of conventional chemotherapeutic agents, such as adriamycin (Fujita et al., 1982), and to reduce the toxicity and improve therapeutic gain of radiation therapy (Okunieff, 1991). There also is evidence that some of the severe toxicity associated with interleukin-2/LAK cell therapy may result from the drastic reduction in plasma vitamin C levels that this therapy causes (Marcus et al., 1987). Thus, these examples suggest that the use of vitamin C or other nutrients as adjuncts to therapy may reduce toxicity and thereby permit the use of more effective doses of the therapeutic agent.

Coenzyme Q10. Recently, Lockwood and colleagues (1994) treated 32 breast cancer patients with antioxidants, fatty acids, and 90 mg of coenzyme Q10 (CoQ10) per day and reported partial tumor regression in six patients. In one of the cases, the dosage was increased to 390 mg per day and, reportedly, within two months the tumor was no longer detectable by mammography. Encouraged by this, Lockwood and colleagues treated another patient with a verified breast tumor with 300 mg per day, and after three months they could find no sign of remaining tumor. Folkers reported that administration of this enzyme increases levels of immunoglobulin G, an antibody that is known to participate in antibody-dependent cellular toxicity against virally infected cells and, possibly, against cancer cells (Folkers et al., 1982, 1993). The same studies also showed increases in T4 lymphocytes—the immune cells targeted and destroyed by HIV infection—when CoQ10 was given with pyridoxine to AIDS patients.

Arteriosclerosis, Heart Attacks, Arrhythmias, Sudden Cardiac Death, Strokes, and Toxemias of Pregnancy.

Vitamin E. Postoperative thromboembolism, a major complication of surgery, involves the formation of blood clots in the deep veins of an extremity. The clots can break off and travel to blood vessels in the lungs, causing a pulmonary embolism that can be fatal. This is often a major postoperative complication despite the use of various treatments that are partially effective in preventing it. As far back as the late 1940s, Alton Ochsner repeatedly advocated the administration of vitamin E to prevent postoperative thromboembolism. His vitamin E regimen consisted of 200 to 600 IU of alpha-tocopherol per day, administered intramuscularly or by mouth, beginning no later than the day of surgery and continuing through the postoperative period (Kay et al., 1950; Ochsner, 1964, 1968; Ochsner et al., 1950a, 1950b, 1951). As late as 1968 he wrote, "For 15 years I have used alpha-tocopherol (vitamin E) routinely in the treatment of patients who have been subjected to trauma of any magnitude. None of these patients have had pulmonary embolism" (Ochsner, 1968).

In 1981, Kanofsky and Kanofsky completed a search of the American and British literature, which disclosed six studies comparing a vitamin E-treated group with a control group (Coon and Whitrock, 1951; Coon et al., 1952; Crump and Heiskell, 1952; Ochsner et al., 1951; Kawahara, 1959; Moorman et al., 1953; Wilson and Parry, 1954). All these controlled studies were published between 1951 and 1959. That none of the studies used a double-blind design is unfortunate, since the diagnosis of deep-vein thrombosis or pulmonary embolism was primarily based on the observations of clinicians, which can be easily influenced by bias. However, Kanofsky and Kanofsky analyzed the data from the six studies and found a highly statistically significant effect from the vitamin E treatment. There was a twofold greater risk of deep vein thrombosis, a six-fold greater risk of all pulmonary embolism, and a nine-fold greater risk of fatal pulmonary embolism in the control group than in the vitamin E-treated group (Kanofsky and Kanofsky, 1981). The authors postulated that the physiological mechanism that might explain these results involved the ability of vitamin E to inhibit platelet aggregation.

Magnesium. Magnesium also has anticoagulant activity, acting directly on the steps involved in blood coagulation, counteracting the procoagulant effect of calcium (Greville and Lehmann, 1944; Herrmann et al., 1970; Seelig, 1993), and decreasing platelet clumping. In the 1950s there were reports of use of magnesium to prevent and treat clinical thrombotic conditions (Hackethal, 1951; Heinrich, 1957, Schnitzler, 1957). Animal studies demonstrated that magnesium supplements prevented formation of coronary artery thromboses when the animals were fed a thrombogenic diet (Savoie et al., 1973; Szelenyi et al., 1967). Case reports have been published of patients with magnesium deficiency characterized by neuromuscular disorders and whose thromboemboli were prevented from recurring by magnesium supplements; when the supplements were discontinued, the thromboemboli recurred (Dupont et al., 1969; Durlach, 1967). Recent findings have demonstrated that magnesium inhibits blood coagulation and arterial constriction by increasing the production of factors with antithrombotic and vasodilating activities by the inner lining (endothelium) of blood vessels. These findings have shed light on magnesium's usefulness in both eclampsia and heart attacks.

The anticoagulant activity of magnesium has found practical application in microsurgery, in which local application during the surgical procedure prevented thrombotic and subsequent scarring lesions (Acland, 1972). When used intravenously in dogs and rabbits with partially constricted coronary arteries, magnesium prevented formation of microthrombi distal to the partial occlusion, a finding considered pertinent to human angina with and without blockage of coronary arteries (Gretz et al., 1987).

Since the 1920s, large doses of magnesium (producing blood levels as high as two to three times normal) had been shown to be effective in the treatment of preeclampsia (hypertension with proteinuria or edema, or both, due to the influence of pregnancy or recent pregnancy) (Lazard, 1925). Diuretics and anticonvulsants eventually replaced magnesium as the preferred treatment for this condition, until studies showed that magnesium treatment resulted in better outcomes, including more live births (Zuspan and Ward, 1965) and was the more appropriate treatment (Sibai, 1990).

198

It appears that adequate magnesium is necessary to maintain the integrity of the inner lining of the blood vessel and to increase its production of the vasodilating, anti-platelet-aggregating (antithrombosis) substance (Briel et al., 1987; Watson et al., 1986). This activity of magnesium in inhibiting thrombosis has provided the rationale for its use in patients who have had a heart attack. In a large, double-blind study of 2,300 patients, called the second Leicester Intravenous Magnesium Intervention Trial, half of the patients received an intravenous injection of magnesium within three hours of a heart attack. This was followed by a 24-hour magnesium infusion in a dose sufficient to raise the blood level of magnesium to twice that of normal levels. This treatment, which was given in conjunction with the standard treatment for a heart attack, reduced heart failure and mortality by 25 percent in comparison with patients who received only the standard treatment (Woods et al., 1992; Woods and Fletcher, 1994).

However, a much larger "megatrial" of magnesium therapy in heart attack victims failed to find such an effect (Casscells, 1994; Unsigned Commentary, 1994). It has been proposed that the failure of the megatrial (called ISIS-4) to find the lifesaving effect of magnesium in heart attack patients may have been due to the institution of magnesium treatment only after use of a clot-dissolving treatment. This resulted in a delay of almost eight hours before the magnesium was given. In contrast, in the earlier study, the magnesium was given immediately upon hospitalization. Thus, in ISIS-4, the magnesium may have been given after the damage to the heart muscle was done (Casscells, 1994; Woods and Fletcher, 1994).

Lymphedema.

Lymphedema, a swelling of the arms or legs resulting from pathology in the lymphatic system, often can be disabling or even crippling. It has been estimated that 32 to 75 percent of women who undergo surgery for breast cancer will have some chronic lymphedema of the arm on the affected side (Casley-Smith and Casley-Smith, 1986). Unfortunately, the treatment of this side effect of breast cancer surgery is often neglected (Farncombe et al., 1994). Recently, however, there has emerged an orthomolecular treatment for this condition using benzopyrones. An overview of the studies utilizing this compound for the treatment of lymphedema is presented below.

Benzopyrones. Since the mid-1980s, J.R. Casley-Smith has recommended the use of large doses of benzopyrones for the treatment of lymphedema. The benzopyrones, though now frequently synthesized, were originally derived from plants. The coumarins and flavonoids, such as rutin, are benzopyrones. Szent-Gyorgi, the Nobel prize winner who isolated vitamin C, discovered that a lack of benzopyrones caused greatly increased capillary fragility and permeability (Casley-Smith and Casley-Smith, 1986). Since then, benzopyrones have sometimes been called "vitamin P" or "P factors."

Casley-Smith and colleagues believe that large doses of benzopyrones alleviate lymphedema by stimulating macrophage cells to break down unwanted proteins in the edema fluid (Piller et al., 1988). Once excess protein is eliminated, the edema fluid that it causes is no longer retained. Thus, they believe that the benzopyrones safely change a slowly worsening condition into a slowly improving one. There now are at least six double-blind studies demonstrating that the benzopyrones are a safe and effective treatment for lymphedema (Casley-Smith et al., 1986, 1993; Cluzan and Pecking, 1989; Desprez-Curely et al., 1985; Piller et al., 1985, 1988).

Unfortunately, no benzopyrones are available as pharmaceuticals in the United States. Approval for drugs containing rutin and other bioflavonoids was withdrawn in 1970 by FDA on the grounds that there was no substantial evidence of the effect they were purported to have. However, Casley-Smith has argued that FDA used old, greatly outmoded data, which allegedly showed that these drugs could not be absorbed (Casley-Smith and Casley-Smith, 1986). He and others are emphatic that more recent data show that the benzopyrones are absorbed and are effective. Moreover, Casley-Smith and others believe that because benzopyrones possess specific immune-stimulating properties and can reduce every type of high-protein edema, they eventually will become extremely valuable therapeutic agents in a wide variety of clinical conditions (Casley-Smith and Casley-Smith, 1986).

Mental and Neurological Disorders.

Despite continued widespread skepticism among mainstream psychiatric professionals about the effectiveness of vitamin therapy in the treatment of neurological disorders, a small but growing number of researchers persist in studying the use of vitamins for such conditions. In fact, reports continue to surface on the effectiveness of vitamins such as folic acid as well as a variety of antioxidant vitamins in treating various mental and neurological disorders.

Folic acid. Low serum folate has been reported in 10 to 33 percent of psychiatric patients. In one retrospective survey, psychiatric patients treated with folic acid spent less time in the hospital and made significantly better social recoveries than those in whom low serum folates were not treated (Carney and Sheffield, 1970). Godfrey and colleagues recently demonstrated that 41 (33 percent) of 123 patients with depression or schizophrenia had borderline or definite folate deficiency. These patients took part in a double-blind, placebo-controlled trial of methylfolate (the actively transported form of folate), taking 15 mg daily for six months in addition to standard psychotropic medication. Among both depressed and schizophrenic patients, methylfolate significantly improved clinical and social recovery (Godfrey et al., 1990). These researchers speculate that folate or methylfolate may have a direct pharmacological action irrespective of whether the subjects were folate deficient.

Antioxidant therapy. Antioxidant therapy with nutrients such as vitamin C, vitamin E, and beta-carotene has been hypothesized as a treatment for schizophrenia (Lohr, 1991). The hypothesis is based on evidence that the serum of schizophrenics has high levels of lipid peroxides and the enzyme superoxide dismutase. Both these substances are indicators of unwanted oxidative products (mainly free radicals).

Just focusing on vitamin C, there is a substantial body of animal and clinical data that ascorbic acid may have an antipsychotic effect (Beauclair et al., 1987; Giannini et al., 1987; Heikkila et al., 1983; Kanofsky et al., 1988, 1989a; Milner, 1963; Rebec et al., 1984; Thomas and Zemp, 1977; Tolbert et al., 1979a, 1979b), which seems to be most apparent when ascorbic acid is given in combination with antipsychotic medication. A double-blind study showed that vitamin C increases the antipsychotic effects of haloperidol in treating PCP psychoses (Giannini et al., 1987). Observational studies and one double-blind study have indicated a similar adjunctive role for vitamin C in treating schizophrenia (Beauclair et al., 1987; Kanofsky et al., 1989a, 1989b; Milner, 1963). No one has studied the simultaneous use of several antioxidants in the treatment of schizophrenia, which seems a worthwhile avenue of research (Kanofsky and Sandyk, 1992; Lohr, 1991).

Double-blind studies have shown that tardive dyskinesia (a late-occurring, movement-disorder side effect of antipsychotic medication) can be treated with vitamin E supplementation. The therapeutic effect of vitamin E seems most likely when it is introduced within several years after the onset of the disorder (Adler et al., 1993; Egan et al., 1992; Elkashef et al., 1990). Several studies of patients with Alzheimer's disease have been performed in which brain tissue at autopsy showed evidence of increased brain lipid peroxidation (Farooqui et al., 1988; Hajimohammadreza and Brammer, 1990; Subbarao et al., 1990). Conceivably, antioxidants such as vitamin C and vitamin E might prevent this increase; however, much more research needs to be done before this treatment could be seriously considered (Lohr, 1991). In view of current evidence that vitamin E, either alone or in combination with deprenyl (an inhibitor of monoamine oxidase in the brain), fails to delay continued neurological deterioration in Parkinson's disease (Parkinson Study Group, 1993), it is also possible that to be most effective, antioxidant therapy must be introduced very early in the development of neurological and psychiatric disorders—prior to the point at which irreversible cell damage has occurred. A similar argument can be made with regard to the effectiveness of orthomolecular therapy in schizophrenia itself.

Magnesium. A condition known as "latent tetany" syndrome, which is seen in some patients with slight magnesium deficiency, is characterized by depressive anxiety, weakness, irritability, fatigue, and many ill-defined complaints (Durlach, 1988; Fehlinger et al., 1987; Galland, 1991-1992). This syndrome has characteristics that resemble premenstrual syndrome as well as chronic fatigue syndrome, both of which have responded favorably to supplementation with magnesium compounds alone or with other nutritional supplements (Abraham and Lubran, 1981; Stewart and Howard, 1986; London et al., 1991; Facchinetti et al., 1981).

There is evidence suggesting that magnesium deficiency participates in the abnormalities of migraine headaches and that migraines will respond to treatment with magnesium (Swanson, 1988; Weaver, 1990). Transient ischemic attacks, another disorder which like migraine is associated with cerebral arterial spasms, has also been found to respond to magnesium (Fauk et al. 1991). These clinical findings of magnesium's protective effects against ischemia (loss of blood flow) and hypoxia (oxygen deprivation) make it worthwhile to examine the considerable animal evidence that magnesium deficiency increases susceptibility to brain damage caused by cerebral arterial spasm, arterial blockage (i.e., stroke), or trauma (McIntosh et al., 1988; Blair et al., 1989; Okawa, 1992) and that magnesium treatments offer the potential for minimizing such brain damage (McIntosh et al., 1989; Vink, 1991-1992; Smith et al., 1983).

Clinicians in Japan have shown in a small pilot study that intravenous magnesium infusions improved the cerebral flow of stroke victims (who before treatment had low magnesium levels in their cerebrospinal fluid) (Iwasaki et al., 1989). Indeed, 10 patients who received magnesium therapy had a better return of normal cerebral functioning than did ten control patients who did not receive magnesium after a stroke. Whether prompt magnesium treatment after a stroke and/or after brain trauma will improve the prognosis of such patient deserves further investigation.

Selenium. In certain regions of the world, including Great Britain and parts of the United States and Canada, selenium levels in food are so low that the possibility of subclinical deficiency (and a possibly related adverse effect on mood) exists. Benton and Cook (1991) conducted a double-blind, crossover trial of 50 subjects in ostensibly good health. They were randomly assigned to receive a 100-microgram selenium tablet or placebo each day for five weeks. After a 6-month washout, they received the alternate treatment for five weeks. Benton and Cook concluded that the intake of selenium tablets was associated with an elevation of mood, particularly in subjects whose diets were relatively deficient in the trace element.

Amino acids. A double-blind, randomized study showed S-adenosylmethionine—the physiologically active form of the amino acid methionine—to be a more rapidly acting antidepressant than the pharmaceutical drug imipramine in treating major depression (Bell et al., 1988). At the end of this 2-week study, 66 percent of the S-adenosylmethionine patients had a clinically significant improvement in depressive symptoms versus 22 percent of the imipramine patients. If S-adenosylmethionine does turn out to be a more rapidly acting drug—taking days rather than weeks to achieve results—this characteristic may offer a considerable advantage in light of the known risk of suicide during the early non-responding phase of treatment with most, if not all, other antidepressants.

Clinical trials of the amino acid glycine given orally to schizophrenic patients have yielded conflicting results. However, in the most recent double-blind study, Javitt and colleagues (1994) showed a statistically significant improvement in negative symptoms of schizophrenia when glycine was added to conventional antipsychotic drug regimens. This suggests that glycine may serve as a distinctive and valuable adjunctive treatment for schizophrenia.

Essential fatty acids. Vaddadi and colleagues (1989) reported the results of a double-blind crossover trial of essential fatty acid supplementation in 48 predominantly schizophrenic psychiatric patients. Active treatment produced highly significant improvements in total psychopathology scores and a significant improvement in memory.

Food and Macronutrient Modification Diets as a Method for Controlling and Treating Chronic Illnesses

This section is an overview of the theoretical basis and available research on a variety of diets that are advocated for the treatment of chronic conditions such as cancer, cardiovascular disease, and food allergies. Virtually all of these dietary interventions emphasize the intake of much more produce (fresh and freshly prepared vegetables, fruits, whole grains, and legumes), providing high nutrient density while at the same time restricting such "empty" calories as those provided by sweets, fats, and over-processed foods. In these diets, moreover, overall caloric intake tends to be lower than that of the general U.S. population.

Nutrient Modification for the Treatment of Cancer.

Cancer accounts for one of every five deaths in the United States (American Cancer Society, 1990). More than one million cases of new cancers are diagnosed every year, and about 75 million, or one in three Americans now living, will eventually have cancer (Public Health Service, 1990). Cancer is not one disease but a constellation of more than 100 different diseases, each characterized by the uncontrolled growth and spread of abnormal cells. Cancer may strike at any age, though it does so more frequently with advancing age. Although corroborative intervention data are not yet available, it is estimated that 35 percent of cancer deaths may be related to diet (Eddy, 1986).

The rationale behind most dietary regimens for the treatment of cancer—and for vegetarian, low-fat, high-fiber dietary regimens in particular—is that if dietary excesses can lead to the development of certain cancers, then such cancers may be susceptible to dietary manipulation as well. These diets, for the most part, share certain characteristics with the kinds of foods currently recommended by mainstream groups, such as the American Cancer Society (ACS), for lowering the risk of developing cancer and heart disease. Recent ACS guidelines for cancer prevention suggest reducing the intake of fat, alcohol, and salt-cured and smoked foods while increasing the intake of fruits, vegetables, and whole grains (Nixon, 1990). One way these alternative dietary regimens for cancer differ, however, from mainstream preventive recommendations is that they may emphasize a few particular foods and limit or totally eliminate others.

In September 1990 the U.S. Congress Office of Technology Assessment (OTA) completed a study of a number of unconventional cancer treatments. Among these was a variety of dietary regimens developed for the treatment of cancer and/or the support of patients undergoing conventional cancer therapy. This report, Unconventional Cancer Treatments, focused on three of the most well-known dietary interventions for cancer: the Gerson therapy, the Kelley regimen, and the macrobiotic diet. These three regimens and a few others are reviewed below. Findings from the OTA report as well as studies done since that report was released are covered.

Gerson therapy. The Gerson therapy was developed by physician Max Gerson in the early part of this century. Gerson was born in Germany in 1881 and immigrated to the United States in 1936. He received his New York medical license in 1938 and his U.S. citizenship in 1944. He opened a private medical practice in New York City and in 1946 also began treating patients at nearby Gotham Hospital.

He gained renown in Germany through his success in treating tuberculosis of the skin through low-salt dietary management (Gerson, 1929). He then began testing modifications of this regimen in other conditions, including pulmonary tuberculosis (Gerson, 1934). He first used his diet for cancer in 1928, reportedly after a woman with a bile duct cancer that had spread to her liver insisted that he put her on his diet despite his reluctance to do so (Lerner, 1994). Much to his surprise, Gerson wrote, the woman recovered (Gerson, 1958). Afterward, Gerson tried variations and combinations of foods and other agents on his patients, noted the ones who reacted favorably, and adjusted subsequent patients' regimens accordingly (Gerson, 1978). By the time he came to America, he was focusing on treating cancer patients.

In 1946 Gerson testified before a subcommittee of the Senate Committee on Foreign Relations, which was holding a hearing on a proposed bill to authorize increased Federal spending for cancer research. Gerson reported to the Senate committee that he had developed a dietary regimen that was effective for the treatment of advanced cancer. According to the historian Patricia Spain Ward, Gerson's testimony was supported by the director of the Gotham Hospital, with which Gerson was affiliated, as well as others in attendance (Ward,

1988). Gerson described five patients in clinical detail and submitted written case histories of those and five more patients who had been treated with his regimen, in whom he had observed improvements in "general body health" and, in some cases, tumor reduction. In a later publication, Gerson noted that in six additional patients his treatment appeared to reduce inflammation around the tumors, relieve pain, improve psychological condition, and provide at least temporary tumor regression (Gerson, 1949). In the mid-1950s, Gerson first published explanations of the components of his regimen and the rationale for their use, along with some of the outcomes he observed.

Gerson believed that his treatment regimen reversed the conditions he thought necessary to sustain the growth of malignant cells. He attached great importance to the elimination of "toxins" from the body and the role of a healthy liver in recovery from cancer. Gerson noted that if the liver was damaged (e.g., by cancer or cirrhosis) the patient had little chance of recovery on his or her treatment regimen (Gerson, 1949, 1986). He observed that cancer patients who died during treatment showed a marked degeneration of the liver, which he presumed was due to the release of unspecified toxic factors into the bloodstream by the process of tumor regression. He believed that these toxic tumor-breakdown products poisoned the liver and other vital organs (Cope, 1978).

Another central point of Gerson's approach concerned the balance of potassium and sodium in the body. He believed that an imbalance in the concentration of these substances contributes to cancer-induced edema, a condition in which cellular damage leads to infiltration by excess sodium and water, failure of cellular transport mechanisms, subsequent failure of cellular energy production, and, finally, loss of resistance to cancer. Therefore, he sought to eliminate sodium in patients' diets, supplement it with potassium, and thereby alter the internal environment supporting the tumor (Gerson, 1954a, 1954b, 1954c).

At present, the Gerson therapy is an integrated set of treatments that include the restriction of salt in combination with potassium supplementation of the diet. Thyroid supplements also are given to stimulate metabolism and cell energy production. Hourly feedings of fresh, raw juices of vegetables and fruits are given in addition to a basically vegetarian diet. Fat intake is restricted (to lower intake of potential tumor promotors), and protein is temporarily restricted (to promote nonspecific, cell-mediated immunities). Coffee enemas are provided to manage pain and to stimulate bowel and liver enzymes that may increase the release of toxins (Gerson Institute, undated-a).

Other treatments beyond the ones specified by Gerson have been added to the current protocol in recent years. Gerson gave patients raw liver juice several times daily, but the practice has been abandoned by current practitioners because of bacteria in the liver juice that caused major infections in some patients (Office of Technology Assessment, 1990).

Critics of the Gerson therapy point to the fact that it is based on the beliefs of a physician who practiced many years ago and whose knowledge of the cause of cancer was rudimentary (Green, 1992). Proponents of the therapy argue, rather, that Gerson was far ahead of his time; however, they also note that many of Gerson's original assumptions and therapies have been updated to take into account the latest scientific evidence (Hildenbrand, 1986). Because of such misconceptions about Gerson and how his therapy is currently administered, proponents contend that it has never been given a fair evaluation by mainstream science. Furthermore, they argue that such myths and misconceptions about the Gerson therapy are perpetuated by major medical journals that routinely publish articles attacking the basic tenets of the therapy while refusing to publish rebuttals to such attacks (Lechner and Hildenbrand, 1994).

Research base. There have been several attempts by a number of groups and individuals to assess the clinical effects of the Gerson regimen. However, none have yet offered any definitive results (Office of Technology Assessment, 1990). The following is an overview of early and more recent cases.

In 1959, NCI reviewed 50 case histories presented in Gerson's book, A Cancer Therapy: Results of Fifty Cases. NCI concluded that in the majority of cases a number of basic criteria were not met. NCI also concluded overall that Gerson's data provided no demonstration of benefit (Avery, 1982; U.S. Department of Health and Human Services, 1987). The Gerson Institute, however, disputed NCI's findings and charged that NCI had dismissed legitimate evidence on the basis of technicalities. In addition, the Gerson Institute claimed that even though NCI had indicated six cases were acceptable for further review and another 20 needed further documentation, NCI's own records indicate that such reviews were never done (Gerson Institute. undated-b).

More recently, an exploratory study of the clinical effects of some components of the Gerson regimen was conducted by Peter Lechner, M.D., at the University Hospital of Graz, Austria. This study used a modified Gerson therapy (i.e., liver juice and thyroid supplements were omitted, the number of coffee enemas was limited, and a high-calorie beverage was added to double energy consumption) as an adjunctive treatment. Lechner reported that patients following the modified Gerson regimen showed no side effects attributable to the treatment and did not become malnourished. One of the patients with inoperable liver metastases who followed the Gerson treatment showed a temporary regression. In Lechner's opinion, there were subjective benefits from the modified Gerson regimen: patients needed less pain medication, were in better psychological condition, and experienced less severe side effects from chemotherapy than did control patients (Lechner and Kronberger, 1990).

Lechner's study also suggested that a modified Gerson regimen might be effective in lowering rates of post-surgical complications and secondary infections, increasing tolerance of conventional radiotherapy and chemotherapy, reducing reliance on analgesics, providing for an improved overall psychological profile, retarding progress of liver metastases, and improving the state of malignant effusions (Lechner and Kronberger, 1990).

A research team from the University of London that visited the Mexican clinic offering the Gerson therapy (see below) in 1989 on behalf of a British insurance company studied 27 cases in detail. Of those cases, 20 were considered not assessable. Of the seven assessable cases, three showed progressive disease, one showed stable disease, and three (43 percent of the accessible cases) were in regression. Moreover, the therapy clearly provided a subjective benefit for the patients and their families. In light of the poor prognosis of most of the patients they observed at the clinic, the British team concluded that the example of the Gerson therapy demonstrated a "way forward" for the treatment of cancer (Sikora et al., 1990).

The Gerson Research Organization of San Diego is currently conducting large retrospective reviews of treatment outcomes of more than 5,400 patient charts, including 5-year survival rates by stage (Hildenbrand et al., 1993), for patients treated by the Mexican medical group Centro Hospitalario Internacional del Pacifico, S.A. This facility, a semi-intensive care hospital, has offered Gerson's treatment since 1976. The review will include patients who either had no previous treatment or failed previous treatment as well as patients who received complementary conventional treatments.

Kelley regimen for cancer. In the 1960s, William Donald Kelley, an orthodontist by training, developed and publicized a nutritional program for cancer after reportedly being told by his doctor that he had metastatic pancreatic cancer and had only two months to live (Office of Technology Assessment, 1990). By trial and error, he self-administered doses of enzymes, vitamins, and minerals to treat his cancer. After his recovery, he applied his dietary program to his family; he also believed that his wife and two of his three children had developed cancer (Kelley, 1969). The Kelley regimen clearly derives from Gerson's. Common elements include carrot juice, a basically vegetarian diet, coffee enemas, and pancreatic enzymes, although pancreatic enzymes play a more emphatic role in the Kelley treatment. The Kelley regimen for cancer became one of the most widely known unconventional cancer treatments. Although Kelley is no longer practicing his treatment, the regimen has been continued in a variety of forms by his followers.

One of the people who adopted the Kelley regimen for the treatment of cancer patients was New York physician Nicholas Gonzalez, M.D. Gonzalez has examined the Kelley regimen and provided his own analysis of Kelley's individual metabolic profiles. According to Gonzalez, Kelley believed that human beings are of three genetically based types: sympathetic dominants, parasympathetic dominants, and balanced types. Sympathetic dominants, who have highly efficient and developed sympathetic nervous systems but inefficient parasympathetic nervous systems, evolved in tropical and subtropical ecosystems, eating plant-based diets. Parasympathetic dominants, in which the opposite is the case, evolved in colder regions, eating meat-based diets. Balanced types, whose nervous systems are equally developed, evolved in intermediate regions, eating mixed diets (Office of Technology Assessment, 1990).

Kelley developed a diet for each type according to the type's hypothesized historical origins. He had also traced a characteristic path of "metabolic decline" for each group when it consumed the wrong diet. He associated "hard tumors" with severely compromised sympathetic dominants, and "soft tumors" (cancers of the white blood cells and lymph system) with severely compromised parasympathetic dominants (Office of Technology Assessment, 1990).

As offered by Gonzalez, the Kelley program stresses biodiversity, tailoring diets to individual needs and ranging from purely vegetarian to diets requiring fatty red meat several times daily. Patients consume many supplements—vitamins, minerals, and trace elements—in 130 to 160 capsules daily.

Research base. In his 1987 manuscript *One Man Alone: An Investigation of Nutrition, Cancer, and William Donald Kelley*, Gonzalez presented case histories of 50 patients he selected from his files (Gonzalez, 1987). This case series has been singled out by proponents as one of the most convincing in support of an unconventional cancer treatment (Office of Technology Assessment, 1990).

In 1990, OTA attempted to find out whether the information presented in these cases would be convincing to the medical community by asking six physicians on its advisory panel to review the cases; three of the physicians supported some unconventional treatments, though none was associated with Kelley or Gonzalez, and the other three were mainstream oncologists. Fifteen cases were judged by the reviewers generally supportive of some unconventional medicine as definitely showing a positive effect from the Kelley program; in contrast, the mainstream oncologists found that 13 of these 15 were unconvincing and that 2 were unusual (Office of Technology Assessment 1990).

Another nine cases were judged unusual or suggestive by the supportive group, and unconvincing by the mainstream group. Another 14 cases were judged by the supportive physicians as having been helped by a combination of the Kelley regimen and mainstream cancer therapy; the mainstream group found 12 of these cases unconvincing and 2 unusual. Finally, 12 cases were considered unconvincing by both groups of physicians. The different interpretations of these cases by physicians who are open to unconventional medicine and those who are not illustrates the difficulty in evaluating therapies that fall out of the bounds of conventional medical wisdom.

Gonzalez recently submitted to NCI a meticulously documented best case series (Friedman, 1993). At least 6 of the 24 cases reportedly document complete remissions of cancers, 5 of them metastatic to various sites including liver, pleura, brain, and bone. Two additional cases reportedly document partial remissions.

Macrobiotic diet for cancer. The philosophy and general components of the "standard macrobiotic diet" are described below in the "Alternative Dietary Lifestyles and Cultural Diets" section of this chapter. In the area of cancer management and treatment, the macrobiotic philosophy holds that the development of cancer is determined by dietary, environmental, social, and personal factors; by extension, existing cancers may be influenced by the same factors. The development of cancer is described as a long-term, multi-step process that begins well in advance of actual tumor formation (Kushi and Jack, 1983).

According to macrobiotic teachings, accumulated toxins result from over-consumption of milk, cheese, meat, eggs, and other fatty, oily, or greasy foods. Also included in this list are foods with a cooling or freezing effect, such as ice cream, soft drinks, and orange juice (Kushi and Jack, 1983). Macrobiotics uses the traditional oriental concepts of yin (expansive) and yang (contractive) to devise a framework for explaining and formulating a set of dietary recommendations to treat each type of cancer.

A macrobiotic approach to treating cancer would first classify each patient's illness as predominantly yin or yang, or sometimes a combination of both, partly on the basis of the location of the primary tumor in the body and the location of the tumor in the particular organ. In general, tumors in peripheral or upper parts of the body or in hollow, expanded organs are considered yin; examples include lymphoma, leukemia, Hodgkin's disease, and tumors of the mouth (except tongue), esophagus, upper stomach, breast, skin, and outer regions of the brain. Tumors in lower or deeper parts of the body or in more compact organs are considered yang; examples include cancers of the colon, rectum, prostate, ovaries, bone, pancreas, and inner regions of the brain. Cancers thought to result from a combination of yin and yang forces include melanoma (skin cancer) and cancers of the lung, bladder, kidney, lower stomach, uterus, spleen, liver, and tongue (Kushi and Jack, 1983).

For cancers classified as predominantly yang, the standard macrobiotic diet is recommended, with slight emphasis on yin foods. The same diet is recommended for yin-classified cancers, with a slight emphasis on yang foods. Patients with cancers resulting from both yin and yang imbalances are advised to follow "a central way of eating," as suggested in the standard macrobiotic diet. Different cooking styles also are recommended on the basis of this disease classification (Kushi and Jack, 1983).

Research base. The available information on the effectiveness of the macrobiotic diet for treating cancer comes from retrospective case reviews and anecdotal reports, some of which come from the popular literature, and two unpublished retrospective studies (Office of Technology Assessment, 1990). A number of individual accounts of patients who attributed their recovery from cancer to their adherence to a macrobiotic diet have been written in recent years.

In one unpublished retrospective study, Carter and colleagues (1990) compared survival times between 23 pancreatic cancer patients maintained on a macrobiotic diet and similar patients who received conventional cancer therapy. The authors reported that the mean survival (the average) and the median survival (the point in time after diagnosis by which half the group died) was significantly longer for the macrobiotically maintained patients. A follow-up study by Carter also showed improved survival time for 11 patients with prostate cancer on a macrobiotic diet. However, OTA pointed out that the studies had design flaws that may have overstated the effect (Office of Technology Assessment, 1990).

In another unpublished manuscript, Newbold (undated) presented six case histories of patients with advanced cancer who adopted a macrobiotic diet in addition to using mainstream treatment. These cases were well described medically, including references to appropriate diagnostic tests (all but one case was definitely biopsy proven) and follow-up scans and tests (Office of Technology Assessment, 1990).

As in the review of the Kelley regimen, when OTA asked its independent advisory panel of six physicians to review Newbold's cases the three mainstream reviewers did not find any of the cases compelling, while two physicians who were open to unconventional therapies were more positive about the outcomes. One concluded that five of the six cases (all except the one without the biopsy-proven diagnosis) showed positive effects from the macrobiotic diet. The remaining physician found two cases that seemed "legitimate," two "highly suggestive," one "suggestive," and one not convincing (Office of Technology Assessment, 1990).

The retrospective studies presented by Carter and Newbold's case histories were later combined and published in the Journal of the American College of Nutrition (Carter et al., 1993). Although the design flaws noted by OTA were still extant in the study, an accompanying editorial suggested that these findings may provide clues to a new approach to the dietary management of cancer (Weisburger, 1993). The editorial stated that the macrobiotic diet has "been construed by classical nutritionists as inadequate . . . Yet, the application to control the growth of cancer may actually be based on the fact that it is an inadequate diet." The editorial continued by stating that "Perhaps the time has come to teach nutritionists that, in some instances, a nutritional regimen clearly deficient in growth promoting substances might actually be helpful in controlling otherwise untreatable diseases."

Additional Cancer Diets.

Additional cancer diets reviewed by the Office of Technology Assessment included the Livingston/Wheeler regimen and the Wigmore treatment.

Livingston/Wheeler regimen. This regimen is mentioned here because its practitioners advocate diet as a means of potentiating antitumor immunity. Based on Dr. Virginia Livingston's observation of a putative cancer-causing microorganism, the treatment combines vaccines, bacterial reagents, a patented retinoic acid, intravenously administered vitamins, long-term use of antibiotics, and a modified Gerson diet with coffee enemas. Her San Diego-based clinic has continued, after her death, to offer her treatment.

Wigmore treatment. This treatment is an empirically developed dietary regimen (Wigmore, 1985) that uses seed sprouts, wheat grass juice, and uncooked vegetables and fruits. The available literature contains accounts of positive outcomes in cancer, but they are presented without conventional documentation, making it impossible to confirm or deny them. Although advocates have gone to considerable lengths to present supportive literature for their practices (Wigmore, 1993), formal clinical testing has been limited to studies of the reversible, short-term effects of the diet on serum lipids, lipoprotein, and apolipoprotein (W. Ling et al., 1992), which findings are consistent with, if less extensive than, those of similar fat-restricted, basically vegetarian diets (Walford et al., 1992).

Fat-modified diets for treatment of cardiovascular disease and diabetes. Coronary artery disease is the leading cause of death and disability in the United States. Seven million people, nearly 3 percent of the U.S. population, have clinical coronary heart disease. Every year, 1.5 million Americans have acute heart attacks, which kill approximately 520,000 persons, 247,000 of whom are women (American Heart Association, 1991). In fact, cardiovascular diseases—primarily coronary heart disease and stroke kill nearly as many Americans each year as all other diseases combined (National Center for Health Statistics, 1990). Furthermore, more than 60 million Americans, or 30 percent of the adult population, currently have high blood pressure (National Heart, Lung, and Blood Institute, 1985), which makes them prime candidates for stroke and heart or kidney disease.

Balloon angioplasty (inserting a tiny balloon into the circulatory system and inflating it to open up a plaque-blocked artery) is performed approximately 300,000 times a year in the United States. Although angioplasty provides immediate and possibly lifesaving relief for many patients, it is not a long-term solution. There is no evidence that angioplasty does anything to prevent future angina (severe chest pain) or heart attacks, and about 30 to 40 percent of all angioplasty-treated vessels block up again within six months, meaning another angioplasty must be performed (Becker, 1991). Each angioplasty procedure costs about $20,000.

For the most severe cases of heart disease, surgeons remove veins (usually from the legs) and use them to "detour," or bypass, around the clogged arteries of the heart. Even though people who undergo bypass operations experience a reduction in chest pain, the benefits of this surgery, which costs approximately $30,000, often wear off (Myrmel, 1993)

Researchers have known for several decades that a proper diet may prevent the onset of cardiovascular disease. However, once an individual develops this chronic condition, surgery and drugs have been considered the only available methods in mainstream medicine for trying to reverse its effects (Califf et al., 1989). Only recently has diet been considered an alternative to drugs and surgery for treating cardiovascular disease. In the mid-1970s, Nathan Pritikin began using an extremely low-fat, high-fiber diet along with exercise to treat heart disease patients and showed that he could lessen their clinical symptoms. Then in the late 1980s, San Francisco physician Dean Ornish set out to do the same. However, Ornish was armed with a powerful new tool: the angiogram, which is an interior picture of patients' blood vessels. Using "before" and "after" angiograms, Ornish was able to see how changes in diet and lifestyle affected the status of the blockage, or plaque, in the artery. The Pritikin and Ornish diets are described below.

Pritikin diet. The diet is named after the man who developed it, Nathan Pritikin, who had been told by his cardiologist that he was at great risk of death from myocardial infarction. Therefore, he patterned for himself a diet modeled after a vegetarian diet followed by the people of Uganda, who were shown to be essentially free from death by heart attacks (Martin, 1991). In the late 1960s, after a few years on this diet, Pritikin decided that it had saved his life and founded his clinic in Santa Monica to treat cardiac patents.

The Pritikin diet is basically vegetarian, high in complex carbohydrates and fiber, low in cholesterol, and extremely low in fat (less than 10 percent of daily calories). The Pritikin diet also requires 45 minutes of walking daily. Although this diet and exercise program can be followed completely on an outpatient basis, the Pritikin Longevity Center in Santa Monica recommends that patients attend a 26-day program to learn how to prepare their new type of meals and practice new daily exercise and living habits.

Ornish diet. This diet was developed by Dean Ornish, M.D., an assistant clinical professor of medicine at the University of California, San Francisco. The Ornish diet is basically vegetarian, allowing no meat, poultry, or fish, and permitting only the white of eggs. Also, no nuts, caffeine, or dairy products, except a cup a day of nonfat milk or yogurt, are allowed, and no oil or fat is permitted—not even for cooking. Two ounces of alcohol a day are allowed. Providing an average of about 1,800 calories a day, the diet provides 75 percent of its calories from carbohydrates and less than 10 percent from fat (Ornish, 1990). The American Heart Association's recommended adult "prudent diet" calls for total fat of less than 30 percent, which Ornish feels is not really low enough, even for healthy adults, but especially not for people trying to reverse atherosclerosis (Ornish, 1990). Ornish provides his patients all their lunch and dinner meals, precooked, packed in Tupperware, and handed out a week's worth at a time.

In many ways, the Ornish diet is similar to the Pritikin diet. Both are basically vegetarian (although Pritikin does allow 85 grams of chicken or fish per week), high in complex carbohydrates, high in fiber, low in cholesterol, and extremely low in fat (less than 10 percent of daily calories). However, Ornish's program—run on an outpatient basis—calls for stress reduction practices in addition to the diet and emphasizes emotional social support systems, particularly between members of the group. It also requires daily stretching and an hour's walk three times a week.

Research base. The following is an overview of the available research on these two ultra-low-fat dietary regimens.

Pritikin diet. In a study of men taking the Pritikin 26-day course, all 21 participants reduced their cholesterol level, 19 reduced their triglyceride level, and 16 had a reduction in their estradiol level (Rosenthal et al., 1985).

In another study assessing the effectiveness of the Pritikin diet and exercise program on cardiovascular hemodynamics, 20 subjects were divided in two groups (active/treatment and control). These data were compared to a group of 10 healthy individuals not involved in the program. Hemodynamic parameters were collected at admission and at the end of the 26-day program. In obese and hypertensive subjects not on medication who followed the Pritikin program, the cardiac index increased by 10 percent, mean arterial pressure decreased by 5 percent, and the systemic vascular resistance index decreased by 18 percent. Little change was seen in controls. There also was an improvement in ventricular performance (Mattar et al., 1990)

The Pritikin diet has also been studied in connection with adult-onset diabetes mellitus and peripheral vascular disease. Studies suggest that it may show promise in controlling newly diagnosed cases of adult-onset diabetes without drugs. One study (Barnard et al.,1982) evaluated 60 patients who had completed the Pritikin 26-day program. Of the 23 who were taking oral hypoglycemic agents upon entry, all but two were off medication by the end of the program. Of the 17 patients who were taking insulin, all but four were off medication at discharge. Two of those four had their insulin reduced by 50 percent, while the remaining two had no major change in their insulin dosage. Fasting blood glucose levels were significantly reduced in all patients; serum cholesterol levels were similarly reduced, as were triglyceride levels. The group as a whole lost an average of 4.3 kg of body weight and achieved 40.5 percent of their desired weight loss. Maximum work capacity increased significantly, while daily walking increased from approximately 11.7 minutes a day to approximately 103 minutes.

In another study, University of California, Los Angeles (UCLA) investigator Dr. James R. Barnard put 650 diabetic patients on the Pritikin diet. After three weeks, some 76 percent of the newly diagnosed diabetics, along with 70 percent of those on oral agents, had normal glucose levels (Barnard et al., 1992). However, only 40 percent of those already receiving insulin responded to the diet. According to Barnard, muscles, which may become severely insulin resistant during drug treatment, respond to exercise and a low-fat diet. In contrast, drugs may eventually weaken the pancreas while failing to reduce physically and financially devastating vascular complications (e.g., deterioration of eyes and kidneys).

Ornish diet. In what is now known as the Lifestyle Heart Trial, in the late 1970s and early 1980s Ornish conducted a series of trials in which patients with confirmed heart disease were placed on a diet and lifestyle modification program. In the first study, after 30 days people reported a substantial reduction in frequency of angina (heart pain), and many were pain free. Cholesterol levels were down about 20 percent, and high blood pressure was reduced (Ornish et al., 1979). In a follow-up study in the early 1980s, Ornish reported that 30 days of his regimen were enough to improve blood flow to the heart in some patients and that patients could exercise almost 50 percent more, on average, than they could before beginning the treatment (Ornish et al., 1983).

Finally, in a prospective, randomized, controlled trial to determine the effectiveness of his program over a longer time, Ornish and his colleagues put 28 men and women whose arteries were partially blocked on his program for a full year. Twenty other patients were assigned to a "usual care" group. After 1 year, without the use of lipid-lowering drugs, patients in the experimental group (i.e., receiving the Ornish treatment) reported a 91-percent reduction in the frequency of angina, a 42-percent reduction in the duration of angina, and a 28-percent reduction in the severity of angina. In contrast, control group patients reported a 165-percent rise in frequency, a 95-percent rise in duration, and a 39-percent rise in severity of angina (Ornish et al., 1990).

Patients in the experimental group also showed a significant overall regression, or reduction, of coronary atherosclerosis (blocked arteries) as measured by angiograms. In contrast, patients in the usual care group had a significant overall progression, or worsening, of their coronary atherosclerosis. This finding led Ornish to conclude that the conventional recommendations for patients with heart disease, such as a 30-percent fat diet, are not sufficient to bring about an improvement in many patients.

Ornish has never tested separately each component of his multi-faceted program, so it is impossible to be sure which component contributed most to the improvements. If it was the dietary regimen that led to the improvements, it is a regimen that most Americans would have a hard time following, admits Ornish (Schardt, 1993). However, some researchers believe that it does not take such a radically restricted diet to start reversing the effects of heart disease. In a study in Germany, 56 men suffering from angina caused by partially blocked arteries were placed on a reduced-fat diet (less than 20 percent of calories from fat, 7 percent of calories from saturated fat, and 200 mg of cholesterol a day). As in the Ornish program, they also participated in an exercise program. After a year, angiograms showed that the blockages in 32 percent of the men on the low-fat diet had improved, compared with just 17 percent in the control group (Schuler et al., 1992).

In addition, in the late 1980s, researchers in Britain placed 26 men with partially blocked arteries and elevated blood cholesterol on carefully monitored diets and reduced their fat intake to 27 percent of calories—about three-fourths of what the average American eats. The diet's saturated fat and cholesterol amounts also were substantially less than most Americans eat, while its fiber content was slightly higher. Over the next three years, the men on the fat-restricted diet suffered only one-third as many deaths, heart attacks, and strokes as men in the control group—who were not told what to eat, and whose diets were not monitored (Watts et al., 1992). Furthermore, angiograms showed that the openings in the arteries of 38 percent of the men who changed their diets became slightly larger.

Food Elimination Diets for Treatment of Food Allergies

Allergies to food, or food intolerance, have become a major area of research in recent years. Many of the researchers involved in this research specialize in environmental medicine (see the "Alternative Systems of Medical Practice" chapter), which is the science of assessing the impact of such environmental factors as chemicals, foods, and inhalants on health. It provides an understanding of the interface between the external environment and the biological function of the individual.

Dietary management of food allergies is based on avoidance of food antigens and the 4-day rotary diversified diet. With the rotary diet and avoidance of repetitive food exposures, it is possible to reduce sensitivity to foods and hasten recovery from food allergies. Nutritional supplements are prescribed as indicated by objective nutritional testing and the symptoms of the patient.

Research base. Miller (1977) studied eight chronically ill food-sensitive patients who were tested with provocation-neutralization techniques. The patients were treated with injections of allergy extracts and compared to those treated with placebos. In a rigidly controlled study, King (1988) showed a correlation between oral food challenge and provocation-neutralization testing. Treatment using results from this testing showed significant symptom relief. Using neutralization therapy, Rea and colleagues (1984) found significant improvement in 20 patients with known food sensitivity in signs and symptoms of allergy reactions to certain foods.

Food intolerance is also being studied as a causal or contributing factor in rheumatoid arthritis. In a clinical trial in Norway, Kjeldsen-Kragh and colleagues (1991) found that fasting followed by dietary restriction could relieve the symptoms of rheumatoid arthritis on a long-term basis. They subjected 27 rheumatoid arthritis patients to a 7- to 10-day fast (except for herbal teas, garlic, vegetable broth, a decoction of potatoes and parsley, and extracts from carrots, beets, and celery) followed by 1 year of an individually adjusted vegetarian diet. The diet-restricted patients stayed on a Norwegian health farm the first four weeks of the study. A control group of 26 patients stayed in a convalescent home for four weeks but ate an ordinary diet throughout the trial.

218

After 4 weeks, the diet group showed a decrease in pain score; a significant decrease in pain, morning stiffness, and the number of tender and swollen joints; and improved grip strength and ability to articulate the joints. There was also a significant improvement in a number of biochemical markers associated with inflammation. These improvements were maintained throughout the year. In contrast, the control group showed a decrease in pain score after its stay in the convalescent home, but none of the other indices improved. At the end of the study the conditions of the control patients had deteriorated.

This study suggests that there is a food allergy component to rheumatoid arthritis and that food restriction appears to be a useful supplement to the conventional medical treatment of rheumatoid arthritis. Darlington and colleagues (1986) and Beri and colleagues (1988) obtained similar results, but their studies lasted only three months.

There is also evidence that food elimination diets may benefit many children with hyperactivity (Kanofsky, 1986). Several research teams have used double-blind designs to demonstrate this point. The Institute of Child Health and Hospital for Sick Children in London undertook a randomized, crossover, placebo-controlled trial to evaluate the effect of diet on the development of hyperactivity (Egger et al., 1985). The first phase of the study consisted of placing 76 hyperactive children on a food elimination diet. The presupposition was that individuals can be sensitive to a food or food additive in their diet and that improvement occurs when the offending foods or food additives are removed from the diet. At the end of the first phase of the study, 62 of the 76 children (82 percent) improved on the diet, and a normal range of behavior was achieved in 21 (29 percent) of them. In addition to overactivity, other symptoms such as headaches, abdominal pain, antisocial behavior, and fits were also often alleviated.

In all, 48 foods were implicated as contributing to hyperactivity in the young patients. However, 34 of the 50 children for whom full data are available reacted to fewer than seven foods. Two reacted to 30 foods. Five patients were also noted with symptoms from such inhalants as pollen, perfume, and house dust. Foods that frequently caused problems included cow's milk (64 percent of subjects tested), chocolate (59 percent), wheat (49 percent), and oranges (45 percent).

The second phase of the study included 28 children from the original group, who entered into a double-blind, crossover, placebo-controlled trial that reintroduced one incriminated food. Symptoms returned or were exacerbated much more often when patients were on active material than on placebo. One of the most interesting findings of the study is that the artificial food coloring tartrazine and the preservative benzoic acid were the commonest food items causing a reaction. The behavior of 79 percent of the 34 children tested deteriorated when tartrazine or benzoic acid was reintroduced into their diet. These findings are compatible with the work of Dr. Benjamin Feingold, the San Francisco allergist who implicated tartrazine and other artificial food additives in children's diets as contributors to hyperactivity. It is worth noting that the same London group also published a study stating that 93 percent of 88 children with severe, frequent migraines recovered on a diet that eliminated foods and food additives that had been shown to cause symptoms (Egger et al., 1983).

Some confirmation for the food elimination treatment for hyperkinesis was provided by Kaplan and colleagues (1989). In their study, 10 of 24 hyperactive children exhibited approximately a 50-percent improvement in behavior when placed on an elimination diet that was not as restrictive as the London diet.

Alternative Dietary Lifestyles in Prevention and Treatment of Chronic Illness

A number of alternative dietary lifestyles throughout the United States and the world are believed to increase resistance to illness. Although some diets, such as macrobiotics, have been intentionally developed in the past half century, others have evolved more naturally over the centuries.

An "alternative lifestyle" diet can be described as any diet that differs from the mainstream American diet. Such diets include various forms of vegetarianism and diets with emphasis on "natural," "organic," "unrefined," "unprocessed," and/or other health foods in varying degrees. Others are drawn from other societies around the world, such as the "Mediterranean" diet.

Historically, there has been much skepticism among some health professionals about such diets. For example, when the vegetarian movement started in the United States about 50 years ago, people questioned whether adults subsisting on such diets could even do a full day's work and still survive (Krey, 1982). However, generations of people around the world have now grown up on these diets, helping to dispel such myths. Furthermore, many individuals and population groups have practiced vegetarianism on a long-term basis and have demonstrated excellent health (American Academy of Pediatrics, 1977). Indeed, the case against such diets has been largely cultural and economic (see the section "Barriers and Key Issues Related to Diet and Nutrition" in this chapter).

Vegetarian Diets

Vegetarian diets are among the most common of alternative diets in the United States today. The degree of vegetarianism can vary widely, ranging from those who eat red meat infrequently to those who totally exclude any animal-derived foods, such as dairy products or eggs, from their diet. Vegetarianism is often categorized according to the extent of these restrictions. For example, people who consume dairy products and eggs but not other animal foods are referred to as lacto-ovo-vegetarians, while people who avoid all animal products are referred to as vegans. Studies of vegetarians in the United States and other industrialized nations probably provide the most extensive support for the idea that alternative dietary habits can favorably influence the incidence and pathology of disease.

This section focuses on the nutritional aspects of the two most widely studied variations on the vegetarian diet: the one followed by adherents of the Seventh-Day Adventist Church, and the macrobiotic diet. The health-related data from people eating these diets are compared with data taken from individuals in the general U.S. population. Seventh-Day Adventists. The Seventh-Day Adventists are a Protestant sect that among other things preaches a clean, wholesome lifestyle and admonishes against eating animal flesh (i.e., red meat, poultry, fish). Thus, Seventh-Day Adventists are for the most part lacto-ovo-vegetarians. They also abstain from alcohol, tobacco, and caffeine-containing beverages, such as coffee and tea. Even though they avoid meat, Seventh-Day Adventists' diets are not substantially lower in fat intake than the typical American diet. For example, in one survey of lacto-ovo-vegetarian Seventh-Day Adventists, total fat intake averaged 36 percent of energy versus 37 percent for the average American (Phillips et al., 1983).

Macrobiotic Diet

Along with Seventh-Day Adventists, people who consume a macrobiotic diet have been studied extensively to examine associations with disease risk factors. In addition, macrobiotic diets are among the most popular alternative dietary therapies for cancer and other chronic diseases (Cassileth et al., 1984).

The earliest version of the macrobiotic diet, termed the "zen macrobiotic diet," originated with the lecturer-philosopher Georges

221

Ohsawa (1893-1966), the pen name for Yukikaza Sakurazawa, a Japanese teacher who studied the writings of Japanese physician Sagen Ishikuzuka (1850-1910). Ohsawa is said to have cured himself of serious illness by changing from the modern refined diet then sweeping Japan to a simple diet of brown rice, miso soup, sea vegetables, and other traditional foods. He initiated the development of macrobiotic philosophy, reportedly integrating elements of Eastern and Western perspectives with "holistic" perspectives on science and medicine. Ohsawa made his first of several visits to the United State in 1959

Ohsawa outlined 10 stages of diet (designated by numbers -3 to +7). Diet -3 consists of 10 percent cereal grains, 30 percent vegetables, 10 percent soups, 30 percent animal products, 15 percent salads and fruits, 5 percent desserts, and beverages "as little as possible." With each higher number diet, Ohsawa reduced the percentages of foods from some categories or eliminated the category entirely and increased others, so that in the +3 diet, for example, 60 percent was cereals, 30 percent was vegetables, and 10 percent was soups.

Since the early 1970s, the macrobiotic movement in the United States has been under the leadership of Michio Kushi. Kushi, who studied with Ohsawa and came to the United States from Japan in 1949, preserved elements of Ohsawa's philosophy while incorporating a variety of broader and more complex components into macrobiotic philosophy and practice. Most notably, Ohsawa's 10-phase dietary levels were replaced with the general "standard macrobiotic diet," which Kushi described in detail in his 1983 book, The Cancer Prevention Diet (Kushi and Jack, 1983).

Unlike Seventh-Day Adventists, whose vegetarian diets usually include dairy products and eggs, the standard macrobiotic diet as practiced today tends to minimize consumption of all animal products except fish (M. Kushi, 1977, 1983). Thus the macrobiotic diet is predominantly vegan, with an emphasis on whole cereal grains and vegetables, preferably organically grown. As a result, it tends to be relatively high in complex carbohydrates and low in fat content (and, therefore, calories) in comparison with the standard American diet. One survey of 50 adults consuming a macrobiotic diet demonstrated that fat intake averaged 23 percent of energy, saturated fat intake averaged 9 percent of energy, and carbohydrate intake averaged 65 percent of energy (L. Kushi et al., 1988).

Research base. The following is an overview of the available research on the health-promoting and disease-preventing effects of the Seventh Day Adventist and macrobiotic diets.

Seventh-Day Adventist diet. Despite their relatively high fat intake, Seventh-Day Adventists have less heart disease and incidence of some cancers than occurs in the general U.S. population. For example, Seventh-Day Adventists who eat little or no red meat have a lower death rate from heart disease than the general U.S. population (Phillips et al., 1978; Snowdon et al., 1984a). Indeed, studies on Seventh-Day Adventist males have shown that their serum cholesterol levels were lower and that the first heart attack occurred almost a decade later than average. The incidence of heart disease was only 60 percent as high as that of a control group in California (Register and Sonnenberg, 1973). Abstinence from tobacco and alcohol also may have contributed to this effect. Studies comparing Seventh-Day Adventists with non-Adventists demonstrate that the former tend to have lower blood pressure levels as well. For example, in one study in which age, sex, and body size were taken into account, blood pressure levels for vegetarian Seventh-Day Adventists averaged 128.7 mm Hg systolic and 76.2 mm Hg diastolic versus non-vegetarians' average levels of 139.3 mm Hg systolic and 84.5 mm Hg diastolic (Armstrong et al., 1977). Similar findings were seen in other studies comparing vegetarian and non-vegetarian Seventh-Day Adventists (Melby et al., 1989).

Another study comparing blood pressure levels of vegetarian Seventh-Day Adventists with non-vegetarian Mormons, who similarly avoid tobacco and alcohol, demonstrated that the Seventh-Day Adventists still had lower blood pressure levels (Rouse et al., 1982). Comparisons of California Seventh-Day Adventists with their non-Adventist neighbors also demonstrated that the Adventists had lower LDL cholesterol levels (Fraser, 1988).

The overall cancer death rate of male Seventh Day Adventists is only about half that of the overall cancer death rate of the U.S. general population, and the overall cancer death rate of female Seventh-Day Adventists is about 70 percent of that of the general population (Phillips et al., 1980). The lower death rates apply not only to those cancer sites known to be associated with cigarette smoking (e.g., lungs), but also to other sites such as the breast. In fact, Adventists have 80 to 90 percent of the general population's breast cancer death rate and only 50 to 60 percent of the colon and rectal cancer death rate (Phillips et al., 1980). These observations suggest that smoking habits alone cannot explain the difference between cancer death rates of Seventh-Day Adventists and those of the general population.

The results of other prospective dietary studies among Seventh-Day Adventists are mixed when vegetarians are compared with non-vegetarians. For instance, there appears to be little relationship between such dietary variables as total fat or animal fat intake with risk of breast cancer (Mills et al., 1988, 1989a). However, in two prospective cohort studies, Seventh-Day Adventists who rarely consumed meat, poultry, or fish appeared to have a lower risk of breast cancer than those who consumed these foods at least once a week (Mills et al., 1989a; Phillips and Snowdon, 1983). In neither of these studies was this association statistically significant.

However, a study of 35,000 California Seventh-Day Adventists, covering a follow-up period from 1976 to 1982, did indicate an increased risk of colon cancer with increasing animal fat intake (Morgan et al., 1988). Indeed, those individuals in the highest third of animal fat intake rates had a risk of developing colon cancer that was 1.8 times that of individuals in the lowest third of animal fat intake rates; people with intermediate animal fat intakes were intermediate in their risk (Morgan et al., 1988).

In another study of cancer among 25,000 California Seventh-Day Adventists covering 20 years (1960-80), men who consumed meat at least four times a week experienced a prostate cancer death rate of 41.9 deaths per 100,000 person-years versus 29.7 deaths per 100,000 person-years for men who did not consume meat (Phillips and Snowdon, 1983). In the study begun in 1976, daily consumption of meat was associated with a risk of developing prostate cancer 1.41 times greater than that of men who never ate meat (Mills et al., 1989b). In the earlier, study, meat intake was also associated with increased risk of prostate cancer (Snowdon et al., 1984b).

On the other hand, increased consumption of beans and lentils appeared to decrease the risk of colon cancer in the Seventh-Day Adventist population (Morgan et al., 1988). In fact, among the people who ate the highest amounts of these foods, the risk of developing colon cancer was one-third that of people who ate the lowest amounts (Morgan et al., 1988). Furthermore, consumption of beans and lentils at least three times per week was associated with approximately 50 percent lower risk of developing prostate cancer than consumption of beans and lentils less than once a month (Mills et al. 1989b).

The association of vegetarianism with decreased risk of certain cancers appears to have correlates with biological parameters in Seventh Day Adventists. Vegetarian Seventh-Day Adventists appear to have less colonic mucosal cell turnover than non-vegetarians and those at increased risk of colon cancer (Lipkin et al., 1985). This point is significant, because it is believed that decreased cell proliferation of the colonic mucosa may be a hallmark of decreased risk of colon cancer (Lipkin, 1974). Macrobiotic diet. No studies to date have examined directly the role of a macrobiotic diet in chronic disease prevention. However, a number of studies have examined associations between macrobiotic diets and biological Ask parameters such as blood pressure, cholesterol levels, and estrogen metabolism. The earliest of these studies were surveys of blood pressure and blood lipid levels, which were conducted in the Boston macrobiotic community. One of these studies showed that young adults eating a macrobiotic diet had blood pressure levels of 106 mm Hg systolic and 60 mm Hg diastolic, which was significantly lower than would be expected in the general population (Sacks et al., 1974). In fact, in comparison with people of similar age and sex in Framingham, MA, the subjects'systolic blood pressure was an average of 11 mm Hg lower and diastolic blood pressure 14 mm Hg lower (Sacks et al., 1975). In addition, those in the macrobiotic community who ate some animal food tended to have higher blood pressures than others in the macrobiotic community who did not (Sacks et al., 1974).

Blood lipid levels, a general indicator of coronary heart disease risk, also were substantially lower among the people eating macrobiotically than in the Framingham comparison group. In fact, average plasma total cholesterol levels among the macrobiotic vegetarians was 126 mg/dL versus a total average plasma cholesterol level of 184 mg/dL in the age- and sex-matched controls in the Framingham population (Sacks et al., 1975). Levels of low-density lipoprotein (LDL) cholesterol—the type of cholesterol that promotes heart disease—also were substantially lower in those eating a macrobiotic diet, averaging 73 mg/dL in the macrobiotic vegetarians and 118 mg/dL in the controls (Sacks et al., 1975). Although levels of high-density lipoprotein (HDL) cholesterol—the type of cholesterol that protects against heart disease—were also lower in the macrobiotic vegetarians (43 mg/dL vs. 49 mg/dL), the ratio of total to HDL cholesterol, a measure of the relative atherogenicity (i.e., ability to form plaques) of the blood lipid profile, was substantially lower among the macrobiotic vegetarians than in the comparison group (2.9 vs. 3.8). These differences persisted even when adjusted for weight differences. The relatively favorable blood cholesterol profile of macrobiotic vegetarians has been confirmed in several other surveys (Bergan and Brown, 1980; Knuiman and West, 1982; L. Kushi et al., 1988; Sacks et al., 1985).

In recent years, there has been increasing interest in the role of fat-soluble antioxidants in atherogenesis. It has been hypothesized that oxidation of LDL particles may be a critical step in the uptake of LDL by macrophages, as well as for some other mechanisms that increase the atherogenicity of LDL cholesterol (Steinberg and Witztum, 1990). The relative proportion of antioxidants to circulating LDL has been suggested as an additional measure of the atherogenicity of blood lipid levels (Berry, 1992). A study of macrobiotic vegetarians demonstrated that they had not only lower LDL levels but also higher plasma levels of antioxidants relative to cholesterol compared to non-vegetarians (Pronczuk et al., 1992).

The favorable cardiovascular disease profile of macrobiotic vegetarians is likely to be largely due to the relative avoidance of meat and dairy products. Indeed, when the diet of macrobiotic vegetarians was supplemented with 250 grams of beef per day, plasma total cholesterol increased by about 19 percent after four weeks, from an average of 140 mg/dL to 166 mg/dL (Sacks et al., 1981). Comparisons of macrobiotic vegetarians with lacto-vegetarians and non-vegetarians also indicate a direct relationship between average blood total cholesterol levels and dairy product intake (Sacks et al., 1985).

In the context of cancer risk, studies comparing women eating a macrobiotic diet with women eating a typical American diet demonstrate substantial differences in estrogen metabolism (Goldin et al., 1981, 1982). In fact, women eating a macrobiotic diet had substantially higher fecal excretion and lower urinary excretion of estrogens, with somewhat lower serum levels of estradiol. This point is significant because many cancers, especially breast cancer, are growth dependent on hormones such as estrogen. The altered estrogen metabolism profile of women eating macrobiotically may reflect a lower risk of breast cancer (Goldin et al., 1981, 1982).

Furthermore, in subsequent studies it was demonstrated that women eating macrobiotically had dramatically higher urinary excretion of lignans, such as enterolactone and enterodiol, and of isoflavonoids, such as daidzein and equol, than women consuming a lacto-ovo-vegetarian diet or an omnivorous diet. Women with breast cancer had the lowest levels of these phytoestrogens (Adlercreutz et al., 1986, 1987). These differences appeared to be related to greater intake of whole grains, legumes, and vegetables by the macrobiotic women.

It has been hypothesized that such a fiber-rich diet may, by the presence of these lignans and other weak estrogens (i.e., phytoestrogens) in the intestinal tract, stimulate the synthesis of sex hormone binding globulin in the liver and may thus decrease levels of free estradiol in the plasma (Adlercreutz et al., 1987). This may, in turn, reduce the risk of breast as well as other hormone-dependent cancers. It has also been suggested that these phytoestrogens (see the

"Herbal Medicine" chapter) may actually compete with endogenous estradiol on the cellular level, further reducing the cellular proliferation and, hence, the potentially carcinogenic effects of estradiol (Price and Fenwick, 1985; Tang and Adams, 1980).

In addition to the general macronutrient differences (lower fat, higher complex carbohydrate intake) between macrobiotic diets and the standard American diet, certain foods in the standard macrobiotic diet may have specific anticancer effects. Examples of such foods, which are absent in the typical American diet, include various soy foods, such as miso and tofu, and sea vegetables (see the "Diets of Other Cultures" section for a discussion of the health benefits of these foods).

Health Risks Associated with Strict Vegetarian Diets

Except for vitamin B12 deficiency, diets that exclude meat or animal products do not produce deficiencies in adults if they are correctly followed. Nevertheless, there are reports in the literature that have associated some forms of vegetarianism with high risks of deficiencies in children and pregnant women (Debry, 1991). The nutrition of children on a vegetarian diet is considered to be adequate and well balanced when the diet contains dairy products and eggs. It has been suggested that a severe or strict vegetarian diet is not suitable for infants or toddlers. For example, serious deficiency states (e.g., rickets, osteoporosis, anemia, growth retardation) have been described in children subsisting on such regimens (Lentze, 1992). However, it is interesting to note that in a study that examined the maternity care records of 775 vegan mothers living on a commune in southern Tennessee, there was only one case of preeclampsia (Carter et al., 1987). The authors concluded that it is possible to sustain a normal pregnancy on a vegan diet, and the source of protein (i.e., animal or vegetable) does not seem to affect birth weight, as long as vegan mothers receive continuous prenatal care, supplement their diets with prenatal vitamins, calcium, and iron, and apply "protein-complementing" nutritional principles.

Diets of Other Cultures

A cultural diet is defined as the diet of any group of people who share beliefs and customs. By this definition, everyone in the United States is a member of some cultural group. For many cultural groups, food plays an important role in maintenance of both spiritual, and physical health. The following is a brief overview of several cultural diets—Asian, Mediterranean, and traditional Native American Indian—that are thought to provide some protection against many of the nutritionally related chronic illnesses prevalent among users of the mainstream diet in the United States today. Although there are many more cultural diets than are covered here, solid scientific research has not yet been collected to establish whether they provide any particular health benefits.

Asian diet. This diet is consumed predominantly by people living in China, Southeast Asia, Korea, and Japan. Rice is a staple and the center of the meal, and there is little or no use of dairy products. Soybean products are important sources of protein and calcium. Dishes incorporate many different ingredients and may be stir fried or steamed. This diet, in its traditional form, is low in fat and high in carbohydrates and sodium (Kittler and Sucher, 1989).

Mediterranean diet. The Mediterranean Basin is geographically defined as an inland sea that touches three continents—Europe, Asia, and Africa—and is surrounded by 15 almost contiguous countries: Spain, France, Italy, the former Yugoslavia, Albania, Greece, Turkey, Syria, Lebanon, Israel, Egypt, Libya, Tunisia, Algeria, and Morocco. Divided by language and, historically, by political and religious conflict, the Mediterranean countries have for centuries been joined by a similar diet of daily staples.

The Mediterranean diet consists of a daily intake of grains, potatoes, pasta, greens and other vegetables, fruit, beans and other legumes (e.g., lentils, split peas), nuts, cheese, and yogurt. Fish, poultry, eggs, sweets, and red meat are eaten less frequently. However, olive oil and garlic are almost always consumed in abundance (Spiller, 1991). In the case of Spain, France, and Italy, it is their southernmost parts that are considered Mediterranean, defined by their use of olive oil.

Another important aspect of the Mediterranean diet is its emphasis on less refined complex carbohydrates (e.g., pasta) in place of sugar and the highly refined starches generally consumed in the United States, even though direct evidence for benefit in reducing disease risk is limited. Anticipated reductions in colon cancer by diets high in grain fiber diets have been difficult to document epidemiologically, although inverse associations with vegetables have been seen repeatedly. However, reduced constipation and reduced risk of colonic diverticular disease are clear benefits (Willett et al., 1990).

It is interesting to note that in the northern areas of many of the European Mediterranean countries, where there is more use of butter, other animal fats, and meat, there is also a higher incidence of cancer (La Vecchia, 1993).

Traditional Native American Indian diet. Many foods used throughout the world today were probably first used by Indians of North, Central, and South America—for example, beans, corn, cranberries, peanuts, peppers, potatoes, pumpkin, squash, and tomatoes. Today, Native American Indians live in areas that are vastly different from one another, so there is no single typical diet. In fact, traditional diets are prepared infrequently except for ceremonial occasions. This is true even for the Arizona Hopi, who still live in old villages that their ancient ancestors inhabited (Kuhnlein and Calloway, 1977). Nevertheless, in many American Indian diets, corn is the staple food. It is eaten fresh roasted or boiled, as hominy, or as cornmeal in a variety of dishes. Meat is eaten when it can be obtained by hunting or fishing, but because it is so expensive to buy, it is used sparingly. Milk and dairy products are not used often because of a high incidence of lactose intolerance (lactose is the primary sugar in milk). Berries, wild plants, and roots are used when available (Robinson and Lawler, 1982).

Research base. The following provides an overview of research on the effectiveness of some components of the Asian, Mediterranean, and traditional Native American Indian diets in lowering some risk factors for disease.

Asian diet. In a cohort study of 265,000 people in Japan, consumption of miso soup (a food made from soybeans) appeared to reduce the risk of breast cancer (Hirayama, 1986) and stomach cancer (Hirayama, 1981). A similar inverse association was seen between stomach cancer and tofu intake (Hirayama, 1971). Furthermore, miso has been observed to inhibit formation of mammary tumors in rodents (Baggott et al., 1990) and may have antioxidant properties as well (Santiago et al., 1992).

Antioxidant properties have been proposed as a principal mechanism by which dietary compounds such as beta-carotene, vitamin E, indoles, and others exert cancer-preventive effects (Steinmetz and Potter, 1991a, 1991b). It has also been suggested that sea vegetables, perhaps through their high concentration of alginic acid, a type of dietary fiber, may decrease the risk of breast cancer (Teas et al., 1984;

229

Yamamoto et al., 1987). Beans and bean products, especially those derived from soybeans (e.g., miso, tofu, tempeh), also contain protease inhibitors (Messina and Barnes, 1991), isoflavonoids (Adlercreutz et al., 1987), and other compounds that may play roles in cancer prevention (Axelson et al., 1984).

Mediterranean diet. The high consumption of olive oil is considered a major contributor to the disease-preventive aspects of this diet. Olive oil is a monounsaturated fat, meaning that somewhere along the fat, or fatty acid, molecule there is a single site not completely "saturated" with hydrogen atoms. Substituting monounsaturated fats, such as olive oil, for saturated fat in the diet has been shown to reduce LDL cholesterol without affecting HDL cholesterol, thus providing an improved ratio (Mensink and Katan, 1992). In addition, monounsaturated fats in the diet have been found to reduce blood sugar and triglycerides in adult-onset diabetics (Garg et al., 1992).

In one of the first studies of its kind, researchers in France placed approximately 300 patients who had recently had a heart attack (myocardial infarction) on a Mediterranean type of diet and compared their incidence of having a second myocardial infarction with that of a control group of patients who were placed on the standard therapeutic diet. The experimental group consumed significantly more bread and fruit, a margarine with a fatty acid composition comparable to that of olive oil, and significantly less butter, cream, and meat than the control group. After a follow up of about 27 months, there were only 3 cardiac deaths and 5 nonfatal myocardial infarctions in the experimental group versus 16 cardiac deaths and 17 nonfatal myocardial infarctions in the control group (de Lorgeril et al., 1994). It is interesting to note that the patients on the Mediterranean type of diet had increases in blood levels of vitamin E and C while controls did not.

Garlic, a staple of the Mediterranean diet, also has been implicated as a major disease-preventive food. A growing number of reports in the medical literature suggest that garlic supplementation may be effective in decreasing serum cholesterol levels by as much as 15 to 20 percent and thus may have a protective effect against cardiovascular disease (Kleijnen et al., 1989; Turner, 1990). Many of these studies have been faulted for having methodological problems, although a recent meta-analysis of the various studies reporting a cholesterol-lowering effect found that garlic did appear to significantly reduce total serum cholesterol (Silagy and Neil, 1994).

There are also reports suggesting that garlic may prevent the development of cancer in humans (Dorant et al., 1993). Lin and colleagues

(1994) reported that processed garlic effectively reduced the amount of DNA damage caused by N-nitroso compounds, which are found in many foods such as cooked meat and have been implicated as carcinogens (cancer-causing compounds).

Traditional Native American Indian diet. In the case of the Hopi and Papago tribes, studies have shown that traditional foods have mineral content superior to federally provided commodity foods (Calloway et al., 1974). Followers of traditional Native American diets have found ways of maximizing available nutrients; an example is in the techniques of processing the corn used in tortillas, a staple in diets derived from the Mexican and Central American tradition. The corn is soaked in lime, which softens the skin of the corn kernels as well as increasing the calcium content of the resulting tortillas (Katz, 1987). Traditional lime soaking also liberates bound niacin in the corn. Because milled corn has been substituted for lime-soaked corn in Native American Indian diets, niacin deficiency has become a problem, and incidences of niacin-deficiency-induced pellagra have increased. Although few studies have been done on the possible disease-preventive aspects of the traditional Native American Indian diet, health surveys have found that heart disease and cancer, two diet-related diseases, are virtually nonexistent in some Indian populations, such as the Navajo (Reese, 1972).

The Trouble with Margarine

Margarine starts out as a liquid vegetable oil. However, it is converted to a form that will remain solid at room temperature, and thus resemble butter in texture, by a process called hydrogenation. The hydrogenation of vegetable oils changes the three dimensional structure of the fatty acids that make up the oil, converting the naturally occurring cis fatty acids to trans fatty acids. Oils composed primarily of hydrogenated fats typically melt at higher temperatures than those composed of non-hydrogenated (polyunsaturated) fats.

Over the past few decades many American physicians and nutrition experts have advised people to eat margarine in place of butter and lard, which contain "saturated" animal fats and are associated with an increased risk of developing coronary heart disease (CHD) However, recent evidence suggests that consuming significant amounts of margarine may pose health risks of its own, unrelated to problems caused by saturated animal fats. This is because trans fatty acids have been found to increase blood levels of low-density lipoprotein cholesterol; which is associated with an increased risk of developing CHD. At the same time, trans fatty acids also lower blood levels of high-density lipoprotein cholesterol, which has a protective effect against CHD. In addition, recent epidemiological studies have found a positive association between the consumption of trans fatty acids and CHD. Thus, it now appears that consuming margarine may not offer any health advantages over consuming butter (Willett and Ascherio, 1994).

In fact, because the average American takes in approximately 4-7 grams of these trans fatty acids daily by eating margarine and processed foods containing partially hydrogenated vegetable oils, the number of excess deaths in the United States attributed to the consumption of such food products is likely to be substantial.

Barriers and Key Issues Related to Alternative Diet and Nutrition Research

This chapter has so far dealt primarily with basic and clinical research relating to diet and nutrition interventions either for preventing or treating illness. However, to discuss such research without mentioning outside factors that will affect how research results are evaluated or disseminated to the public provides only a small part of the overall picture. Because nutritional and dietotherapy interventions affect an array of biochemical and physiological processes in the body, evaluating the interventions' effectiveness requires equally complex methodologies. Also of concern to those who work in this field is to research and develop "alternatives" to institutionalized nutrition and feeding programs that directly contribute to diet- and nutrition-related chronic disease. Finally, there is the issue of dissemination; no matter how good the research, it is valuable only if it reaches those who will benefit from it. Research data should be disseminated not only to the doctors or other health personnel who may prescribe such therapies, but also to the eventual target audience (i.e., the patients). Some of those issues are discussed below

Study Design

In most instances, it is virtually impossible to conduct a double-blind study of a dietary regimen. Patients obviously will know whether they are being fed a normal diet or a modified diet. Therefore, a single-blind design (in which the evaluator of the data is "blind" to who receives which treatment) is more appropriate for most dietary studies.

However, in some instances a double-blind study is appropriate, such as when all subjects are given a tasteless, colorless pill. Also, investigators must consider the possibility of a negative placebo ("nocebo") effect in the control group as well as a placebo effect in the treatment group. In other words, patients who think they are not getting the therapy may not get better because of this knowledge—just as patients who think they are receiving an effective treatment may get better spontaneously, independent of the therapy. (See the "Mind-Body Interventions" chapter for a discussion of placebo and nocebo effects.)

The recommendation of the recent OTA report Unconventional Cancer Treatments offers an example of one possible methodological approach to evaluating many nutritional interventions. As a practical approach to evaluating the treatments they had examined, the OTA report's authors proposed a "best case review" conceptually similar to approaches used by NCI for evaluating biological response modifiers (BRMs) (Office of Technology Assessment, 1990). Best case reviews are discussed in detail in appendix F.

BRMs are agents that exert anticancer effects in a novel manner. Unlike conventional cytoxic therapy, which kills tumor cells with slightly less chemical toxicity than chemotherapy, BRMs stimulate, or potentiate, the body's immune system to overcome or at least restrain the invading tumor. Most BRMs currently being investigated are genetically engineered copies of peptides found naturally in the human body; among them are tumor necrosis factor, interleukins, and interferons. At an early stage in this clinical research, NCI researchers recognized that because BRMs act biologically and not chemically, they had to be evaluated using a procedure that is significantly different from the one used for standard cytotoxic agents (Oldham, 1982). With this in mind, in 1978 NCI created a special Biological Response Modifiers Program to coordinate research to identify, study, and clinically evaluate BRMs.

Clinical evaluation of BRMs is difficult because determining the optimal dose or dosing schedule for the agent is critically important. Also important is the identification of responsive tumor types and even of the stage of disease and metabolic condition of patients who are treated (Creekmore et al., 1991; Hawkins et al., 1986; Oldham, 1985). Consequently, experts in BRM research advise against testing BRMs in large, controlled clinical trials (Phase III trials) until after these parameters have been optimized in careful individual tests of the proposed therapy in patients believed to be the most likely to show a favorable response (Creekmore et al., 1991; Hawkins et al., 1986; Oldham, 1985). This type of evaluation is inherently exploratory and observational; therefore, it cannot be conducted in the same rigidly stipulated way as a Phase III trial.

Because such studies demand the continual application of good clinical and scientific judgment, they are demanding of the time and energy of investigators, who typically are experts keenly interested in the therapy under evaluation. This time-consuming process is necessary because the consequence of proceeding prematurely to a Phase III trial is an inconclusive or falsely negative result. Since dietary and nutritional interventions often affect biology in ways at least as complicated as the anticancer BRMs currently being evaluated by NCI, recommendations concerning the evaluation of BRMs should apply to the evaluation of many diet and nutrition interventions.

Furthermore, careful scientific judgment is needed as to when sufficient evaluation has gone on and confirmation is in order. For example, there is general agreement in the scientific community that the time is now at hand to "confirm" the efficacy of megadose antioxidants in the prevention of coronary artery disease progression in a large Phase III trial (Steinberg, 1993). This assessment is correct even though such trials are costly, and there is always a risk of a false negative result if all the relevant parameters have not yet been fully optimized. The interaction of a variety of factors in producing a therapeutic outcome would be expected to be of particular importance in biological or nutritional therapies (Christensen, 1993; Weglicki et al., 1993).

An excellent example of the superiority of good scientific judgment over the premature use of the controlled clinical trial is the discovery by George C. Cotzias that L-dopa is an effective treatment for Parkinson's disease (Cotzias et al., 1967). When Cotzias began his studies, L-dopa was regarded as an interesting therapeutic idea that had been determined to be without utility in a series of careful clinical trials that included controlled double-blind, Phase III methodology (Fehling, 1966; Lasagna, 1972). Had Cotzias not used good scientific judgment and persistent curiosity by testing L-dopa in careful, uncontrolled protocols that included larger doses than in the earlier, methodologically flawed trials, it is entirely possible that recognition of L-dopa's enormous value would have been delayed for decades or never recognized at all.

Phase III trials of orthomolecular therapy, for example, may also require a similarly innovative approach. One possibility, after preliminary, dose-optimization studies have been completed, is to randomly allocate suitable patients to conventional or orthomolecular programs. Much of the evaluation would have to be "open"; however, symptom-rating scales could be scored by observers unaware, or "blinded," to which patients received which treatment.

First and foremost, however, is the requirement for an open-minded approach by intelligent and skeptical clinical investigators whose effort is respected by their peers. Such studies also will require good-faith cooperation from academic medical units and the support provided by adequate research funding. Evaluation of the research will have to include a recognition that initially negative results do not prove a therapy valueless: the therapy may merely have been incorrectly tested. Investigators should strive to develop hypotheses that can be objectively tested. Even when testing mechanisms are novel, they must be rigorous and reproducible by independent investigators, and their results must be convincing to open-minded but skeptical reviewers. These objectives can and must be achieved. The cost of not achieving them may be the unnecessary delay or, worse, the complete dismissal of an effective treatment for a previously untreatable debilitating illness.

Alternatives to Federal and Other "Institutionalized" Programs That Influence Diet and Contribute to Chronic Disease

Not even increased openmindedness in mainstream research or increased Federal funds for research may be enough to get effective alternative diet and nutrition prophylactic and therapeutic treatments into more general use. Indeed, without some significant changes in Americans' beliefs and expectations about food and nutrition, promising research results—whether alternative or conventional—will have little impact. For example, studies indicate that Americans are quite aware of the relationship between nutrition and health (Cotugna et al., 1992). However, during the past two decades they have made little apparent progress toward meeting the RDAs (U.S. Department of Agriculture and U.S. Department of Health and Human Services, 1990), which recent research indicates may already be too low for many vitamins and nutrients. Although there has been an increase in consumption of low-fat milk and a decrease in the consumption of meat and eggs during the past decade, USDA's 1987-88 national food consumption survey (U.S. Department of Agriculture, 1988) indicated that Americans, on average, eat only one serving of fruit or fruit juice and two servings of vegetables per day. This amounts to roughly half the recommended Federal Government minimum (Patterson et al., 1990) and much less than the minimum advocated by many others. Furthermore, the consumption of saturated fat by women has consistently remained around 13 percent of total calories (Welsh, 1991).

Numerous Government programs and information dissemination channels exist that potentially could have a major positive influence on American dietary habits. Unfortunately, many, if not most, are having a negative rather than a positive impact on Americans' dietary knowledge, beliefs, and practices. These programs and channels include:

- Government feeding and food support programs,
- Public education and the mass media,
- School-based and worksite programs, and
- Health care provider settings.

Government feeding and food support programs. The Food and Nutrition Service of USDA administers 14 food assistance programs that aim to "provide needy people with access to a more nutritious diet, to improve the eating habits of the Nation's children, and to stabilize farm prices through the distribution of surplus foods" (U.S. Department of Agriculture, 1993a). More than 25.4 million people participated in the Food Stamp Program in 1992, and more than 5.6 million participated in the Special Supplemental Food Program for Women, Infants, and Children (WIC). In addition, approximately 25 million children participate in the National School Lunch Program (NSLP) each day, and an average of 900,000 people participate daily in the Nutrition Program for the Elderly.

Studies have reported that participation in the Food Stamp Program or the size of the food stamp benefits, or both, have had a positive impact on the availability of nutrients. However, the effect of these programs on nutrient intake is negligible. Only WIC was found to increase intake of numerous nutrients, including iron, calcium, and vitamin C, among pregnant women (Rush et al., 1988) and preschool children (Rush et al., 1988). Moreover, when participants in NSLP were compared to nonparticipants, increased nutrient intakes of vitamin A, vitamin B6, calcium, and magnesium (Hanes et al., 1984)—vitamins typically deficient in the school-aged population (Nelson et al., 1981)—were observed in the NSLP participant population.

Whether these various feeding programs provide adequate nutrition for Americans deserves critical analysis. For example, NSLP has been criticized for maintaining its outdated purpose of preventing nutritional deficiencies without including food patterns that would prevent such prevailing chronic diseases as heart disease, hypertension, cancer, and atherosclerosis (American School Food Service Association, 1991; Citizens' Commission, 1990). In light of the findings on the positive effects of fruits and vegetables (Steinmetz and Potter, 1991a, 1991b) and the negative effects of saturated fats (Willett, 1990) on health and chronic disease, it may be necessary to modify NSLP to at least meet the Dietary Guidelines for Americans (U.S. Department of Agriculture and U.S. Department of Health and Human Services, 1990).

In September 1993, assistant secretary of agriculture Ellen Haas announced plans to improve NSLP by doubling the amount of fresh fruits and vegetables supplied to schools and reducing the amount of fat in commodity foods (U.S. Department of Agriculture, 1993b). This modification is urgently needed to update NSLP so that it will be in line with the current scientific findings on diet and disease. Similar modifications should be made across all USDA feeding and food assistance programs to help Americans consume a better diet.

Furthermore, for the agricultural system to meet even the current USDA dietary guidelines, adjustments are required in the mix and output of farm products. Appropriate new food policies need to be in place to support such changes. For example, in the commodity area, the price and income support programs put a premium on milk fat, and surplus disposal operations are designed to increase the supply of high-fat butter and cheese on the market at artificially low prices. This system runs counter to encouraging better diet and nutrition in the population.

Public Education and Role of the Mass Media

The primary goal of public nutrition education is to bring about behavioral changes in individuals', groups', and populations' dietary patterns presumed to be detrimental to health. The educational program is designed to provide enough knowledge so that healthy choices in nutrition can be made. The mass media, including magazines, newspapers, and television, are a major source of nutrition information for the public (American Dietetic Association and International Food Information Council, 1990). An analysis of mass initiatives in the area of promoting healthy diet and nutrition choices indicates that such campaigns can be useful in setting the stage for behavior change (DeJong and Winsten, 1990). One example is a joint NCI-Kellogg (the cereal manufacturer) initiative that promoted consumption of a high-fiber diet through advertising and food labeling on cereal boxes. On the basis of purchase data from supermarkets in the Baltimore and Washington, D.C., metropolitan area, the purchase of high-fiber cereals increased 37 percent in the 48 weeks of the initiative (Levy and Stokes, 1987).

Mass media-based education programs not only affect the intermediary steps to behavior change but also have proved to have a more direct influence on health, such as affecting changes in eating patterns and disease risk factors. For instance, the Finnish North Karelia Project showed that education programs using mass media strategies can markedly reduce certain coronary heart disease risk factors (Vartiainnen et al., 1991).

In recent years, the social marketing approach, which draws marketing techniques from the private sector and focuses on the thorough understanding of consumer needs and opinions, has been used increasingly in health promotion campaigns (J. Ling, 1992). This approach can yield promising new insights into consumer behavior and into product and strategy design (Walsh et al., 1993), thereby enhancing the efficacy of a health promotion initiative.

The National Heart, Lung, and Blood Institute's (NHLBI's) National High Blood Pressure Education Program (NHBPEP) and National Cholesterol Education Program are examples of Federal public education programs that extensively use mass media and social marketing strategies to convey health messages to the public. Both programs employ the strategy of focusing on raising knowledge and awareness on two tiers: among the public and among health care professionals. From NHBPEP's inception in 1972, awareness, treatment, and control rates for high blood pressure have increased dramatically (Rocella and Lenfant, 1992), and age-adjusted stroke mortality has fallen nearly 57 percent (Rocella and Horan, 1988).

Unfortunately, few nutrition messages in the mass media promote a healthy diet. Indeed, advertisements for foods that are high in sodium, fat, or sugar often compete directly against nutrition messages designed to help people make better food choices. For example, breakfast cereals, snacks, and fast foods are among the most heavily advertised products on television programs aimed at children (Cotugna, 1988), and the television "diet" consists of foods primarily of low nutritional value (Story and Faulkner, 1990). Television viewing also appears to affect food consumption. Studies have reported, for instance, that the amount of time spent watching television directly correlates with the request, purchase, and consumption of foods advertised on television (Clancy-Hepburn et al., 1974; Gorn and Goldberg, 1982; Taras et al., 1989). Consequently, the mass media, the food industry, the Government, and health professionals should collaborate to broadcast health promotion messages more extensively. One such example is the airing of public service announcements on Saturday morning children's television by a major fruit-processing company, which was prompted by the "Five-a-Day for Better Health" campaign initiated by NCI and the Produce for Better Health Foundation.

School-based and Worksite Programs

Schools are an ideal setting in which to model and encourage healthy lifestyle behaviors. More than 95 percent of American youth aged 5 to 17 are enrolled in schools (U.S. Department of Education, 1990). School-based nutrition education and physical activity programs appear to be ideal venues for effecting change in lifestyle-related risk factors for heart disease, cancer, and obesity. Children eat one to two meals per day in school, and the cafeteria can be a learning laboratory where students can practice and experience positive nutrition habits they learn from the school curriculum. Previous studies in school-based cardiovascular research, including the "Know Your Body" program (Walter et al., 1988), have shown that health promotion in schools can have a favorable impact on nutrition knowledge and diet-related skills (Contento et al., 1992) as well as on specific outcomes, such as blood cholesterol level, carbohydrate intake, fitness, blood pressure, and smoking status (Stone et al., 1989). In addition, school-based health promotion programs have had positive impacts on obesity (Resnicow, 1993).

Additional research of longer duration that includes multiple components (school food service, curriculum, family outreach) is needed to determine the degree to which schools can affect the exercise and diet habits of children. These studies could be similar to the ongoing NHLB-funded "Child and Adolescent Trial for Cardiovascular Health" and the "Eat Well and Keep Moving" project at the Tesseract schools in Baltimore, MD.

Worksites are another important channel for promoting nutrition. Nearly 70 percent of adults between the ages of 18 and 65 are employed (U.S. Bureau of the Census, 1986). Thus worksites provide access to large numbers of people and offer the opportunity to make environmental and social norm changes that support healthy eating (Sorensen et al., 1986). Indeed, worksite educational programs have been shown effective in weight control (Sherman et al., 1989), cardiovascular risk reduction (O'Brien and Dedmon, 1990), smoking cessation

(Windsor and Lowe, 1989), and cancer screening (Heimendinger et al., 1990). By modifying cafeteria menus and policy for meals served at corporate functions to support healthier choices and allowing time at work for nutrition education activity, worksites can be promising vehicles in modifying employees' eating habits. However, efforts should be made to overcome low participation rates and high dropout rates in worksite programs (American Dietetic Association, 1986).

Education of Health Care Providers and Patient Counseling

Patients place a great deal of credibility in the nutrition advice given to them by their physicians (American Dietetic Association, 1990). Many physicians, however, fail to provide such advice to their patients. A study by the University of Minnesota found that only 10 percent of surveyed physicians gave nutrition advice to more than 80 percent of their patients (Kottke et al., 1988). Although many physicians view nutrition as an effective tool that should be used in medical practice, there are significant barriers that keep physicians from adequately counseling their patients on issues of diet and nutrition. These barriers include lack of time, adequate staffs, and insufficient insurance coverage (Glanz and Gilboy, 1992). In addition, physicians' perceived inability to effectively alter their patients' lifestyle practices contributes to this problem (Wechsler et al., 1983). Another major contributor to physicians failing to give their patients nutrition counseling may be their own lack of nutrition knowledge. More than one study of practicing physicians has found that only about half of those surveyed felt prepared to provide dietary counseling to their patients (Kimm et al., 1990).

This lack of adequate nutrition knowledge among physicians may be partly due to a deficient nutrition curriculum in U.S. medical schools. In fact, a survey of 45 U.S. medical schools by the National Academy of Sciences found the state of nutrition education in medical schools to be largely inadequate to meet the needs of patients and the medical profession (National Research Council, 1985). Improved standards for nutrition education in U.S. medical schools appear to be necessary if the vast preventive and therapeutic role of nutrition in health care is to be exploited to the fullest.

In the context of alternative diets or therapies, an additional barrier to effective counseling by conventional health care providers is the sometimes outright hostility toward alternative therapies held by these providers. For example, surveys have indicated that many cancer patients do not tell conventional providers that they are pursuing alternative therapies, in part, because the conventional health care provider is often unsupportive or skeptical of such therapies (Eisenberg et al., 1993). In extreme cases, some conventional providers will refuse to treat a patient whom the provider knows is seeing an alternative practitioner for the same condition. Such attitudes are substantial hurdles to overcome for both the adequate and objective evaluation and dissemination of effective alternative therapies.

Another problem physicians may encounter when trying to give nutrition counseling to patients is that American society is becoming increasingly multicultural. Health professionals often have difficulty communicating with clients whose cultural heritage is different from their own. This problem is particularly acute when a physician is dealing with someone who comes from a cultural group or society where health and religion are intertwined (Kittler and Sucher, 1989). For example, "looking good" is a common goal in many technologically developed societies, but various cultural groups have a different view. Mexican Americans, African Americans, and other ethnic groups do not share the typical American concepts of appropriate body size, particularly for adult women (Massara, 1980; Schreiber and Homiak, 1981; Stern et al., 1982). It has been suggested that the "mainstream" standards for weight in adult women are, in fact, based more on the value of thinness—which is related to youth and higher socioeconomic status (Cassidy, 1991; Sobal, 1991)—than on science or epidemiology (Ritenbaugh, 1982).

Therefore, successful nutritional counseling depends on culturally sensitive communication strategies; health care practitioners must be both knowledgeable about general ethnic, regional, and religious food habits and aware of individual practices and preferences. Health care professionals can improve cross-cultural counseling through a four-step process of self-evaluation, preinterview research, in-depth interviewing, and unbiased data analysis. A detailed description of the rationale for these steps can be found in Kittler and Sucher (1990).

However, the success of cross-cultural counseling cannot always be measured by a patient's adherence to a diet. Differences in worldview, traditional food habits, and factors that influence dietary adaptation may be of greater consequence to a client than the health implications of the diet. The best chances of compliance occur when the health care practitioner is aware of personal cultural assumptions and is knowledgeable about the cultural heritage of a patient and its specific influences on the patient's food habits, and when diet modifications are made with consideration for individual cultural and personal preferences.

241

There are some examples of successful intervention programs that have been based on in-depth studies of the total context of ethnic food consumption. Hall (1987) noted that materials designed for Mexican-American diabetics not only had to be translated into Spanish but also had to be redesigned, incorporating culturally relevant concepts, methods, meal plans, and activities, to be effective. The same study also found it advisable to incorporate recommendations for traditional home remedies that have been shown scientifically to be of value in the treatment of diabetes. For example, a diabetes intervention directed toward Mexican Americans may include the use of cooked prickly pear cactus (nopales), which has long been used in Mexican folk medicine to control diabetes (Frati-Munari et al., 1983). Traditional remedies, however, are encouraged only as complements to biomedical treatments; the Hall program suggests that prescribed diabetes medications be taken with traditional herbal teas (Hall, 1987).

Another excellent intervention program is a physician-based system of dietary risk assessment and intervention, designed for use with low-literacy, low-income southern populations (Ammerman et al., 1991, 1992). This program focuses on the top 20 contributors of saturated fat and cholesterol that, based on the National Health and Nutrition Examination Survey II (NHANES II) data, are commonly found in the diets of African-American populations in the South. Attention is also given to traditional southern food preparation practices, such as baking with lard, frying with vegetable shortening, and seasoning vegetables with meat fat (Ammerman et al., 1991). All assessment and intervention materials are based on food rather than on nutrients. Diet change recommendations are linked with recipes in a southern-style cookbook.

For those who do little cooking at home (a growing population), information is provided on how to eat sensibly at fast-food restaurants. Low-cost dietary alternatives and southern food preferences are emphasized throughout the materials, which are written at the fifth- to sixth-grade reading level. The goal of the program is to reduce saturated fat and cholesterol intake while preserving ethnic eating patterns—that is, to adapt the traditional diet rather than introduce a radical transformation of eating patterns (Ammerman et al., 1992). Evaluation of the program shows promising results, both in the physicians' administration of the program and in changes in patients' attitudes. Currently underway is a 5-year, randomized clinical trial of the effectiveness of the program in lowering cholesterol among patients in rural Virginia and North Carolina (Ammerman et al., 1992). In addition, a "northern" version of this approach and these materials is being tested. Programs of the type described by Hall and Ammerman cannot be developed in the absence of the necessary data specific to the ethnic group being targeted. Multidisciplinary research with a nutritional-anthropological focus is necessary to explore these issues further.

Research Needs and Opportunities in Diet and Nutrition

It is virtually impossible to list all of the research opportunities in diet and nutrition that should be pursued more extensively and vigorously. Rather, this section presents broad areas where the data indicate that more intense efforts might yield significant results.

Optimal Levels of Vitamins, Minerals, and Other Nutritional Supplements

Although there have been many studies to determine the effect of a single vitamin deficiency, few studies have attempted to determine the optimal dietary requirement for most vitamins and minerals. There is increasing evidence that the consumption of nutrients at RDA levels is not adequate for promoting optimal health. Thus, nutritional supplementation above the RDAs for many vitamins and minerals may be indicated. The following areas of research in vitamin and nutritional supplementation are likely to yield significant results:

- Research is needed to determine how and at what levels such antioxidants as vitamins E and C and beta-carotene provide optimal immune enhancement.

- There is growing evidence that some carotenoids can directly affect cancer cells. Mechanisms may include free radical and other charged particle quenching, which would result in less damage to DNA; decreased adenylate cyclase activity, which would decrease proliferation of the cancer; generation of regulatory proteins that could alter cell cycles and metabolism; and other mechanisms as yet unknown (Bendich, 1991). Carotenoids have been shown to protect cells from mutagens. Further, research into the direct effects of antioxidants on cancer cells and on DNA repair mechanism is needed.

- Research is needed into the role that many vitamins play aside from being enzyme cofactors. In view of the interest in free radicals or reactive molecular intermediates in the pathogenesis of

243

a variety of medical and neurological diseases, there is a wealth of opportunities for research on the ability of vitamins and other nutritional supplements to prevent or reverse the effects of these types of molecules.

- Research is needed in the United States to provide data from controlled studies to verify mostly European work on the clinical efficacy of minerals such as magnesium and selenium in the treatment of disease. More extensive intervention studies are needed to determine whether adding mineral supplements will improve the preventive effects of other dietary interventions (e.g., salt and fat restriction) against cardiovascular disease, and to verify the promising effects from Europe in prevention of abnormalities in pregnancy. In particular, the extended study of magnesium treatment of bronchial asthma is also indicated. There are already many clues on magnesium's mechanisms of action, and there are many data on clinical efficacy in a number of clinical diseases or complaints. It would be more feasible, not to mention less expensive—to set up double-blind intervention studies supplementing subjects' existing diets with magnesium or selenium, rather than try to get them to completely change their diet to include more foods containing these minerals.

- A recent National Institutes of Health (NIH) report (1994) on calcium recommended that optimal levels of intake by women to prevent osteoporosis should be 1,500 mg per day. Because the usual American intake of magnesium is no more than 300 mg per day, such a level of calcium intake would constitute a calcium-magnesium ratio of 5:1. It is noteworthy that in Finland, where the prevalence of osteoporosis is high (Simonen, 1991), the average calcium-magnesium intake ratio is 4:1, a ratio that has been associated with the highest death rate in young to middle-aged men from ischemic heart disease in the world (Karppanen et al., 1978). An NIH consensus development conference on magnesium, similar to the one held recently on calcium, would provide a much-needed forum for elucidating other avenues of research that may be warranted on this important mineral.

Alternative Dietary Lifestyles and Cultural Diets

Studies of Seventh-Day Adventists, macrobiotic vegetarians, and populations eating Asian and Mediterranean types of diets indicate that these groups are at lower risk of heart disease and some cancers.

Likewise, studies usually demonstrate that blood pressure and blood lipid levels fall when participants follow a vegetarian diet (Cooper et al., 1982; Kestin et al., 1989; Margetts et al., 1986; Rouse et al., 1986). Prospective studies of vegetarian groups other than California Seventh-Day Adventists have found a decreased risk of heart disease and cancer as well as a decreased risk of death from all causes (Burr and Butland, 1988; Burr and Sweetnam, 1982; Chang-Claude et al., 1992; Frentzel-Beyme et al., 1988). Vegetarian populations, including Seventh-Day Adventists, also appear to be at decreased risk of other diseases such as gallbladder disease (Pixley et al., 1985) and diabetes mellitus (Snowdon and Phillips, 1985). Furthermore, such vegetarian diets as advocated under the Pritikin program appear to improve control of diabetes (Barnard et al., 1983).

Accordingly, studies of populations eating vegetarian and some cultural diets provide evidence that alternative dietary patterns may have a major impact on disease risk. Specifically, such studies show evidence of potentially profound implications for the risk of developing heart disease, certain cancers (such as colon or prostate cancer), and other chronic illnesses, such as diabetes. For example, in addition to containing large amounts of antioxidants, beans, leafy green vegetables, whole grains, many fruits, and fish are very rich in magnesium (Seelig, 1980). The Pritikin, Mediterranean, Seventh-Day Adventist, and macrobiotic diets are, thus, rich in magnesium. Studies have shown that magnesium supplementation of animals on atherosclerosis inducing diets protects against arterial damage. Animal studies also have shown that magnesium deficiency increases hypercholesterolemia (especially the LDLs) and increases vulnerability to oxidative damage (Rayssiguier et al., 1989, 1993). It has recently been shown that magnesium repletion and vitamin E are mutually enhancing in protecting against magnesium deficiency- and stress hormone-induced cardiac necrosis (Freedman et al., 1990, 1991; Guenther et al., 1992, 1994a; Weglicki et al., 1992), and that vitamin E and magnesium deficiency shortens the time needed to induce atherosclerosis (Guenther et al., 1994b).

There is experimental evidence that magnesium deficiency (at least in very young rodents) can cause leukemias and lymphomas (Averdunk and Guenther, 1985; Battifora et al., 1968, 1969; Bois, 1968; Bois and Beaulnes, 1966; Bois et al., 1969; Hass et al., 1981a, 1981b; Jasmin, 1963; McCreary et al., 1967), especially when there is also deficiency in such antioxidants as vitamins C and E, and in selenium (Aleksandrowicz, 1975). The protective role of magnesium against certain diseases may be supported by epidemiological findings about geographic areas low in magnesium where there is a high prevalence of human and cattle lymphoid neoplasms, leukemias, and gastric cancers (Aleksandrowicz, 1973; Aleksandrowicz and Skotnicki, 1982; Seelig, 1979, 1993).

The studies of vegetarian groups and Asian and Mediterranean populations are congruent with the growing body of studies in other populations that indicate a potentially profound role for dietary factors in the etiology of various chronic illnesses. These include growing evidence of the undesirable health effects of meat and high-fat dairy intake and the health promotion effects of abundant consumption of vegetables, fruits, monounsaturated fats, garlic, and whole cereal grains.

The translation of the findings of these animal and human studies into therapeutic approaches may alleviate the burden of some of these diseases. Equally important are measures that are being taken by industry and the Federal Government to support healthful dietary habits. Studies need to be undertaken on a wide variety of alternative diets that have been found to be beneficial, including:

- vegetarian diets,

- ultra-low-fat diets,

- high-polyunsaturated-fat diets,

- Mediterranean-type diets, and

- diets rich in soy foods, such as East Asian diets.

Initiatives also are needed along the following lines:

- There is a need for a more critical examination of dairy products on health, especially regarding fractures.

- There is a need for a more critical look at the effects of meat consumption on health—for example, on coronary heart disease, colon cancer, and fractures.

- More detailed data are needed on the effects of fruits, vegetables, monounsaturated fats, and garlic on cancer, coronary heart disease, cataracts, stroke, and so forth.

- There is a need for more information on the long-term effects of overrefined carbohydrates (e.g., sugar) on the human metabolism and immune functioning.

246

Qualitative research is needed on various aspects of cultural diets and the effects of cultural beliefs on health and illnesses. Such studies might include the following:

- Qualitative research on ethnic concepts of appropriate body shape and size by gender, age, and socioeconomic status.

- Qualitative research on ethnic definitions of health and approaches to health.

- Qualitative research on ethnic attitudes and approaches to dieting.

- Research on how the types of programs described by Hall and Ammerman can be adapted for use with other ethnic populations, and evaluation of such programs in meeting biomedical and nutritional goals (e.g., reduction of cholesterol levels).

The goal in all this research should be to elucidate categories and concepts of importance to members of the public and to determine which of their traditions should be encouraged. These data are critical in achieving the larger biomedical nutritional goal of a well-nourished and healthy population by using terms that can be understood by the lay public, especially members of minorities.

Studies on the Relationship Between Energy Consumption and Disease

Data that have been accumulating since the early part of this century indicate that over consumption of energy may contribute to chronic illness, while restriction of energy may promote health and prolong life. Moreschi (1909) demonstrated that underfeeding could impede the growth of tumors. Rous (1914) confirmed and expanded those findings, but no further progress occurred until 1935 when McKay demonstrated a broad disease preventive effect, as well as extension of lifespan, as a result of caloric restriction (McKay et al., 1935).

In 1940, Albert Tannenbaum demonstrated that energy restriction per se in rodents can inhibit tumor initiation and growth, that increased caloric use stimulated by exogenous thyroid may inhibit certain cancers and metastases, and that fats can promote the growth, in many circumstances, of already initiated tumors (Tannenbaum, 1940, 1942a, 1942b, 1945a, 1945b). Later, Jose reported that Australian

Aborigines who became malnourished upon weaning, and who regularly developed a decreased ability to produce antibodies, unexpectedly showed increased proliferative responses of T lymphocytes upon stimulation with certain phytomitogens (Jose et al., 1969).

As research progressed, it was demonstrated that protein-energy restriction could cause in animals the same enhanced response to phytomitogens seen in Australian Aborigines. In addition, experiments revealed that even at presumably dangerously low protein levels (3 to 5 percent), cell-mediated immunity remained intact and in some cases appeared to be greatly increased, as in the development of cell-mediated responsiveness to stimulation with minute doses of antigen. Additional effects were augmentation of delayed allergic reactions, increased capacity for lymphoid cells to initiate graft-versus-host reactions, up-regulated cellular immune responses against syngeneic and allogeneic tumor cells, and increased capacity to resist certain types of viral infections (Good et al., 1977, 1980).

A direct attempt to follow a high-quality energy-restricted diet as a health measure has been advocated for a number of years by R.L. Walford, M.D. at UCLA (Walford and Crew, 1989). Recently Walford participated in a 2-year experiment in which he monitored the health of eight humans growing and recycling all food in the 3.15-acre hermetically sealed experimental ecological enclosure called Biosphere 2 in Oracle, AZ. The eight Biosphere 2 subjects underwent 24 months of moderate caloric restriction (1,700 to 2,400 kcal per day, despite a heavy work load) with a very high quality semi-vegetarian diet in rigidly controlled circumstances. Physiologic changes in the eight volunteers over the 2-year stay were dramatic, with blood glucose dropping 15 percent, cholesterol dropping to an average of 125 mg/ dL, and blood pressure dropping to low normal (Walford et al., 1992). Blood white cell counts also decreased, which, along with the decrease in glucose, mirrored changes seen in restricted monkeys and restricted rodents. Further tests are ongoing, but preliminary results thus suggest that humans respond, at least initially, much like all other mammals tested on dietary energy restriction. A great deal more study is needed to see if the immune-enhancing, life-prolonging effect of an energy-restricted diet in lower animals also is manifest in humans.

Patient Education Issues

Research shows that physicians can have a beneficial impact on their patients' lifestyle practices (Inui et al., 1976; Leon et al., 1987; Russell et al., 1979). For example, brief anti-smoking advice given to patients by general practitioners has been shown to reduce patients' smoking rates by as much as 7 percent (Russell et al., 1979), which is a potentially huge public health impact given the prevalence of smoking. Similar changes in populations' eating patterns, such as reduction in saturated fat intake, could also have a huge impact on decreasing the rates of diseases, such as coronary heart disease and certain cancers, where diet has been implicated in causation. What is lacking, however, are incisive screening questions that physicians can use to quickly assess a patient's nutritional risk within the time constraints of a visit to or by a physician. Research is necessary into this issue to determine what screening questions would be both timely and effective in identifying points of dietary intervention to reduce risk.

Broadening the Database on Intervention Information

Something that became apparent during the development of this chapter was the wealth of diet and nutrition information outside the regular electronic databases, such as MEDLINE. There is a great deal of social science and agriculture literature relating to diet and nutrition, as well as in the world literature, that is often overlooked. Furthermore, literature from before 1965 is not routinely stored in electronic databases; if it is, abstracts are not included. For example, dietary modification and the use of vitamins to prevent and affect disease was the subject of intense research in pre-World War II Germany (Gerson, 1929, 1935; Sauerbruch and Herrmannsdorfer, 1928) and, to a lesser extent, in the rest of Europe (Hval, 1932) and even in the United States (Banyai, 1931; Emerson, 1929; Mayer and Kugelmass, 1929). However, much of this information has been lost to many contemporary nutrition researchers because it is not cataloged in present-day electronic databases.

Much of this older information, as well as information from such countries as China, India, and Japan, is university-based clinical research that, if made more widely available, might be of enormous value to researchers investigating similar phenomena today. A fruitful research project could be to screen the older data, the social science and agricultural data, and the world data that are available in foreign databases to develop a bibliography of references that might be added to nationwide databases such as MEDLINE. The World Health Organization literature, for example, would be a good starting point in looking for information relating to databases on diet and nutrition research in other countries.

Attention should be given to examining many of the widespread popular and folk dietary suggestions for maintaining health or controlling illness. For example, cranberry juice has long been known as a folk remedy for controlling or curing bladder infections in women. Recent analyses of this popular treatment show that it actually is effective (Walsh, 1992). As noted previously, the prickly pear has long been used by Mexican Americans as a treatment for diabetes. Biochemical studies have shown that it does have a mild glucose-lowering effect, which is due to its content of glucose-6-phosphate isomerase (FratiMunari et al., 1983; Ibanez-Camacho and Roman-Ramos, 1979). Laboratory testing of the efficacy of ethnic foods used as remedies, as was done with the prickly pear cactus, might provide interesting results.

Moreover, there are literally hundreds of popular folk sayings that might warrant serious scrutiny, first with literature, then with appropriate laboratory and clinical tests. Some examples are "When people feel weak, they should eat meat"; "People with lung disorders should avoid dairy products" (especially common in traditional medical systems such as Ayurveda); "An apple a day keeps the doctor away."

Such research should be supplemented by in-depth qualitative research on how and when these remedies are used.

Specific Disease Areas

AIDS. AIDS is a chronic disease characterized by progressive decline in immunocompetence. Because many vitamins and nutritional supplements are biological response modifiers that have been shown to stimulate or enhance immune response, the potential areas of fruitful research in this area are limitless.

There is at least preliminary evidence that vitamin A or beta-carotene (its precursor) decreases the immune deficiency that results when animals are exposed to a wide variety of immuno-compromising conditions such as trauma, infection, irradiation, and treatment with cytotoxic agents (Seifter et al., 1982, 1983a, 1983b, 1984). There is evidence suggesting that vitamin A supplementation in immune-compromised individuals may be necessary to replace a vitamin A deficiency caused by HIV infection (Lack et al., 1993; Semba et al., 1993). Many other vitamins and nutritional supplements that have been shown to affect immune status also may be potentially potent tools for fighting this deadly infection. This area is ripe for intensive research.

Cancer. It is well accepted that cancer and its treatment can cause malnutrition and that malnutrition itself predicts a poor outcome (DeWys et al., 1980). In general, however, oral dietary treatments for cancer have not been evaluated by mainstream medicine for the possible prevention of malnutrition or for the possible effect on the course of the disease in cancer patients. There are no nutritional recommendations per se for the cancer patient in mainstream oncology (Office of Technology Assessment, 1990), and no diet is currently recommended publicly by NCI or the American Cancer Society for use in cancer treatment. Those nutritional support measures that are offered usually come only after patients have reached advanced stages of cancer and have become malnourished, often as a result of side effects of their treatment (e.g., chemotherapy)(American College of Physicians, 1989; Shike and Brennan, 1989).

Little is understood about the nutritional requirements of cancers. However, there is growing evidence that many types of tumors have an increased need for iron in order to grow (Elliott et al., 1993; Weinberg, 1992). Red meat is one of the best sources of iron, and iron from red meat continues to be absorbed even if body stores of iron are plentiful (Ascherio and Willett, 1994). Therefore, there is at least a theoretical basis for proposing that cancer patients eat a primarily vegetarian diet to slow the growth of their tumors. Furthermore, although the epidemiological data provide solid support for recommendations to consume an abundance of vegetables and fruits or vitamin supplements to prevent cancer, there is a need for research on the effects of such nutritional interventions on individuals who already have cancer. Immunological parameters such as certain immune cell activity or levels of certain cytokines (immune-cell-activating compounds) would provide information about whether such diets do or do not increase the body's ability to attack cancer cells.

The 1990 OTA report Unconventional Cancer Treatments suggested that at least certain aspects of most of the unconventional dietary regimens for cancer it reviewed (e.g., intake of fresh fruits and vegetables and reduction or elimination of sodium and fat) are consistent with current Federal dietary recommendations about reducing the risk of contracting certain types of cancer and other illnesses (Office of Technology Assessment, 1990). The controversial aspects of these therapies, according to OTA, is the idea that dietary treatment can cause the regression of cancer. It is possible that the earlier such dietary regimens are begun, the more effective they are. It would be informative to look at various aspects of some of these regimens to determine whether they conform to basic biochemical and immunological research relating micronutrient manipulation to improving immune function or the inhibition of cancer cell growth. For example, Simone (1983) suggested that coffee enemas may increase absorption of vitamin A. There is evidence that vitamin A may play a vital role in boosting immune function (see the section on orthomolecular medicine in this chapter). The Gerson diet is estimated to provide approximately 100,000 IU of vitamin A daily (Seifter, 1988). Further studies are needed to confirm the ability of such measures to increase the absorption of micronutrients.

Heart disease and diabetes. Studies such as those using fat-restricted or fat-modified diets (i.e., intake of greater amounts of monounsaturated fats) have produced quite credible evidence suggesting not only that cardiovascular disease may be stabilized through such methods, but also that death rates from cardiovascular disease can be greatly reduced. Dietary intervention for coronary heart disease may find broader application if attempts are made to further both clinical research and use. A systematic review of the literature, broader clinical evaluations, and the development of clinical guidelines could lead to general acceptance. Efforts to disseminate information and transfer technology may be essential. Cost comparisons with conventional treatments may be instructive.

The following are specific areas that are likely to yield fruitful results:

- Sufficient evidence now exists to compel larger scale, multi-center, randomized clinical trials of modified diets such as the Ornish regimen, the Mediterranean-type diet, and high-soy-content diets.

- Dean Ornish's program relies heavily on relaxation techniques as well as fat restriction. It would be informative to know which aspect of his regimen contributes most to the regression of heart disease. If the relaxation component turns out to be a significant factor, this knowledge could potentially save the overall health care system billions of dollars.

- The Pritikin diet and other diets that require low fat, low cholesterol, high fiber, and high complex carbohydrate consumption should be tested and evaluated (in terms of all their components) for the treatment of adult-onset diabetes. Even if a small percentage of the nation's 11 million diabetics could control their disease with diet, the savings—in health improvement, delayed mortality, and financial costs—would be enormous.

Food allergies. Despite the large body of literature on food allergies, there is still a need to further study the approach taken by environmental medicine in a variety of other conditions commonly encountered. A mechanism similar to that proposed for arthritis has been proposed in asthma, ulcerative colitis, migraines, hyperactivity, recurrent infections, and other common conditions. The testing techniques need further validation, as does treatment with immunotherapy, environmental control units, and basic biochemical understanding of the causes of chemical hypersensitivity and other "20th century" diseases.

More work needs to be done in the area of food intolerance and neuropsychiatric disorders. Egger and colleagues (1992) have recently implicated an immune system effect as being the mechanism by which incriminated foods produce hyperactivity. Work from other investigators is sorely needed.

Conclusion

This chapter has demonstrated that the more we learn about the potential influences of dietary factors on health, the more we must realize the need for maintaining an open mind. There are numerous examples where medical consensus—even when it represents the honest opinions of the most knowledgeable, leading scientists in the field—has clearly been wrong. For example, not long ago, the medical community strongly advised pregnant women to avoid taking vitamin supplements. Today pregnant women are advised to do exactly the opposite, especially with regard to taking folic acid to prevent neural tube defects. Another widespread erroneous consensus medical recommendation was the use of margarine rather than butter to reduce risk of coronary heart disease. It now seems, that at least some margarines, which are made from partially hydrogenated vegetable oils, are no better, if not worse, than butter in reducing the risk of heart disease.

Each of these cases was based on limited or no direct evidence. Further, many of the most promising research topics of today, such as the role of dietary antioxidants or alternative dietary lifestyles in preventing coronary heart disease and specific cancers, were topics dismissed by most nutritionists only a few years ago as practices of misguided vitamin and food faddists. Given the extreme complexities of the interrelationships between diet and human health and the relatively meager directly relevant data, an element of humility is appropriate in evaluating "alternative" dietary practices. Lack of data, such as from randomized trials, should not be confused with evidence of no benefit. However, a willingness to consider possible benefits of alternative diets does not imply blind acceptance of them, but rather should foster a rigorous scientific evaluation of potentially beneficial practices.

Unfortunately, nutritional therapies or dietary practices that do not readily fit into the "norm" previously have too often been routinely dismissed without such a rigorous examination. An ample investigation of a diet or nutritional intervention should test it in an appropriate model, under the appropriate conditions, and using appropriate research methodologies. In particular, potential study subjects must be selected with extreme care; that is, they should be individuals in which the dietary or nutritional modification, if truly beneficial, is likely to produce an effect. Moreover, if a study involves a micronutrient or vitamin or mineral supplementation, the dosage must be optimized to ensure that the intervention will have the opportunity to display an effect. Also, any evaluation of an alternative diet or nutrition research experiment will have to include a recognition that initially negative results do not prove any therapy is valueless; rather, the therapy may merely have been incorrectly tested. Thus, going the extra step is an imperative in conducting this type of research. Finally, more efforts are needed in translating findings related to specific micro- and macronutrients to whole foods and practical, attractive diets. Only by doing this can physicians and public health officials adequately disseminate important diet and nutrition information to all sectors of the public.

Chapter 17

Nutritional Therapies

"Nutritional therapies" is an umbrella term, covering a vast range of treatments and philosophies. For example, there are disciplines such as nutritional medicine, defined as "the study of the interactions of nutritional factors with human biochemistry, physiology and anatomy and how the clinical application of a knowledge of these interactions can be used in the prevention and treatment of disease as well as in the improvement of health."[1] There is also macrobiotics, "the art of choosing food according to a set of principles, with the objective that man, in order to live naturally, actively and healthily, must eat natural foods"[2]

The first of these does not seem too far removed from orthodox medicine, while the second, in which foods are classified according to their yin and yang characteristics, has elements that simply cannot be understood in terms of Western science.

These examples demonstrate how wide an area nutritional therapies cover, and it continues to expand, as the briefest examination of the shelves marked "complementary medicine" in a large bookshop or library will show: authors with impressive credentials, and others with none, apparently promise to cure everything from coryza to cancer by advising extra intake of some nutrients and/or reduced intake of others. If texts concerning slimming are included it becomes almost impossible to keep up with the claims—diets that burn up only certain types of fat or will lead to weight loss in specific areas of the body,

©1993 *Nursing Times* September 15, 1993. Volume 89, Number 37. Reprinted with permission.

leaving the rest unchanged, are just two that have challenged beliefs fundamental to nutritional science.

Yet despite evidence that interest in nutritional therapies is growing, they receive only a passing mention in the recent British Medical Association report on complementary therapies, and the survey it contains, of which the authors say "it is . . . likely that the main therapies currently available in the UK are represented", appears to have excluded them altogether[3]. The reasons for this are not clear, but it may be a reflection of how nebulous the whole area has become.

Historical Background

For as long as medicine has been practiced, food has been recognized as providing more than nutritional needs. The original nutritional therapist was probably the first person who found that eating something made him or her feel better or worse and passed the information on.

Over the centuries, different foodstuffs were valued for their medicinal properties: according to one author, garlic was prescribed in ancient Egypt, Babylonia and Greece as a cure for many disorders, while cabbage was recommended by Hippocrates for cardiac problems and was used as a wound dressing in 19th-century France[4].

A more widely known example is the administration of lime juice to British sailors in the 18th century as prophylaxis for scurvy (scorbusis), which led to the slang term "limey". It was only in this century that the active ingredient in citrus fruits was isolated.

A Polish biochemist working in London, Casimir Funk, proposed in 1912 that there were substances in some foods that fell into the class of proteins called amines and were essential to life; he named them vital amines or "vitamines". The first of these had been discovered 20 years earlier, and by 1915 several diseases were found to be preventable if extracts from certain foods were given. Increasingly efficient analytic techniques made it possible to isolate the active substances, and the foundations were laid for the system we have today—the fat-soluble vitamins A, D, E and K and the water-soluble B complex and vitamin C.

Many nutritional therapies were based on the use of these newly identified substances, and later advances in scientific knowledge, such as the discovery of possibly tissue-damaging "free radicals" and the anti-oxidant properties of some vitamins, have led to claims that vitamin supplements may slow the ageing process[5].

Other nutritionally based theories of health promotion in recent years have included the role of minerals and micronutrients, dietary fibre, cholesterol and other lipids, food additives, "complex" carbohydrates and salt. A critical review of the evidence put forward for these theories and several others can be found in a book by Yetiv[6].

How Nutritional Therapies Work

All nutritional therapies are, without exception, based on the belief that diet is inextricably linked with health. Individual therapies seek to identify an excess or deficiency of a nutrient or nutrients, either in intake or excretion, and correct it.

Examples of Nutritional Therapies

Nutritional medicine identifies four factors that influence nutritional status[1]:

* The quality of food we eat
* The quantity of the food we eat
* The efficiency of digestion, absorption and utilization
* Biochemical individuality.

Nutritional medicine aims to correct problems in one or more of these areas. So, for example, a therapist who believes that hyperactivity in a child might be due to chemical additives (such as coloring agents) or residues (for example, pesticides) would be looking at food quality when seeking a cause for abnormal hyperactivity. But each child is different, so biochemical individuality would also be a crucial consideration. An exclusion diet might be used here: the person fasts or starts—a fairly bland diet regime, and if the symptoms subside the likely cause is nutritional. Different foodstuffs can then be reintroduced to identify those that trigger a reaction[14].

The Gerson therapy[15], which its practitioners say has benefits for people with cancer, arthritis and many other conditions, is based on the theory that toxicity results from pollution, particularly in food, building up in the body and causing alterations in the body's cells related to biochemical individuality. The regime involves eating only organic vegetables, supplemented with hourly vegetable or calves' liver juice; some dairy products may be added later. Coffee enemas, which practitioners believe will boost the liver's detoxification rate, are also given.

257

Megavitamin therapy has been hotly debated for some years. Linus Pauling, a highly respected US chemist, became interested in vitamin C in the 1960s and went on to develop a theory that an optimum mental state could be achieved biochemically using substances such as vitamins; to describe this state, he coined the adjective "orthomolecular". Other researchers seized on this concept, and the disciplines of orthomolecular psychiatry and orthomolecular medicine were born.

Put simply, the idea behind megavitamin treatment is that for some reason the body cannot utilize enough of the vitamins in the diet and deficiency results. To get round this, doses many times higher than the recommended daily minimum are given[16].

Pauling went on to claim that giving very high doses of vitamin C could prolong the life of terminally ill cancer patients[17], but the methodology used in the trial was claimed to have several problems that invalidated the results[6].

Complementary Nutritional Therapy

Usually just called "nutritional therapy", the adjective "complementary" is sometimes used to avoid confusion with the blanket term used for all other treatments. The Society for the Promotion of Nutritional Therapy defines this as "a therapeutic approach which aims to explore all possible avenues whereby a patient's nutrition can be manipulated to obtain maximum health promotion".

When looking for the cause of a health problem, three possible diagnoses are examined:

- Allergy or intolerance to food or environmental factors

- Toxicity arising from heavy metals or chemicals, because of environmental exposure, lowered eliminative ability, poor liver function (or any combination of these factors)

- Deficits of nutrients because of insufficient intake, malabsorption or "special needs".

One diagnosis does not, of course, exclude either or both of the others.

If any of these diagnoses can be made, provisionally, confirmation comes from a "therapeutic trial", which involves education about nutrition, a modified diet and, where necessary, nutritional supplements[7].

Optimum Nutrition

Optimum nutrition is based on three principles:

- Every person is biochemically unique and therefore each person's nutritional need is also unique to him or her

- There is an intimate connection between nutrition and the environment

- The human race's nutritional needs must be considered in the light of the fact that they have been shaped over many thousands of years[8].

Practitioners working along optimum nutrition lines believe that four analyses—of diet, biochemical status, symptoms and lifestyle—can, when the results are collated, indicate whether an individual's diet is deficient in any way and what supplements are necessary.

This is a very small selection of the nutritional therapies available; a more detailed list can be found in Olsen[4].

What Nutritional Therapy Claims to Do

There are few health problems that nutritional therapists do not feel able to help with. A brief list can be found in a book by Ward and others[9], but much more detail is given by Davies and Stewart[1].

Contraindications

A Swedish study[10] looking at problems arising where "alternative" therapies had supplanted conventional treatment found that the majority of deaths or serious complications occurred when catabolic diseases had been treated by the institution of a vegetarian diet or regimes involving fasting.

Some nutritional supplements may interact with other medication, so it is important that when a person seeking nutritional advice is having concurrent medical treatment his or her medical practitioner should be kept informed of the therapy.

Research

Critical analyses of the most important papers can be found in Yetiv's work[6].

One research paper that led to a great deal of controversy in recent years concerned the Bristol Cancer Help Centre (BCCH)[11]. This establishment, set up in 1980, lays great emphasis on holistic care and counselling and used to prescribe the "Bristol diet", a whole-food regime with vitamin supplements. A comparative study was set up in which women at the BCCH were compared with others receiving treatment at three conventional centers. When the results were published in 1990 it seemed as though the BCCH was obtaining systematically worse results than the hospitals, but the findings were challenged and the dispute continues today[12].

Implications for Nursing

Writing in *Nursing Times* recently, Sue Holmes, a senior lecturer in nutrition, said: "Nutrition should be regarded as a positive contribution to treatment. Its success or failure is largely dependent on the nurse's interest, knowledge and understanding"[13]

If a patient or client has been receiving some form of nutritional therapy before he or she comes into a nurse's care, it is important that this be discussed with medical staff, the pharmacist and a dietitian, as the person may wish to continue the nutritional regime alongside other prescribed treatment.

References

1. Davies, S., Stewart, A. Nutritional Medicine. London: Pan Books, 1987.

2. Mayes, A. The Dictionary of Nutritional Health. Wellingborough: Thorsons, 1986.

3. British Medical Association. Complementary Medicine.—New Approaches to Good Practice. Oxford: Oxford University Press, 1993.

4. Olsen, K. The Encydopaedia of Alternative Health Care. London: Piatkus, 1989.

5. Passwater, R.A. The New Supernutrition. New York: Pocket Books, 1991.

6. Yetiv, J. Sense and nonsense in Nutrition. Harmmondsworth: Penguin, 1988.

7. Lazarides, L. Personal communication. June 1993.

8.   Holford, P. Optimum Nutrition. London: ION Press, 1992.

9.   Ward, B., Tripp, P., Evans, M. Your Diet. Bromley: Harrap, 1990.

10. Bostrom, H., Rossner, S. Quality of alternative medicine: complications and avoidable deaths. Quality Assurance in Health Care 1990; 2:2, 111-117.

11. Bagenel, F.S., Easton, D.F., Harris, E. et al. Survival of patients with breast cancer attending the Bristol Cancer Help Centre. Lancet 1990; 2: 606-610.

12. Buckman, R., Sabbagh, K. Magic or Medicine? An Investigation into Healing. London: Macmillan, 1993.

13. Holmes, S. Building blocks. Nursing Times 1993; 89:21,28-31.

14. Brostoff, J., Gamlin, L. The Complete Guide to Food Allergy and Intolerance. London: Bloomsbury, 1989.

15. Holmes, P. The Gerson therapy. Nursing Times 1988;84:14,41-42.

16. Stanway, A. Alternative Medicine.—A Guide to Natural Therapies. London: Bloomsbury, 1992.

17. Cameron, E., Pauling, L. Supplemental ascorbate in the supportive treatment of cancer: prolongation of survival times in terminal hum, cancer. Proceedings of the National Academy of Science 1976; 73: 3685.

— by Brian Booth, RGN, is
assistant clinical editor
of Nursing Times

When therapeutic techniques are described, it is purely for illustration and not intended to act as a guide to practice. No therapeutic interventions should ever be carried out by nurses, midwives or health visitors who have not undergone the appropriate training

Chapter 18

Is Organic More Nutritional?

Getting at the Truth Behind a Claim for Organically Grown Produce

The rich, healthy soils on organic farms produce fruits and vegetables with superior... nutritional value.

So goes the marketing copy in a pamphlet from Bread & Circus, a popular health food supermarket chain. Other sellers of organic food also make claims about its nutritional superiority. But does organically grown produce, which costs some 20 to 50 percent more than other produce, really contain higher levels of vitamins and minerals than fruits and vegetables that are grown with conventional farming techniques?

No one knows. "We just don't have enough data," says Kate Clancy, PhD, of the Henry Wallace Institute for Alternative Agriculture. 'That's because it's extremely difficult to conduct studies that control for all the variables that could affect nutrient content: seeds, soil type, and climate, for instance.

Whatever reliable research has been conducted has been sparse, and results have often been conflicting. Even when minor differences in protein and certain vitamins have been noted between organic and conventionally produced foods, scientists have found little overall distinction.

An international conference on agricultural production and nutrition hosted this year by Tufts's School of Nutrition Science and Policy yielded a fresh crop of research findings but again, few definitive results. Various studies examining spinach, broccoli, winter squash, carrots, and potatoes showed little to no nutritional differences between organic and conventionally grown crops.

Joan Dye Gussow, EdD, professor emeritus of nutrition and education at Columbia University who has been studying organic foods for more than 30 years, says a lack of nutritional difference between the different types of crops doesn't matter. "It is not the issue," she states emphatically. "My feeling is that the environmental, social, and political issues are more important when considering organic farming."

Even critics of the organic movement agree: nutrition aside, the methods used to farm organically are better for the environment and, by extension, society at large.

How Growing Foods Organically Serves the Environment

During the last 50 years, agriculture output has exploded. The United States now grows and produces more food than any other nation in the world. But the tradeoff has been high. Fertilizer use on the country's 300 million acres of farmland has increased fivefold since 1950. The use of pesticides, including insecticides, herbicides, and fungicides, has also increased dramatically. Not only is that potentially harmful for the food supply, it also threatens the environment by causing toxic runoff of pesticides into water supplies.

Another problem inherent in conventional farming techniques is decreased biodiversity. Simply put, certain food varieties have become extinct. "That's because farmers have developed and come to rely almost solely on seeds which produce crops that ripen simultaneously and therefore can lie harvested more efficiently. 'The result: while there were almost 300 varieties of carrots grown at the turn of the century, only 21 remain. Tomatoes once boasted 408 varieties. The number has shrunk to 79. Winnowing down vegetables and fruits to just a few varieties increases the potential for vulnerability to blight. That is, if a plant disease became rampant and wiped out a significant portion of a particular vegetable crop, resistant varieties might not be available to grow in its place.

For these reasons, a move back in the direction of organic farming is called for. We could never revert totally to organic agricultural practices. At least some use of pesticides and other non-organic techniques is necessary in order to produce enough food to feed the ever-expanding population. In addition, a large-scale shift toward organic farming couldn't be accomplished overnight. Most of the farms in this Country are set up for conventional agriculture and would need to change their methods gradually.

But the value of organic farming—using one species of insects to prey on a crop-destroying species rather than spraying synthetic pesticides; planting many different varieties of a particular food; rotating crops more often to replenish the soil—is becoming more and more well recognized. The Clinton Administration, in fact, has called for widespread adoption by the year 2000 of integrated pest management—an approach that uses many organic farming principles to cut down on the application of pesticides.

The bottom line: Eating more foods grown organically might not put more nutrients into your body. But the techniques used to grow them will certainly help keep the planet in the best shape possible, which, of course, is best for your health in the long run.

Chapter 19

Vitamin and Nutritional Supplements

Sorting out fact from fiction amid a storm of controversy

"The most powerful nutritional force in the universe, a super-powered, full-spectrum liquid organic supplement with 72 bioelectrical minerals, 16 vitamins, and 18 amino acids."

You've seen advertisements like these in magazines and health food stores. The hype is unavoidable—white oak helps you live longer, melatonin prevents cancer, magnesium eases migraines, and essence of flowers can reverse hot flashes.

Since 1994, when Congress changed Food and Drug Administration (FDA) regulation of "nutritional" supplements, there's been an explosion of "health-enhancing" megavitamins, magic pills and potions. Almost every mall in America has a health food store, shelves lined with products that promise to relieve pain, help you sleep better and give your health, vitality and virility a boost.

It's a $6 billion-a-year business, and it's booming as people search for a fast fix—an easy way to feel better and stay healthy. One-quarter to one-third of Americans now take daily vitamin supplements. Seventy percent take nutritional supplements at least occasionally, and one in three people with chronic disease looks to herbal remedies for help.

Now, more than ever, people are focusing on nutrition to help them remain healthy and active. That's good. But do you need supplements? Do they work? And perhaps most important, are they safe?

267

The answers to these questions are not always clear-cut. There's disagreement, even within the medical community, as researchers continue to uncover new information about how nutrition affects your health. Further clouding the issue is an almost daily barrage of media reports on new studies—some suggesting benefits from supplements, others indicating harm. And then there are those advertisements, promising health in a capsule or in a steaming herbal brew.

So how do you sort out fact from fiction from outright fantasy amid the swirl of information about vitamin and nutritional supplements? We hope this chapter will help. In it, we'll discuss what's known about supplements and what's not. We'll talk about who may need a supplement and who doesn't. And, we'll address critical safety issues surrounding what has become a largely unregulated industry.

What is a vitamin?

For centuries, sailors on long voyages battled not only the high seas, but a disease that can cause bones to become brittle, gums to bleed and even death. That disease is scurvy.

It had long been suspected there might be a relationship between the lack of fresh food and the development of scurvy, but it wasn't until 1747 that a carefully planned trial showed that lemons and oranges would prevent the disease. It took until 1928, when the science of chemistry was more advanced, for a researcher to identify the substance in lemons and oranges (and many other fruits and vegetables) that prevents or cures scurvy. The substance was given the name "vitamin C."

Most vitamins and minerals were discovered this way—scientists identifying substances you need because a shortage causes a health problem.

Vitamins and essential minerals are substances required in tiny amounts to promote essential biochemical reactions in your cells. Together, vitamins and minerals are called micronutrients. Lack of a micronutrient for a prolonged period causes a specific disease or condition, which can usually be reversed when the micronutrient is re-supplied.

Your body can't make most vitamins and minerals. They must come from food or supplements.

Vitamin and Mineral ABCs

There are 13 vitamins. Four—vitamins A, D, E and K—are stored in your body's fat (they're called fat-soluble vitamins). Nine are water-soluble and are not stored in your body in appreciable amounts. They are vitamin C and the eight B vitamins: thiamin (B-1), riboflavin (B-2), niacin, vitamin B-6, pantothenic acid, vitamin B-12, biotin and folic acid (folate).

Vitamins in the right amounts are needed for normal growth, digestion, mental alertness and resistance to infection. They enable your body to use carbohydrates, fats and proteins. They also act as catalysts in your body, initiating or speeding up a chemical reaction. However, you don't "burn" vitamins, so you can't get energy (calories) directly from them.

Your body strives to maintain an optimal level of each vitamin and keep the amount circulating in your bloodstream constant. Surplus water-soluble vitamins are excreted in urine. Surplus fat-soluble vitamins are stored in body tissue. Because they're stored, excess fat-soluble vitamins can accumulate in your body and become toxic. Your body is especially sensitive to too much vitamin A and vitamin D.

Therefore, whether you're taking water-soluble or fat-soluble vitamin supplements, more is not necessarily better and can even be harmful.

Your body also needs 15 minerals that help regulate cell function and provide structure for cells. Major minerals include calcium, phosphorus and magnesium. In addition, your body needs smaller amounts of chromium, copper, fluoride, iodine, iron, manganese, molybdenum, selenium, zinc, chloride, potassium and sodium.

Do you need a vitamin-mineral supplement?

Vitamin hucksters spend millions planting the fear, "Are you getting enough vitamins?" They recommend vitamin, mineral and nutritional supplements as "vitamin insurance." But there's no need for most people to bank on vitamin insurance. The American Dietetic Association, the National Academy of Sciences, the National Research Council and other major medical societies all agree that you should get the vitamins and minerals you need through a well-balanced diet. Although certain high-risk groups may benefit from a vitamin-mineral supplement, healthy adults can get all necessary nutrients from food.

Experts favor food, rather than supplements, because food contains hundreds of additional nutrients, including phytochemicals. Phytochemicals are compounds that occur naturally in foods and may contain important health benefits. Scientists have yet to learn exactly what role phytochemicals play in nutrition, and there's no RDA established for them. However, if you depend on supplements rather than trying to eat a variety of whole foods, you miss out on possible health benefits from phytochemicals.

In addition, only long-term, well-designed studies can sort out which nutrients in food are beneficial and whether taking them in pill form provides the same benefit. In the meantime, it's best to concentrate on getting your nutrients from food, not supplements.

However, many people don't get all the nutrients they need from their diets because they don't eat properly. For example, only one person in 10 regularly consumes the recommended five servings a day of fruits and vegetables. Skipping meals, dieting and eating meals high in sugar and fat all contribute to poor nutrition. For these people, taking supplemental vitamins would be reasonable, although the best course of action would be to adopt better eating habits.

Vitamin-mineral supplements shouldn't substitute for a healthful diet. However, there's probably no harm in taking a multiple vitamin-mineral supplement with dose levels no higher the 100 percent of the Daily Value (see "Choosing a vitamin and mineral supplement," and "Use DVs as a guide.") Doses above that don't give extra protection, but do increase your risk of encountering toxic side effects.

For example, taking large amounts of vitamin D can indirectly cause kidney damage, while large amounts of vitamin A can cause liver damage. Even modest increases in some minerals can lead to imbalances that limit your body's ability to use other minerals. And supplements of iron, zinc, chromium and selenium can be toxic at just five times the RDA. Virtually all nutrient toxicities stem from high-dose supplements.

When you may need a supplement

Although most people can get all the vitamins and minerals they need from a balanced diet, there are situations where a supplement may be appropriate. Even if you don't have a documented deficiency, your doctor or dietitian may recommend a vitamin-mineral supplement if:

- **You're older.** Lack of appetite, loss of taste and smell, and denture problems can all contribute to a poor diet. If you eat alone or are depressed, you also may not eat enough to get all the nutrients you need from food.

  In addition, if you're age 65 or older, you may need to increase your intake of vitamin B-6, vitamin B-12 and vitamin D because your body may not be able to absorb these as well. And women, especially those not taking estrogen, may need to increase their intake of calcium and vitamin D to protect against osteoporosis.

There's also evidence that a multivitamin may improve your immune function and decrease your risk for some infections if you're older.

- **You're on a strict weight-loss diet.** If you eat less than 1,000 calories a day, or your diet has limited variety due to intolerance or allergy, you may benefit from a vitamin-mineral supplement.

- **You have a disease of your digestive tract.** Diseases of your liver, gallbladder, intestine and pancreas, or previous surgery on your digestive tract, may interfere with your normal digestion and absorption of nutrients. If you have one of these conditions, your doctor may advise you to supplement your diet with vitamins and minerals.

- **You smoke.** Smoking reduces vitamin C levels and causes production of harmful free radicals (see "Vitamin and mineral supplements in the headlines"). The RDA for vitamin C for smokers is higher—100 milligrams (mg) compared to 60 mg for nonsmokers. Still, you can easily get this much by eating foods rich in vitamin C. If you smoke, try to stop. And don't depend on high-potency supplements to provide necessary nutrients. Two studies of beta carotene have shown an increased risk of lung cancer in smokers who take these supplements.

- **You drink alcoholic beverages to excess.** If you regularly consume alcohol to excess, you may not get enough vitamins due to poor nutrition and alcohol's effect on the absorption, metabolism and excretion of vitamins.

- **You're pregnant or breast-feeding.** If you're pregnant or breast-feeding, you need more of certain nutrients, especially folic acid, iron and calcium. Your doctor can recommend a supplement.

- **You're in another high-risk group.** Vegetarians who eliminate all animal products from their diets may need additional vitamin B-12. And if you have limited milk intake and limited exposure to the sun, you may need to supplement your diet with calcium and vitamin D.

Supplement Safety

For the millions of healthy Americans who want to take a daily multivitamin supplement with no more than 100 percent of the Daily Value, the risks of side effects are probably small. But if you're tempted to take high-dose vitamins, thinking that "more is better," think again. High doses of some vitamins can have serious side effects.

And if you're considering herbal and other types of supplements, be particularly cautious (see "Clues to quackery"). Quality and dose potency may not be well-regulated.

For example, in 1989, a sudden illness outbreak that affected more than 1,500 people and caused 38 deaths was linked to L-tryptophan, an amino acid sold as an over-the-counter dietary supplement to treat insomnia. The supplements, manufactured by a foreign pharmaceutical company, were contaminated during the manufacturing process.

Today, experts are concerned about reported health problems linked to popular herbal supplements containing ephedrine. Although the FDA has linked the supplements to more than 600 reports of adverse events and 15 deaths since 1993, they're still on the market (see "Buyer beware—there's no guarantee dietary supplements are safe," and "Herbs can have many health effects").

Reported side effects have included abnormal heart rhythm, seizure, stroke, psychosis, heart attack, hepatitis and death. The FDA is considering a ban on ephedrine-containing Supplements because no safe level has been identified for its use in dietary supplements.

Play it Safe with Your Diet and Your Health

The L-tryptophan and ephedrine deaths are tragic consequences of the largely unregulated health-supplement industry and our desire for easy ways to feel better, boost energy, reduce stress, lose weight and stave off disease. But despite the dangers, supplements are proliferating.

If you want to improve your nutritional health, look first to a well-balanced diet. in most cases, making changes in your diet has a far greater chance of promoting health than taking supplements.

Choosing a Vitamin and Mineral Supplement

Supplements are not substitutes. They can't replace the hundreds of nutrients in whole foods needed for a balanced diet. But if you do decide to take a vitamin supplement, here are things to consider:

- **Stick to the Daily Value.** Choose a vitamin-mineral combination limited to 100 percent DV or less. Take no more than the recommended dose. The higher the dose, the more likely you are to have side effects.

- **Don't waste dollars.** Synthetic vitamins are the same as so-called "natural" vitamins. Generic brands and synthetic vitamins are generally less expensive and equally effective. Don't be tempted by added herbs, enzymes or amino acids—they add nothing but cost.

- **Read the label.** Supplements can lose potency over time so check the expiration date on the label. Also look for the initials USP (for the testing organization U.S. Pharmacopeia) or words such as "release assured" or "proven release," indicating that the supplement is easily dissolved and absorbed by your body.

- **Store them in a safe place.** Iron supplements are the most common cause of poisoning deaths among children.

- **Don't self-prescribe.** See your doctor if you have a health problem. Tell him or her about any supplement you're taking. Supplements may interfere with medications.

Vitamin and Mineral Supplements in the Headlines

New claims for vitamins and minerals are in the news almost every day. Here's a look at some of the most widely publicized supplements:

- **Beta carotene.** This nutrient, widely found in plants, is converted in your body into vitamin A. Beta carotene (and vitamins C and E) are antioxidants. Antioxidants neutralize harmful substances called free radicals that result from your cells' ordinary metabolism. Scientists think damage from free radicals may contribute to cardiovascular disease and cancer.

  But, several well-designed studies have found that beta carotene supplements offer no protection against cardiovascular disease. And two studies found an increased risk of lung cancer in smokers who took beta carotene supplements.

- **Folic acid.** The big news in B vitamins is folic acid (folate), which may help during pregnancy to prevent spinal cord birth defects. For this reason, the RDA for folic acid is expected to be roughly doubled this summer. In addition, the FDA is requiring manufacturers of breads, cereal, pasta and other grain products to fortify their products with folic acid by January 1998.

The increased fortification may also carry certain benefits—or a slight risk—for older adults. Folic acid has been linked to possible cardiovascular benefits, but it also carries a small risk of masking a vitamin B-12 deficiency (see our April 1996 edition), However, experts say masking is unlikely if your intake of folic acid stays below 1,000 micrograms (1 mg) a day. Fortification is designed to keep intake below that.

• **Niacin.** Another B vitamin, niacin, can reduce fats (lipids) in your blood. Niacin can lower LDL ("bad") cholesterol and triglycerides and raise HDL ("good") cholesterol. Studies show niacin can slow and even reverse the progression of atherosclerosis when used with other cholesterol-lowering drugs, diet and exercise.

However, in the doses typically needed for these effects (usually greater than 1,000 mg), niacin is being used as a medication, not a vitamin. At doses of higher than 2,000 mg, niacin has potentially serious side effects that can include liver damage, high blood sugar and irregular heartbeats. As little as 50 mg can cause flushing, headaches, cramps and nausea. So take increased doses only with your doctor's advice.

• **Vitamin C.** Studies have shown that people who eat diets high in vitamin C have lower rates of cancer and cardiovascular disease. However, it's unclear—and controversial —whether taking vitamin C supplements produces similar benefits.

Adequate levels of vitamin C may help strengthen your resistance to viral infections and act as a mild antihistamine to help relieve cold symptoms. But vitamin C can't "cure" colds.

Doses above 250 mg appear to have diminishing returns, and above 500 mg most additional vitamin C is excreted in urine and less is absorbed.

A recent National Institutes of Health (NIH) study has proposed raising the current RDA of 60 mg to 200 mg, and the National Cancer Institute concurs. Two-thirds of Americans consume much less than 200 mg a day, and about one-third consume less than 60 mg. Still, the 200-mg recommendation can be achieved with just five servings a day of fruits and vegetables.

- **Vitamin D and calcium.** This vitamin/mineral team may be the exception to the no-need-for-supplements advice because some people may not get enough through their diets.

  In 1994, NIH scientists reviewed new information about calcium's role in preventing osteoporosis. They recommended increasing the RDA of calcium from 800 mg to 1,500 mg for people—older than age 65. That's the equivalent of five 8-ounce glasses of milk a day. Most women consume only about 600 mg a day. The new recommendation stems from studies showing that age affects your ability to use vitamin D and calcium.

  In addition to getting vitamin D from dietary sources, your body makes it when sunlight converts a chemical in your skin into a usable form of, the vitamin. Vitamin D then helps your body absorb dietary calcium and deposit the mineral in your bones. But as you age, your intestine absorbs: less dietary calcium. In addition, many older people don't get enough vitamin D due to lack of exposure to sunlight (15 minutes a day is sufficient), less efficient conversion of the vitamin in their skin, and reduced liver or kidney function.

  For these reasons, supplements may be appropriate for people who don't get enough calcium and vitamin D in food, or who live in cloudy environments or rarely go outside. Studies show that people who supplement their diets with calcium and vitamin D slow bone loss and reduce the number of fractures.

  However, be cautious. Prolonged intake of vitamin D above 2,000 International Units (IU) a, day poses the risk of toxic effects. Side effects can include nausea, headache, excessive urination, high blood pressure, kidney damage and other problems. Most doctors recommend that older adults consume 400 IU of vitamin D every day.

- **Vitamin E.** Of all the antioxidants, vitamin E shows the most promise for protecting against cardiovascular disease.

  Vitamin E is a potent antioxidant that attaches directly to LDL ("bad") cholesterol in your blood and helps prevent damage from free radicals. Studies show vitamin E might prevent or slow progression of atherosclerosis in people with cardiovascular disease and diabetes. In addition, the vitamin may even slow the effects of Parkinson's disease and Alzheimer's disease.

However, any benefit vitamin E offers against cardiovascular disease is much less than you get from exercise and a healthful diet. And at high doses (above 1,080 IU) vitamin E can cause side effects that can include bleeding, especially for people on blood-thinning medications, and gastrointestinal complaints.

Although initial data appear promising, there isn't enough evidence yet to recommend vitamin E supplements for the general population. But if you have cardiovascular disease, the benefits of taking vitamin E—no more than 400 IU a day—probably outweigh the risks.

- **Chromium.** Although chromium work with insulin to help your body use blood sugar, preliminary studies assessing the effect of chromium in the treatment of diabetes are controversial, and there's no proof chromium can prevent the disease. There's also no proof of the popular claims that taking chromium supplements can increase your muscle mass, help you lose weight, reduce cholesterol and prevent osteoporosis.

- **Iron.** Certain groups can be at risk of having low iron levels. These include young children and early teens, menstruating women and people with conditions that cause internal bleeding, such as ulcers or intestinal diseases.

  But for healthy men and postmenopausal women, iron deficiency is rare. In fact, one study suggested that high iron levels may increase risk of heart attack and atherosclerosis, although a link hasn't been proven. In addition, if you have the uncommon—but not rare—genetic disease hemochromatosis, iron supplements could cause a hazardous iron buildup in your body.

- **Selenium.** Selenium is an antioxidant mineral that has been claimed to help prevent cancer and cardiovascular disease. One recent study did suggest that selenium supplements may decrease cancer risk. However, more research is needed. Taking excessive amounts of selenium may cause hair and nail loss.

- **Zinc.** Many people began taking zinc supplements when a 1996 study published in the *Annals of Internal Medicine* showed that dissolving one particular formulation of a zinc lozenge in your mouth could reduce the severity of cold symptoms and shorten the duration of a cold by up to three days. Some studies have also shown that taking a daily multivitamin-mineral supplement containing zinc may increase immune response in older people. However, other studies have shown just the opposite—that zinc may weaken the immune status of older people.

  What is known is that megadoses of zinc can interfere with the way your body uses other essential minerals, such as iron and copper. And, excess zinc (more than 10 times the RDA) can lower HDL ("good") cholesterol levels. Until the effects of taking supplemental zinc are known, stick to 100 percent of the Daily Value.

Clues to Quackery

Even well-informed consumers can be duped by health quackery. Here are some tips to help you sort out dubious claims:

- **Be cautious about claims to treat diseases.** Vitamins can treat a few rare diseases caused by a vitamin deficiency. In addition, the B vitamin niacin is used to treat high cholesterol levels in some people. But studies show that vitamin and nutritional supplements can't cure diseases such as cancer and arthritis.

- **Beware of testimonials.** One person's story can't help you distinguish a true benefit from chance or a "placebo effect." In one study of vitamin C, people who thought they were given vitamin C but had been given a placebo, reported that they felt unusually well.

- **Avoid "tests" that can determine your body's overall nutritional status.** There's no single test that can measure your nutritional well-being and overall health.

- **Don't assume all advertising is truthful.** The Federal Trade Commission (FTC), doesn't have resources to halt much fraudulent advertising. Be suspicious of words such as "miraculous," "amazing" and,"powerful," or products that claim to "strengthen," "rebuild" or "rejuvenate."

- **Be cautious about buying a nutritional supplement by phone or mail order.** These products are often very expensive and frequently a waste of money. Sometimes promotions are a scam.

Buyer Beware—There's No Guarantee Dietary Supplements Are Safe

When you buy a product in a store, particularly something you eat, you naturally assume it's safe. Some government agency has checked to make sure it's not harmful, right?

Not any more. In 1994, Congress passed and President Clinton signed the Dietary Supplement Health and Education Act. That act removed dietary supplements from premarket safety evaluations required of food ingredients and drugs.

Drugs and food ingredients still undergo lengthy FDA safety review before they can be marketed. Drugs are also tested for effectiveness. But the 1994 legislation eliminated the FDA's authority to regulate the safety of nutritional supplements before they're on the market. Now, the FDA can intervene only after an illness or injury occurs.

The FDA can still restrict the sale of an unsafe dietary supplement when there's evidence the product presents a significant or unreasonable safety concern. But now the agency must wait for complaints about a product before acting.

Consumers can report problems through a "consumer complaint coordinator" at FDA district offices in cities across the country (listed in the "government" pages of your phone book).

But even after complaints are received, the FDA is required to prove the supplement caused harm when taken "as directed" on the label before a product can be restricted. Harm is usually difficult to prove because people may not take supplements as directed. They often exceed the recommended dose and take different types of supplements simultaneously.

Since passage of the legislation three years ago, the FDA hasn't been able to "prove" harm in a single case, despite reports of illness and even death from supplements.

The 1994 legislation also changed guidelines for marketing supplements. Marketing representatives can make unproven claims, such as saying a product "cures" cancer, as long as they're not selling the product at the same time.

And, while it's illegal to make false or misleading health or nutritional claims on a product label, government agencies lack resources to pursue the multitude of dubious claims that have swept the marketplace.

In addition, since the nutritional supplement industry is now largely unregulated, you can't be sure of product purity or the amount of active ingredient in a supplement—even from one package to the next of the same product.

What all this means for you is that you can't automatically assume the safety and effectiveness of any of the nutritional supplements sold today. If you have questions about a supplement, talk to your doctor or registered dietitian. Or, call the American Dietetic Association's consumer hotline at 1-800-366-1655.

Use DVs as a Guide

You've no doubt seen "Percent Daily Value" listings on food labels.

Daily Values (DV) have their origin in the Recommended Dietary Allowances (RDA) that tell how much of each vitamin and mineral you need, on average, each day to maintain health. The percent DV tells you what percent of the DV one serving of a food or supplement supplies. Use it to compare the nutritional value of products.

Herbs Can Have Many Health Effects—Some Beneficial, Some Dangerous

Herbs are the basis for many of our most helpful medicines, such as aspirin, morphine and digitalis. And scientists are still discovering medicinal mysteries in plants. For example, the new anticancer drug paclitaxel (Taxol) is derived from the bark and needles of the Pacific yew tree.

But while some herbal remedies may show promise, there's little evidence that most of the herbal remedies Americans spend $700 million a year on provide any health benefits. Some have significant health risks. In addition, there's no guarantee that product purity or potency will be consistent, let alone safe.

At a minimum, use these precautions: Don't use herbal remedies for serious illnesses, don't give herbs or other "dietary supplements" to children, and don't use herbal supplements if you're pregnant or trying to get pregnant. And, to avoid interactions with other medications, tell your doctor about all supplements you take.

Here's a list of health effects of some widely promoted herbal supplements:

- **Comfrey.** Also called borage and coltsfoot, it can cause liver and kidney disease.

- **Chaparral.** Nontoxic when used in a tea, chaparral can cause acute toxic hepatitis (liver disease) when taken in pill form.

- **Echinacea.** May increase resistance to upper respiratory infections, but continued use decreases effects. Some allergic reactions have been reported.

- **Ephedrine-containing compounds.** Ephedrine is a drug that stimulates heart rate. It can cause stroke and dangerous increases in blood pressure. Products are sold under the names Ma Huang, Ephedra, Ultimate Xphoria and others.

- **Germanium.** Long-term use can lead to kidney damage and death.

- **Ginkgo biloba.** May dilate blood vessels and improve blood flow to your brain and aid circulation in your legs, but side effects can include gastrointestinal problems, headaches and allergic skin reactions.

- **Ginseng.** Ginsenosides, the active ingredients found in ginseng root, may enhance immunity, but many "ginseng" products contain little or none of the active ingredient. Ginsenosides can increase blood pressure.

- **Jin bu huan.** A sedative that has caused hepatitis in adults and drowsiness, slow heartbeat and slow breathing in children.

- **Kombucha tea.** This "herbal tea," also called mushroom tea, kvass tea, kwassan and kargasok, is really a colony of yeast and bacteria. It can cause liver and other organ damage, gastrointestinal upset and death.

- **Lobelia.** Also called Indian tobacco, low doses act like a mild stimulant to help open airways and ease breathing. Large doses can cause convulsions, coma and death.

- **St. John's wort.** May be an effective treatment for mild to moderately severe depression. Further studies for possible side effects are needed.

- **Saw palmetto.** May improve urinary flow in men with noncancerous enlarged prostate. Teas made from saw palmetto aren't effective. Use with a doctor's supervision, not as a substitute for conventional medical treatment.

- **Stephania.** Also called magnolia. Used in weight-loss preparations, this herb has caused kidney disease and resulted in kidney transplants and dialysis in Europe.

- **Yohimbine.** Sold as an aphrodisiac (for which it's ineffective), yohimbine can cause tremors, anxiety, high blood pressure and rapid heartbeat.

Non-herbal Supplements

Not all supplements come from herbs or vitamins and minerals. Here are three that have been widely promoted: a DHEA (dehydroepiandrosterone)—Banned before 1994, DHEA is a hormone. It's been promoted as a treatment for everything from heart disease to cancer and Alzheimer's disease. But none of these claims has been proven. Side effects may include acne, increased facial hair and deepened voice in women, and, theoretically, increased risk of breast and prostate cancer.

- **DMSO.** Dimethyl sulfoxide is an industrial solvent not approved by the FDA for human use. It may relieve pain from sore muscles when rubbed on skin, but it's no more effective than products like BenGay or MenthoRub. Taken internally, DMSO can lead to cataracts.

- **Melatonin.** Melatonin is a hormone produced in your brain. It's thought to set your body's sleep cycle. Supplements may reduce effects of jet lag when taken for short periods. There's less evidence to support claims it will increase immune function and aid sleep.

    Claims that melatonin lowers cholesterol and prevents breast cancer are unproven. Melatonin prevents ovulation, so don't use it if you want to become pregnant. Avoid it if you have severe allergies or immune disease, and don't give it to children.

Part Five

Herbal Medicine

Chapter 20

Herbal Therapies

Overview

History of Herbal Medicine

Early humans recognized their dependence on nature in both health and illness. Led by instinct, taste, and experience, primitive men and women treated illness by using plants, animal parts, and minerals that were not part of their usual diet. Physical evidence of use of herbal remedies goes back some 60,000 years to a burial site of a Neanderthal man uncovered in 1960 (Solecki, 1975). In a cave in northern Iraq, scientists found what appeared to be ordinary human bones. An analysis of the soil around the bones revealed extraordinary quantities of plant pollen that could not have been introduced accidentally at the burial site. Someone in the small cave community had consciously gathered eight species of plants to surround the dead man. Seven of these are medicinal plants still used throughout the herbal world (Bensky and Gamble, 1993). All cultures have long folk medicine histories that include the use of plants. Even in ancient cultures, people methodically and scientifically collected information on herbs and developed well-defined herbal pharmacopoeias. Indeed, well

Extracted from NIH Publication No. 94-066 from the Office of Alternative Medicine. December 1994. Due to space considerations, bibliographic data have not been reprinted in this chapter. However, to aid readers who wish to consult the original document or do further research, the in-text references have been retained.

into the 20th century much of the pharmacopoeia of scientific medicine was derived from the herbal lore of native peoples. Many drugs, including strychnine, aspirin, vincristine, taxol, curare, and ergot, are of herbal origin. About one-quarter of the prescription drugs dispensed by community pharmacies in the United States contain at least one active ingredient derived from plant material (Farnsworth and Morris, 1976).

Middle East medicine. The invention of writing was a focus around which herbal knowledge could accumulate and grow. The first written records detailing the use of herbs in the treatment of illness are the Mesopotamian clay tablet writings and the Egyptian papyrus. About 2000 BC, King Assurbanipal of Sumeria ordered the compilation of the first known *materia medica*—an ancient form of today's United States *Pharmacopoeia*—containing 250 herbal drugs (including garlic, still a favorite of herbal doctors). The Ebers Papyrus, the most important of the preserved Egyptian manuscripts, was written around 1500 BC and includes much earlier information. It contains 876 prescriptions made up of more than 500 different substances, including many herbs (Ackerknecht.1973).

Greece and Rome. One of the earliest materia medica was the Rhizotomikon, written by Diocles of Caryotos, a pupil of Aristotle. Unfortunately, the book is now lost. Other Greek and Roman compilations followed, but none was as important or influential as that written by Dioscorides in the 1st century A.D., better known by its Latin name *De Materia Medica*. This text contains 950 curative substances, of which 600 are plant products and the rest are of animal or mineral origin (Ackerknecht, 1973). Each entry includes a drawing, a description of the plant, an account of its medicinal qualities and method of preparation, and warnings about undesirable effects.

Muslim world. The Arabs preserved and built on the body of knowledge of the Greco-Roman period as they learned of new remedies from remote places. They even introduced to the West the Chinese technique of chemically preparing minerals. The principal storehouse of the Muslim materia medica is the text of Jami of Ibn Baiar (died 1248 A.D.), which lists more than 2,000 substances, including many plant products (Ackerknecht, 1973). Eventually this entire body of knowledge was reintroduced to Europe by Christian doctors traveling with the Crusaders. Indeed, during the Middle Ages, trade in herbs became a vast international commerce.

East India. India, located between China and the West, underwent a similar process in the development of its medicine. The healing that took place before India's Ayurvedic medical corpus was similar to that of ancient Egypt or China (i.e., sickness was viewed as a punishment from the gods for a particular sin). Ayurvedic medicine emerged during the rise of the philosophies of the Upanishads, Buddhism, and other schools of thought in India. Herbs played an important role in Ayurvedic medicine. The principal Ayurvedic book on internal medicine, the *Characka Samhita*, describes 582 herbs (Majno, 1975). The main book on surgery, the *Sushruta Samhita*, lists some 600 herbal remedies. Most experts agree that these books are at least 2,000 years old.

China and Japan. The earliest written evidence of the medicinal use of herbs in China consists of a corpus of 11 medical works recovered from a burial site in Hunan province. The burial itself is dated 168 BC, and the texts (written on silk) appear to have been composed before the end of the 3rd century BC. Some of the texts discuss exercise, diet, and channel therapy (in the form of moxibustion—see the "Alternative Systems of Medical Practice" chapter). The largest, clearest, and most important of these manuscripts, called by its discoverers *Prescriptions for Fifty-Two Ailments*, is predominantly a pharmacological work. More than 250 medicinal substances are named. Most are substances derived from herbs and wood; grains, legumes, fruits, vegetables, and animal parts are also mentioned. Underlying this entire text is the view that disease is the manifestation of evil spirits, ghosts, and demons that must be repelled by incantation, rituals, and spells in addition to herbal remedies.

By the Later Han Dynasty (25-220 A.D.), medicine had changed dramatically in China. People grew more confident of their ability to observe and understand the natural world and believed that health and disease were subject to the principles of natural order. However, herbs still played an important part in successive systems of medicine. The *Classic of the Materia Medica*, compiled no earlier than the 1st century A.D. by unknown authors, was the first Chinese book to focus on the description of individual herbs. It includes 252 botanical substances, 45 mineral substances, and 67 animal-derived substances. For each herb there is a description of its medicinal effect, usually in terms of symptoms. Reference is made to the proper method of preparation, and toxicities are noted (Bensky and Gamble, 1993).

Since the writing of the *Classic of the Materia Medica* almost 2,000 years ago, the traditional Chinese materia medica have been steadily increasing in number. This increase has resulted from the integration into the official tradition of substances from China's folk medicine as well as from other parts of the world. Many substances now used in traditional Chinese medicine originate in places such as Southeast Asia, India, the Middle East, and the Americas. The most recent compilation of Chinese materia medica was published in 1977. *The Encyclopedia of Traditional Chinese Medicine Substances (Zhong yao da ci dian)*, the culmination of a 25-year research project conducted by the Jiangsu College of New Medicine, contains 5,767 entries and is the most definitive compilation of China's herbal tradition to date (Bensky and Gamble, 1993).

Traditional Chinese medicine was brought to Japan via Korea, and Chinese-influenced Korean medicine was adapted by the Japanese during the reign of Emperor Ingyo (411-453 A.D.). Medical envoys continued to arrive from Korea throughout the next century, and by the time of the Empress Suiko (592-628 A.D.), Japanese envoys were being sent directly to China to study medicine. Toward the end of the Muromachi period (1333-1573 A.D.) the Japanese began to develop their own form of traditional oriental medicine, called kampo medicine. As traditional Chinese medicine was modified and integrated into kampo medicine, herbal medicine was markedly simplified.

Herbal Medicine in the United States

In North America, early explorers traded knowledge with the Native American Indians. The tribes taught them which herbs to use to sharpen their senses for hunting, to build endurance, and to bait their traps. In 1716, French explorer Lafitau found a species of ginseng, *Panax quinquefolius L.*, growing in Iroquois territory in the New World. This American ginseng soon became an important item in world herb commerce (Duke, 1989). The Jesuits dug up the plentiful American ginseng, sold it to the Chinese, and used the money to build schools and churches. Even today, American ginseng is a sizable crude U.S. export.

As medicine evolved in the United States, plants continued as a mainstay of country medicine. Approaches to plant healing passed from physician to physician, family to family. Even in America's recent past, most families used home herbal remedies to control small medical emergencies and to keep minor ailments from turning into chronic problems. During this period there was a partnership between home folk medicine and the family doctor (Buchman, 1980). Physicians often used plant and herbal preparations to treat common ills.

Until the 1940s, textbooks of pharmacognosy—books that characterize plants as proven-by-use prescription medicines—contained hundreds of medically useful comments on barks, roots, berries, leaves, resins, twigs, and flowers.

As 20th-century technology advanced and created a growing admiration for technology and technologists, simple plant-and-water remedies were gradually discarded. Today, many Americans have lost touch with their herbal heritage. Few Americans realize that many over-the-counter (OTC) and prescription drugs have their origins in medicinal herbs. Cough drops that contain menthol, mint, horehound, or lemon are herbal preparations; chamomile and mint teas taken for digestion or a nervous stomach are time-honored herbal remedies; and many simple but effective OTC ache- and pain-relieving preparations on every druggist's and grocer's shelf contain oils of camphor, menthol, or eucalyptus. Millions of Americans greet the morning with their favorite herbal stimulant—coffee.

Despite the importance of plant discoveries in the evolution of medicine, some regulatory bodies such as the U.S. Food and Drug Administration (FDA)—the main U.S. regulatory agency for food and drugs—consider herbal remedies to be worthless or potentially dangerous (Snider, 1991). Indeed, today in the United States, herbal products can be marketed only as food supplements. If a manufacturer or distributor makes specific health claims about a herbal product (i.e., indicates on the label the ailment or ailments for which the product might be used) without FDA approval, the product can be pulled from store shelves.

Despite FDA's skepticism about herbal remedies, a growing number of Americans are again becoming interested in herbal preparations. This surge in interest is fueled by factors that include the following:

- Traditional European and North American herbs are sold in most U.S. health food stores. The same is true for Chinese and, to a lesser extent, Japanese herbal medicinals. Ayurvedic herbals are available in most large U.S. cities, as are culinary and medicinal herb shops called botanicas that sell herbs from Central and South America and Mexico. The reemergence of Native American Indian cultural influences has increased interest in Native American Indian herbal medicines.

- Pharmaceutical drugs are seen increasingly as overprescribed, expensive, even dangerous. Herbal remedies are seen as less expensive and less toxic.

- Exposure to exotic foreign foods prepared with non-European culinary herbs has led many Euroethnic Americans to examine and often consider using medicinal herbs that were brought to the United States along with ethnic culinary herbs.

- People increasingly are willing to "selfdoctor" their medical needs by investigating and using herbs and herbal preparations. Many Americans—especially those with chronic illnesses such as arthritis, diabetes, cancer, and AIDS—are turning to herbs as adjuncts to other treatments.

The next section discusses the regulatory status of herbal medicine in various countries around the world, particularly in Europe and Asia, as well as in less developed countries. It is followed by an overview of promising European and Asian herbal medicine research and recommendations for making herbal medicine a more viable health care alternative in this country.

Regulatory Status of Herbal Medicine Worldwide

The World Health Organization (WHO) estimates that 4 billion people—80 percent of the world population—use herbal medicine for some aspect of primary health care (Farnsworth et al., 1985). Herbal medicine is a major component in all indigenous peoples' traditional medicine and is a common element in Ayurvedic, homeopathic, naturopathic, traditional oriental, and Native American Indian medicine (see the "Alternative Systems of Medical Practice" chapter).

The sophistication of herbal remedies used around the world varies with the technological advancement of countries that produce and use them. These remedies range from medicinal teas and crude tablets used in traditional medicine to concentrated, standardized extracts produced in modern pharmaceutical facilities and used in modern medical systems under a physician's supervision.

Europe

Drug approval considerations for phytomedicines (medicines from plants) in Europe are the same as those for new drugs in the United States, where drugs are documented for safety, effectiveness, and quality. But two features of European drug regulation make that market more hospitable to natural remedies. First, in Europe it costs less and takes less time to approve medicines as safe and effective. This is especially true of substances that have a long history of use and can be approved under the "doctrine of reasonable certainty." According to this principle, once a remedy is shown to be safe, regulatory officials use a standard of evidence to decide with reasonable certainty that the drug will be effective. This procedure dramatically reduces the cost of approving drugs without compromising safety. Second, Europeans have no inherent prejudice against molecularly complex plant substances; rather, they regard them as single substances.

The European Economic Community (EEC), recognizing the need to standardize approval of herbal medicines, developed a series of guidelines, *The Quality of Herbal Remedies* (EEC Directive, undated). These guidelines outline standards for quality, quantity, and production of herbal remedies and provide labeling requirements that member countries must meet. The EEC guidelines are based on the principles of the WHO's *Guidelines for the Assessment of Herbal Medicines* (1991). According to these guidelines, a substance's historical use is a valid way to document safety and efficacy in the absence of scientific evidence to the contrary. The guidelines suggest the following as a basis for determining product safety:

A guiding principle should be that if the product has been traditionally used without demonstrated harm, no specific restrictive regulatory action should be undertaken unless new evidence demands a revised risk-benefit assessment. . . . Prolonged and apparently uneventful use of a substance usually offers testimony of its safety.

With regard to efficacy, the guidelines state the following:

For treatment of minor disorders and for nonspecific indications, some relaxation is justified in the requirements for proof of efficacy, taking into account the extent of traditional use; the same considerations may apply to prophylactic use (WHO, 1991).

The WHO guidelines give further advice for basing approval on existing monographs:

If a pharmacopoeia monograph exists it should be sufficient to make reference to this monograph. If no such monograph is available, a monograph must be supplied and should be set out in the same way as in an official pharmacopoeia.

To further the standardization effort and to increase European scientific support, the phytotherapy societies of Belgium, France,

291

Germany, Switzerland, and the United Kingdom founded the European Societies' Cooperative of Phytotherapy (ESCOP). ESCOPs approach to eliminating problems of differing quality and therapeutic use within EEC is to build on the German scientific monograph system (below) to create "European" monographs.

In Europe, herbal remedies fall into three categories. The most rigorously controlled are prescription drugs, which include injectable forms of phytomedicines and those used to treat life-threatening diseases. The second category is OTC phytomedicines, similar to American OTC drugs. The third category is traditional herbal remedies, products that typically have not undergone extensive clinical testing but are judged safe on the basis of generations of use without serious incident.

The following brief overviews of phytomedicine's regulatory status in France, Germany, and England are representative of the regulatory status of herbal medicine in Europe.

France, where traditional medicines can be sold with labeling based on traditional use, requires licensing by the French Licensing Committee and approval by the French Pharmacopoeia Committee. These products are distinguished from approved pharmaceutical drugs by labels stating "Traditionally used for . . . " Consumers understand this to mean that indications are based on historical evidence and have not necessarily been confirmed by modern scientific experimentation (Artiges, 1991).

Germany considers whole herbal products as a single active ingredient; this makes it simpler to define and approve the product. The German Federal Health Office regulates such products as ginkgo and milk thistle extracts by using a monograph system that results in products whose potency and manufacturing processes are standardized. The monographs are compiled from scientific literature on a particular herb in a single report and are produced under the auspices of the Ministry of Health Committee for Herbal Remedies (Kommission E). Approval of such remedies requires more scientific documentation than traditional remedies, but less than new pharmaceutical drug approvals (Keller, 1991).

In Germany there is a further distinction between "prescription-only drugs" and "normal prescription drugs." The former are available only by prescription. The latter are covered by national health insurance if prescribed by a physician, but they can be purchased over the counter without a prescription if consumers want to pay the cost themselves (Keller, 1991). OTC phytomedicines—used for self-diagnosed, self-limiting conditions such as the common cold, or for simple symptomatic relief of chronic conditions—are not covered by the national health insurance plan.

England generally follows the rule of prior use, which says that hundreds of years of use with apparent positive effects and no evidence of detrimental side effects are enough evidence—in lieu of other scientific data—that the product is safe. To promote the safe use of herbal remedies, the Ministry of Agriculture, Fisheries, and Food and the Department of Health jointly established a database of adverse effects of nonconventional medicines at the National Poisons Unit.

Asia

In more developed Asian countries such as Japan, China, and India, "patent" herbal remedies are composed of dried and powdered whole herbs or herb extracts in liquid or tablet form. Liquid herb extracts are used directly in the form of medicinal syrups, tinctures, cordials, and wines.

In China, traditional herbal remedies are still the backbone of medicine. Use varies with region, but most herbs are available throughout China. Until 1984 there was virtually no regulation of pharmaceuticals or herbal preparations. In 1984, the People's Republic implemented the Drug Administration Law, which said that traditional herbal preparations were generally considered "old drugs" and, except for new uses, were exempt from testing for efficacy or side effects. The Chinese Ministry of Public Health would oversee the administration of new herbal products (Gilhooley, 1989).

Traditional Japanese medicine, called kampo, is similar to and historically derived from Chinese medicine but includes traditional medicines from Japanese folklore. Kampo declined when Western medicine was introduced between 1868 and 1912, but by 1928 it had begun to revive. Today 42.7 percent of Japan's Western-trained medical practitioners prescribe kampo medicines (Tsumura, 1991), and Japanese national health insurance pays for these medicines. In 1988, the Japanese herbal medicine industry established regulations to manufacture and control the quality of extract products in kampo medicine. Those regulations comply with the Japanese government's Regulations for Manufacturing Control and Quality Control of Drugs.

Developing Countries

Herbal medicines are the staple of medical treatment in many developing countries. Herbal preparations are used for virtually all minor ailments. Visits to Western-trained doctors or prescription pharmacists are reserved for life-threatening or hard-to-treat disorders.

Individual herbal medicines in developing regions vary considerably; healers in each region have learned over centuries which local herbs have medicinal worth. Although trade brings a few important herbs from other regions, these healers rely mainly on indigenous herbs. Some have extensive herbal materia medica. A few regions, such as Southeast Asia, import large amounts of Chinese herbal preparations. But the method and form of herb use are common to developing regions.

In the developing world, herbs used for medicinal purposes are "crude drugs." These are unprocessed herbs—plants or plant parts, dried and used in whole or cut form. Herbs are prepared as teas (sometimes as pills or capsules) for internal use and as salves and poultices for external use. Most developing countries have minimal regulation and oversight.

Research Base

The professional literature of Europe and Asia abounds with efficacy and safety studies of many herbal medicines. It is beyond this report's resources to investigate the validity of this vast literature. The following is an overview of some of the more promising research on herbal remedies around the world.

Europe

European phytomedicines, researched in leading European universities and hospitals, are among the world's best studied medicines. In some cases they have been in clinical use under medical supervision for more than 10 years, with tens of millions of documented cases. This form of botanical medicine most closely resembles American medicine. European phytomedicines are produced under strict quality control in sophisticated pharmaceutical factories, packaged and labeled like American medicines, and used in tablets or capsules.

Examples of well-studied European phytomedicines include Silybum marianum (milk thistle), Ginkgo biloba (ginkgo), Vaccinium myrtillus (bilberry extract), and Ilex guayusa (guayusa). Their efficacy is well documented. Herbs of American origin, such as Echinacea

294

(purple coneflower) and Serenoa repens (saw palmetto), are better studied and marketed in Europe than in the United States. Below is an overview of recent research on these phytomedicines and American herbs.

- **Milk thistle (*Silybum marianum*).** Milk thistle has been used as a liver remedy for 2,000 years. In 1970s studies, seed extracts protected against liver damage and helped regenerate liver cells damaged by toxins (alcohol) and by diseases such as hepatitis (Bode et al., 1977) and cirrhosis (Ferenci et al., 1989). More recently, a 6-month treatment of milk thistle significantly improved liver function in 36 patients with alcohol-induced liver disease (Feher et al., 1990). Animal studies show that it may protect against radiation damage caused by x rays (Flemming, 1971), and it gave "complete protection" to rats against brain damage caused by the potent nerve toxin triethyltin sulfate (Varkonyi et al., 1971). European hospital emergency rooms use intravenous milk thistle extract to counteract cases of liver poisoning from toxins such as those in the Amanita phalloides mushroom.

- **Bilberry extract *(Vaccinium myrtillus*).** Bilberry extract is believed to help prevent or treat fragile capillaries. Capillary fragility can cause fluid or blood to leak into the tissues, causing hemorrhage, stroke, heart attack, or blindness. Less serious effects include a tendency to bruise easily, varicose veins, poor night vision, coldness, numbing, and leg cramping. Bilberry extract may protect capillaries and other small blood vessels by increasing the flexibility of red blood cell membranes. This action allows capillaries to stretch, increasing blood flow, and red blood cells can deform into a shape that eases their way through narrow capillaries.

  European clinical trials have shown the effectiveness of bilberry extract for venous insufficiency of the lower limbs in 18- to 75-year-old subjects (Corsi, 1987; Guerrini, 1987). It has been used to treat varicose veins in the legs, where it significantly improved symptoms of varicose syndrome such as cramps, heaviness, calf and ankle swelling, and numbness (Gatta, 1982). These trials revealed no significant side effects, even at 50 percent over the normal dose. In two clinical trials, a standardized bilberry extract was given to 115 women with venous insufficiency and hemorrhoids following pregnancy. Both studies documented improvements of symptoms, including pain, burning, and pruritus, all of which disappeared in most cases (Baisi, 1987; Teglio et al., 1987).

* **Ginkgo biloba extract.** Though this oriental herb has a different traditional use in Asia, Ginkgo biloba is one of Europe's most lucrative phytomedicines (Duke, 1988). In Europe, ginkgo is used mainly against symptoms of aging. It is believed to stimulate circulation and oxygen flow to the brain, which can improve problem solving and memory. It was shown to increase the brain's tolerance for oxygen deficiency and to increase blood flow in patients with cerebrovascular disease (Haas, 1981). No other known circulatory stimulant, natural or synthetic, has selectively increased blood flow to disease-damaged brain areas. In a French study, "the results confirmed the efficacy of [ginkgo extract] in cerebral disorders due to aging" (Taillandier et al., 1988). In another experiment, those given ginkgo showed consistent and significant improvement over the control group on all tests, including mobility, orientation, communication, mental alertness, recent memory, and other factors (Weitbrecht and Jansen, 1985). A "digit copying test" and a computerized classification test confirmed the improved cognitive function related to use of this herb (Rai et al., 1991).

Ginkgo extracts also stimulate circulation in the limbs, reducing coldness, numbness, and cramping. In elderly people, ginkgo improved pain-free walking distance by 30 percent to 100 percent (Foster, 1990). It also lowered high cholesterol levels in 86 percent of cases tested and prevented oxygen deprivation of the heart (Schaffler and Reeh, 1985). The extract seems to affect neurons directly, as shown by a recent French study (Yabe et al., 1992). Another French study proved protection against cell damage, this time by ultraviolet light (Dumont et al., 1992).

A German study documented benefits of long-term ginkgo use in reducing cardiovascular risks, including those associated with coronary heart disease, hypertension, hypercholesterolemia, and diabetes mellitus (Witte et al., 1992). By maintaining blood flow to the retina, ginkgo extracts inhibited deteriorating vision in the elderly. An adequate amount of extract may reverse damage from lengthy oxygen deprivation of the retina. The assessment by doctors and patients of the patients' general condition showed a significant improvement after therapy. These results show that visual field damage from chronic lack of blood flow is reversible (Raabe et al., 1991).

- **Ilex guayusa (*guayusa*).** In animal studies, a concentrated aqueous herbal preparation from guayusa leaves significantly reduced uncontrolled appetite, excessive thirst, and weight loss associated with diabetes (Swanston-Flatt et al., 1989). Although guayusa's active principles are not established, guayusa contains guanidine, a known hypoglycemic (blood sugar-lowering) substance (Duke, 1992b).

- **Echinacea (*purple coneflower*).** The subject of more than 350 scientific studies, most conducted in Europe, *Echinacea* seems to stimulate the immune system non-specifically rather than against specific organisms. In laboratory tests, *Echinacea* increased the number of immune system cells and developing cells in bone marrow and lymphatic tissue, and it seemed to speed their development into immunocompetent cells (cells that can react to pathogens). It speeds their release into circulation, so more are present in blood and lymph, and increases their phagocytosis rate—the rate at which they can digest foreign bodies. *Echinacea* also inhibits the enzyme hyaluronidase, which bacteria use to enter tissues and cause infection. This inhibition helps wounds to heal by stimulating new tissue formation. *Echinacea* exhibits interferon-like antiviral activity documented through extensive experiments in Germany. For example, in a double-blind, placebo-controlled study of 180 volunteers, *Echinacea*'s therapeutic effectiveness for treating flu-like symptoms was "good to very good" (Braunig et al., 1992). Another study showed that orally administered *Echinacea* extracts significantly enhanced phagocytosis in mice (Bauer et al., 1988). Water-soluble *Echinacea* components strongly activated macrophages (Stimpel et al., 1984), enhanced immune system cell motility, and increased these cells' ability to kill bacteria. Other immune system cells were stimulated to secrete the disease-fighting tumor necrosis factor and interleukins 1 and 6 (Roesler et al., 1991). Another study showed that *Echinacea* polysaccharides increased the number of immunocompetent cells in the spleen and bone marrow and the migration of those cells into the circulatory system. The authors said these effects resulted in excellent protection of mice against consequences of lethal listeria and candida infections (Coeugniet and Elek, 1987).

- **Saw palmetto (*Serenoa repens*).** These berries have been used to treat benign prostatic hypertrophy (BPH). The standardized extract was clinically evaluated as effective, has no observed side effects, and costs 30 percent less than the main prescription drug marketed in the United States for BPH (Champpault et al., 1984).

- ***Prunus africanum.*** Another effective herbal drug for treating BPH is made from *Prunus africanum* and is widely prescribed in France. It is interesting to note that the U.S. government is funding a multicenter study on BPH treatment to find the most cost-effective criteria for surgical versus medical treatment. However, because the study includes neither saw palmetto nor *Prunus africanum*, it may not reflect the "state of the art" in clinical medicine worldwide.

China

Since the early 19th century, attempts have been made to understand the actions and properties of traditional Chinese medicine through scientific research. Nearly all of this work has been conducted during the past 60 years, primarily in laboratories in China, Korea, Japan, Russia, and Germany. It was also during this time that most of the drugs used in modern biomedicine were developed. It is therefore not surprising that most of the biomedical research into the effects and uses of traditional Chinese medicinal substances has attempted to isolate their active ingredients and to understand their effects on body tissues.

Several institutions and laboratories at the forefront of medicinal plant research in China are working to identify and study the active ingredients in traditional Chinese herbal remedies. Researchers at the Institute of Materia Medica in Beijing study the use of herbal remedies to prevent and treat the common cold, bronchitis, cancer, and cardiovascular disease and to prevent conception. The institute has isolated compounds such as bergenin from *Ardisia japonica*, traditionally used to treat chronic bronchitis, and monocrotaline from *Crotalaria sessiliflora*, used in folk medicine to treat skin cancer. Most of China's 5,000 medicinal plant species are represented in the institute's herbarium. Other Chinese research organizations with major programs on medicinal herbs are the Institute of Chinese Medicine, Beijing; the Institute of Materia Medica, Shanghai; the Institute of Organic Chemistry, Shanghai; the Municipal Hospital of

Chinese Traditional Medicine, Beijing; the College of Pharmacy, Nanking; and the Department of Organic Chemistry and Biochemistry, Beijing University (Duke and Ayensu, 1985).

Many herbs in China have been extensively studied by using methods acceptable from a Western perspective. For example, a 1992 article in the *Journal of Ethnopharmacology* reported that during the preceding 10 years more than 300 original papers on Panax ginseng had been published in Chinese and English (Liu and Xiao, 1992). Ginseng is one of the world's most thoroughly researched herbs. Following is an overview of recent research on ginseng and other herbs in China. Unless otherwise indicated, the data on specific herbs are taken from *Chinese Herbal Medicine: Materia Medica*, revised edition, compiled and translated by Dan Bensky and Andrew Gamble (1993).

- **Ginseng root (*Panax ginseng* [ren shen]).** The Chinese first used oriental ginseng (*Panax ginseng*) more than 3,000 years ago as a tonic, a restorative, and a specific treatment for several ailments. By the 10th century, oriental ginseng had traveled the Silk Road to the Arabic countries (Kao, 1992), and during the next 4 centuries it spread to Europe, where the French, among others, used it to treat asthma and stomach troubles (Vogel, 1970).

  In modern times, ginseng has been extensively studied in China, Japan, and Korea and, to a lesser degree, in the United States. In its various forms, ginseng or its compounds have various physiological effects. These include antistress capabilities (Cheng et al., 1986; Yuan et al., 1988), antihypoxia effects (Cheng et al., 1988; Han et al., 1979; Qu et al., 1988), alteration of circadian rhythms by modifying neurotransmitters (Lu et al., 1988; Zhang and Chen, 1987), cardiac performance effects (Chen et al., 1982), protection against myocardial infarction in animals (Chen, 1983; Fang et al., 1986), histamine response effects (Zhang et al., 1988), inhibition of platelet aggregation (Shen et al., 1987; Yang et al., 1988), alteration of circadian variation of plasma corticosterone (Li et al., 1988), modulation of immune functions (Qian et al., 1987; Wang et al., 1980), and delay of the effects of aging (Tong and Chao, 1980; Zhang, 1989).

- **Fresh ginger rhizome (*Zingiber officinale* [sheng jiang]).** In one study, preparations of sheng jiang and brown sugar were used to treat 50 patients with acute bacillary dysentery. A cure rate of 70 percent was achieved in 7 days. Abdominal pain and tenesmus (an urgent but ineffectual attempt to urinate or defecate) disappeared in 5 days, stool frequency returned to normal in 5 days, and stool cultures were negative within 4 days, with no side effects.

In another study, 6 to 10 thin pieces of sheng jiang placed over the testes were used to treat acute orchitis (inflammation of the testicles). The ginger was changed daily or every other day. All participants felt a hot-to-numbing sensation in the scrotum, while a few reported local erythema and edema. Among 24 patients in the study, average cure time was 3 days. In a control group of four patients, average healing time was 8.5 days. This technique is not recommended for patients with scrotum lesions.

- **Chinese foxglove root (*Rehmannia glutinosa* [sheng di huang]).** A preparation of this herb and *Radix glycyrrhiza uralensis* (*gan cao*) was used to treat 50 cases of hepatitis in various stages. Within 10 days, 41 cases showed improved symptoms, reduced liver and spleen size, and improved liver function tests. Experiments from the 1930s seemed to show that sheng di huang, given to rats via gastric lavage or injection, lowered serum glucose levels. Later studies of this problem showed variable results. Work in Japan showed that the herb is useful in treating experimental hyperglycemia in rats. In other studies, decoctions of sheng di huang have been used to treat rheumatoid arthritis in adults and children. In one uncontrolled study, 12 subjects all showed reduced joint pain and swelling, increased function, improved nodules and rash, and lowered temperature. Follow up over 3 to 6 months showed only one relapse, which was treated successfully with the same preparation.

- **Baical skullcap root (*Scutellaria baicalensis* [huang qin]).** Huang qin was shown to inhibit the skin reaction of guinea pigs to passive allergic and histamine tests. It has been shown to be effective in treating guinea pigs with allergic asthma. Huang qin also prevented pulmonary hemorrhage in mice subjected to very low pressure. Huang qin has an inhibitory effect against many kinds of bacteria in vitro, including *Staphylococcus aureus*, *Corynebacterium diphtheriae*, *Pseudomonas aeruginosa*, *Streptococcus pneumoniae*, and *Neisseria meningitidis*. In one report, one strain of bacteria (*Staph. aureus*) that was resistant to penicillin remained sensitive to this herb. According to one study, 100 patients with bacillary dysentery received a prescription composed mainly of huang qin. Mean recovery times were 2.5 days until symptoms disappeared, 3.3 days until normal stool examination, and 4.3 days until negative stool cultures.

- **Coptis rhizome, or yellow links (*Coptis chinensis* [huang lian]).** Huang lian and one of its active ingredients, berberine, have broad effects in vitro against many microbes. It strongly inhibits many bacteria that cause dysentery; it is more effective than sulfa drugs but less effective than streptomycin or chloramphenicol. Decoctions of huang lian have been effective against some bacteria that developed resistance to streptomycin and other antibiotics. The herb's antimicrobial ingredient is generally considered to be berberine. Experiments on chicken embryos show that huang lian has an inhibitory effect against flu viruses and the Newcastle virus.

  Huang lian preparations have a strong inhibitory effect in vitro against many pathogenic fungi. Capsules of powdered huang lian were given to patients with typhoid fever, with good results. In one report, two cases that were resistant to antimicrobials responded to this herb. In another study, 30 cases of pulmonary tuberculosis were treated with huang lian for 3 months; all improved.

  A 10-percent solution of huang lian also was used to treat 44 cases of scarlet fever. It was as effective as penicillin or a combination of penicillin and a sulfa drug. Huang lian also has been successfully used to treat diphtheria; in one study, the fever subsided in 1 to 3 days. Huang lian ointments or solutions promoted healing and reduced infections in first- and second-degree burns. It also has positive effects on blood pressure, smooth muscle, lipid metabolism, and the central nervous system; is effective as an anti-inflammatory; and has been used successfully in gynecology, ophthalmology, and dermatology patients.

- **Woad leaf (*Isatis tinctoria* [da qing ye]).** Da qing ye kills some kinds of bacteria, including some strains resistant to sulfa drugs. It was reported effective in hundreds of cases of encephalitis B, with cure rates of 93 percent to 98 percent. In most cases the fever subsided in 1 to 4 days, and symptoms disappeared 3

301

to 5 days later. Da qing ye has been effective by itself in mild and moderate cases; other herbs, acupuncture, and Western drugs should be added in severe cases.

In a study of 100 subjects, only 10 percent of the group given a da qing ye decoction twice daily had upper respiratory infections during the study period versus 24 percent of the control group. When a mixture of decoctions of da qing ye and *Herba taraxaci mongolici cum radice* (*pu gong ying*) was given to 150 children with measles, signs and symptoms disappeared in 4 to 5 days. In 68 of 100 cases, da qing ye was used successfully to treat infectious hepatitis.

- **Wild chrysanthemum flower (*Chrysanthemum indicum* [ye ju hua]).** Ye ju hua has been used to treat hypertension, either alone as an infusion or with *Elos lonicerae japonicae* (jin yin hua) and *Herba taraxaci mongolici cum radice* (pu gong ying) in a decoction. Ye ju hua preparations have an inhibitory effect in vitro against some bacteria and viruses. Preparations given orally or as injections lowered blood pressure. Preparations made from the whole plant had more toxicity and less efficacy than those made from the flower alone.

One study was performed with 1,000 subjects to see whether ye ju hua would prevent colds. The subjects were compared with their own histories and against a matched set of 261 controls. A ye ju hua decoction was taken once a month by people with histories of infrequent colds, twice a month by those with three to five colds a year, and weekly by those with frequent colds. Comparison with their own histories showed a 13.2-percent reduction in frequency, but a greater frequency in comparison with the controls. At the same time, another clinical series of 119 cases of chronic bronchitis was observed. Using the same preparation, this group experienced a 38-percent reduction in acute attacks in comparison with their seasonally adjusted rate for the previous year.

- **Bletilla rhizome (*Bletilla striata* [bai ji]).** Bai ji, in powdered form or in a powder made from starch and a decoction of bai ji, helped control bleeding in seven of eight cases of surgical wounds to dogs' livers. Pure starch was much less effective. Similar results have been achieved with sponges soaked in a sterile water-extraction solution of the herb. In anesthetized dogs with 1-mm-diameter stomach perforations, washing the perforations with 9 g of powdered bai ji through a tube closed the perforations in 15 minutes. Eight hours after the procedure the abdomens were opened, and no trace of gastric contents was found. When the dogs' stomachs were full or the perforations were larger, powdered bai ji had no effect.

In another study, powdered bai ji was used to treat 69 cases of bleeding ulcers, and in all cases the bleeding stopped within 6.5 days. In another series of 29 perforated ulcer cases, the powdered herb was successful in 23 cases, 1 required surgery, and the other 4 died (1 went into hemorrhagic shock while under treatment, and the other 3 were in precarious condition on admission). In other studies, powdered bai ji was given to 60 chronic tuberculosis patients who had not responded to normal therapy. After taking the herb for 3 months, 42 were clinically cured, 13 significantly improved, and 2 showed no change. A sterile ointment made from decocted bai ji and petroleum jelly was used in a local application to treat 48 cases of burns and trauma (less than 11 percent of total body area). Dressings were changed every 5 to 7 days, and all patients recovered within 1 to 3 weeks.

- **Salvia, or cinnabar root (*Salvia miltiorrhiza* [dan shen]).** Dan shen caused coronary arteries to dilate in guinea pig and rabbit heart specimens. In one study of 323 patients given a dan shen preparation for 1 to 9 months, there was marked improvement in 20.3 percent of clinical cases and general improvement in 62 percent of cases. Results were best when patients had coronary artery disease and no history of myocardial infarction. In a clinical series of more than 300 patients with angina pectoris, a combination of dan shen and *Lignum dalbergiae odoriferae* (*jiang xiang*) given intramuscularly or intravenously improved symptoms in 82 percent and electrocardiograms in 50 percent of cases.

- **Corydalis rhizome (*Corydalis yanhusuo* [yan hu suo]).** Yan hu suo is widely used to treat pain. Powdered yan hu suo is a very strong analgesic, about 1 percent the strength of opium. In one clinical study of 44 patients with painful or difficult menstruation, 50 mg of the yan hu suo active ingredient, dihydrocorydaline, given 3 times a day brought significant relief in 14 cases and reduced pain in another 18 cases. Side effects included reductions in menstrual flow, headaches, and fatigue.

- **Root of Szechuan aconite (*Aconitum carmichaeli* [fu zi]).** Fu zi's toxicity has always been a major concern. It is usually prepared with salt to reduce its toxicity. Anesthetized dogs or cats given fu zi preparations showed a sharp drop in blood pressure. In another experiment, fu zi caused blood vessels to dilate in lower extremities and coronary vessels. In normal dosage for humans, fu zi slightly lowers blood pressure, while a large overdose can cause rapid heartbeat or ventricular fibrillation. This herb seems to have some cardiotonic function and a regulatory effect on heart rhythm. Administered with herbs such as *Cortex cinnamomi cassiae (rou gui), Panax ginseng (ren shen), Rhizoma zingiberis officinalis (gan jiang),* and *Radix glycyrrhiza uralensis (gan cao),* fu zi raised blood pressure in animals with acute hemorrhage. In one study, patients with congestive heart failure were treated by intramuscular injections of a fu zi preparation. In all cases, including one of cardiogenic shock, the result was increased cardiac output as well as decreased breathing difficulty, liver swelling, and general edema. A few cases showed temporary side effects of flushing and slight tremors.

- **Licorice root (*Glycyrrhiza uralensis* [gan cao]).** Gan cao preparations have been used with common antituberculosis drugs in many large clinical studies among patients who did not respond to standard treatment. In most cases, symptoms improved or disappeared and x rays improved markedly. In many clinical studies using gan cao for ulcers with groups of 50 to 200 subjects, effectiveness was around 90 percent. It was especially useful to treat the pain, which disappeared or improved within 1 to 3 weeks. The more recent the onset of disease, the better the results. In almost all cases the powdered herb was most effective.

In rats with experimentally induced atherosclerosis, gan cao lowered cholesterol levels and stopped progression of lesions. In several experiments, the herb reduced the toxicity of some substances, including cocaine, and moderately reduced the toxicity of others, including caffeine and nicotine. When decocted with fu zi, it sharply reduced fu zi's toxicity.

- **Dryopteris root, or shield fern (*Dryopteris crassirhizoma* [guan zhong]).** *Dryopteris crassirhizoma* is called *dong bei guan zhong* because it is found in northeastern (*dong bei*) China. In recent times this herb has been prescribed as a preventive measure during influenza epidemics. Guan zhong preparations strongly inhibit the flu virus in vitro. In one clinical trial, 306 people took twice-weekly doses of guan zhong and 340 served as controls. In the treatment group, 12 percent became ill versus 33 percent of the controls. Local versions of guan zhong from Guangdong, Hunan, and Jiangxi provinces have mildly inhibitory effects in vitro against many pathogenic bacteria. Guan zhong also is effective against pig roundworms in vitro, and it expels tapeworms and liver flukes in cattle.

  In other studies, decoctions and alcohol extracts of dong bei guan zhong strongly stimulated the uterus of guinea pigs and rabbits. It increased the frequency and strength of contractions. Intramuscular injections of dong bei guan zhong preparations were used with more than 91-percent success to treat postpartum, post-miscarriage, and post-surgical bleeding.

- **Garlic bulb (*Allium sativum* [da suan]).** Da suan preparations have a strong inhibitory effect in vitro against amebae. In one study, concentrated da suan decoctions were used to treat 100 cases of amebic dysentery. The cure rate was 88 percent, and the average hospital stay was 7 days. In this clinical study, purple-skinned bulbs were more effective than white-skinned bulbs. Patients were discharged on a regimen that included purple-skinned da suan in the daily diet.

  When used with Chinese leek seeds, da suan juice and decoctions have a strong inhibitory effect in vitro against many pathogenic bacteria. Da suan can be effective against bacteria that resist penicillin, streptomycin, and chloramphenicol. In one clinical study, 130 patients with bacillary dysentery were given da suan enemas. Of the follow up colonoscopies, 126 showed that pathological changes were resolved within 6.3 days. In other studies with hundreds of patients, da suan's effectiveness against bacillary dysentery was more than 95 percent. Again, purple-skinned garlic seemed more effective than white-skinned, and fresh bulbs were more effective than old ones. In one clinical study, 17 cases of encephalitis B were treated with

305

an intravenous drip of da suan preparations and supportive care. Except for one fatality, all other cases recovered.

India

Ayurveda, the oldest existing medical system, is recognized by WHO and is widely practiced. The word comes from two Sanskrit roots: ayus means life or span; veda means knowledge or science. India recently increased research on traditional Ayurvedic herbal medicines after observations that they are effective for conditions to which they have traditionally been applied. For example, the ancient Sanskrit text on Ayurveda, the *Sushruta Samhita*, noted that *Commiphora mukul* was useful in treating obesity and conditions equivalent to hyperlipidemia, or increased concentrations of cholesterol in the body. The plant has been used by Ayurveda practitioners for at least 200 years and may have been in use since the writing of the *Sushruta Samhita* more than 2,000 years ago. In a recent study, the crude gum from *Commiphora mukul* significantly lowered serum cholesterol in rabbits with high cholesterol levels. The plant substance also protected rabbits from cholesterol-induced atherosclerosis (hardening of the arteries). This finding led to pharmacological and toxicological studies that showed this herbal remedy to be effective in humans, with no adverse side effects. Approval was obtained from the national regulatory authority in India for further clinical trials (Verma and Bordia, 1988). The drug is marketed in India and other countries for treatment of hyperlipidemia (Chaudhury, 1992).

The following other Ayurvedic herbs have recently been studied in India under modern scientific conditions:

- **Eclipta alba.** In Ayurvedic medicine, *Eclipta alba* is said to be the best drug for treating liver cirrhosis and infectious hepatitis. *Eclipta alba* and *Wedelia calendulacea* are widely used in India for jaundice and other liver and gall bladder ailments. One recent study showed that a liquid extract from fresh *Eclipta* leaves was effective in vivo in preventing acute carbon tetrachloride-induced liver damage in guinea pigs. Clinically, the powdered drug is effective against jaundice in children (Wagner et al., 1986).

- **Common teak tree (*Tectona grandis*).** Trunk wood and bark of the common teak tree are described in Ayurvedic medicine as a cure for chronic dyspepsia (indigestion) associated with burning pain. Teak bark forms an ingredient of several Ayurvedic preparations used to treat peptic ulcer. Pandey et al. (1982) experimentally screened teak bark and its effect on gastric secretory function and ulcers in albino rats and guinea pigs. The solution reduced gastric ulcers in restrained albino rats and significantly inhibited gastric and duodenal ulcers in guinea pigs.

- **Indian gooseberry (*Emblica officinalis* [*amla*]).** Jacob et al. (1988) studied the effect of total serum cholesterol by using amla to supplement the diets of normal and hypercholesterolemic men aged 35-55. The supplement was given for 28 days in raw form. Normal and hypercholesterolemic subjects showed decreased cholesterol levels. Two weeks after the supplement was withdrawn, total serum cholesterol levels of the hypercholesterolemic subjects rose almost to initial levels.

- ***Picrorhiza kurroa.*** *P. kurroa* rhizomes are main ingredients of a bitter tonic used in fever and dyspepsia (indigestion). This drug occupies a prestigious position in Ayurveda. It often substitutes for *Gentiana kurroo*, the Indian gentian. Powdered rhizomes also are used as a remedy for asthma, bronchitis, and liver diseases. Other researchers have reported that a P. kurroa-derived mixture called *kutkin* exhibits hepatoprotective activity; that *P. kurroa* acts as a bile enhancer; that it has antiasthmatic effects in patients with chronic asthma; and that it has immunomodulating activity in cell-mediated and humoral immunity. Another study (Bedi et al., 1989) shows that *P. kurroa* works to boost the immune system as a supplement to other treatments in patients with vitiligo, a skin disease that causes discolored spots.

- **Articulin-F.** This herbomineral formula contains roots of *Withania somnifera*, stem of *Boswellia serrata*, rhizomes of Curcuma longa, and a zinc complex. Kulkarni et al. (1991) performed a randomized, double-blind, placebo-controlled crossover study of articulin-F to treat osteoarthritis, a common progressive rheumatic disease characterized by degeneration and eventual loss of articular cartilage. Articulin-F treatment produced a significant drop in pain severity and disability score, whereas radiological assessment showed no significant changes.

- **Abortifacient plants.** Nath et al. (1992) organized a survey program in Lucknow and Farrukhabad, two towns in Uttar Pradesh, India, from March to July 1987. During the survey, they recorded the common folk medicine used by women and consulted Ayurvedic and Unani drug encyclopedias for the antireproductive potential of the following medicinal plants: leaves of *Adhatoda vasica*, leaves of *Moringa oleifera*, seeds of *Butea monosperma*, seeds of *Trachyspermum ammai*, flowers of *Hibiscus sinensis*, seeds of *Abrus precatorius*, seeds of *Apium petroselinium*, buds of *Bambusa arundensis*, leaves of *Aloe barbadensis*, seeds of *Anethum sowa*, seeds of *Lepidium sativum*, seeds of *Raphanus sativus*, seeds of *Mucuna pruriens*, seeds of *Sida cordifolia*, seeds of *Blepharis edulis*, flowers of *Acacia arabica*, and seeds of *Mesua ferrea*. Plant materials were collected, authenticated, chopped into small pieces, air dried in shade, and then ground to a 60-mesh powder. During the survey, female rats were given aqueous or 90-percent ethanol extracts of the plants orally for 10 days after insemination by males, with special attention to effects on fetal development. Leaf extracts of *Moringa oleifera* and *Adhatoda vasica* were 100-percent abortive at doses equivalent to 175 mg/kg of starting dry material.

- **Neem (*Azadiractica indica*) and turmeric (*Curcuma longa*).** In the Ayurveda and Sidha systems of medicine, neem and turmeric are used to heal chronic ulcers and scabies. Charles and Charles (1991) used neem and turmeric as a paste to treat scabies in 814 people. Ninety-seven percent of cases were cured within 3 to 15 days. The researchers found this to be a cheap, easily available, effective, acceptable mode of treatment for villagers in developing countries, with no adverse reactions.

- **Trikatu.** Trikatu is an Ayurvedic preparation containing black pepper, long pepper, and ginger. It is prescribed routinely for several diseases as part of a multidrug prescription. These herbs, along with piperine (alkaloid of peppers), have biological effects in mammals, including enhancement of other medicaments. Of 370 compounds listed in the *Handbook of Domestic Medicines and Common Ayurvedic Remedies* (Handbook, 1979), 210 contain trikatu or its ingredients. Trikatu is a major decoction used to restore the imbalance of *kapha*, *vata*, and *pitta*, the body's three humors (see the "Alternative Systems of Medical Practice" chapter). *Piper* species are used internally to treat fevers, gastric and abdominal disorders, and urinary difficulties.

Externally they are used to treat rheumatism, neuralgia, and boils. *P. Iongum* and *P. nigrum* are folklore remedies for asthma, bronchitis, dysentery, pyrexia, and insomnia (Akamasu, 1970; Chopra and Chopra, 1959; Perry, 1980; Youngken, 1950). In Chinese folklore, *P. nigrum* is mentioned as a treatment for epilepsy (Pei, 1983). The efficacy of *P. Iongum* fruits in reducing asthma in adults (Upadhyaya et al., 1982) and children has been reported (Dahanukar et al., 1984). *P. nigrum* promoted digestive juice secretion (Shukla, 1984) and increased appetite (Sumathikutty et al., 1979). *P. Iongum* was reported useful in patients with gastric disorders accompanied by clinical symptoms of achlorhydria (Kishore et al., 1990).

Native American Indian Herbal Medicine

In 1977 and 1978, Croom (see Kirkland et al., 1992) spent 2 years documenting plant remedies among the Lumbee Indians, the largest group of Native American Indians east of the Mississippi River. Following are some often-used medicinal plant remedies of the Lumbee:

- **Rabbit tobacco (*Gnaphalium obtusifolium*).** These annual herbs reach a height of 1 to 3 feet and have erect stems with brown, shriveled leaves persisting into winter and stems covered with felt-like hairs in summer. The leaves are 1 to 3 inches long, and alternate. The flowers, minute in whitish heads, appear in late summer to fall. Fields, pastures, and disturbed areas are the sites of this common native plant of the eastern United States. It is used to treat colds, flu, neuritis, asthma, coughs, and pneumonia. This is one of the most popular plants used by the Lumbee. The decoction is drunk hot, like most medicinal teas, and is said to cause profuse sweating.

- **Poke (*Phytolacca americana*).** Also a common native plant of the eastern United States, poke is a robust, perennial herb that reaches a height of 9 feet. It has a large white root; a green, red, or purple stem; alternate leaves up to 1 foot long; and white flowers in a drooping raceme. The fruit is a dark purple to black berry, round, soft, and juicy. Poke is found in waste areas, road sides, disturbed habitats, fields, and pastures. It is used to treat asthma, spring tonic, boils (risings), sores, intestinal worms in people or chickens, cramps, and stomach ulcers. Poke is said to inhibit gram-positive and gram-negative bacteria and is listed as a parasiticide in the British Herbal Pharmacopoeia.

309

- **Pine (*Pinus echinata, P. palustris, P. virginiana*).** Pines are resinous evergreen trees with needlelike foliage leaves in bundles of two to five. The male and female reproductive structures are in separate cones on the same tree; the female cone matures to a large woody cone with winged seeds; pollen sheds in the spring. Pine is used to treat colds, flu, pneumonia, fever, heartburn, arthritis, neuritis, and kidney problems.

- **Oak (*Quercus laevis, Q. phellos*).** These deciduous trees have alternate, unlobed, or variously lobed leaves and minute flowers; the fruit is an acorn. Oak is used to treat kidney problems (including Bright's disease), bladder problems, virus, menstrual bleeding, diarrhea, sores, sprains, and swellings. It is also used as a booster for other remedies.

- **Sassafras (*Sassafras albidum*).** These deciduous, aromatic, small trees or shrubs have green twigs and—when mature thick, furrowed bark. The leaves are 2.5 to 5 inches long; alternate; and either unlobed, lobed on one side, or three-lobed. Flowers are small and yellow in clusters at the end of twigs. The fruit is a dark blue, fleshy drupe on a bright red stalk and cup. This common native plant of fencerows, woodland borders, and old fields of the eastern United States is used to treat measles, chicken pox, colds, flu, and fever. It is also used as a "shotgun heart remedy," a blood purifier, and a spring tonic.

According to the *Handbook of Northeastern Indian Medicinal Plants*, Native American Indians used about 25 percent of the flora of Maryland for medicinal purposes (Duke, 1986). A few examples of medicinal plant species in Maryland are as follows:

- **Sweetflag or calamus (*Acorus*).** The root has been used to treat flatulence, colds, coughs, heart disease, bowel problems, colic, cholera, suppressed menses, dropsy, gravel, headache, sore throat, spasms, swellings, and yellowish urine. Some tribes considered the root a panacea: others thought it had mystic powers.

- **Bloodroot (*Sanguinaria*).** This very poisonous plant is emetic, laxative, and emmenagogue. It has been used to treat chronic bronchitis, diphtheria, sore throat, uterine and other cancers, tetterworm, deafness, and dyspepsia; it has also been used as a pain reliever and sedative. In Appalachia it is carried as a charm to ward off evil spirits.

- **Yellowdock.** Contains anthraquinones of value in the treatment of ringworm and some types of psoriasis. Rumicin from the roots reportedly destroys skin parasites. The anthraquinones are proven laxatives.

- **Coneflower (*Echinacea, Rudbeckia*).** *Echinacea* (purple coneflower) reportedly increases resistance to infection, bad coughs, dyspepsia, venereal disease, insect bites, fever, and blood poisoning.

- **Witch hazel.** A proven astringent and hemostat (to stop bleeding).

- **Lobelia (*lobelia cardinalis*).** Cardinal flower was used to indurate ulcers and to treat stomachache, syphilis, and worms. The leaf tea was used for cold, croup, epistaxis (nosebleed), fever, headache, rheumatism, and syphilis. *Lobelia inflata* (Indian tobacco) yields lobeline sulfate, used in antitobacco therapy. It is used as an antiasthmatic, an expectorant, and a stimulant for bronchitis; it also is used to treat aches, asthma, boils, croup, colic, sore throat, stiff neck, and tuberculosis of the lungs. Some smoked the herb to break a tobacco habit.

- **Mayapple (*Podophyllum peltatum*).** Early Native American Indians used the roots as a strong purgative, liver cleanser, emetic, and worm expellant. A resin made from the plant has been used to treat venereal warts and exhibits antitumor activity; it also is used for snakebite and as an insecticide for potato bugs.

- **Wild cherry (*Prunus virginiana*).** The bark has been used to treat sores and wounds, diarrhea, cold and cough, tuberculosis, hemoptysis, scrofula, sore throat, stomach cramps, and piles. Native American Indians treated snow blindness by leaning over a kettle of boiling bark "tea." Some smoked the bark for headache and head cold.

- **White willow (*Salix alba*).** The bark is astringent, expectorant, hemostatic, and tonic. It is used to treat calluses, cancers, corns, tumors, and warts. Salicylic acid (used to make aspirin) is found in white willow. Leaves and bark of different willows are used in a tea to break a fever. Some Native American Indians burned willow stems and used the ashes to treat sore eyes

311

Barriers to Herbal Medicine Research in the United States

The regulatory lockout of natural remedies has crippled natural products research in U.S. universities and hospitals. There is no dedicated level of support by the Federal Government for herbal medicine research. Herbalists may apply under existing guidelines for approval of new pharmaceutical drugs, but this burden is unrealistic because the total cost of bringing a new pharmaceutical drug to market in the United States is an estimated $140 million to $500 million (*Wall Street Journal*, 1993). Because botanicals are not patentable (although they can be patented for use), an herbal medicine manufacturer could never recover this expenditure. Therefore, herbal remedies are not viable candidates for the existing drug approval process: pharmaceutical companies will not risk a loss of this magnitude, and herb companies lack the financial resources even to consider seeking approval.

Another major barrier is that the academic infrastructure necessary for proper study of ethnomedical systems has seriously eroded in recent decades and must be reinvigorated to accommodate the newly recognized need for preserving traditional medical systems and biological diversity. Pharmacognosy and other academic studies of medicinal plants have declined alarmingly in the United States. North American scientists, once at the forefront of this research, lag behind their European and Japanese colleagues, reducing the likelihood that they will discover useful new medicines from plants. This problem is exacerbated by the fact that much of the discipline of botany has moved away from field studies and into molecular and laboratory approaches. Today only a handful of active full-time ethnobotanists are trained to catalog information on the medicinal properties of plants.

In contrast to the United States, many European and Asian countries have taken a more holistic approach to researching the efficacy of herbal remedies. In Germany, France, and Japan, the past 20 years have seen a rapid increase in research into and use of standardized, semipurified (still containing multiple individual chemicals) herbal extracts called phytomedicines. In Europe and Japan, phytomedicines treat conditions ranging from serious, life-threatening diseases such as heart disease and cancer to simple symptomatic relief of colds, aches and pains, and other conditions treated by OTC drugs in the United States. Phytomedicines include preventive medicines, an often-neglected area of medicine in the United States. The FDA has approved many plant-derived "heroic" cures, but never a plant-derived preventive medicine.

Research Needs and Opportunities

Much modern-day medicine is directly or indirectly derived from plant sources, so it would be foolish to conclude that plants offer no further potential for the treatment or cure of major diseases. Worldwide, the botanical pharmacopoeia contains tens of thousands of plants used for medicinal purposes. Hundreds, perhaps thousands, of definitive texts, monographs, and tomes on herbal remedies exist. But most of this information is outside current databases and remains unavailable to physicians, researchers, and consumers.

Globally, herbal remedies have been researched under rigorous controls and have been approved by the governments of technologically advanced nations. The scientific validation is good to excellent, and the history of clinical use is even stronger. Many phytomedicines have been used by thousands of physicians in their practices and are consumed under medical supervision by tens of millions of people.

A great deal of literature exists on the use of phytomedicines in Europe and within native medical systems in China, Japan, India, and North America. Much of this literature can be found in a unique database developed and maintained by the University of Illinois at Chicago, College of Pharmacy. The database, NAPRALERT (Natural Products Alert), holds references for more than 100,000 scientific articles and books on natural products (plant, microbial, and animal extracts). NAPRALERT includes considerable data on the chemistry and pharmacology (including human studies) of secondary metabolites of known structure, derived from natural sources. About 80 percent of the references are from post-1975 literature, the rest from pre-1975 literature.

In 1981 the U.S. Department of Agriculture (USDA), in conjunction with the National Cancer Institute, concluded a 25-year study of plants with possible anticancer properties. One result is published in the *Handbook of Medicinal Herbs* (Duke and Ayensu, 1985). This work lists 365 folk medicinal species and identifies more than 1,000 pharmacologically active phytochemicals. Toxicity estimates are given for many of these biologically active compounds. More recently, Dr. James Duke of USDA published databases on biologically active compounds of more than 1,000 species of plants with potential medicinal uses (Duke, 1992a, 1992b). Duke proposed to FDA a computer-calculated toxicity index to parallel the Ames Human Exposure Rodent Potency

(HERP) index for carcinogenicity. He calls his index the Better Understanding of Relative Potency (BURP) index.

Much of the literature on traditional Chinese and other Asian countries' herbal medicine is only now beginning to be translated into English. While much of this information is in the form of folklore, there is a growing body of data from scientifically valid literature on herbal medicine research in China as well as India and Japan. In 1986, the book *Chinese Herbal Medicine: Materia Medica* was published by Dan Bensky and Andrew Gamble, both of whom are fluent in Chinese dialects and studied herbal medicine in Asia. Revised in 1993 (Bensky and Gamble, 1993), it presents an in-depth study of 470 herbs used in traditional Chinese medicine. Each entry details the traditional properties, actions and indications, principal combinations, dosage, and contraindications of the herbs, as well as summaries of abstracts regarding pharmacological and clinical research conducted in Asia. The revised edition also provides a brief description of the appearance of each herb.

Although very little laboratory or clinical research has been performed on Native American Indian herbal remedies, extensive listings of herbs and their uses have been compiled by ethnobotanists for several tribes. One source, *American Indian Medicine* (Vogel, 1970), cites references in the professional ethnobotanical literature on herbal medicines for the following tribes: Alabama-Koasati, Arakara, Algonquian, Arapaho, Aztec, Catawba, Cheyenne, Chickasaw, Choctaw, Comanche, Congaree, Creek, Dakota, Delaware, Hoh, Hopi, Houma, Huron, Illinois-Miami, Iroquois, Kwakiutl, Lake St. John Montagnais, Mayan, Menomini, Mescalero Apache, Malecite, Meswaki, Michigan, Mohawk, Mohegan, Natchez, Navajo, Nebraska, Oglala Sioux, Ojibwa, Omaka, Pawnee, Penobscot, Ponca, Potawatomi, Quileute, Rappahannock, San Carlos Apache, Seminole, Sioux, White Mountain Apache, Ute, Winnebago, Yuma, and Zuni. Moerman's database (Moerman, 1982) lists more than 2,000 species of Native American Indian medicinal plants, and Duke (1986) lists more than 700 eastern ones.

These sources—the NAPRALERT database, USDA laboratory research, the Bensky and Gamble book, and the Native American Indian herbal medicinal books—are the foundation on which the U.S. Government, particularly the National Institutes of Health (NIH), can begin substantial research into herbal medicines.

Much unwritten knowledge resides in the hands of healers in many societies where oral transmission of information is the rule. Unfortunately, in many regions this information is endangered because there are no young apprentices to whom elderly healers can pass on their unwritten wisdom; the knowledge that has been refined over thousands of years of experimentation with herbal medicine is being lost. A major research opportunity in this area would be to catalog information on herbal medicines from thousands of traditional healers in cultures where these skills are normally transmitted through an apprentice system. Some organizations have recently increased their efforts to catalog endangered herbal knowledge from traditional medical systems in Latin America, such as those practiced in the rain forests of Belize (Arvigo and Balick, 1993) and Peru (Duke and Martinez, in press).

Basic Research Priorities

Basic research into characterizing these plant products and compounds in terms of standardized content and potential toxicity is needed to allow safe and replicable research to document clinical efficacy. Basic science research should be conducted to evaluate research on the biochemical effects of traditional herbal prescriptions from Western, Ayurvedic, oriental, and other traditions (see the "Alternative Systems of Medical Practice" chapter).

Clinical Research Priorities

Research in phytomedicines in the United States could follow on the results of existing high-quality European and Asian research on plant medicines and should focus on replicating results of key studies or addressing weaknesses in those studies. Reviews of foreign literature and translations of non-English literature would be helpful. Current widespread use of herbal medications as "food supplements" in the United States provides a ready base of users, producers, and practitioners for clinical research in traditional and modern applications of botanical medicine.

Research Issues

Before a comprehensive research agenda is developed, several key issues must be addressed, including the following: the impending loss of knowledge about traditional healing in many societies; the impending loss of large numbers of plant species of potential medicinal value; impediments to the use of herbal remedies outside the cultures in which they originated; and determination of the conditions under

315

which herbal medicines are most appropriate, safe, and effective. Additionally, several regulatory issues hamper research into herbal medicines.

Loss of Knowledge

The knowledge of traditional healers in remote Amazonian or Central American regions may have the potential to make a significant contribution to Western society. But few, if any, practitioners of these lesser known medical systems practice outside their native range, and those who still practice within these regions are elderly and often have not found younger disciples.

Loss of Plant Species of Potential Medicinal Value

This loss of knowledge from traditional healers comes at a time when native flora in many areas, especially tropical regions, are being destroyed at an alarming pace. In the United States alone, an estimated 10 percent of all species of flowering plants will be extinct by the year 2000, including an estimated 16 species of medicinally useful plants (Farnsworth et al., 1985).

One hopeful sign is that the U.S. Government recently formed a cooperative biodiversity group including representatives from NIH, the National Institute of Mental Health, the National Science Foundation (NSF), and the U.S. Agency for International Development. This group intends to fund research to locate and catalog medicinally active substances that can be analyzed and used for new pharmaceutical drug development, while working to preserve biological diversity in developing countries.

Use in Practice

Basic to the use of medicinal herbs in many societies is the practice of using whole, unrefined plant material. The material may be leaves, buds, flowers, bark, or roots, separately or in combination. In some cases an herbal remedy is a complex mixture of many plants. There is an age-old belief that whole-plant medicines have fewer dangerous side effects and provide a more balanced physiological action than plant-derived pharmaceutical drugs whose single ingredient has been isolated, concentrated, and packaged as a pill or liquid.

Herbs and herbal preparations generally are self-administered. Often they are purchased through native herbalists who prescribe one or more herbs or preparations on the basis of medical and health approaches that often include concepts of attaining balance in the client's body, psychology, and spirit (see the "Community-Based Medical Practices" section of the "Alternative Systems of Medical Practice" chapter). Consequently, it is often difficult to assess the relative value of herbal remedies versus prescription drugs on a one-to-one basis.

Indeed, herbal remedies of all types, including those from China, are composed of a multitude of ingredients whose interactions with the body are exceedingly complex. A high level of sophistication of research methodology is necessary to describe the interaction between the human body and substances as complex as those contained in many herbal remedies. Only recently has such a rigorous methodology begun to be developed. For example, the Chinese herb Herba hedyotidis diffusae (bai hua she she cao) has been shown clinically effective in the prevention and treatment of a variety of infectious diseases. However, it has not been demonstrated to have a significant inhibitory effect in vitro against any major pathogen. Only as techniques became available to test the immunological system did it become apparent that at least part of the herb's effect was due to its enhancement of the body's immune response (Bensky and Gamble, 1993).

Another complicating factor in researching traditional Chinese herbal medicine is the fact that Chinese medicine characteristically tries to treat the whole body to alleviate disease stemming from one body organ. Therefore, it rarely relies on a single herb to treat an illness. Instead, formulas usually contain 4 to 12 different herbs (Duke and Ayensu, 1985).

Beyond the problem of trying to test herbal preparations that may contain many active ingredients is the question of whether the research eventually will lead to the isolation of single active ingredients that can be packaged and sold separately. Intense debate surrounds the issue of how to conduct clinical trials of herbal medicines according to Western pharmaceutical clinical standards. Critics say there is an inherent problem with the single-active-ingredient approach preferred by pharmaceutical companies that are actively involved in herbal medicine research. The problem, they say, is that isolating a single compound may not be the most appropriate approach in situations where a plant's activity decreases on further fractionation (separation of active ingredients by using solvents) or where the plant contains two or three active ingredients that must be taken together to produce the full effect (Chaudhury, 1992). Beckstrom-Sternberg and Duke (1994) have documented several cases where synergy has been lost by using the single-ingredient approach to developing drugs from plants.

317

A good example of this single-active-ingredient versus whole-plant debate is illustrated by intense interest among pharmaceutical companies in the compound called genistein. Genistein is part of a class of compounds called flavonoids that occur naturally in plants such as kudzu, licorice, and red clover. Soybeans contain high concentrations of genistein, and lima beans reportedly are even higher in genistein than soybeans (Duke, 1993). There is increasing evidence that genistein may inhibit the growth of cancers of the stomach (Yanagihara et al., 1993), pancreas (Ura et al., 1993), liver (Mousavi and Adlercreutz, 1993), and prostate (Peterson and Barnes, 1993). Genistein is believed to inhibit the growth of cancers because of its antiangiogenetic properties (i.e., it prevents the growth of new blood vessels—a process known as angiogenesis—to tumors).

Genistein is being intensely studied as a possible preventive or treatment for breast cancer, which kills an estimated 44,000 women in the United States each year (Duke, 1993). Studies indicate a correlation between a high intake of foods containing genistein (soy products) and a low incidence of hormone-dependent cancers such as breast cancer (Hirayama, 1986) and prostate cancer (Baker, 1992). The growth of certain cancers, especially breast cancers, has been shown to depend on the female sex hormone estrogen. Genistein exhibits estrogen-like activity in plants and is often called a phytoestrogen. In humans it binds to estrogen receptors (Baker, 1992). It has been suggested that these phytoestrogens may compete with endogenous estrogen on the cellular level, further reducing the cellular proliferation and the potentially carcinogenic effects of estrogen (Tang and Adams, 1981). Thus, it may prevent the growth of estrogen-dependent cancer by competing for estrogen sites on the tumor cells.

If genistein is developed as an isolated pharmaceutical drug, it may have some action against cancer, but the purified compound may not be as potent as genistein in its natural state, and trials may give misleading results. The reason is that all plant species containing genistein also contain other flavonoid compounds, which may have synergistic effects when ingested with genistein. Formononetin—a precursor of equol, which also occurs with genistein—is said to be more active estrogenically than genistein (Spanu et al., 1993). Although genistein clearly inhibits angiogenesis, several other compounds are pseudoestrogens. With this in mind, the question arises: Is a mixture of genistein, formononetin, and other flavonoids, as occurs in many plants, more estrogenic (and antiangiogenic) than an equivalent quantity of any one of these components? If so, the herbal or dietary approach may make more sense than a genistein "silver bullet" approach.

Safety, Efficacy, and Appropriateness

Opinions about the safety, efficacy, and appropriateness of medicinal herbs vary widely among medical and health professionals in countries where herbal remedies are used. Some countries' professionals accept historical, empirical evidence as the only necessary criterion for herbal medicine's efficacy. Others would ban all herbal remedies as dangerous or of questionable value.

The problem is further complicated by the fact that many "patent medicines" available in world trade often are sold as herbal medicinal preparations when they include nonherbal substances. These nonherbal additives often include toxic metals (cinnabar, i.e., mercury) (Kang-Yum and Oransky, 1992), poisonous substances (powdered scorpion), or refined prescription drugs (Catlin et al., 1993). Usually labeled "Chinese herbal medicine," many of these products are manufactured in Thailand, Taiwan, or Hong Kong and exported to the United States, where they are sold in retail outlets. The California Department of Health Services, in conjunction with the Oriental Herbal Association, recently published a list of 20 popular Asian patent medicines that contain toxic ingredients.

Regulatory Issues

The increased use of plant medicines has potential for improving public health and lowering health care costs. Phytomedicines, if combined with the preventive model of medical practice, could be among the most cost-effective, practical ways to shift the focus of modern health care from disease treatment to prevention. But drug regulatory policy prevents the United States from taking advantage of these phytomedicines for two reasons. The first is the exorbitant expense involved in investigating each chemical compound in a given plant extract before it can be tested for clinical usefulness. Hence there is an urgent need to rework current research guidelines to allow the whole plant material or combination mixture (an herbal remedy containing more than one plant) to be evaluated instead of requiring separate evaluations of each chemical component of the therapeutic ingredients.

The second reason is that regulatory requirements for proof of safety and efficacy constitute an economic disincentive for private industry to conduct additional scientific studies. Relaxing regulatory requirements for efficacy for herbal products might make it economically feasible for more private companies to pursue research into issues of safety and quality control. Even with such regulatory change, some public funding of research is needed to confirm the remedies' validity. Public funds are needed because private industry has no incentive to develop an herbal product that might displace a patented drug from an approved treatment regime.

Recommendations

The Panel on Herbal Medicine recommends the following:

- OAM should hold a research organizational conference to facilitate planning in herbal medicine research. The conference would help to identify state-of-the-art questions in ethnomedical research, existing databases, and research personnel needed to support basic and clinical research needs in this area.

- Federal funding agencies such as NSF and NIH must begin to support the training of ethnobotanists—specifically in the field of ethnomedicine—and to offer funding opportunities to foster the rebirth of this field at U.S. universities and research institutions. This is a critical priority because much traditional knowledge in herbal remedies is in danger of disappearing, as are the plant species used in these systems of medicine.

- The bias against plant medicines must be eliminated by restructuring the requirements for proof of efficacy and concentrating on safety, and by removing the need for extensive analyses of chemically complex natural product medicines (thus eliminating the "monosubstance bias"). Several international regulatory models exist to guide the United States in this direction. For example, the German "Kommission E" (expert committee for herbal remedies) monographs give a good example of how the United States might simplify the approval of natural products without sacrificing safety or quality standards. (The "doctrine of reasonable certainty" that influences the approval of drugs under this system was previously mentioned.)

  Adopting a more realistic standard of evidence for established plant medicines would eliminate much of the expense required for approval of new and unknown chemical drugs. Doing so would be similar to having standardized the crude drug senna leaf, used in the United States as an OTC laxative and documented for safety, effectiveness, and quality.

Another option might be to require pharmaceutical companies that are testing a plant-derived, single-ingredient pharmaceutical on a specific condition to demonstrate that it is more effective than the natural product. For example, before a patent could be issued to a pharmaceutical company for an isolated compound such as genistein, the company would first have to prove that the isolated compound is more effective than genistein consumed in context (as a food). But some market incentive, such as exclusive prescriptive marketing rights, might be needed to allow the pharmaceutical company to recoup its research costs.

- Legislative action may be required to restate FDA's mandate with respect to herbal products and traditional medications. The current regulatory mandate puts FDA in a difficult position. It is expected to "protect the public" but has no expertise or resources to evaluate the global herbal medicine inventory. If a crisis such as the contaminated tryptophan affair (see the "Diet and Nutrition" chapter) were to occur with a popular herbal product, FDA might attempt to prohibit the sale of medicinal herbs altogether. Instead of expecting FDA to be an omnipotent protector, Congress should legislate a more educational, informational role.

With respect to herbs used in popular health care, a proactive FDA role in establishing quality and safety standards would benefit the public and industry. A certification system for herbal content and potency of marketed products could be set up by FDA with USDA and the herbal industry. Such a system could draw on the existing global database and other countries' regulatory experiences. Participation in a voluntary product certification system would be a marketing advantage for ethical producers, allowing them, for example, to make a statement such as "This product meets U.S. government purity and potency standards." New statutory authority also would be necessary to establish a category that would allow traditional usages to be listed on labels according to criteria similar to WHO guidelines.

Finally, if herbal remedy producers were given the option to apply for specific health condition label indications based on new FDA phytomedicine standards, the United States would have the same three-tiered regulatory system adopted by other developed countries. Such a voluntary system would let consumers make intelligent personal choices about the use of medicinal herb products while mandating safety standards consistent with existing OTC practices for potentially toxic drugs such as aspirin and ibuprofen.

• OAM should review the TRAMIL approach [Traditional Medicine for the Islands; see www.idrc.ca/books/reports/1997/22-01e.html], in which distinguished Caribbean botanists, chemists, ethnologists, and physicians review promising herbs and label them as reasonably safe and effective for people who cannot afford the prescription alternatives.

Chapter 21

Herbal Supplements

Natural Doesn't Mean Safe

They come in capsules, tablets, liquids and powders. Their names are often strange and difficult to pronounce. They promise to heal or enhance your health—naturally.

And they're selling like hot cakes.

They're herbal supplements. Americans spend almost $700 million a year on herbal remedies sold in health food stores.

Yet there's scanty proof that the supplements can actually help you. Worse, scientists know little about the ingredients in some products.

Shred of Truth Isn't Proof

The popularity of herbs often stems from testimonials or exaggerated bits of scientific evidence.

Echinacea (ek i NAY see ah), a member of the daisy family, is touted as a remedy for cold or flu. Echinacea does contain substances capable of strengthening the immune system to fight infection.

Yet scientists haven't determined its practical usefulness. And it hasn't been approved by the Food and Drug Administration (FDA).

Studies show ginkgo biloba extract can stimulate blood flow in the brains of older adults. In Germany, the herb is sold as a prescription

©1994 Reprinted from the *Mayo Clinic Health Letter,* June 1994 with permission of the Mayo Foundation for Medical Education and Research, Rochester, Minnesota 55905. For subscription information, please call 1-800-333-9038. Reprinted with permission.

drug. Because its complete chemical makeup hasn't been analyzed, it hasn't been approved as a drug in the United States.

It's likely some herbs improve certain conditions. Many of today's pharmaceuticals originated from plants. Digitalis, used to treat congestive heart failure, initially came from the leaves of the foxglove plant.

Taxol, a drug originally from the yew tree, is a promising medication for ovarian and breast cancer.

Yet what separates these plant-derived drugs from herbal supplements is careful scientific study. Many herbs are sold in drug-like formulas and potencies without having been evaluated for safety and effectiveness, which is required by the drug-approval process.

Known Hazards

Lack of regulation doesn't mean all herbs are dangerous. Yet taking them is risky. Here are several supplements to avoid because they can have serious side effects:

- **Comfrey, borage and coltsfoot**. Toxic chemicals called pyrrolizidine alkaloids contained in these herbs may cause liver disease.

- **Chaparral**. Five cases of liver disease (acute toxic hepatitis) have been linked to the use of this medicinal herb. Although word of mouth touts chaparral as a cure for cancer, no evidence supports the claim. FDA also has no evidence that chaparral slows aging, "cleanses" the blood or helps treat skin problems.

- **Ma huang**. You'll find this herb mainly in "weight loss" teas. Not only is it ineffective for helping you lose weight, but Ma huang acts on the central nervous system and can cause a dangerous rise in blood pressure. It's particularly unsafe if you have heart disease, diabetes or thyroid disease.

- **Germanium**. This substance has no properties of a food or nutrient, yet it's claimed to promote overall health. Proponents also claim germanium neutralizes heavy metal toxicity. Long-term use of this supplement may lead to kidney damage and death.

- **Yohimbe (yo HIM be)**. Used to enhance sexual performance, it generally lacks practical use due to its serious side effects, including tremors, anxiety, high blood pressure and rapid heart rate.

324

A *Game of Russian Roulette*

When you take an herbal supplement, you do so at your own risk. At a minimum, use these precautions:

- Don't use herbal remedies for serious illnesses like heart disease, cancer or arthritis.

- Tell your doctor about all supplements you take, to avoid interactions with other medications.

- Don't give herbs or other "dietary supplements" to children.

New Regulations

Effective in July 1994, the supplement industry must abide by the same food labeling laws that govern packaged foods.

The laws require any supplement bearing a health claim to support the claim with scientific evidence that meets government approval.

Any product marketed as a way to cure, modify, treat or prevent disease, will continue to be regulated by the Food and Drug Administration as a drug.

The regulations won't drastically change the availability of supplements. But they will make it more difficult for companies to promote unproven health benefits on a product's label or accompanying literature.

The regulation won't affect books and pamphlets about herbs and other "dietary supplements" not associated with a particular product.

Chapter 22

The Efficacy and Politics of Medicinal Plants

Herbal medicine is the oldest and most widely used form of medicine in the world today. Yet medicinal herbs that formerly were held in esteem now are commonly dismissed as placebos. This chapter reviews the state of plant-derived drug research and discusses the efficacy and safety of herbal medicines within the context of the contemporary political and regulatory framework. The chapter also explores the relationship between medicinal plant use and temporally changing disease pattern.(*Alternative Therapies in Health and Medicine.* 1996,—2(4)36-41)

Throughout history medical practitioners have used as remedies plants and other materials taken from nature. Although some of the therapeutic proper ties attributed to plants have proven to be erroneous, medicinal plant therapy is based on the empirical findings of hundreds and thousands of years. For example, ancient Egyptians used the fruits and leaves of the bishop's weed (*Ammi majus*) to treat vitiligo, a skin condition characterized by a loss of pigment. More recently, a drug (ß-methoxypsoralen) has been produced from this plant to treat psoriasis and other skin disorders, as well as T-cell lymphoma. Claims made in the 18th century that pokeroot (*Phytolacca decandra*) is effective against cancer have been discounted, though this plant has been shown to kill cancer in mice.

327

One quarter of all medical prescriptions are formulations based on substances derived from plants or plant-derived synthetic analogs, and 80 percent of the world's population—primarily those in developing countries—rely on plant-derived medicines for their healthcare. During the last 40 years at least a dozen potent drugs have been derived from flowering plants including *Dioscorea* spp-derived diosgenin, from which all anovulatory contraceptive agents have been derived; reserpine and other antihypertensives and tranquilizing alkaloids from *Rauwolfia* species; pilocarpine to treat glaucoma and "dry mouth," derived from a group of South American trees (*Pilocarpus* spp) in the citrus family; two powerful anticancer agents from the rosy periwinkle (*Catharantus roseus*); laxative agents from *Cassia* species and a cardiotonic agent to treat heart failure from *Digitalis* species. Although discovered through serendipitous laboratory observation, three of the major sources for anticancer drugs on the market or completing clinical trials were derived from North American plants used medicinally by Native Americans: the papaw, *Asimina* spp; the Western yew tree (*Taxus brevifolia*), effective against ovarian cancer; and the mayapple (*Podophyllum peltatum*), used to combat leukemia, lymphoma, lung, and testicular cancer.

The scientific literature is replete with studies indicating the antiviral, antimicrobial, anti-inflammatory, antifungal, antibiotic, and anticarcinogenic activity of specific plants. For the most part, however, these findings are not followed up, due to the lengthy and expensive procedures involved in testing and developing a drug for regulatory approval. In fact, research investment in plant-derived drugs by pharmaceutical companies has been dwindling for much of the 20th century, and by the end of the 1970s had virtually ground to a halt. One reason is that after a 20-year, multimillion-dollar plant screening effort by researchers for the National Cancer Institute, not a single agent of general use in the treatment of human cancer was identified. It should be noted, however, that the screening program used a mouse leukemia cancer as the only screen, whereas cancer comprises some 200 disease types. Japan, France, China, and many other countries are actively studying and developing plant-derived medicines, while the US is lagging behind.

With developments in biotechnology; molecular receptor- binding bioassays; and automated, assembly line screening facilities and analytical techniques, thousands of plant extracts can be tested daily for a spectrum of diseases. In order to keep this highly sophisticated technology in operation, drug companies once again are actively collecting plants and other natural products such as marine organisms;

insects; leech anticoagulants; and spider, snake, and frog venom. Biochemical research on plants is expected to lead to the discovery of direct therapeutic agents and new leading structures that facilitate the synthesis of more complex compounds or novel analogs. Two results of this chemical prospecting are alkaloids from a Cameroonian rain forest vine and an Australian chestnut tree showing activity against the AIDS virus. These advances in separation and structural elucidation technology make it advisable to reevaluate many scientifically discarded plants. Issues that have arisen as a result of this renewal of biochemical prospecting are whether the plants should be collected randomly or on the basis of local ethnobotanical knowledge, intellectual property rights and equitable remuneration to the indigenous population and host nation for any drugs derived from native plants, and environmental protection. Plant-derived drug research is competing with other drug discovery methods such as microbial fermentation; intercellular receptor-based drugs; receptor cloning; directed molecular evolution; peptide selectide; partial, Furka-split, and combinatorial synthesis; drug-producing plant tissue cultures with directed biosynthesis; and transgenically engineered plants to produce oral vaccines. Whether synthetic or natural research will first be successful is far from clear.

The therapeutic efficacy of botanical drugs depends on several factors including purity, potency, and correct dosage. A low dose might be ineffective and the margin of safety between dosages that are correct and fatally excessive—as with *Digitalis* drugs—is at times quite small. To achieve this accuracy, crude drug plants must be standardized in terms of chemical races, growing conditions, harvesting periods, drying and storage conditions, and precise dosage. These standardized procedures, however, are frequently lacking. Pharmaceutical disparagement of herbal medicines is based on more than scientific criteria. The scientific discovery of a plant grown in a flower pot that will prevent an ailment from which drug companies make large profits is obviously an economic threat. The chemical constituents of plants, if published, cannot be patented and generate profit. With no profit incentive, drug companies are unwilling to investigate and develop plant-based drugs. In some cases, the synthetic analogs of unpatentable chemical constituents do not reproduce their biological activity. Some $6 billion is spent annually on herbal medicines in Europe. Given the popularity and marketing opportunities, drug companies are aggressively buying up smaller herbal medicine companies, though they have no allegiance to the philosophy of green medicine.

The Efficacy and Safety of Herbal Medicines

The prevailing scientific theory of drug discovery is that all disease causation occurs on a molecular level. The imbalances or derangements of molecules set in motion a cascade of malfunctions called disease. Cholesterol molecules, for example, cause heart disease by forming obstructions in the lining of the blood vessels. Similarly, a chemical drug produces its effect on the body by entering a cell through a portal or receptor that conforms to the shape of the drug molecule. Each molecular receptor is uniquely designed to grab hold of a specific chemical. All drug discovery procedures entail finding particular molecules that stimulate or block the activity of cell receptor molecules by fitting into them, like a lock and key. In contrast, medicinal plants are described as having activities on a higher, physiological level (e.g., antispasmodics relieve irregular and painful action of muscles or muscle fiber; astringents, applied to the body, render the solids dense and firm; diaphoretics promote or cause perspirable discharge by the skin). A plant that increases the secretion of urine can be used to treat kidney and bladder ailments or to eliminate body poisons. Tannins, for example, are plant compounds that can bind with proteins in the skin and mucous membranes and convert them into insoluble and resistant tissues. Hence, plants high in tannins such as bilberry and oak bark are used for a number of ailments including diarrhea, wounds, inflamed gums, hemorrhoids, and frostbite.

Herbal medicines, preparations, and extractions represent the major portion of the traditional, preindustrial pharmacopoeia. In the 1800s, medical doctors commonly had a comprehensive knowledge of botany, which is no longer the case. Following the coal-and-tar revolution at the turn of the century, the use of synthetic drugs increasingly dominated medical practice. With the development of chemistry, active plant constituents could be isolated and produced synthetically. Synthetically derived chemicals were considered to have improved activity and considered superior to the natural active ingredients. The remaining material in the plant was termed ballast, until it was learned that the isolated substances frequently showed toxic activity, and that these secondary substances, perceived as inactive impurities, displayed a certain moderating activity in the body. Taking vitamin C pills is not the same as eating an orange, and there are marked differences in effect between taking a drug such as caffeine, cocaine, or mescaline, and taking the plant from which the drug is derived.

Medicinal plants, unlike pharmacological drugs, commonly have several chemicals working together catalytically to produce a combined effect that surpasses the total activity of the individual constituents. The combined action of these substances increases the activity of the main, medicinal constituent by speeding up or slowing down its assimilation in the body. Secondary substances might increase the stability of the active compound, minimize the rate of undesired side effects, and have an additive, potentiating, or antagonistic effect. Secondary constituents might contribute to the overall effect, as do the polysaccharides in chamomile, which increase the anti-inflammatory activity of apigenin, luteolin, and other flavones. Saponins increase the bioavailability and permeability of secondary substances, which might influence the strength of action of the active components. Bitters and aromatic compounds might improve metabolic function and facilitate the dissolution and absorption of the active principles by stimulating gastrointestinal secretions. Saponins, tannins, and organic acid salts also facilitate absorption of the active principles by inhibiting intestinal movements or modifying bile secretion. By influencing bioavailability, absorption, and the excretion of the active ingredients, secondary substances might determine the strength of action, minimize side effects, and act in a synergistic, additive, or antagonistic manner.

Herbal medicines commonly are mixtures of several plants that might act synergistically, a phenomenon that is viewed by molecular oriented bioscientists as "voodoo." Herbal combinations are formulated in a precise way to increase or promote therapeutic effectiveness, alter the actions of substances, or reduce toxicity or side effects. Two or more plant drugs with similar properties mutually reinforce therapeutic action in an additive or synergistic manner. Mixtures or formulations may act in different ways and on different parts of the body to yield an overall effect. In traditional Chinese medicine, combinations of plant drugs also are formulated to minimize or eliminate the toxicity or undesirable side effects of one substance, diminish or neutralize each other's action, inhibit the action of one drug, lead the principal therapeutic ingredients to their appropriate sites, and change the action or effect of the individual herbs.

The therapeutic activity of medicinal plants greatly depends on their proper use and application. Simply dipping an herbal tea bag into hot water is insufficient and in many cases herbal medicines must be taken in sufficient strength and over an extended period of time in order to obtain therapeutic benefit. The method of preparation and strength will have different results. A hot infusion of boneset, for example, yields a diaphoretic, a cold infusion acts as a mild laxative, and in large doses boneset acts as an emetic and cathartic. A highly promising anticancer alkaloid from the Chinese plant *Camptotheca acuminata* was quickly discarded during clinical trials when it was discovered to be toxic to the liver. Later, it was found that this side effect was the result of changing the mode of administration from oral to intravenous. Research on this plant drug subsequently has been revived. The content and effectiveness of the active principles in plants, moreover, are reduced when the fresh plant materials are dried. Herbal medicines commonly are prepared by extraction with boiling water, which in certain instances produces yields that are higher than those in other extraction methods. Chemists commonly work with organic solvents that yield enzymes producing destruction of certain constituents and the nondetection of relevant pharmacological activity.

Reasons for official misgivings regarding plant medicines include the unsubstantiated and oftentimes extravagant claims made by herbal advocates and the uncritical manner in which herbal books are compiled. For example, one popular herb book ascribes, on the average, 23 different medicinal uses to each plant (e.g., *Angelica* is prescribed for cancer, electric shock, epilepsy, tuberculosis, and so on). Many herbs have a long history of medicinal use, and the lists of ailments treated with them therefore are quite extensive. Medicinal plant use changes over time, and many of the diseases found in herbal books are indicative of ailments that were widespread during earlier time periods. Moreover, plants commonly exhibit a wide range of pharmacological activities. Nut grass (*Cyperus rotundus*), for example, shows hypotensive, antihistamine, antiemetic, smooth muscle relaxant, antipyretic, and anti-inflammatory activities in experimental animal studies. A plant may contain several natural compounds that cause a single biochemical effect, a chemical substance may affect some aspects of two diseases sharing a common biochemical mechanism, or a substance may possess two biochemical activities that contribute to its effect in several therapeutic areas. A compound such as gingkolide B, which inhibits the platelet activating, factor—an important inflammatory mediator—has potential clinical utility in treating a broad spectrum of illnesses including psoriasis, lupus, bronchoasthma, allergic inflammations, anaphylaxis, graft rejection, Alzheimer's disease, and immunocomplex disorders like toxic shock. Herbal preparations made from the gingko tree containing gingkolide have a commercial value of $500 million annually in Europe, where it is used to treat circulatory disorders, improve metabolism in the brain, and prevent oxidative damage to the cerebral membranes. Gingko constituents improve cerebral capillary flow and are used to treat sleep disturbances, depression, and other symptoms of cerebral insufficiency in the elderly. Chemical constituents of gingko also expand the blood vessels, increase circulation—especially in deep-lying arteries—and prevent blood platelet clotting.

Plato's definition of the Greek word *pharmakon* as meaning both "cure" and "poison" suggests an early recognition of the hidden property of many plants: that they contain medicinal and potentially toxic substances. Taken in excessive dosages, plants, like virtually all substances, are toxic. Prune juice taken as a laxative may produce diarrhea, and licorice root, active against gastric ulcers, in large doses causes heart failure. Castor oil (Ricinus communis) seeds yield a strong laxative but are highly toxic. Several common medicinal plants including chamomile, marigold, and yarrow may produce minor allergic reactions, and mistletoe, sassafras bark, comfrey, coltsfoot, and calamus contain carcinogenic chemicals. Phytotherapeutic drugs show mutagenic activity and severe illnesses and deaths have been reported from pyrrolizidine alkaloid-containing medicinal herbs and dietary exposure to cyanogenic glycosides and lectins.

Advocates of herbal medicines tend to minimize potential dangers, whereas pharmacologists and health authorities magnify out of proportion the actual adverse effects. Although pepper mint and some other herbs may contain toxic elements in trace amounts, the toxins are only dangerous if taken in pure form. Cases of adverse reactions to herbal medicines are rare and often due to misidentified or incorrect plant admixtures, adverse interaction of the herbal medicine with a prescription drug, inadequate evaluation and quality control, and overconsumption or prolonged use of an herbal remedy. Contamination by microorganisms, the Chernobyl reactor accident, and metal pollutants such as lead, cadmium, and magnesium, is often due to a lack of good quality control in the cultivation and production of herbal products. Compared with the dangerous side effects of many pharmaceutical products and the thousands killed or maimed by biomedical intervention each year, the overall risks of herbal medicines are quite low.

The advanced herbal medicines marketed in Europe ar generally safe, though certain imported herbal products distributed by mail or sold in health food stores are sources for concern. One such product for asthma was found to contain arsenic cockroach extract, stramonium, and strychnine. Although there are dangers to uninformed consumers of botanical drugs four cases of herbal poisoning in 2 years is not very startling considering that tons of most every kind of herb have been consumed over the years. In contrast, there are three million severe pesticide poisonings each year, with 220,000 deaths worldwide. Health authorities avidly institute projects to document toxicological problems resulting from exposure to herbal medicine and food supplements; yet no clinical trials are set to determine the safety of the billions of tons of more than 100,000 foreign chemicals released into the environment annually.

Although many diseases such as pyorrhea and arthritis have always been with us, the mortality patterns due to disease have changed dramatically throughout history. It is important to understand this process in order to evaluate medicinal plants used under different historical and cultural conditions. Medicinal plant therapy, though equipped to treat a formidable number of diseases, was developed under preindustrial conditions and is largely unprepared to deal with cancer and the other diseases of civilization that were little known and almost nonexistent until recently. Although the use of plants, animals, and mineral matter constitutes a major component of all medical systems, they are combined with bloodletting, cauterization, diet, enemas, fumigation, heat, music and incantation, and shamanic and mediumistic exorcisms. Medicinal plants are more than simply objects with chemical and symbolic aspects: they are living organisms that are functionally imbedded in a complex, interrelated cultural fabric of social groups, institutions, and ideas of balance and cosmological order that often reflect a sophisticated medical theory of the body, the symptoms it experiences, and the underlying causes of those systems. The elements that comprise this medicinal plant-related nexus include a broad network of kin and friends; diverse medical specialists; a health-seeking process of therapeutic resort; patient-healer relationships; specific times of the year and days that a plant may be gathered, and prayers and offerings associated with their collection; modes of preparation; and dietary, sexual, or other restrictions associated with specific plants. The constituents of this medicinal plant-related complex vary from culture to culture and form a rich and diverse array of medical systems.

Hunting and gathering populations generally are healthy and highly fit, with developed coordination, vision, and acute learning capacities. Viral infections are infrequent and limited to those, such as herpes simplex and chicken pox, that are marked by latency or recurrence. Low population density and a scattered mobile existence cannot indefinitely support measles and other viral infections characterized by subsequent recovery and immunity. Many agriculturist skeletal samples from the New World display elevated disease and/ or nutritional stress, when compared with skeletal material from hunting and gathering groups. Cancer and chronic and cardiovascular diseases are infrequent and mortality is predominantly a result of venomous organisms, wild beasts, trauma, warfare, and other forms of social mortality, all of which are reflected in the diseases treated by hunters and gatherers with plant medicines. The Andaman Islanders have only 20 herbal remedies, limited to colds, fever, malaria, sepsis, various injuries and bone fractures, gastrointestinal disorders, toothache, body pain, swellings, hydrocele and gynecological disorders. Of the 35 medicinal plants used by the Alawa people of northern Australia, 44 percent are used to treat skin ailments and the rest are used for intestinal, respiratory, and other ailments. The ethnopharmacopoeia of agricultural populations is more complex and reflects marked ecological and cultural changes. One agriculturist group, the Shuar of the Ecuadorian Amazon, possesses 245 medicinal plants, 104 of which are for gastrointestinal disorders and 98 of which are for skin ailments, reflecting the impact of tropical rain forest conditions on health. Similarly, of 99 plant species used medicinally by the agricultural population of New Guinea, 53 percent are used for various types of wounds and aches, with the rest employed for first aid, intestinal problems, skin conditions, fevers, natal care, and tonics. Changes in the use of herbal remedies are clear indicators of evolving disease patterns, but often occur rapidly and are difficult to detect. During a recent 40-year period, medicinal plant use among rural Mexicans in Texas shifted from remedies for work-related traumas and infections to herbal treatments for cancer, hypertension, and diabetes. Although treatments for the common cold, gastrointestinal disorders, and skin irritations remained the same, these simultaneous changes in diseases and treatment indicate a rural-to-urban shift in lifestyle.

The domestication of plants and animals, which took place approximately eight thousand years ago, resulted in settled communities and increased population density. These new conditions permitted the rapid transmission of infectious viral, bacterial and protozoan microorganisms, worms, and constant reinfection. Contaminated water supplies, inadequate disposal of human excreta and sewage, the housefly, and the use of human offal as fertilizer witnessed the advent of cholera and many other viral and bacterial diseases. Domestic animals served as hosts for agents of typhoid fever, anthrax, and tuberculosis. Malaria and schistosomiasis increased dramatically through irrigative practices, and deforestation was responsible for the spread of yellow fever, dengue, and scrub typhus. Specific nutritional disorders such as beriberi, sprue, and kwashiorkor also appeared when humans began living on diets consisting largely of grains.

335

Widespread epidemics of infectious diseases intensified with the growth of preindustrial cities and the proliferation of flocks, crops and human populations.

During the 19th century the Industrial Revolution—a period of urbanization and rapid population growth—was marked by the prevalence and severity of infectious diseases. The transmission of typhus, diphtheria, smallpox, cholera, and other infectious diseases was aided by intense squalor, poverty, and overcrowding. Tuberculosis, occupational diseases of miners and tanners, and diseases of the respiratory tract were a result of the same condition, as were position, confinement, long hours of work, malnutrition, and the use of toxic industrial materials. Great reliance was placed on herbal remedies sold in factory town markets by rural villagers, because physicians did not tend to working class families who were too poor to pay for treatment. The decline in mortality toward the end of the century was more a consequence of improvements in sanitation, diet, and general standards of living than vaccination and other medical advances.

Today the leading causes of death are cardiovascular disease and cancer, caused by synthetic chemicals, radiation, and industrial pollutants such as lead and pesticides; overconsumption of high-fat diets, tobacco, and alcohol; and inadequate exercise. Despite billions of dollars spent on research, the overall incidence of cancer increased in industrial countries by 18 percent between 1973 and 1990. Although the proximate cause of cancer is tumor-producing genes such as p16, the ultimate causes are imbedded in the socioeconomic fabric of our industrial environment. Many of today's incredibly sophisticated and costly bio-medical services were developed largely to treat diseases that are a consequence of our contemporary lifestyle and industrial, urban development. Although cancer is attributed to the increased longevity of the population, the mutation theory of cancer and aging does not account for the high incidence of prostate and breast cancers among the middle-aged. It is estimated that as much as 80 percent to 90 percent of all cancer could be avoided if people changed their smoking and eating habits and the environment were cleaned of harmful chemicals.

Plants and Politics

The concern for environmental degradation; the trend to stay green and lead a healthier lifestyle; the esteem for natural, alternative products; and the negative reactions toward the over specialized, dehumanized, and excessively technological aspects of biomedicine have revitalized the use of herbal medicines. Although herbal medications are a thriving, multimillion dollar business, phytotherapy is in an economically, legally, and politically adversarial and subaltern position with respect to scientific medicine. The success of scientific biomedicine lies not in its capacity to confront and refute alternative therapies, but in the power to push subjected or rejected knowledge to the margins of rational discourse. Recognition of alternative therapies has been blocked in France, for example, because 11 percent of the parliamentary deputies are members of the medical profession (*New York Times*. April 11, 1994:4). Because one in five households in Paris uses herbal medicines, the French, like most other people, resort to divergent, pluralistic medical traditions.

Regulatory policies regarding herbal medicines vary from country to country. In France and England plant medicines that have a long record of use are considered safe and effective. Germany has a regulatory commission that reviews all plant medicines for approval. In Canada, medicinal plants are reviewed by an expert committee for safety, but not for clinically proven efficacy, and sold under the category of "folklore medicine." In France, Germany, Italy, and Japan, prescriptions for herbal medications are covered by health insurance systems. In Germany, medical students take exams in the field of phytotherapy. In one survey of German physicians, 61 percent reported the use of one or more alternative methods of healing. Similarly, in Japan 37 percent of the physicians surveyed reported using traditional herbal medications (kanpo).

In the United States all drugs must be proven safe and effective. Because this is a costly and time-consuming process, and because herbal medicines are unpatentable, most herbal products are sold in health food stores without accompanying information regarding properties, usage, dosage, or precautions. Ideally, the Food and Drug Administration (FDA) would like to have every chemical in a single plant or herbal extract evaluated for safety and efficacy; this would, in essence, remove herbal from the marketplace. The passage of the Dietary Supplement Health and Education Act in 1994 placed the burden of proving that an herb is unsafe on the FDA, rather than on the herbal products industry, and prohibited the FDA from treating herbs as food additives. Scientific information can be used in connection with herbal products, which are now labeled as "dietary supplements." Because herbal products are sold without accompanying instructions, consumers attempting to treat minor self limiting conditions are deprived of basic knowledge regarding properties, proper use, dosage, and precautions. Given the uncritically compiled, variable, and outdated nature of at least some herbal literature, adequate knowledge is lacking, which could have detrimental consequences. Because recommending or providing herbal medications can lead to raids and arrests, many herbal practitioners are afraid to share their knowledge. Many specialists in the field have advised adopting, as a model, the regulatory policies established in other industrial countries for assessing the safety and efficacy of herbal products.

Because they contain a complex of active principles, single plants and formulations are difficult to assess by laboratory methods. Bioactive compounds, however, can be studied within the particular chemical environment characterizing their traditional preparation. In order to evaluate the efficacy of herbal medications, clinical observations should be conducted using traditional preparations and dosages for their symptomatic usages. Herbal vitamins, minerals, and phytochemicals have a wide range of therapeutic actions that strengthen the ailing body in the gradual reestablishment of its defense system. Only a few powerful plant drugs would come up to the standards of the FDA drug review process, which is geared toward the single drugs of pharmaceutical companies. Given the adversarial posture of the FDA—which currently is embroiled in legislation reducing the regulations of food safety, proposing the registration of food engineered with biotechniques, and dealing with drug companies desiring the marketing of drugs sold in Europe—any change in the regulation of herbal products will be delayed for several years.

— by Frank J Lipp, PhD

Frank J. Lipp is a research associate at the Foundation for Shamanic Studies in Mill Valley, Calif. is the author of Herbalism: Living Wisdom and coauthor (with Siri von Reis) of New Plant Sources for Drugs and Foods.

Chapter 23

Review and Critique of Common Herbal Alternative Therapies

Patients' uses of herbal therapies warrant close scrutiny by providers. With the current proliferation of lay literature on herbal remedies and the wide availability of such products in health foods and other such stores, more people are relying on herbal and less conventional therapies for a wide variety of problems. Guidance in safe and effective use is needed. Only nine herbs are approved by the Food and Drug Administration for selected applications, so that any lay press book or article that touts the benefits of an herbal remedy must be considered in light of the scientific literature for patient safety. Judging safety and efficacy becomes particularly difficult with the current lack of standardization and regulation of herbal products. German Commission E provides a review of some of the more than 1,400 herbal drugs; this review may be useful in evaluating such therapies. This chapter provides an overview of the current status of herbal therapies in the United States, a review of selected commonly used herbs by popular claims and scientific information, and relevant safety and efficacy data.

"Can a Berry Fight the Flu?" (*Good Housekeeping*, February 1996). "Herbs That Ease the Mind." (*Prevention*, January 1996). "Uncommon Remedies for the Common Cold." (*Ladies' Home Journal*, December 1995). These are but a few of the explosion of headlines of articles about herbal therapies in lay press magazines, books, and newspapers that have bombarded the American public in the past year. It behooves today's clinician to have some understanding of the safety of such remedies as patients seek answers to questions stimulated by such literature.

The purpose of this chapter is to explore selected common herbal therapies and provide some guidance for safe and effective use. The renewed interest in herbal therapies today is due in part to the changing health care system's focus on preventive care [1], as well as resurgence of interest in natural therapies, such as herbal medicines. Although a healthy lifestyle is the primary promoter of good health, and conventional medicine may be the best therapy for many problems, selected herbal therapies may have a place among options for health and illness management.

Alternative Therapies

Alternative or unconventional therapies are gaining public attention and are more widely used than most health care professionals may realize. "In a given year about a third of all American adults use unconventional medical treatments . . . The most frequent users are educated, upper income white Americans in the 25-to 49-year age group . . . " [2, p. 282-83]. These therapies include but are not limited to megavitamin treatments, relaxation and biofeedback techniques, massage therapy, therapeutic touch, guided imagery, chelation therapy, acupuncture, and herbal medicine. The National Institutes of Health was instructed by Congress in 1992 to establish an Office of Alternative Medicine, which is supporting studies of alternative therapies [4].

The lay press is replete with articles that tout the benefits of alternative therapies, yet their efficacy may not be well studied [5]. Unfortunately, the value of these alternative treatments generally has been determined by anecdotal reports, and, in fact, many can be harmful and even fatal. For example, in February 1995, the Food and Drug Administration (FDA) issued a warning against nutritional products containing *Ma huang* (ephedrine) and kola nut. In 1994, there had been more than 100 reports of irregular heartbeats, heart attack, stroke, seizure, psychosis, and several deaths likely due to the combination of ephedrine and the caffeine in the kola nut [6]. In another example, the blossoms of germander (*Teucrium chamaedrys*) have been used in folk medicine to treat obesity. Seven cases of hepatitis after taking germander in herbal teas or capsules were reported in one investigation [7]. Hepatitis also has been reported after ingestion of preparations containing valerian, asafetida, hops, skullcap, gentian, senna fruit extracts, Chinese herbs, mistletoe, and chaparral leaf [8]. Given the high rate of self-medication by patients, health-care professionals should attempt to ascertain their patients' ingestion of unconventional therapies when taking a medication history as these therapies may be causing or exacerbating ill health [3].

Judging Safety and Efficacy

The Food and Drug Administration (FDA) regulates drugs, foods, and cosmetics in this country. Currently, only nine herbs have been judged by the FDA to be both safe and have effective therapeutic actions [8]. There are more than 1,400 remaining herbs sold commercially and promoted for various unproven medicinal merits [6]. Any product that makes a therapeutic claim is considered to be a drug. Herbs used in food for reasons such as flavoring, with no therapeutic claims, still must be safe for consumption [9]. Herbs used in cosmetics (hundreds) do not require FDA approval, but the FDA may take action if a product is found to be harmful.

Prior to 1962, herbs were considered to be drugs. In 1962, the FDA required that all drugs on the market be evaluated for safety and efficacy, so manufacturers began marketing herbs as "food" products sold in health food stores [6]. The FDA made no moves to regulate these so-called "foods" as long as no claims of efficacy were made. More recently, the passage of the Dietary Supplement Health and Education Act in 1994 ruled that herbs can be labeled with information on their effects on the structure and function of the body. These labels must be accompanied by a disclaimer stating that the FDA has not reviewed the herb and it is not intended to be used as a drug [6]. Canada banned some 57 herbs in 1984 after safety concerns led to an advisory committee review. Also, warning labels were required on five others that could be harmful in pregnancy [10].

In Europe and Great Britain, herbal medicines have a longer history of being accepted alongside more conventional drug therapy [11]. The German government established a panel, Commission E, in 1988 to review the clinical literature on more than 1,400 herbal drugs, including clinical trials and case reports. This effort has resulted in some 300 monographs on the most popular herbal remedies. Even with the latest information from Germany's Commission E and the steps made by passage of the Dietary Supplement Act in the United States (U.S.), determining safety and efficacy of herbal products is difficult because the FDA, manufacturers, and herbal experts disagree on how to interpret the varying evidence available for many types of herbal remedies [11].

An additional note of caution is advised. There are currently no government standards on the quality of herbal products sold in the United States. Herbs may be sold to manufacturers as whole plants or plant parts, cut pieces or finely ground particles. The only definitive way to truly know the purity and concentration of a particular product is to perform assays. However, herbal manufacturers have little incentive to do potentially costly assays since there is no pressure from the government for quality control. Adulteration and substitution of the active ingredient(s) are more likely to occur with the more expensive plant materials. For example, analysis of 54 ginseng products revealed that 25 percent contained no ginseng at all, while 60 percent of these products were worthless [11].

Some general comments about herbal teas are in order. This is a multimillion dollar business in the United States. In 1990, $118.6 million was spent by consumers for herbal teas in supermarkets alone [10]. The concern is safety, and one may conclude from the large number of herbal teas sold without untoward reactions reported that commercially packaged herbal teas are safe when consumed in moderate amounts or less. It is when a product is consumed in excess amounts, to render some perceived medicinal effect, or is consumed without knowledge of possible adverse reactions, that problems arise. For instance, comfrey tea is popular because people believe that it has healing properties. However, one woman drank up to 10 cups a day for her stomach pains, and developed liver disease [10]. Comfrey has since been dropped from commercial leaders' repertoires.

The FDA says that regulation of teas comes somewhere between food and drugs and thus is a "gray" area. However, there are no regulations for herbal teas since any herb thought safe by the FDA for food use is considered safe in tea [10]. Major commercial tea manufacturers avoid any herbs that have the least question of safety, and avoid making therapeutic claims. However, home-grown herbs and the foreign imported herbs are of great concern to the FDA—Many herb lovers grow their own and may use much-too-much in brewing teas or in other preparations. The basic premise, "the dose makes the poison," is not well understood by the lay public [10]. A medical report in the March 1996 issue of *Glamour* magazine tells a frightening story of a woman who used two bags of the Laci Le Beau Super Dieter's Tea that she purchased at a health food store. The woman died during the night from cardiac arrest. Since her death, the article states that the FDA has convened advisory committees to consider if herbal diet products that contain senna (a potent laxative in the Laci Le Beau Tea) and ephedra (ephedrine found in some herbal products sold as

342

energy boosters) should carry warning labels. No decision had been made when the magazine article was written. However, the message should be clear that consumers need to be cautious, even if the herb is purchased in a health food store and is labeled "natural."

The other problem is that people may not be sure what they are using. In one reported case, a woman died after drinking a tea made from leaves she had identified as eucalyptus. They were, in fact, oleander leaves, and very poisonous. Additionally, many foreign herb preparations include herbs about which little is known, especially Oriental and Indian herbs. Differences in climate, soil conditions, the part of the plant from which the product is derived, and extraneous matter added all affect the pharmacologic activity of an herbal substance. Of grave concern is the fact that many imported products contain strong prescription drugs or toxic substances that are not declared as drug substances when the products are sent to this country. This is extremely dangerous, particularly since many people—especially the elderly—are searching for remedies for ailments not responsive to conventional measures [12].

Selected Common Herbs and Relevant Data

The remainder of this chapter presents tables for use by clinicians in determining safety of selected herbal therapies that their patients may be using or want to use. Table 23.1 provides definitions of common terms used by herbalists. Table 23.2 provides lay press claims as compared to safety and efficacy data derived from the German Commission E and other biomedical literature for selected commonly used herbs. Data from human studies takes precedence over information available from animal studies, given the inherent difficulties in extrapolating animal data results to effects in adult humans. Difficulty arises in interpreting the medical studies since many are written in German. The authors of this paper have relied on experts in this field for the interpretation and translation of these studies. Additionally, readers should be aware that controversy exists among these "experts" on the scientific merit of many of these herbs. These differences are listed in Table 23.2. Other discrepancies exist between the scientific references concerning dosage recommendations, also shown in Table 23.2. Health care professionals are referred to references in Table 23.2 for specific dosage information. Table 23.2 further presents information about the herbs' actions, and adverse effects or warnings. Readers should be aware that approval of an herb by the German Commission E does not mean that the drug is approved for use in the United States, though most of these herbs are available in health food stores.

Of the 56 herbal therapies presented in this chapter, only seven are FDA approved; thirty-six are considered by the German Commission E to be effective for one or more specified complaint, and only four are approved by both groups. Clinicians must be cautious in supporting use of any herbal therapy, recognizing that some substances may be dangerous. What advice should the clinician give to patients regarding herbal use? The following guidelines have been recommended and pertain to all patients [13].

- Do not take herbs if pregnant or attempting to become pregnant.

- Do not take herbs if nursing.

- Do not give herbs to your baby or young children.

- Do not take a large quantity of any one herbal preparation.

- Do not take any herb on a daily basis.

- Buy only preparations when the plants and their quantities are listed on the packet (no guarantee of safety).

- Do not take anything containing comfrey.

Engebretsen and Wardell, in reviewing alternative therapies, advise providers to use the guidance of "knowledgeable herbalists" in considering safe and effective herbal alternatives [14].

As an additional caution clinicians should investigate carefully in the scientific literature any herb that the patient is taking. This review should be conducted as carefully as one might review a drug in a reputable drug reference. An open mind tempered with science must be maintained [15]. It is essential to consider herbs as drugs with active ingredients and weigh the scientific information against the lay reputation in making decisions with the patient. As Eisenberg restates from Hufford in a 1993 review, "conventional medicine will neither assimilate nor 'stamp out' folk practices. Clinicians, therefore, must learn 'an effective diplomacy' in order to deal responsibly with a variety of medical models and practices" [16]. It becomes increasingly clear in this era of more diverse patient populations that health professionals must understand and respect the cultural beliefs and practices of their patients [17].

Table 23.1. Definitions of Common Terms Used by herbalists [18,19]

Abortifacient	An agent that induces expulsion of a fetus
Adaptogen	An agent that strengthens organs or the entire organism (synonym for "tonic")
Alterative	An agent that produces a gradual beneficial change in the body
Antihydrotic	An agent that reduces or suppresses perspiration
Antispasmodic	An agent that relieves spasms or cramps
Aphrodisiac	An agent that increases sexual desire or potency
Astringent	An agent that contracts organic tissue, thus reducing secretions
Calmative	An agent with mild sedative or tranquilizing properties
Carminative	An agent for expelling gas from the intestines
Cholagogue	An agent that stimulates the release and secretion of bile from the gallbladder
Demulcent	An agent that soothes irritated tissue, especially mucous membranes
Diaphoretic	An agent that promotes perspiration
Diuretic	An agent that increases the expulsion of urine
Emmenagogue	An agent that promotes menstrual flow
Emollient	An agent used externally to soften and soothe
Expectorant	An agent that promotes discharge of mucus from respiratory passages
Febrifuge	An agent that helps the body reduce fevers
Galactagogue	An agent that increases secretion of milk
Mucilaginous	An agent characterized by a gummy or gelatinous consistency
Rubefacient	An agent that, when applied to the skin, causes a local irritation that increases circulation, which relieves internal pains
Sialogogue	An agent that stimulates the secretion of saliva from the salivary glands
Stimulant	An agent that excites or quickens the activity of a physiological process
Stomachic	An agent that strengthens or tones the stomach
Tonic	An agent that strengthens organs or the entire organism (synonym for adaptogen)

Table 23.2. Summary of Herbs and their Properties; continued on next page.

Common Name (Scientific Name) Part of plant used [18-20]	Other Names [18]	Popular Laypress Claims [11,18-24]	Scientific Information Scientific Properties/ FDA Approval	German Commission E Recommendations	Adverse Effects/ Warnings	Additional Comments/ Contraindications
Agrimony (Agrimonia eupatoria) leaves	common agrimony	astringent, inflammation of the throat, cystitis, gastroenteritis, gall bladder disorders, incontinence, hemostatic agent, analgesic, antiviral and anti-inflammatory agent	astringent [24]	Internally: mild, acute diarrhea; inflammation of mouth and throat Externally: mild, superficial inflammation of the skin [24]	No known adverse effects [24]	
Aloe (Aloe barbadensis) fresh gel, dried juice	Barbados aloe, Curacao aloe	emollient, laxative, minor burns, insect bites, skin irritations, minor cuts, wrinkles, regulates liver function, PMS, emmenagogue	FDA approved as a laxative	acute constipation [24]	may bring about abortion or premature birth; loss of electrolytes with chronic use [24]	avoid use if ileus present; do not use if pregnant or lactating
Angelica (Angelica archangelica) root, fruit, leaves	garden angelica, European angelica	emmenagogue, flavoring agent, abortifacient, carminative, stomachic, expectorant, relieves menstrual cramps and nervous insomnia, diuretic, diaphoretic	conflicting evidence: possible spasmolytic properties and effects on secretion of gastric juice [24]; others stating there is no scientific evidence to support claims [20]	approved for lack of appetite; dyspepsia [24]	photosensitivity [20,24]; dermatitis [20] may be carcinogenic [20]	used as a flavoring in alcoholic beverages such as gin [20]
Anise (Pimpinella anisum) fruits (commonly called seeds)	anise plant, aniseed, common anise	antispasmodic, aromatic, expectorant, tonic, carminative, aphrodisiac, emmenagogue, galactagogue	expectorant, weakly spasmolytic, antibacterial [24]	Internally: dyspeptic complaints Internally & Externally: catarrh of the respiratory tract [24]	allergic reactions of the skin, respiratory and gastrointestinal tract [24]	contraindication: allergy to aniseed or anethole [24]
Bayberry Bark (Myrica pensylvanica and M. cerifera) root bark, berries		astringent, circulatory stimulant, diaphoretic, colds, hemorrhoids, diarrhea	mineralocorticoid activity, choleretic [20]	no information		potential carcinogen therefore its use cannot be recommended [20
Balm (Melissa officinalis) leaves	balm mint, bee balm, blue balm, cure-all, dropsy plant, garden balm, lemon balm	antispasmodic, calmative, carminative, diaphoretic, hypotensive, stomachic, emmenagogue, insomnia, depression, relief of menstrual cramps, asthma, migraine, relief of toothache & cold sores	sedative, carminative [24]	useful for nervous disorders that cause problems with sleep and for gastrointestinal disorders [24]	no known adverse effects [24]	
Black Cohosh (Cimicifuga racemosa) rhizome, root	black snakeroot, rattleweed, rattleroot, squawroot, cimicifuga	dysmenorrhea, antispasmodic, astringent, diuretic, expectorant, promotes labor, sedative, rheumatism, PMS, menopausal symptoms	may reduce secretion of luteinizing hormone [11,20]	premenstrual discomfort, dysmenorrhea, and climacteric symptoms [8]	stomach upset; no other information on toxicity [11,20]	long-term safety requires verification [8]

Table 23.2. Summary of Herbs and their Properties; continued from previous page, continued on next page.

Common Name (Scientific Name) Part of plant used [18]	Other Names [18]	Popular Laypress Claims [11,18-24]	Scientific Properties/ FDA Appoval	German Commission E Recommendations	Adverse Effects/ Warnings	Additional Comments/ Contraindications
			Scientific Information			
Blessed Thistle (Cnicus benedictus) leaves, seeds	holy thistle	bitter tonic, astringent, diaphoretic, antibacterial, expectorant	promotes secretion of saliva and gastric juice [24]	lack of appetite, dyspeptic complaints [24]	allergic reactions possible [24]	
Boneset (Eupatorium perfoliatum) leaves, tops	agueweed, crosswort, feverwort, Indian sage, sweating plant, wood boneset	diaphoretic, cathartic, emetic, tonic, febrifuge, useful in "breaking up" mucus associated with the common cold and flu	contains no compounds known to have therapeutic value, though this herb does appear to increase sweating [20]	no information	causes nausea [20]	caution in consumption of this herb is advised due to the possible presence of toxic alkaloids
Borage (Borago officinalis) leaves, tops	bugloss, common bugloss, burage	diuretic, astringent, febrifuge, tonic, galactagogue, antipyretic, pleurisy, peritonitis, diaphoretic, expectorant, laxative, anti-inflammatory	astringent properties due to presence of tannin and mild expectorant action but no truly therapeutic effect has been found with this herb [20]	no information	slight constipating effects [20]	contains low levels of pyrrolidine alkaloids which are potentially hepatotoxic and carcinogenic therefore consumption of this herb should only be done under medical supervision [20]
Capsicum or Cayenne Pepper (Capsicum spp.) fruits	chile pepper, red pepper	stimulant, carminative, tonic, antiseptic, rubefacient, sialogogue, reduces symptoms of common cold, stomachic	FDA approved as a topical analgesic. It is marketed as a cream that may be effective when used topically for herpes zoster, diabetic neuropathy [11,20]	no information	avoid touching eyes or mucus membranes after applying product [11,20]	
Cascara (Rhamnus purshiana) dried bark	sacred bark, bitter bark	laxative, bitter tonic, gallstones, liver ailments	FDA approved as a laxative; stimulates peristalsis [24]	constipation [24]	chronic use: increased loss of electrolytes [24]	contraindicated if ileus present; avoid use during pregnancy or lactation [24]
Catnip (Nepeta cataria) leaves, tops	catnep, catmint	bronchitis, antidiarrheal agent, antiflatulent, digestive aid, astringent, antispasmodic, sedative, diaphoretic, mind-altering effects (smoked)	No scientific evidence to support claims [11,20]	no information	no adverse effects reported [11,20]	patients may be able to drink the tea safely, though the safety of smoking this herb is not known [20]
Chamomiles (Matricaria recutita, Chamaemelum nobile) flowering heads	German chamomile, Hungarian chamomile	carminative, anti-inflammatory, antispasmodic, anti-infective, anti-anxiety, diaphoretic, analgesic, local healing	antiinflammatory and antispasmodic effects [11,20,24]	useful as antispasmodic anti-flatulent agents; inflammation of the mouth and throat [24]	contact dermatitis, anaphylaxis, hypersensitivity reactions [11,20]	persons allergic to ragweed, asters or chrysanthemums should use this herb with caution [11,20]

Table 23.2. Summary of Herbs and their Properties; continued from previous page, continued on next page.

Common Name (Scientific Name) Part of plant used [18-20]	Other Names [18]	Popular Laypress Claims [11,18-24]	Scientific Properties/ FDA Approval	German Commission E Recommendations	Adverse Effects/ Warnings	Additional Comments/ Contraindications
				Scientific Information		
Chaste Tree Berry (*Vitex agnus-castus*) fruit	monk's pepper	PMS, dysmenorrhea menopause symptoms	Inhibits secretion of prolactin by the pituitary gland [20]	useful for a variety of menstrual disorders [24]	very limited toxicity data; may cause an itchy rash [20]	
Comfrey (*Symphytum officinale*)	blackwort, bruise-wort, gum plant, healing herb, slippery root	astringent, demulcent, emollient, expectorant, hemostatic, refrigerant, hoarseness, intestinal problems, bronchitis, pleurisy, rheumatism	antiinflammatory action, promotes callus formation; contains pyrrolizidine alkaloids that may be hepatotoxic and carcinogenic [11,20,24]	**Externally:** contusions, sprains, dislocations [24]	hepatotoxicity [11,20,24]	The drug should only be applied to intact skin and used for no longer than 4 to 6 weeks in a year [24]; internal use of comfrey should be avoided and comfrey should not be used in young children or pregnant or lactating women [11]
Damiana (*Turnera aphrodisiaca*) leaves, stems	blowball, canker-wort, lion's tooth, priest's crown, puffball, swine snout, white endive, wild endive	aphrodisiac, laxative, antianxiety, urinary antisepetic, antidepressant	No scientific evidence to support claims [20]	no information	no information available [20]	considered an "herbal hoax" [20]
Dandelion (*Taraxacum officinale*) rhizome, roots, leaves	tang kuei, dang qui	digestive aid, laxative, diuretic, liver and gallbladder protectant, prevents iron-deficiency anemia, PMS, breast tenderness	According to Wichtl, this herb has choleretic and diuretic actions along with appetite stimulating properties [24]; Tyler states roots may aid digestion and have a slight laxative effect but there is no evidence to support a significant therapeutic benefit [11,20]	useful in biliary disorders, as a carminitive, and to stimulate diuresis [24]	skin rash, no other significant side effects or toxicities noted [11,20,24]	preparations of dandelion may be taken for a period of up to 4 to 6 weeks [24]
Dong quai (*Angelica sinensis*) root		antispasmodic, dysmenorrhea, laxative, PMS, amenorrhea, hot flashes, insomnia, high blood pressure, prevents anemia, vaginal lubricant	No scientific evidence to support claims. [20]	no information	photosensitization, contains coumarin derivatives [20]	it is recommended to avoid all unnecessary exposure to this drug [20]

348

Table 23.2. Summary of Herbs and their Properties; continued from previous page, continued on next page.

Common Name (Scientific Name) Part of plant used [18-20]	Other Names [18]	Popular Laypress Claims [11,18-24]	Scientific Information — Scientific Properties/ FDA Approval	Scientific Information — German Commission E Recommendations	Adverse Effects/ Warnings	Additional Comments/ Contraindications
Echinacea (Echinacea angustifolia E. pallida, E. purpurea) rhizome, roots, leaves, tops	Sampson root, purple coneflower	antiseptic, digestive, eczema, acne, migraine, antipyretic, antiflatulent, wound healing, immune stimulant to help fight colds, influenza	immune-stimulant effect [11,20]	used to enhance resistance to infectious conditions in the upper respiratory tract [24]	allergies (infrequent) [11,24]	use of Echinacea root does not exclude concomitant administration of antibiotics [24]; this herb should not be used by persons with conditions such as tuberculosis, AIDS, collagen diseases, multiple sclerosis [11,24]
Ephedra (Ephedra spp.) stems	ma huang	antiasthmatic, nasal decongestant, vasodilator, anti-allergic, hypertensive, circulatory stimulant, anorexant	effective nasal decongestant [20]	no information	increases blood pressure and heart rate, may cause insomnia, palpitations, dizziness, headaches, nervousness [11,20]	Persons with heart disease, thyroid disease, hypertension and diabetes should use this herb with caution [11,20]; FDA advisory in 1995 issued warning against products containing this herb [6]
Eucalyptus (Eucalyptus globulus) leaves	blue gum	antiseptic, deodorant, expectorant, stimulant, indigestion, respiratory ailments	secretomotor, expectorant, weakly spasmolytic [24]	catarrhal disorders of the respiratory passages [24]	nausea, vomiting, diarrhea [24]	
Evening Primrose (Oenothera biennis) seed oil	fever plant, field primrose, night willow-herb, king's cureall	astringent, demulcent, depression, stimulating effect on liver, spleen and GI tract, skin rashes, PMS, weight loss	conflicting evidence on efficacy of this herb; no data to support safety of prolonged consumption [11,20]	no information		
Fennel (Foeniculum vulgare) root, fruit (commonly called seed)	large fennel, sweet fennel, wild fennel	demulcent, stomachic, antispasmotic, aromatic, carminative, diuretic, expectorant, stimulant, galactagogue, aromatic, rubefacient	spasmolytic, increases gastrointestinal motility, secretolytic action in the respiratory tract; antiflatulent [20,24]	dyspeptic complaints, such as feelings of distension, flatulence; catarrh of the upper respiratory tract [24]	fennel fruit: allergic reaction of the skin & respiratory tract [24]; fennel volatile oil: skin irritation, vomiting, seizures, respiratory problems, thus self-medication with oil is not recommened [20]	Do not use in pregnancy [24]

Table 23.2. Summary of Herbs and their Properties; continued from previous page, continued on next page.

Common Name (Scientific Name) Part of plant used [18-20]	Other Names [18]	Popular Laypress Claims [11,18-24]	Scientific Information		Adverse Effects/ Warnings	Additional Comments/ Contraindications
			Scientific Properties/ FDA Approval	German Commission E Recommendations		
Fenugreek (*Trigonella foenum-graecum*) seeds	trigonella, Greek hay seed	aphrodisiac, antidiabetic, expectorant, gout, demulcent, restorative, neuralgias, skin irritations, menstrual cycle stabilizer	studies in small animals point to a number of potential applications but no data available in humans to support claims [20]	**Internally:** anorexia **Externally:** local inflammation [24]	adverse skin reactions with repeated local applications [11]	
Garlic (*Allium sativum*) bulb	clove garlic	antihelmintic, antispasmodic, diuretic, carminative, digestive, expectorant, treatment of atherosclerosis and high blood pressure, blood clotting disorders	garlic appears to provide some protection against atherosclerosis and stroke and may reduce blood cholesterol and blood pressure [20]	no information	allergic reactions; reduction of clotting time; consumption of (25 cloves/day) may cause heartburn, flatulence. [20]	avoid large amounts in persons taking aspirin or other anticoagulant drugs [20]
Ginger (*Zingiber officinale*) rhizome	Jamaica ginger, African ginger, black ginger, race ginger	appetizer, carminative, diaphoretic, stimulant, prevention of motion sickness, rubefacient	antiemetic, promotes salivary and gastric secretion; increases intestinal peristalsis [11,20,24]	dyspeptic complaints; prevention of symptoms of motion sickness [24]	no known adverse effects [24]	in patients with a history of gallstones, use only after consultation with a health care professional [24]
Ginkgo (*Ginkgo biloba*) leaf extract	maidenhair tree	enhanced cerebral blood flow, tinnitus, vertigo, Alzheimer's, hemorrhoids, slows aging process, prevents cancer, antidepressant, improves memory	ginkgo promotes vasodilation and improved blood flow in arteries and capillaries; acts as a free radical scavenger [11,20,25]	effective in treatment of circulatory disturbances and treating symptoms such as vertigo, weakened memory, mood swings [11,20,25]	GI disturbances, headache, allergic skin reactions, restlessness [11,20,25]	May interact with anticoagulants [11,20]
Ginseng (*Panax ginseng*-Oriental) (*Panax quinquefolius*-American) Siberian ginseng (*Eleutherococcus senticosus*) roots	American ginseng; five-fingers, five-leafed ginseng	Asiatic ginseng, Chinese ginseng, wonder-of-world	adaptogen, demulcent, cure-all, antistress agents, aphrodisiac, menopausal symptoms, reduces cholesterol, increases energy, inhibits tumors	solid clinical data supporting claims is lacking though some studies have shown some beneficial pharmacologic effects [11,20]	useful for conditions manifested by lack of energy or poor concentration and during periods of convalescence [24]	insomnia, diarrhea, skin eruptions [11,20,24]; menopausal bleeding [24]	concern exists over lack of standardized products, differences between Oriental and American plants [11,20]; recommended for use for only 3 months (Commission E) [24]]
Goldenseal (*Hydrastis canadensis*) rhizome, roots	eye balm, eye root, ground raspberry, Indian plant, yellowroot, jaundice root, yellow puccoon	bitter tonic, digestive aid, genitourinary conditions, menorrhagia, upper respiratory ills, irritated gums, canker sores, ringworm treatment, atrophic vaginitis	this herb may have some astringent and weak antiseptic properties but there is no scientific evidence to support claims [20]	no information	no safety or efficacy data available when this herb is used internally [20]	

Table 23.2. Summary of Herbs and their Properties; continued from previous page, continued on next page.

Common Name (Scientific Name) Part of plant used [18-20]	Other Names [18]	Popular Laypress Claims [11,18-24]	Scientific Information — Scientific Properties/ FDA Approval	Scientific Information — German Commission E Recommendations	Adverse Effects/ Warnings	Additional Comments/ Contraindications
Gotu Kola (*Centella asiatica*) leaves	Indian pennywort, hyrocotyle	promote longevity, aphrodisiac, phlebitis, episiotomy healing, expectorant, leprosy, hypertension, ulcers, rheumatism, hot flashes, improves memory, antidepressant	may have some antiinflammatory effects and may promote wound healing; no other claims have been substantiated [20]	no information	data not available [20]	do not confuse with kola (which) contains caffeine [20]
Hawthorn (*Crataegus monogyna, C. laevigata*) fruits, leaves, flowers	May bush, May tree, thorn-apple tree, whitehorn	antispasmodic, sedative, vasodilator, myocarditis, atherosclerosis, antihypertensive	positive inotrope and chronotrope; increased coronary and myocardial circulation [11,20,24]	cardiac insufficiency corresponding to NYHA stages I and II; a feeling of pressure and tightness in the chest, mild bradycardia [24]	not known [24]	self-medication with this herb is not recommended [11,20]
Hops (*Humulus lupulus*) strobile (floral part)	hop vine	sedative, mind-altering action, appetite stimulant, antiflatulent agent, antiseptic, astringent	studies have failed to confirm any of the claims [11,20]	no information	data not available [11,20]	
Iceland Moss (*Cetraria islandica*) whole plant	cetrari	antiemetic, demulcent, galactogogue, tonic catarrh, gastroenteritis, anemia	demulcent, weakly antibacterial [24]	irritation of mucus membranes of mouth and throat; lack of appetite [24]	none known [24]	use of this herb in large quantities over extended periods of time is not recommended due to possible lead content [11]
Juniper (*Juniperus communis*) fruit	juniper berries	diuretic, antiseptic, carminative, stomachic, tonic, rubefacient, antirheumatic, gastrointestinal infections	In animals, an increase in urinary output has been observed as well as smooth muscle contractions [24]	dyspeptic complaints (belching, heartburn, distension) [24]	renal damage may occur with prolonged use [24]	do not take during pregnancy or if renal disease present; do not take for longer than 4 weeks without consulting health care professional [24]
Lady's-Mantle (*Alchemilla xanthochiora*) leaves, flowering shoot		astringent, anorexia, diuretic, rheumatism, diarrhea, enteritis, menstrual problems, decreases menstrual flow, leucorrhea	astringent [24]	useful for mild, non-specific diarrhea and gastrointestinal complaints [24]	may cause liver damage in rare cases [24]	

Table 23.2. Summary of Herbs and their Properties; continued from previous page, continued on next page.

Common Name (Scientific Name) Part of plant used [18-20]	Other Names [18]	Popular Laypress Claims [11,18-24]	Scientific Information		Adverse Effects/ Warnings	Additional Comments/ Contraindications
			Scientific Properties/ FDA Approval	German Commission E Recommendations		
Licorice (*Glycyrrhiza glabra*) rhizome, roots	licorice root, sweet licorice, sweet wood	expectorant, demulcent, flavoring agent, rheumatism, prevents cavities, prevents growth of certain cancerous tumors, stabilizes menstrual cycle, antiinflammatory effects	has expectorant, antitussive, antiinflammatory, and antiallergic properties	treatment of peptic ulcers, as a cough suppressant and expectorant [11,20]	headache, lethargy, sodium/water retention, heart failure, hypertension, cardiac arrest [11,20]	avoid in elderly and those with history of cardiovascular disease, kidney or liver problems [11,20] do not take longer than 4 to 6 weeks without consulting a health-care professional [11]
Life Root (*Senecio aureus*) entire plan	ragwort, golden senecio, false valerian, squaw weed, cocash weed, grundy swallow	emmenagogue, uterine diseases, diaphoretic, diuretic, abortifacient, urinary tract problems, various menstrual problems, expectorant	this drug is not safe to use due to presence of a toxic alkaloid [12,15]	no information	hepatotoxicity [11,20]	
Marshmallow root (*Althaea officinalis*) root		diarrhea, cystitis, demulcent, diuretic, emollient	inhibits mucociliary activity, stimulates phagocytosis [24]	inflammation of mucus membranes of mouth and throat, upper respiratory tract and gastrointestinal tract [24]	no known side effects [24]	may delay the absorption of other drugs taken at the same time [24]
Milk Thistle (*Silybum marianum*) fruit (commonly called seeds)	St. Mary's thistle, blessed thistle	liver protectant, galactogogue, demulcent	contains silymarin, which exerts a protectant effect on the liver [20]	**Crude drug:** dyspeptic conditions **Preparations:** used as supportive treatment for chronic inflammatory conditions of the liver and liver cirrhosis [24]	no known side effects [24]	
Myrrh (*Commiphora spp.*) oleo-gum resin	gum myrrh	astringent, fragrance, antiseptic, carminative, stomachic, asthma, antimicrobial, anti-catarrhal, emmenagogue	mild astringent and antiseptic properties [20,24]	inflammation of the gums and mucus membranes of the mouth (gingivitis and stomatitis); pressure spots from prosthesis [24]	no known side effects [24]	used in commercial mouthwashes, as a fragrance in soaps, cosmetics, perfumes and as a flavoring in food products [20]

Table 23.2. Summary of Herbs and their Properties; continued from previous page, continued on next page.

Common Name (Scientific Name) Part of plant used [18-20]	Other Names [18]	Popular Laypress Claims [11,18-24]	Scientific Properties/ FDA Approval	German Commission E Recommendations	Adverse Effects/ Warnings	Additional Comments/ Contraindications
Nettle (*Urtica diocia*) above the ground plant, root	common nettle, stinging nettle, great stinging nettle	relief of heavy bleeding, endometriosis, cystitis, diuretic, astringent, antiasthmatic, tonic, antirheumatic, hair growth stimulator, treatment of BPH (root)	nettle herb and root have well-established diuretic properties and there is some clinical evidence to support use of the root in the treatment of benign prostatic hypertrophy [11,20]	urinary difficulties due to BPH [11,20]	local irritation and rash [11,20]	
Passion flower (*Passiflora incarnata*) flower, fruit top	maypops, passion vine, purple passion flower	sedative, hypnotic, decreases muscle tension, relieves headaches, Parkinson's, epilepsy, neuralgias, shingles, antispasmodic	conflicting data exists; plant constituents may have both stimulant and sedative effects [11,20]	nervous conditions, mild sleeping problems, gastrointestinal complaints of nervous origin [24]	no information available [24]	
Peppermint (*Mentha x piperita*) leaves, flowering tops	lamb mint, American mint	stomachic, carminative, flavoring agent, antispasmodic, diaphoretic, antiseptic, analgesic	direct spasmolytic action on the smooth muscles of digestive tract, carminative, choleretic [11,20,24]	gastrointestinal and biliary complaints [24]	No known side effects [24]	If gallstones present, consult a health care professional prior to use [24]; caution in giving peppermint tea to infants or small children due to possible choking sensation from the menthol [11,20]
Psyllium (*Plantago psyllium, P. ovata, P. spp*) seed	plantago seed	laxative, decreases blood cholesterol	**FDA approved as a laxative:** increases intestinal peristalsis [12]	constipation [24]	allergic reactions (rare) [24]	contraindications: intestinal obstruction
Red Raspberry (*Rubus idaeus* or *R. strigosus*) leaves	Wild red raspberry, garden raspberry	astringent, uterine stimulant, menstrual cramps, antiemetic, laxative, controls frequent and excessive menstrual bleeding	may be effective as an antidiarrheal agent or for use in sore throats but claims have not been substantiated [11,20,24]	therapeutic use of this herb is not advocated due to lack of clinical trials [24]	avoid in pregnancy—no data on teratogenicity [11,20]	
Sage (*Salvia officinalis*) leaves	garden sage	astringent, antihydrotic, flavoring agent, antispasmodic, relief of hot flashes, dries up mother's milk, epilepsy, insomnia, measles, seasickness, venereal disease, rheumatism	antiseptic and local antiinflammatory due to the presence of tannins [11,20]	mouth wash or gargle for inflammations of mouth and throat; internally for use for digestive complaints and excessive perspiration [11,20]	mental and physical deterioration when used for a long period of time in small doses; convulsions and loss of consciousness in larger doses [11,20]	despite Commission E recommendations, others question whether sage should be used internally due to possible adverse effects; use as a spice in cooked foods it is likely safe [11,20]

Table 23.2. Summary of Herbs and their Properties; continued from previous page, continued on next page.

Common Name (Scientific Name) Part of plant used [18-20]	Other Names [18]	Popular Laypress Claims [11,18-24]	Scientific Information — Scientific Properties/FDA Approval	German Commission E Recommendations	Adverse Effects/Warnings	Additional Comments/Contraindications
Sarsaparilla (*Smilax spp.*) roots	Honduras sarsap., Spanish sarsap., Mexican sarsap., Ecuadorian sarsp.	anabolic steroid, diuretic, expectorant, flavoring agent, menstrual stabilizer, carminative, diaphoretic, tonic, rheumatism, colds, fevers	some evidence to support diuretic, expectorant and laxative effects [11,20]	no information		Best use of this herb is as a flavoring agent in soft drinks [11]; no anabolic steroid activity [8]
Saw Palmetto (*Serenoa repens*) ripe fruits		diuretic, BPH, urinary antiseptic, aphrodisiac, GI infections, increase breast size, increase sperm production, reverse atrophy of testes and mammary glands	has antiandrogenic properties and may have antiinflammatory actions [11,20,24]; banned as a drug in the United States by the FDA [11,20]	treatment of BPH [24]		
Skullcap (*Scutellaria lateriflora*) above the ground plant (may be spelled "skullkap" in the popular press)	blue skullcap, blue pimpernel, helmet flower, hoodwort, mad-dog weed, side-flowering skullcap	tonic, tranquilizer, antispasmodic, diuretic, rheumatism, neuralgia, delirium tremens, menstrual promoter, effective against rabies, relieves menstrual cramps, epilepsy	no scientific evidence to support claims [20]	no information	possible hepatotoxicity [20]; hepatotoxicity may be due to adulteration or substitution [8]	ingestion of this drug should be avoided [20]
Senna (*Cassia spp.*) leaflets		cathartic	FDA approved as a laxative	no information	diarrhea, nausea [20]	chronic and/or excessive use of this herb should be avoided [20]
Shepherd's Purse (*Capsella bursa-pastoris*) aerial parts	cocowort, pick-pocket, St. Jame's weed, shepherd's heart	diuretic, vasoconstrictor, blood pressure stabilizer, excessive menstruation, uterine stimulant, astringent	current information lacking	Internally: for treatment of excessive menstruation Topically: nose bleeds and bleeding injuries to skin [24]	no known adverse effects [11]	
Slippery Elm (*Ulmus rubra*) inner bark	red elm	demulcent, emollient, nutrient, astringent	Declared a safe and effective oral demulcent by the FDA	no information		available in some commercial throat lozenges
St. John's Wort (*Hypericum perforatum*) leaves, tops	amber, goatweed, Johnswort, Klamath weed	antidepressant, antiinflammatory, antidiarrheal, astringent, rheumatism, gout, diuretic, gastritis	astringent, mild antidepressant effect [11,20,24]; possible antiviral action [11]	Internally: depression, anxiety, nervous conditions, dyspepsia complaints Externally: contusions, myalgias, first-degree burns [24]	photosensitization, dermatitis [11,20,24]	

Table 23.2. Summary of Herbs and their Properties; continued from previous page.

Common Name (Scientific Name) Part of plant used [18-20]	Other Names [18]	Popular Laypress Claims [11,18-24]	Scientific Information		Adverse Effects/ Warnings	Additional Comments/ Contraindications
			Scientific Properties/ FDA Approval	German Commission E Recommendations		
Valerian (*Valeriana officinalis*) rhizome, roots	wild valerian, garden heliotrope	tranquilizer, carminative, antidepressant, hypotensive	calming and sleep-inducing effects [11,20,24]	effective for treatment of insomnia and restlessness and gastrointestinal cramps [24]		
Witch Hazel (*Hamamelis virginiana*) leaves, bark	snapping hazel, striped alder, tobacco wood, winterbloom	astringent, hemostatic, sedative, tonic, vaginitis, hemorrhoids, menorrhagia, loss of uterine tone, analgesic astringent, antiinflammatory agent	FDA approved as an astringent	useful as supportive therapy for acute, non-specific diarrhea, and inflammation of mouth and gums [24]	stomach irritation, liver damage (rare) [24]	astringent activity of hamamelis water due to added alcohol [8]

Acknowledgments

The authors wish to sincerely thank Dr. Varro E. Tyler, PhD, ScD, Lilly Distinguished Professor of Pharmacology, Purdue University School of Pharmacy and Pharmacal Sciences for his review and consultation. Dr. Tyler is considered to be one of the leading experts in this field.

References

1. Mindell, E: Herb Bible. New York: Simon & Schuster, Fireside, 1992.

2. Campion EW. Why unconventional medicine? N Engl J Med 1993;328:28283.

3. Eisenberg D: Unconventional medicine in the United States. N Engl J Med 1993;328:246-52.

4. Marwick C: Congress wants alternative therapies studied; NIH responds with programs. JAMA 1992;268:9570958.

5. Bachman G: Nonhormonal alternatives for the management of early menopause in younger women with breast cancer. Journal of the National Cancer Institute Monographs 1994;16:61-167.

6. Hurley D: Pharmacists need to increase knowledge of herbal remedies as use skyrockets. Pharmacy Practice News 1995 (May): 24-25.

7. Larrey D, Vial T, Pauwels A, et al: Hepatotoxicity after germander (Teucrium chamaedrys) administration: another instance of herbal medicine hepatotoxicity. Ann Intern Med 1992; 117:129-32.

8. Tyler V. Written communication, 1996.

9. Miller RW. Can herbs really heal? FDA Consumer, Rockville, Md: U.S. Government Printing Office, DHHS Publication No. (FDA) 87-1140, 1987.

10. Snyder S: Herbal teas and toxicity. FDA Consumer, Rockville, Md: U.S. Government Printing Office, DHHS Publication No. (FDA) 92-1185, 1991.

11. Tyler VE: Herbs of Choice: The Therapeutic Use of Phyto-medicinals. New York: Pharmaceutical Products Press, 1994.

12. Napier K: Unproven medical treatments lure elderly. FDA Consumer, Rockville, Md: U.S. Government Printing Office, DHHS Publication, March 1994.

13. Huxtable R: The myth of beneficent nature: the risks of herbal preparations. Ann Intern Med 1992; 117:165-6.

14. Engebretson J, Wardell D: A contemporary view of alternative healing modalities. Nurse Practitioner 1993;18:51-55.

15. Joel LA: Alternative solutions to health problems. American Journal of Nursing July 1995;7.

16. Eisenberg D: Book Reviews: Herbal and Magical Medicine: Traditional Healing Today. N Engl J Med 1993;328:215-16.

17. Autotte PA: Editorial: Folk Medicine. Arch Pediatr Adolesc Med 1995; 149:94950.

18. Lust J: The Herb Book. New York: Bantam Books, 1973.

19. Hoffman D: The New Holistic Herbal. New York: Barnes and Noble, 1990.

20. Tyler VE: The Honest Herbal: A Sensible Guide to the Use of Herbs and Related Remedies 3rd ed. New York: Pharmaceutical Products Press, 1993.

21. Gladstar R: Herbal Healing for Women. New York: Fireside, 1993.

22. Tierra M: The Ways of Herbs. New York: Pocket Books, 1990.

23. Mindell E: Earl Mindell's Herb Bible. New York: Fireside, 1992.

24. Wichtl M: Herbal Drugs and Phytopharmaceuticals: A Handbook for Practice on a Scientific Basis. Stuttgart: Medpharm Scientific Publishers, 1994.

25. KJeijnenj, Knipschild P: Ginkgo biloba. Lancet 1992; 340:1136-39.

*—by Ellis Quinn Youngkin, PhD, RNC, OGNP,
is an associate professor at the School of Nursing,
Virginia Commonwealth University-Medical College
of Virginia, in Richmond.*

*—by Debra S. Israel, PharmD, BCPS,
is an assistant professor at the School of Pharmacy,
Virginia Commonwealth University-Medical College
of Virginia, in Richmond.*

Chapter 24

Drug or Food? Patients Stumble into Gray Area

John Kovarik got a rude shock one day last year when he went to his pharmacy to fill a prescription: His insurance company refused to pay for it.

"I was flabbergasted," said Mr. Kovarik, a lawyer in South Palm Beach, Fla., with a life-threatening genetic disorder known as Wilson's disease. To fight its symptoms, Mr. Kovarik needs an effective treatment to keep copper from accumulating in his body and destroying his vital organs.

He had been taking a drug that could have caused irreversible and sometimes lethal side effects. So, Mr. Kovarik said, he negotiated the maze of his health maintenance organization to find a doctor who would prescribe a newer and safer drug, Galzin. But when his insurance company, Humana Inc., refused to pay for Galzin, Mr. Kovarik angrily called the company from the pharmacy counter.

"I was telling them that I have this life-threatening disease," Mr. Kovarik said, "and that this drug is life sustaining. I told them that the drug I was using was having deleterious side effects. I told them that Galzin is F.D.A. approved." Later, he wrote letter after letter, to no avail.

The problem is that Galzin is zinc acetate, and zinc acetate is sold both as a prescription drug and over the counter as a food supplement. The supplement and the drug are supposed to be the same, but the supplement is not licensed by the Food and Drug Administration, so its manufacture is not regulated and there is no guarantee that the dose on the package is correct.

Humana questioned why it should pay for a prescription drug when the supplement was available. A month's supply of Galzin costs $95, Mr. Kovarik said. If he bought the supplement, it would cost $10 to $15, he said.

"We do not cover nutritional supplements," said Valerie Kennedy, a Humana spokeswoman.

But cost is not the crucial issue, said officials at Teva Pharmaceuticals U.S.A. of Sellersville, Pa., which makes Galzin. "The real issue here is the safety of the patient," said Dr. Carole Ben-Maimon, a senior vice president. "The patients taking a prescription product know what they are getting and how it was made."

A product can be a drug if a company tests it for safety and efficacy, receives approval from the Food and Drug Administration and makes the product according to Federal standards. But under current rules, many of the same products can be sold as supplements if they do not make drug claims.

"The boundary between food and drugs is by no means clear and sharp," said Dr. John Hathcock, the director of nutritional and regulatory science for the Council for Responsible Nutrition, which represents the supplement industry. "It is perfectly legal and, I believe, also legitimate for some products to be on the market both as supplements and drugs."

Patients who need products to treat diseases can take the drugs if their doctors prescribe them, Dr. Hathcock said, while others can buy the supplements.

But patients, their advocates and companies that try to sell drugs like zinc acetate say it is not that simple. Because a substance sold as a supplement is not regulated by the F.D.A., there is no guarantee that it will contain the product on its label or that the dosage stated on the label is accurate. Although only a few products are sold as both drugs and supplements, some are vital to patients, especially those with rare disorders who must take them regularly and in fixed amounts.

"It's a big problem," said Abbey Meyers, the executive director of the National Organization for Rare Disorders, an advocacy group based in Fairfield, Conn. "If your life depends on one of these products, you can't take a chance on buying an over-the-counter supplement that may contain no ingredient or half the ingredient or two or three times more of the ingredient."

Ms. Meyers said her group financed a study in which Duke University scientists analyzed over-the-counter L-carnitine supplements from a variety of companies. They found that doses varied markedly, even in pills coming from the same bottle, with some pills containing no carnitine, others containing more than the label specified and most providing less than 60 percent of the dose promised on the label.

And yet, said Lynn McHenry Morgan of Concord, Calif., when she changed insurance companies last February, her new insurer, Blue Shield, told her it would not pay for prescription L-carnitine for her two children, who need the drug to treat a rare and debilitating disorder involving the mitochondria, which provide energy to cells.

Ms. Morgan said she lobbied Blue Shield for three months before the company agreed to pay.

Dr. Nancy Stalker, the director of pharmacy services at Blue Shield of California, said the company wanted patients to get the care they needed, but had a policy restricting payments for drugs that also were nutritional supplements.

Doctors who treat patients in similar circumstances say they often end up imploring insurance companies to pay for the prescription drugs. Dr. Susan Winters, a geneticist who treats children with rare metabolic disorders, said she aggressively fought for insurance coverage for drugs like L-carnitine, but said she did not always win.

Ms. Meyers said that drug companies realized that testing a drug and getting the F.D.A.'s approval to market it might not be worthwhile if the drug could also be sold as a supplement. With zinc acetate, she said, her group actively sought a company to sell the product as a drug. "Nobody would do it," Ms. Meyers said. "Who wants to put the money into making a pharmaceutical grade zinc when you can buy zinc over the counter?" Finally, she said, Teva agreed to do it.

But the situation can be different when a drug is not urgently needed for patients with an otherwise lethal disease. Dr. Richard J. Wurtman, a co-founder of Interneuron, a small drug company in Lexington, Mass., was convinced that melatonin worked as a sleeping pill if the dose was correct. He wanted to test and market it as a drug. But when he urged this course on his company, he said, he was met with "absolutely zero interest."

"The problem is convincing a company in this country to invest the tens of millions of dollars to get the drug on the market and then have it come out and compete with a supplement," Dr. Wurtman said. "As long as something is available as a dietary supplement, no company will invest in it."

And so Interneuron joined the supplement makers. It is marketing melatonin as a supplement that can induce sleep, through a subsidiary called InterNutria.

—by Gina Kolata

Chapter 25

Judging the Value and Effectiveness of Herbal Remedies

Herbal medicine, the mainstay of therapeutics for centuries before modern purified drugs relegated it to the status of near-quackery, has in the last five years emerged from the fringes of health care with an astonishing flourish and now shows clear signs of joining the medical mainstream. Despite many cautionary tales about adulterated and even dangerous products, herbs formulated as capsules, tinctures, extracts and teas—and increasingly as additions to common foods like potato chips and fruit drinks—are now routinely used by a third of American adults seeking to enhance their health or alleviate their illnesses. Each day the herbal realm wins new converts, particularly among those who have become disillusioned with the cost and consequences of traditional drugs, distrustful of conventional physicians and convinced that "natural" equals "good."

Yet, because herbal products are classified as dietary supplements, not drugs, and face none of the premarket hurdles drugs must clear, consumers have no assurance of safety or effectiveness. Indeed, scores of products sold in the United States are listed by European and American authorities as ineffective, unsafe or both, and manufacturing standards to assure high quality have been proposed but are not yet in force.

Thus, countless consumers are wasting their money on useless products or jeopardizing their health on hazardous ones. Among the serious side effects that have been linked to herbal remedies are high blood pressure, life-threatening allergic reactions, heart rhythm abnormalities, mania, kidney failure and liver damage. A few widely available products, including sassafras and comfrey, contain known carcinogens.

At the same time, according to a report last year in the journal *Psychosomatics*, unsuspecting consumers "have used herbal remedies with good results only to discover that the benefit was actually derived from the presence of undisclosed medicines," including steroids, anti-inflammatory agents, sedatives and hormones.

"The lack of quality standards is the No. 1 problem in the whole industry," said Dr. Varro E. Tyler, emeritus professor of pharmacognosy (the study of active ingredients in plants) at Purdue University. Dr. Tyler has no direct financial connection to herbal products. He holds no equity interest in any maker of such products. However, Dr. Tyler has been paid by a number of herbal companies as a consultant and lecturer. He is perhaps the nation's leading independent expert on herbal medicine. He said: "I feel sorry for the typical consumer. How is he or she to know what is best, what products are reliable and safe? Even when a label says the product has been standardized, the consumer has no way to know if it actually meets that standard." Even if an herbal product has been reliably made in some standard dose, it does not mean that scientific studies have shown it to be effective.

The industry itself is promoting a "good manufacturing practices" doctrine. Annette Dickinson, director of scientific and regulatory affairs for the Council for Responsible Nutrition, a trade organization for producers of dietary supplements, said a consortium of associations submitted a document of manufacturing standards to the Food and Drug Administration two years ago. Although such a standard would say nothing about an herb's safety or effectiveness, it would result in reliable methods that the industry would have to use to insure the identity and quality of its products. The agency has issued a notice of proposed rules but no final ruling as yet.

Nonetheless, botanicals, as herbal products are more accurately known, are enjoying an annual retail market approaching $4 billion, up from $839 million in 1991 and growing about 18 percent a year. Hundreds of products made with virtually no Government oversight are crowding shelves of health food stores, food markets and pharmacies nationwide. Supplements are also widely sold by marketers like Amway, through catalogues and on the Internet.

Now, even major pharmaceutical companies like Warner Lambert, American Home Products, Bayer and SmithKline Beecham are introducing herbal products, adding respectability to this marginalized market.

Some herbs—like echinacea, goldenseal, American ginseng and wild yam—have become so popular that their continued supply from natural sources is in danger. As the plants become scarcer and more expensive, products containing them are increasingly likely to be adulterated and may even contain none of the herb listed on the label. Peggy Brevoort, president of East Earth Herb Inc., a company in Eugene, Ore., that produces botanicals, said that the demand for St. John's wort, used for mild depression, and kava, a calmative said to reduce anxiety, now exceeds their supply, introducing the "danger of adulteration" by "unscrupulous dealers."

At the same time, two major new publications—a 1,244-page *Physicians' Desk Reference for Herbal Medicines*, produced by the same company that publishes the *Physicians' Desk Reference*, and an English-language edition of Germany's therapeutic guide to herbal medicines, *The Complete German Commission E Monographs*—have been issued to help educate physicians, pharmacists and interested consumers about the known uses, proper dosages and safety concerns of more than 600 botanicals now sold in this country. The evaluations in both books are based on studies, most done in Germany and reviewed by teams of experts.

Last month, the National Institutes of Health began listing on the Internet international bibliographic information on dietary supplements, including herbal products. The address is www.nal.usda.gov/fnic/ IBIDS/.

In addition, a few medical and pharmacology schools have recently introduced courses in phytomedicine, the study of botanicals. And next month the American Pharmaceutical Association will conduct a two-day program on herbal medicine as part of its annual meeting. Still, most doctors remain wary of botanicals, especially when patients choose self-medication with plant extracts over established medical remedies.

The Regulations: Law Calls Herbs Food, Not Drugs

The very act of Congress that has fostered this growth—the 1994 Dietary Supplement Health and Education Act—has also permitted chaos to reign in the botanical marketplace, with no mechanism to assure that products are safe or effective. Pushed heavily by Senator Orrin G. Hatch of Utah, the home base of many supplement makers, and passed over the objections of the F.D.A., the law created a new product class, the dietary supplement, that was not subject to regulations applied to drugs. Now any substance that can be found in foods, regardless of amount or action and including substances that act as hormones or toxins, can be produced and sold without any premarket testing or agency approval.

Marketed as neither a food nor a drug, herbal products are not obliged to meet any established standards of effectiveness or safety for medicinal products, which require extensive laboratory and clinical trials before approval. As with other substances classified as dietary supplements, the F.D.A. can restrict the sale of an herbal product only if it receives well-documented reports of health problems associated with it. The agency took four years, and more than 100 reports of life-threatening symptoms and 38 deaths, to act against ephedra, often sold as the Chinese herb ma huang, a stimulant that can prove disastrous to people with heart problems.

With F.D.A. authority limited by the 1994 law, the Federal Trade Commission, which monitors advertising, has taken a more active role in monitoring supplement makers.

The F.T.C. last year took legal action against seven manufacturers that had broken rules requiring advertising be truthful and verifiable. The companies were selling remedies or purported cure-alls for ailments like impotence, cancer and obesity.

The commission also sent E-mail warnings to 1,200 Internet sites that it said had made "incredible claims" for drugs, devices and supplements, including herbal remedies that would supposedly ward off AIDS. Also, the commission late last year issued its first set of advertising guidelines aimed specifically at the supplement industry.

Still, the current regulations have created a quagmire of consumer confusion and set up potential health crises that even industry officials say could ultimately hurt producers as well as users of herbal products. Under the 1994 law, consumers have no assurance that an herbal product contains what the label says it does or that it is free from harmful contaminants. Independent analyses of some products, particularly those containing costly or scarce herbs, revealed that some have little or none of the purported active ingredient listed on the label.

Adding to the confusion is that botanical makers are allowed to describe products only in terms of their effects on the structure or function of the body, not their potential health benefits. Thus, a product label might say "promotes cardiac function" but it cannot say "lowers cholesterol."

Likewise, although the law does allow health warnings on the label, most manufacturers have yet to include them.

Consumers are warned, however, that Federal drug safety officials are not watching the store. All botanicals must display a disclaimer on the label following the description of the product's structural or functional role: "This statement has not been evaluated by the Food and Drug Administration. This product is not intended to diagnose, treat, cure or prevent any disease." To which Dr. Tyler commented, "If that is true, why on earth would anyone use it?"

The Rebirth: With the 90's, Buzzwords and Hype

The seeds of the modern herbal market were sown in the 60's when "green, organic and natural became buzzwords," Dr. Tyler said. But they did not mature until the 90's with the growing consumer interest in "self-care and controlling one's destiny," he said. Many turned to herbs as a gentler way to treat health problems and a potential tool for preserving mental and physical health.

The interest has spawned scores of Internet sites and hundreds of books on various herbs. But much of the literature is replete with poorly documented health claims and, with few exceptions (among them, Dr. Tyler's books), advocacy prevails over objectivity.

Because plants contain a mixture of relatively dilute chemicals, they naturally tend to have milder actions, both in their therapeutic benefits and side effects, than the concentrated, single chemicals in most drugs. Thus, botanicals generally take longer to act than regular pharmaceuticals and few have the potency of a prescription, the one possible exception being saw palmetto, which a well-designed study indicated may be as helpful for an enlarged prostate as the more expensive and riskier drug, Proscar.

The combination of chemicals in botanicals is potentially both a plus and a minus. When two or more chemicals enhance one another's activity, the therapeutic benefit could theoretically exceed that from a isolated substance formulated as a drug. Mark Blumenthal, who heads the American Botanical Council, noted that the herb St. John's wort, widely used in Germany and increasingly in the United States to counter mild depression, is standardized for a substance called hypericin. But, he explained, "hypericin is not directly linked to its antidepressant activity." Rather, other substances in the herb seem to have diverse actions on brain chemicals, all of which work together to counter depression.

But, equally possible when using an herb with two or more active chemicals is that one will cancel the benefits of another or introduce a hazard. Without careful chemical tests and large, well-controlled clinical trials such actions are often hard to detect.

Consumer confidence in herbal medicine is bolstered by the common but erroneous assumption that "natural" equals "safe" and the public's failure to realize that many plants contain chemicals that are potent drugs or outright poisons. Natural laxatives like the herb Cascara sagrada are just as habit-forming and harmful to the colon as laxatives sold as drugs.

Indeed, one quarter of prescription drugs and hundreds of over-the-counter products were originally isolated from plants. Ephedra, for example, contains a natural stimulant that is approved for use as a decongestant and bronchial dilator in some pharmaceutical products. However, when used in uncontrolled dosages or by people with certain underlying health problems, it can cause a dangerous rise in blood pressure and, in its herbal form, has been responsible for serious adverse reactions and dozens of deaths, mainly among people who inappropriately used it as a stimulant or diet aid.

Complicating the safety issue is the fact, shown in several recent surveys, that most patients fail to tell their physicians they use herbal supplements and thus sometimes risk dangerous drug interactions or endure costly tests or treatments when an herb causes an unrecognized side effect. Experts say many patients withhold information about herbal drug use because they fear being ridiculed by their doctors.

Although all German physicians must take courses on herbal remedies, only a handful of American medical and pharmacology schools offer courses in this field.

The Science: Trying to Evaluate Effectiveness

A year ago, the President's Commission on Dietary Supplement Labels recommended that the F.D.A. appoint a committee to evaluate the safety and effectiveness of herbal products. "This could be the most important step in the United States toward legitimizing herbal medicine," Dr. Tyler said.

However, the agency responded that it lacked the budget to support such an effort. American physicians have completed and published only a few well-designed studies of some popular botanicals. Among them were studies showing that saw palmetto can shrink an enlarged prostate and ginkgo biloba can improve memory in patients with early Alzheimer's disease.

The Office of Dietary Supplements at the National Institutes of Health is helping to finance a three-year multicenter study of St. John's wort as a treatment for clinical depression and a study of plant-based estrogens as a preventive for postmenopausal health problems.

However, thousands of studies of botanicals have been completed abroad—mainly in Germany—that strongly suggest a health-promoting role for more than 200 plant products. Germany's Commission E evaluated 380 botanicals, approving 254 as safe and reasonably effective and disapproving 126 as ineffective, unsafe or both.

The Germans use a different criterion to assess an herb's benefits— a doctrine of "reasonable certainty" that the herb has the desired effect and is safe, Mr. Blumenthal said. Whereas standard testing of a drug for approval by the United States F.D.A. can cost as much as $500 million per product—a prohibitive amount for companies to spend on botanicals that cannot be patented—tests to establish "reasonable certainty" would cost only $1 million to $2 million, Dr. Tyler estimated.

In June 1996, Dr. Robert Temple, director of medical policy for the F.D.A.'s Center for Drug Evaluation, suggested that, rather than subjecting botanicals to the extensive tests required for drugs, the agency might consider applying less stringent criteria to assess an herb's effects, at least when a product is to be used only for a short time. He said, "A long history of safe use might provide sufficient safety information for products that are intended for short-term use."

More than four dozen botanicals or botanical formulations have been submitted to the agency as investigational new drugs. If any meet the agency's criteria for safety and effectiveness and are eventually approved as drugs, they would be allowed to make direct health claims—instead of just structure and function statements—on labels and in advertising.

Meanwhile, Dr. Joerg Gruenwald, medical director of a German phytomedicine company and primary editor of the new Physicians' Desk Reference for Herbal Medicines, said professionals can rely on that volume for current, documented information about botanicals. The volume, to be issued annually, updates the Commission E reports and adds several hundred other products sold in the United States, listing effects, side effects and conditions in which their use is inadvisable.

—by Jane E. Brody

Chapter 26

If You Take Herbs, Tell Your Doctor

"When the doctor asks, 'What medications are you taking?' most people don't even think to mention herbs," says Catherine Crone, MD, a psychiatrist at the INOVA Fairfax Hospital in Virginia who has researched the side effects of herbal medicines. It's easy to understand why. Herbs are available over the counter and are thought of as "natural," so they automatically seem safe.

Furthermore, many people who choose to take herbs assume a doctor would pooh-pooh their decision. Robert Hilsden, MD, leader of a Canadian research team that interviewed patients using alternative medicine, says they may be afraid of being criticized. Or they think it's pointless to tell a "medical person" who's not knowledgeable about or even interested in alternative therapies.

That may or may not be a fair assumption, since doctors vary widely in their opinions of herbal medicine's benefits and in their understanding of alternative treatments in general. But either way, when it comes to herbs, two heads—yours and the doctor's—are better than one. Deciding not to tell a physician about herbal remedies can have serious health consequences.

"Many herbs contain very powerful, medically active chemicals," says Fairfax's Dr. Crone, pointing out that a number of prescription medicines, like the cardiac drug digitalis, are derived from herbs or other plants. Thus, like drugs, herbs can have serious side effects, and they can also interact negatively with commonly prescribed medications.

Table 26.1. The Downside of Some Popular Herbs*†, continued on next page.

Herb	Purported Use(s)	Potential Problems
Aloe	Wound healer; laxative	Can cause nausea, vomiting, or diarrhea.
Black cohosh	Alleviates PMS; relieves indigestion	Can cause nausea, vomiting, or uterine contractions.
Chaparral**††	Relieves pain and inflammation	Contains pyrrolizidine, a chemical that can harm the liver. The toxic effect worsens if the herb is combined with medicines like Dilantin or phenobarbital, which increase the activity of liver enzymes.
Comfrey**	Blood purifier; wound healer	Same as for chaparral.
Dandelion Uva ursi (bearberry)	Diuretic	Taking with diuretic medicines like Lasix or hydrochlorothiazide could cause serious dehydration or loss of potassium, which could disrupt the heart's rhythm.
Echinacea	Immune booster	People with autoimmune disorders like lupus or multiple sclerosis who take echinacea in hopes of relieving their symptoms could end up aggravating the illness.
Ginkgo biloba	Memory booster	Acts as a blood thinner. If combined with other anticoagulants, such as aspirin, vitamin E, or the prescription drug warfarin, it could give rise to excessive bleeding.

Table 26.1. The Downside of Some Popular Herbs*†, continued from previous page.

Herb	Purported Use(s)	Potential Problems
Ginseng	Stimulant	Can raise blood pressure. May also cause agitation, anxiety, depression, or insomnia.
Golden seal	Relieves indigestion	Can cause nausea or vomiting if taken in very large amounts.
Kava kava Passion flower Valerian	Sedative	May add to the effect of sedating medications like Valium and could cause oversedation, especially in older people.
Licorice	Anti-ulcer; cough suppressant; diuretic	Can raise blood pressure, lower potassium, and interfere with the action of some medications used to control hypertension.
Pau d'Arco	Blood purifier	May cause nausea, vomiting, anemia, or an increased tendency to bleed.

*This chart is based on research published by Drs. Catherine Crone and T.N. Wise in the Jan/Feb 1998 issue of Psychosomatics.

†Most of the herbs listed are available in health food stores such as GNC or Nature Food Centres.

**This herb appears on the U.S. Food and Drug Administration's list of dietary supplements associated with serious safety problems.

††The FDA issued a warning against chaparral in 1992 after reports that it caused severe liver damage in several users.

For example, if you're already on a sedating medication such as Valium, taking a "nerve-calming" herb like kava kava, valerian, or passion flower adds to the effect of the drug and could cause oversedation, especially in older people. In the same way, herbs such as dandelion, a diuretic, can redouble the effects of some prescription diuretics, causing dehydration or loss of the mineral potassium. And aloe, black cohosh, golden seal, and pau d'Arco, all available in health food stores like GNC or Nature Food Centres, can cause nausea or vomiting if taken in overly large amounts.

Among those most vulnerable to herbs' potential harms are people with chronic illnesses who are frustrated with the inability of conventional medicine to ease their pain or discomfort, says Dr. Hilsden. His research team surveyed patients who have Crohn's disease, a long-term, painful intestinal disorder that is difficult to treat, and found that many of them decided to try alternative therapies as a way of taking health care matters into their own hands when the conventional route didn't relieve their symptoms.

Chapter 27

Aromatherapy

Aromatherapy refers to the therapeutic use of essential oils that have been distilled from plants. The oils are readily absorbed through the skin and are known to interact with our bodies pharmacologically, physiologically and psychologically.

There are many ways in which essential oils can be applied, including with massage, in skin oils and lotions, in douches, in hot or cold compresses, in flower waters, through vaporization (using special burners), through steam inhalation and, in very rare instances, by neat application (for example, lavender oil for burns or tea tree oil for spots).

One of the problems of using essential oils is the quality of the oils themselves because their production is largely unregulated.

Some brands are definitely better than others and it is, therefore, useful to seek a personal recommendation from a qualified aromatherapist before making a purchase.

Essential oils should be stored, sealed, in a cool place away from heat. Some oils, such as jasmine and neroli, should be kept in the fridge. The therapeutic effects of most oils are thought to withstand storage for about two to three years, except citrus oils, where the effects last one year.

Historical Background

The use of plants in medicine has a long history, and oils distilled from them are known to have been prepared as far back as 3000 BC, in the Indus Valley (present-day Pakistan). The ancient Egyptians also used aromatics in their perfumes, medicines and as part of their embalming practices.

The ancient Greeks built on the knowledge accrued by the Egyptians, and as the Romans employed Greek physicians, the use of aromatics spread throughout the Roman empire.

In the Arab world the famous physician Abu Ali Ibn Sina (980-1037), or Avicenna, as he was known in the West, described over 800 plants and their effects on the body. He also developed a method of distilling essential oils. These oils came to Europe with the return of the Crusaders from the Holy Wars. During the Renaissance the distillation process was industrialized and scientific investigation of essential oils began. By the 19th century chemists were identifying the constitutents of plant oils, which contributed to the growth of the pharmaceutical industry.

Aromatherapy is a relatively new discipline. The term was coined by a French chemist called Rene-Maurice Gattefosse in 1928. While working in his laboratory in the family perfume business, he burnt his hand. Noticing some neat lavender oil nearby he plunged his hand into the container. To his surprise the burns healed in hours—without scarring. As a result Gattefosse went on to investigate other oils and to use them in dermatological preparations.

In the 1960s another Frenchman, Jean Valnet, began using essential oils in his medical practice and was instrumental in instigating further research into their properties and their wider use in the French health service. In the UK the popularity of aromatherapy is more recent, and it is still more widely known as a type of beauty treatment than as a therapy.

Claims

According to the International Federation of Aromatherapists, aromatherapy 'enhances well-being, relieves stress, and helps in the rejuvenation and regeneration of the human body'.

Aromatherapists also claim that it can help with premenstrual syndrome, stress-related conditions, moderate anxiety or depression, sleeping problems, minor aches and pains, migraines, digestive disorders, skin problems such as eczema and acne, and minor infections such as thrush and cystitis.

Contraindications

There are some essential oils that should never be used in a therapeutic context as they are known to be toxic or to cause serious skin irritation. For more information on the safety of oils consult, *The Essential Oils Safety Manual*[3].

It is also true that certain essential oils should not be used in particular circumstances. For example:

- Sweet fennel should not be used if a person has epilepsy

- Rosemary, sage and thyme should not be used with anyone suffering from high blood pressure

- Arnica, basil, clary sage, cypress, jasmine, juniper, marjoram, myrrh, sage and thyme should not be used during pregnancy

- Peppermint, rose and rosemary should not be used in the first three or four months of pregnancy, and only well diluted in later months

- Camomile and lavender are described as emmenagogues (encouraging menstruation), so should be used with care in pregnancy if there is a risk of miscarriage or bleeding.

Check with a trained aromatherapist if you are unsure about the safety of using a particular essential oil.

Research

The therapeutic properties of essential oils have been investigated although much of the research was undertaken in France and has not been translated into English. The following papers are selection of those available:

Blackwell, R. An insight into aromatic oils: lavender and tea tree. *British Journal of Phytotherapy* 1991; 2: 1, 25-30.

Bronough, R.L. In vivo percutaneous absorption of fragrance ingredients in rhesus monkeys and humans. *Food and Chemical Toxicology*, 1990; 28: 5, 369-374

Buckle, J. Aromatherapy. *Nursing Times* 1993; 89: 20, 32-35.

Jaeger, W. Evidence of the sedative effect of neroli oil, citronellal and phenylethyl acetate on mice. *Journal of Essential Oil Research* 1992; 4: 387-394.

Koedam, A. *Antimicrobial Activity of Essential Oils*. Stuttgart: Atherische Ole, 1982.

Mishra, A.K. Fungistatic properties of essential oil of cinnamomum camphora. *International Journal of Pharmacognosy*, 1991; 29: 4, 259-262.

Rudzki, E. Essential oils: sensitivity to 35 oils. *Contact Dermatology*, 1976; 2: 196-200.

Evaluations of aromatherapy as a therapy are, however, much thinner on the ground. Most combine the use of particular essential oil with massage. Nurses have been undertaking some research, but this is generally very small scale, involving only a handful of patients. Example of such studies include:

- Registered mental health nurse Mark Hardy found that four elderly patients experiencing sleeping difficulties were able to benefit from a natural and refreshing night's sleep when a vortex air freshener using lavender oil was installed in the dormitory.

Hardy, M. Sweet scented dreams. *International Journal of Aromatherapy*, Spring 1991; 3: 1, 11-13

- A study by Dawn Hewitt, staff nurse at the Royal Sussex Hospital in Brighton, suggests that giving patients in intensive care and coronary care units a 20-minute foot massage with lavender oil reduced heart rate, respiration rate, blood pressure, pain and wakefulness. The reduction was more marked in patients who received the massage with the essential oil than with patients who received massage alone or patients who had an undisturbed rest of 20 minutes.

Hewitt, D. Massage with lavender oil lowered tension. *Nursing Times* 1992 88: 25, 8.

Other studies are in the pipeline. The International Federation of Aromatherapists (IFA) is currently putting the finishing touches to a large research project looking at aromatherapy in the treatment of endometriosis. Leicester University and the University of Ulster are beginning a joint research project on the use of essential oils as adjuncts to behavioral interventions and are looking in particular at sleep patterns in children.

Implications for Nursing

Aromatherapy is immensely popular with nurses, midwives and health visitors, and is already being used in a variety of settings. Its popularity stems from the ease with which nurses believe it can be incorporated into their practice and the positive feedback they receive from patients.

It is important, however, that nurses using essential oils do so in an informed way, undertake a recognized course of study and evaluate their practice. There are nurses using essential oils with no recognized training and some nurse tutors who are teaching aromatherapy to students after completing only a short course.

Nurses who would like their patients to benefit from aromatherapy, but who have not undertaken training, can contact the IFA, which operates the Aromatherapy in Care Project. This is a voluntary service where aromatherapists work alongside health professionals within the NHS. More information is available from the project coordinator, Frances Fewell, at the IFA.

Use of Aromatherapy in Nursing

- In health visiting: Favre Armstrong, a health visitor and qualified aromatherapist working in Bath, regularly uses aromatherapy in her practice. She has found it useful for treating rheumatism, arthritis, backache, sinusitis, catarrh, postnatal depression, menstrual problems and depression.

  Armstrong, F. Scenting relief. *Nursing Times* 1991; 87: 10, 52-54

- In psychiatric nursing: psychiatric nurse Sarah Boden and colleagues have found the following oils useful in reducing seizures among patients with epilepsy: ylang-ylang, lavender, camomile, rosemary, melissa and marjoram.

- In care of the elderly: sister Helen Passant has found that elderly patients massaged with a mixture of comfrey oil and lavender oil in a carrier oil needed fewer drugs and had less pain.

  Passant, H. A holistic approach to the ward. *Nursing Times* 1990; 86: 4, 26-28.

Using Essential Oils at Home

A wide range of books on aromatherapy is available (see resources) and many offer simple remedies for personal use. For example, Patricia Davis in *Aromatherapy: an A-Z*[1] suggests the following oils in a bath as aids to relaxation and sleep: either add four drops of lavender oil and two of bergamot, or four drops of lavender oil and two of marjoram.

Maggie Tisserand, in *Aromatherapy for Women*[2] recommends the following massage oil recipe for muscular aches: 10 drops of juniper oil, seven drops of lavender oil, and eight drops of rosemary in 50ml of a carrier oil. But such remedies should not be used with patients unless administered by a properly trained aromatherapist.

References

[1]Davis, P. *Aromatherapy: An A-Z*. Saffron Walden: C.W. Daniel, 1988.

[2]Tisserand, M. *Aromatherapy for Women*. Wellingborough: Thorsons, 1990.

[3]Tisserand, R. *The Essential Oils Safety Data Manual*. Hove: Tisserand Aromatherapy Institute, 1990.

— by Joanna Trevelyan

Joanna Trevelyan is deputy editor, Nursing Times

Therapeutic techniques are described, it is purely for illustration and not intended to act as a guide to practice. No therapeutic interventions should ever be carried out by nurses, midwives or health visitors who have not undergone the appropriate training.

Chapter 28

Flower Essence Therapy

A New Approach to Mind-Body Wellness

The Pioneering Research of Dr. Edward Bach

Flowers essences are a unique form of vibrational medicine, formulated to address profound issues of emotional well-being and mind-body health. While the use of flowers for healing has many ancient antecedents, the precise application of flower essences for specific emotions and attitudes was first developed by an English physician, Dr. Edward Bach (1886-1936). Dr. Bach initially gained professional recognition as a standard medical doctor in the field of immunology. He developed a series of vaccines which were credited with saving the lives of thousands of World War I soldiers during a virulent flu epidemic in 1918. Bach went on to accept a post at the London Homeopathic Hospital where he refined and reformulated his vaccines into a series of seven bowel nosodes. These homeopathic nosodes rapidly received widespread acclaim for their remarkable healing properties. As Bach developed them, he observed archetypal personality traits associated with each one. Eventually, he developed a protocol for treating according to these fundamental soul expressions, rather than the presenting physical symptoms.

Dr. Bach's increasing sensitivity for the human soul led him to abandon his prominent homeopathic career on prestigious Harley

Street in London and return to the Welsh countryside of his ancestry. Searching for a modality of healing which could work more directly within the realm of the human soul, he developed medicines from flowering herbs and trees, made with careful attention to the elemental influences of earth, air, fire and water. These substances, called flower essences, have unique properties that work primarily in the emotional-mental realm. Unlike pharmaceutical drugs which treat mental and emotional dysfunction by controlling or manipulating physical brain chemistry, flower essences are a form of *vibrational* or *etheric* medicine. Recognizing that the human being consists of more than a dense physical body, vibrational medicines like flower essences are formulated to treat the subtle mental and emotional fields which surround the physical form. The positive archetypes from the flowers stimulate *consciousness rather than blood chemistry*, and by so doing help the individual to recognize harmful and dysfunctional behaviors that need to change. Flower essences are particularly valued for being safe and harmonious, while also being highly efficacious and beneficial.

On the Vanguard of Mind-Body Medicine

Bach's healing philosophy actually anticipated a whole stream of modern mind-body research which has gradually developed since the beginning of this century, and is finally receiving more widespread recognition. In the post World-War II era researchers began to identify personality traits which correlated with certain diseases. One of the most famous of these studies was conducted in the 1950's by Meyer Reidman, M.D. and Raymond Rosenman, M.D., who coined the term "Type A behavior" for the impatient, hostile attitude connected with greater risk of heart disease. Over the years numerous studies have pinpointed the decisive role of many different emotional factors such as anger, grief, depression or self-esteem on the outcome of specific diseases as well as over-all immunity. With the publication of Robert Ader's book *Psychoneuroimmunology* in 1981, an entirely new field of medical research was established (abbreviated as PNI), which provides substantive scientific data to demonstrate that mental and emotional factors affect immunity. These studies identify "biochemical messengers" which transmit emotional responses to and from glands in the body, as well as various neuro-peptides such as endorphins which have pain-killing and euphoric effects.

Despite a growing recognition for the importance of wellness programs which address the whole human being, there are still many wide gulfs in the actual implementation of these new healing paradigms. Few therapies actually interweave physiological and psychological care into one cohesive mind-body component. Mainly developed since World-War II, the wide-ranging field of psychotherapy primarily employs cognitive and *psychological* approaches to wellness, but does not use natural substances which actually impact the body. On the other hand, the medical profession is still largely concerned with the alleviation or suppression of *physical* symptoms of disease through surgical intervention or chemically-based pharmaceutical medicine. Even psychiatric medicine primarily involves the use of psychoactive drugs that alter physical brain chemistry in order to control or suppress human emotions such as depression, fear or anxiety.

Seen from this perspective, flower essence therapy is actually a unique, integrative therapy which uses natural substances acting within the physical matrix of the body to address precise states of psychological consciousness. Yet because the remedies are dilute potentizations which do not act through a bio-chemical mechanism, they have no dangerous side-effects. In fact, they do not suppress or mask physical and emotional symptoms; rather they work as catalysts to stimulate and awaken individual awareness and the inner capacity to make changes. Flower essences have an exceptional ability to enhance other therapeutic modalities; however they are not selected for physical symptoms but rather for archetypal personality traits and accompanying emotional and mental phenomena. Through a change in the inner condition of the human being, a new balance is gradually achieved at all levels, including physical health.

Flower essences are most closely aligned with the field of homeopathy, since both approaches include the use of potentized substances which affect trans-physical levels of the human being. However, Bach prepared the flower essences in a very different way than traditional homeopathic medicines, which are made from a wide range of substances, including human, animal and mineral sources as well as many different parts of plants. These various substances are often desiccated, then pulverized or macerated and extracted into alcohol, and finally diluted and potentized in homeopathic laboratories. By contrast the flower essences work more directly with living forces captured immediately from fresh flowering plants.

Bach had a great respect and familiarity with homeopathic medicine, but he wanted to make another contribution which worked at a further level within the human being. He believed that the flower essences had beneficent properties and that they created their healing effect by a different principle of *polarity* or *resonance*. In an article published in the *Homeopathic World* he explained, "Hahnemann taught that 'Like cures like.' This is true up to a point, but the word 'cures' is misleading. Like repels like might be more accurate . . . The perfect method is not so much to repel adverse influence, as to draw in its opposing virtue; and by means of this virtue flood out the fault. This is the law of opposites, of positive and negative." Qualified homeopathic practitioners observe that flower essences work differently than typical homeopathic medicines. They are more likely to stimulate new patterns of emotional awareness and positivity, and thus work to unblock deep-seated miasmatic layers which often thwart full healing potential.

During the six decades since the early discoveries of Dr. Bach, the use of flower essences has spread throughout the world; they are employed in a wide variety of professional healing modalities as well as home-care. In addition to the 38 remedies first formulated by Dr. Bach, noteworthy essences have also been developed from other indigenous plants throughout the world, including native American wildflowers and herbs. For the last two decades the Flower Essence Society, a non-profit world-wide organization headquartered in Nevada City, California, has brought together a global network of professional health practitioners and interested laypersons who are devoted to the development of flower essence therapy. The Flower Essence Society conducts plant research, collects and publishes case studies, analyzes clinical trends involving flower essences, and administers a variety of educational programs, including an annual certification intensive.

Unique Features of Flower Essence Therapy

Designed for Mental-emotional Healing

Flower essences expand our understanding of health care, recognizing a relationship between body and soul, and the interweaving of spiritual, mental, emotional and physical aspects of wellness. They enjoy a reputation of being both highly effective and very safe to use, since they contain only minute traces of physical substance. Regarded as **potentized remedies,** the essences derive their beneficial powers from the inherent **life forces within substances** affecting transphysical states of being. These remarkable remedies expand our understanding of health care, recognizing a relationship between body and soul, and the interweaving of spiritual, mental, emotional, and physical aspects of wellness. They address the subtle but very important realm of the human psyche, where thoughts and feelings emanate. Just as food nourishes the human body, *flower essences nourish the human soul*, enhancing emotional and psychological well-being. Flower essences should not be misconstrued as cure-alls or simplistic panaceas.

Can Be Integrated with Other Health Modalities

Flower essences are precise tools which can be used by qualified therapists as adjuncts in a wide range of health care programs, or for self-healing by informed and insightful home-care practitioners. The flower essences work most beneficially as part of a holistic program of health enhancement, including exercise, nourishing diet, stress reduction, inner development and appropriate medical care.

What is more, use of the essences can actually enhance other practices by addressing psycho-spiritual issues which may be underlying various health problems. Physicians, nurses, chiropractors, acupuncturists, herbalists, massage practitioners, physical therapists, nutritionists, psychologists, pastoral counselors, social workers, and other professionals find the essences to be an invaluable adjunct to their practices.

Flower essence therapy is not an exclusive answer to all of humanity's ills. It does not substitute for our daily practices of meditation and prayer, physical exercise, healthful diet, social responsibility, and moral development. However, used with sensitivity and understanding, the essences are an important catalyst toward a more health-filled, balanced lifestyle. By stimulating greater awareness of our inner life, the essences build a much needed bridge between the realms of body and soul.

A Spectrum of Metamorphic Responses

Flower essences can produce immediate or dramatic changes, but at other times their effect is quite gradual. The most typical pattern is to discover the gradual effect of the essences over a period of time. These changes can include shifts in relationships, life-style, self-image, stress level, attitude toward work, and state of well-being. It is important to choose flower essences with care and consideration; the more precisely the remedy matches the true inner condition of the soul, the more powerful and beneficial its results will be.

Based upon twenty years of collecting professional clinical data through the Flower Essence Society, four basic levels of outcome have been identified, referred to as the ***Four R's of Flower Essence Response.*** (The original research regarding these stages of soul transformation is outlined in *Flowers that Heal,* by Patricia Kaminski.) These stages do not occur in every case, and while they usually occur in the order listed, several may be operative simultaneously, or in slightly altered sequence.

1. **Release, Relaxation or Rejuvenation:** This is the most immediate and perceptible response to flower essences. It is often felt as a physical release or shift. In this first phase of healing, the energy systems within the physical-soul bodies have been stimulated and are working toward a new center of balance. A general sense of calm, relaxation, or alertness is usually experienced, although a spectrum of other physiological responses can occur, such as changes in breathing, sleeping and eating. While most responses promote a sense of well-being, some may feel unpleasant or unexpected, such as the release of tears if being treated for grief, or pronounced sleepiness for some conditions of stress and overwhelm. These initial physiological responses gradually subside as the stimuli from the flower essences are integrated and balanced with the mind-body complex.

2. **Realization and Recognition:** In this stage the archetypal qualities of the flower essences work more deeply into the soul, producing new cognitive awareness about feelings and behavior. A "witness consciousness" is developed which allows insight into the hidden, or "shadow" aspects of the personality that have been contributing to dysfunctional patterns. By recognizing these parts of ourselves, we change not only *physiologically, but psychologically.* As with Stage One, these initial psychological insights can at times be uncomfortable, but as we come to know our selves more honestly and gain control over previously hidden aspects of our personality, we achieve greater emotional and mental clarity, inner resilience and well-being.

3. **Reaction, Resistance and Reconciliation:** The first two stages deal mostly with present time, and are sufficient for many healing situations in which body-soul issues are not deeply patterned. However, in examining the causes of illness, we can also trace far more profound influences that operate at deeper levels of the psyche, affecting the over-all health, belief

systems, attitudes and creative potential of each individual. These more significant soul wounds usually involve one's early biography, such as childhood experiences at times of great vulnerability, religious, political or other cultural conditioning, traumatic stress which was not fully resolved at the time of occurrence, or karmic patterns inscribed into the soul destiny at birth. Skillful application of flower essences in Stage Three facilitates deep psychological work, combined with complementary modalities like counseling, dream and journal work, meditation and visualization, art therapy and other self-awareness techniques. This stage may appear retrogressive when old patterns leap up to oppose forthright efforts of change. The alchemical stage is set for an "awareness crisis" which releases both physical and psychological residue from the past. By reconciling the buried aspects of self-identity and integrating them with conscious understanding, the soul achieves in-depth healing and transformation.

4. **Renewal and Reconstellation:** While the first two stages operate primarily in present time, and the third stage reaches into the deep past of the human soul, the fourth stage in flower essence therapy points to its future destiny. In Stage Four we are able to identify new possibilities concerning life purpose and the ability to manifest that purpose. One of the profound truths of genuine flower essence therapy is that when soul wounding is addressed in a transformational manner, those very areas of previous pain and limitation become nodal points for new potential and soul evolution. For instance an individual who may have been the victim of social discrimination and suffers from low-self esteem, anger and poor physical vitality can use flower essence therapy to transform these limiting conditions into positive qualities of inner-strength, self-worth and compassionate consideration for the suffering of others. These soul virtues will in turn lead to new possibilities in the destiny and creative potential of such a person.

Practical Considerations in Using Flower Essences

How Flower Essences Are Administered

Flower essences are most commonly taken orally from a dropper bottle directly under the tongue, or in a bit of water. The standard dosage is four drops, four times daily. Flower essences can also be applied topically for direct absorption through the skin. Essences can be added to bath-water, or to cremes, lotions, and oils. Specially prepared *Herbal Flower Oils,* are also available. These formulas are already potentized with flower essences, and are often used as carrier oils for massage and other topical applications.

There are several levels of dilution in the preparation of flower essences. The *mother essence* is derived from fresh blossoms in a bowl of water, infused with the morning sun (or heated by fire, in the case of some of the English essences). The mother essence is generally preserved with brandy. This infusion is then further diluted to the *stock* level, and sometimes again to a *dosage* level. Generally it is the stock level of dilution which is available commercially from flower essence companies, although there are some pre-mixed combinations sold at the dosage level of dilution.

Frequency and Timing of Dosage

Regular, rhythmic use of the flower remedies builds the strength of their catalytic action. Therefore, potency is increased not by taking more drops at one time, but by using them on a *frequent, consistent basis.* In most cases, the essences should be taken *four times daily,* although this may need to be increased in emergency or acute situations to once every hour, or even more often. On the other hand, children or other highly sensitive persons may need to *decrease the frequency* of use to once or twice daily.

The essences address the relationship between the body and soul, and therefore are most effective at the thresholds of *awakening* and *retiring,* since these are the times when the boundaries between body and soul shift. Other transition times of the day are also important, such as just before the noon or evening meals. Even when the essences are used in the midst of a hectic schedule, it is beneficial to allow a quiet moment of receptivity so that the messages of the flowers can be received at a subtle level. Many people find it helpful to remember to take the essences by keeping one bottle of their flower essence formula right on the bed-stand, and another one of the same combination in their purse, briefcase, or in the kitchen.

Although flower essences can be used on a short-term basis for acute situations, their ideal use is for long-term or deep-seated mental-emotional change. At this level, the most common cycle of essence use is four weeks or one month, a time interval which is strongly correlated to the emotional or astral body. Seven-day or 14-day cycles may also be of significance in the growth process. For particularly deep changes, a whole series of monthly cycles may need to be considered. However, in most cases changes will be noticed in about one month. The monthly interval provides a good opportunity to re-assess the flower essence combination, and consider new essences that reflect the ongoing developmental process. It is often beneficial to continue with one more key essences even after some change has been noticed. This allows a possibility for the essences to be "anchored" at deeper levels of consciousness.

Selecting Appropriate Flower Essences

Selecting beneficial flower essences can itself be a process of inner growth and awareness. Through quiet reflection, meditation, self-observation, and consulting and conversation with others, it is necessary to first consider **key issues and challenges** in one's life. These may related to one's work, relationships, or self-image. Next, identify the **positive qualities** and **patterns of imbalance** correlated with each essence, and review supplemental flower essence literature such as the *Flower Essence Repertory*. An *Assessment Guide* is also available from the Flower Essence Society in which questions pertaining to flower essences are grouped according to practical life issues and common mental and emotional problems.

Using one or more of these resources, flower essences that most closely relate to key issues in one's life can be identified. It is important to be aware of positive transformative goals as well as areas of pain and distress when making a selection. It is recommended that one use **no more than three to five essence** at a time, or even just one or two essences. Research through the Flower Essence Society indicates that smaller numbers of essences produce clear, more focused results. Many subsidiary issues or symptoms will clear when core life issues are addressed with flower essences. Essences should also be chosen according to **stages of development and clear time sequences.** A single formula is generally suitable for one-two month's duration, and can be followed by additional flower essences at each stage in the developmental process.

While flower essences are not physically harmful and are intended to be used in self-healing programs, it is also important to receive objective evaluation from professional therapists during any long-term healing process. Many holistic practitioners routinely incorporate flower essence therapy within the spectrum of programs offered to their clients. For those working with chronic health issues, or severe psychological problems it is absolutely necessary to combine the use of flower essences with other qualified health care.

Case Examples

Mariposa Lily (*Calochortus leichtlini),* is an alpine wildflower, native to the Sierra Nevada mountains of North America. Lily family plants have characteristic bulbous roots with three flower petals and three sepals. Many Lilies have a long herbal tradition of being used for feminine healing. The Mariposa Lily is especially used for mothers and children, and seems to stimulate a maternal consciousness of warmth and nurturing. This plant remedy is widely documented and is used by mothers and midwives as well as many professional therapists. The Mariposa Lily is an excellent all purpose remedy for pregnant and nursing mothers but is also used wherever there is a disturbance in the mother-child bond, such as child abuse, abandonment, or for any birth trauma. For example the Centro Infantil Frei Tadeu, a center for impoverished children in Recife, Brazil reports this as a baseline remedy in the care of all their children. The documented studies from this center actually demonstrate that Mariposa Lily helps weight gain and the general improvement of malnutrition, arising from lack of warmth and maternal nurturing.

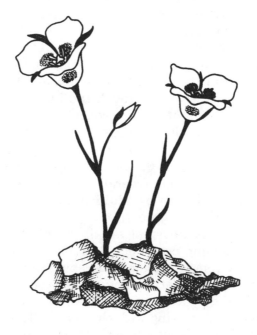

Figure 28.1. *Mariposa Lily*

Borage (*Borago officinalis*) has long been associated in herbal tradition as a heart remedy. It was originally called "Corago," referring to a state of courage, or quality of the heart (*coeur* in French or *cor* in Latin). Borage is particularly indicated for states of intense sadness or depression, what is literally a soul quality of being "discouraged," or "disheartened." A typical case that illustrates the use of Borage involves a middle-aged man who lost his wife suddenly in a car accident. His experience of grief was so profound that he gradually withdrew from many friends and family. A full year after his wife's death he was still unable to perform adequately at his job and was finally dismissed. He sought help from a therapist who used Borage flower essence as a primary remedy along with counseling. This man felt an immediate difference when using this remedy and described it, "as though a weight has been lifted from my heart." He was gradually able to re-build his life and feel new hope and positivity.

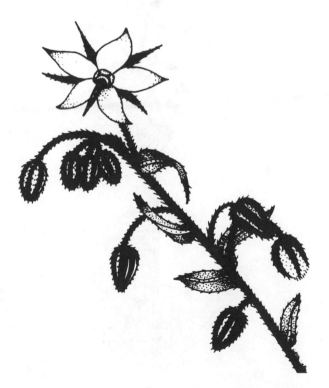

Figure 28.2. Borage

Mimulus (*Mimulus guttatus)* was one of the first flower remedies developed by Dr. Bach, although it is actually native to North America. It flourishes in damp meadows and along riverbanks. As its radiant yellow color suggests, it is a remedy for states of fear and introversion. The Mimulus personality type is very hypersensitive and anxious, thus allowing small everyday challenges to loom much larger than necessary. The Mimulus is an excellent remedy for fretful children and is also very helpful for the elderly. A typical case involves a single woman in her seventies who had gradually become a shut-in following the death of her husband. She feared that her house would be broken into and often imagined that she heard noises in her house. The Mimulus flower essence was chosen for her by a family member. The woman reported that the remedy helped her to feel more calm and better able to sleep at night. She also made gradual changes in her lifestyle, going out of her house more often and accepting social invitations she had previously declined.

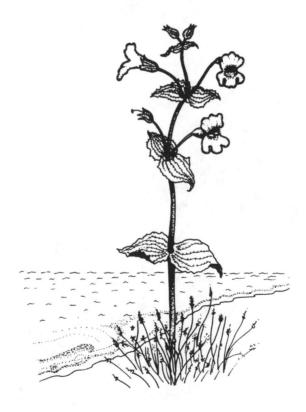

Figure 28.3. Mimulus

Impatiens (*Impatiens glandulifera)* is a vibrant remedy which is naturalized along riverbanks and moist shady, areas in rural England. The deeply invaginated flower and cooling pink color of the Impatiens suggest a quality of interiorization and quiet calming. In fact this plant was named as such in folklore tradition and was associated with impatience. Bach discovered this remedy to help with many states of tension, irritation and anger. This remedy helps calm the overly fiery nature of individuals who rush ahead of themselves, and often have difficulty breathing fully or enjoying quieter moments. The Impatiens is often used for the classic "Type A" personality - a typical case involves a man in his fifties who was diagnosed by his doctor as at risk for a major heart attack. Although the man enrolled in a relaxation program to reduce stress in his life, it was only when he added the Impatiens flower essence that he felt able to fully benefit from the program. He especially noted that the Impatiens seemed to help him with his breathing.

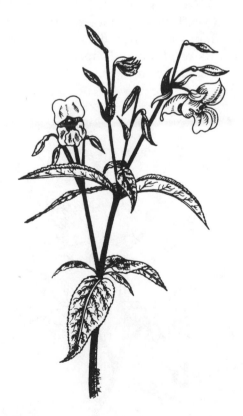

Figure 28.4. Impatiens

California Wild Rose (*Rosa californica*) This simple five-petaled wild rose is native to grasslands and open meadows throughout the foothills of northern California. The rose has a long been associated in both literary and herbal tradition with love. However, the specific soul quality of love which the California Wild rose addresses is that of passionate enthusiasm and interest in life. This flower essence counter-acts many forms of pessimism, alienation, apathy or resignation. It is often used for recovery from severe illness or other hardship, and is especially beneficial for young people. For example, California Wild Rose was used by a mother to help her 16-year-old daughter, whose grades at school deteriorated from above average to barely passing. Her daughter seemed moody and withdrawn and dressed in dark colors. She said she felt "bored with life," and didn't feel she had much future. A recent break-up with a boyfriend coupled with disappointment when she was not chosen for a part in a school play seemed to be precipitating factors in her new behaviors. Her mother noticed a change within about two weeks after taking the California Wild Rose. She was more willing to talk about her hurt feelings, and she found a new friend at school. Within several months her disposition was brighter and more cheerful and her grades at school returned to their former level.

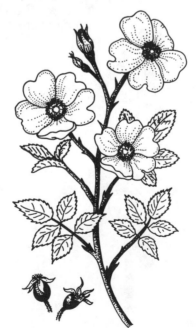

Figure 28.5. California Wild Rose

Star of Bethlehem (*Ornithogalum umbellatum*) is a beautiful six-pointed flower which is a member of the Onion family. Its elegant, harmonious form and pure white color suggest a quality of inner peace and repose. Bach found this remedy to have very soothing, restorative qualities. It is used for many states of shock and trauma and is an important part of Bach's famous emergency combination composed of five flowers(also included are Impatiens, Rock Rose, Clematis, and Cherry Plum). An example of the use of Star of Bethlehem involves a young woman who had been violently attacked and robbed at gunpoint. She developed a severe eating disorder several months later. Despite nutritional therapy and counseling she was only able to make significant improvement when her therapist included Star of Bethlehem to address the initial shock which had precipitated her eating disorder.

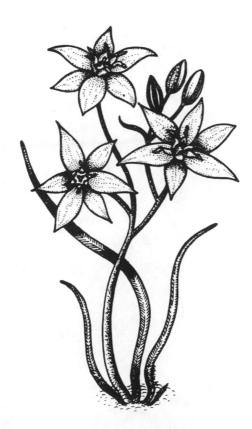

Figure 28.6. *Star of Bethlehem*

For a more detailed listing of flower essences and their positive qualities and patterns of imbalance, see the Flower Essence Society's *Flower Essence Repertory*.

— by Patricia Kaminski

Biographical note: Patricia Kaminski is Director of the Flower Essence Society in Nevada City, California, an international organization affiliated with over 60,000 practitioners. She administrates the Society's research and practitioner training programs, and also maintains a private flower essence therapy practice. She is co-author of the *Flower Essence Repertory* and a new book, *Flowers That Heal*. The **Flower Essence Society** can be reached at www.flowersociety.org or toll-free at 800-736-9222. This non-profit educational organization provides information about practitioners, publications, classes, local networking opportunities, and leading research throughout the world on flower essence therapy.

Part Six

Manual Healing

Chapter 29

Manual Healing Methods:

Osteopathic, Chiropractic, Massage, Pressure Point Therapies, Reflexology, Postural Reduction Therapies, Feldenkrais Method, Structural Integration (Rolfing), Bioenergetical Systems, Biofield, Applied Kinesiology, Quigong, and Craniosacral Therapy

Introduction

Touch and manipulation with the hands have been in use in health and medical practice since the beginning of medical care. Whether in comforting a child by stroking or rubbing a body stiffened by the cold, touch was the first and foremost of all diagnostic and therapeutic devices. Hippocrates discussed the benefits of therapeutic massage and instructed his students in its use and in spinal manipulation. The Chinese also included massage in its ancient healing practices and touch in its diagnostic methods (see "Alternative Systems of Medicine" chapter); the practitioner's taking of the pulse with the fingertips was considered to be the most important diagnostic tool of the ancient Chinese physician (Veith, 1949). Entire healing systems of touch based on the meridian system (see the glossary) were developed centuries ago and remain in use today in the United States as well as in Asia.

The hands once were the physician's greatest and most important diagnostic and therapeutic tool. Today the medical and health practitioner retreats further and further from physical contact with the patient, ever more distanced by banks of diagnostic equipment, legal constraints, and time factors. Psychotherapists are admonished not to touch their clients, and the price of medical doctors' time is now so

Extracted from NIH Publication No. 94-066. December 1994. Due to space considerations, bibliographic data have not been reprinted in this chapter. However, to aid readers who wish to consult the original document or do further research, the in-text references have been retained.

399

high that they cannot even massage the stiffness from a patient's back; instead, the doctor or psychotherapist must write a prescription for a massage therapist, a person with therapeutic skills no longer taught in medical schools. It is skills of this type—ancient traditional healing skills that are now called "alternative"—that this chapter addresses.

All the manual healing methods addressed in this chapter rely on the practitioner's hands as a primary modality both to access information from (that is, to diagnose) and to treat the patient. Nevertheless, many manual healing methods are highly individualized; there is much art in this field, much individualization. Many practitioners have developed unique systems, in some cases teaching them to others. Consequently, there are many more systems than can be discussed here; no slight is intended by the omissions.

This chapter is divided into four sections. The first discusses methods that use physical touch, pressure, and movement. The second discusses those that are described as using a biofield, or "energy." Therapies that appear to rely on both physical and biofield elements are described in the third section. The fourth section illustrates how manual healing methods are becoming included in mainstream health care. Recommendations follow at the end.

Physical Healing Methods

All the biomechanical therapies—grouped here as "physical healing methods"—are based on the understanding that dysfunction of any discrete body part often affects secondarily the function of other discrete, not necessarily directly connected, body parts, both in close proximity and at a distance. The various manual medicines have developed theories and processes that treat these secondary dysfunctions through a variety of methods that manipulate the soft tissues or realign the body parts. Overcoming these misalignments and manipulating soft tissues bring the individual parts back to optimal function and return the body to health.

Osteopathic Medicine

One of the earliest systems of health care in the United States to use manual healing methods was osteopathic medicine. To its practitioners and to much of the public, the manual healing methods of osteopathic medicine are mainstream processes, but some people consider them alternative.

The principles and philosophy of osteopathy integrate health and illness, emphasizing four major areas:

- Structure and function are interdependent. Furthermore, behavior is an intermingled complex in which psychosocial influences can affect both anatomy (structure) and physiology (function). All these relationships are fundamentally designed to work in harmony.

- The body has the ability to heal itself, and the role of the osteopathic physician is to enhance the healing process as much as possible.

- Diseases, impairments, and disabilities arise from disruptions of the normal interactions of anatomy, physiology, and behavior.

- Appropriate treatment is based on the ability to understand, diagnose, and treat—by whatever methods are available—including manually applied procedures. When hands-on procedures are used to identify somatic dysfunction (see the glossary), the practitioner then determines whether the pattern of somatic dysfunction that is observed can be related to any visceral (that is, related to the internal body organs), neuromusculoskeletal, or—occasionally—behavioral dysfunction.

History and context. American osteopathic medicine was begun by Andrew Taylor Still (1828-1917). Still was a physician of his period, trained mainly through apprenticeships. It is said that he attended a medical school in Kansas City, MO, for one semester but found it boring and irrelevant (Gevitz, 1980). As a result of many adverse experiences with then contemporary medical practices, including the death of several family members from untreatable meningitis and pneumonia, Still began a personal search for improved methods to treat diseases and restore health (Gevitz, 1980; Schiotz, 1958). This empirical approach continues to be used by many osteopathic physicians.

Development and use of osteopathically oriented manipulative skills began around the time of Still's search (Carlson, 1975; Gevitz, 1980), but how he developed his system that combined "lightning bone setting" with the magnetic healing concepts of Mesmer is not clear (Hood, 1871).

It seems likely that his knowledge (of manipulation) was derived from simply observing the work of another practitioner in

401

the field. However he learned these methods, Still soon afterwards made an important discovery, namely, that the sudden flexion and extension procedures peculiar to the spinal area were not limited to orthopedic problems; furthermore, they constituted a more reliable means of healing than simply rubbing the spine (Gevitz, 1980).

Whatever the circumstances, Still began his new health profession in 1874, before beginning his use of manipulation, which he was reported to use somewhat later in that decade (Gevitz, 1980). After advertising and working as both a magnetic healer and a lightning bone setter, he began writing about his ideas (Still, 1899). Ultimately, he founded his first school, the American School of Osteopathy, in 1892 at Kirksville, MO, to improve on existing surgical and obstetrical practices. The original emphasis was on observing the relationship between structure and function. He incorporated assumptions that manual restoration of normal anatomic relationships leads to physiological improvements. This reasoning included by definition a spectrum not only of health issues but of specific recommendations for disease and obstetrical interventions. Some examples from osteopathic literature include discussions dealing with labor and delivery, postoperative ileus (bowel) paralysis, asthma, otitis media (middle ear infection), hypertension, coronary artery disease, back pain, neck pain, diabetes, trauma of all kinds, migraine headache, and stress-related illnesses (Downing, 1935; Kuchera and Kuchera, 1990; Sleszynski and Kelso, 1993).

Osteopathy spread to England in the 1920s when John Littlejohn emigrated from Chicago to London, establishing the British School of Osteopathy, the first of several such schools. The expansion continued as continental European practitioners studied at the British schools in the 1930s and 1940s.

Historically, many currently popular manual medical techniques—with the exceptions of "energy" techniques, massage, and high-velocity maneuvers (Hood, 1871)—originated within American osteopathy and spread elsewhere. Among those techniques are manual methods applied in other medically oriented systems and also activities of alternative health care providers. Examples include muscle energy and post-isometric relaxation concepts, which were originally developed and codified by Fred Mitchell, Sr. and Paul Kimberly; fascial-myofascial release and visceral techniques, developed by A.T. Still and others, including Charles Neidner; cranial-craniosacral techniques, William G. Sutherland (Sutherland, 1990); strain and counterstrain,

Lawrence Jones; and thoracic pump and lymphatic techniques, A.T. Still, Gordon Zink, and several contemporaries. (Most of these techniques are described briefly in the "Osteopathic Education" section.)

In many instances, contemporary practices of these methods throughout the world are extensions and refinements of original osteopathic concepts. Other systems, such as chiropractic, Swedish massage, Cyriax (Great Britain), Mennell (Great Britain), Lewit (Czech Republic), Dvorak (Switzerland), and several German systems also have influenced current practices, both in the United States and elsewhere. Two current osteopathically based examples are advances in myofascial release and fascial unwinding maneuvers and in "energy"-based practices arising from basic cranial concepts, codified by both Sutherland and Harold Magoun, Sr. (Magoun, 1976; Sutherland, 1990).

Demographics. As of 1993, this country had more than 32,000 American-educated and licensed doctors of osteopathy (D.O.s), some in every State. They perform all aspects of medical care, including all specialties and family practice. Sixteen colleges and schools graduate approximately 1,500 D.O.s annually. While graduates make up about 5 percent of the country's physician population, the profession is responsible for approximately 10 percent of total health care delivery in the United States. More than 60 percent of osteopathic physicians are involved in primary care areas—family medicine, pediatrics, internal medicine, and obstetrics-gynecology (Annual Directory, 1993).

Many osteopathic physicians from a variety of disciplines regularly incorporate structural diagnosis of abnormalities of musculoskeletal function and manual medical treatments in their day-to-day activities.[1] Ironically, because of current attitudes among third-party payers toward physician use of manual medicine, many are not paid for these services. Much of the reluctance to pay is based on a lack of adequately funded research, particularly relating to outcome measures. From an osteopathic perspective, what is considered "alternative" by most of the medical and research establishment is mainstream for the average D.O. (Gevitz, 1980; Grad, 1979; Schiotz, 1958).

Osteopathic education. Basic American osteopathic education (Gershenow, 1985) includes substantial emphasis on osteopathic philosophy and principles including extensive manually oriented training designed to develop manual medicine diagnosis and treatment skills. The profession generally refers to the latter as structural diagnosis and manipulative treatment. These skills have been used by osteopathic physicians for more than 100 years in a context of total patient care.

The Education Council on Osteopathic Principles, representing the 16 osteopathic colleges, is currently contributing to osteopathic education through three principal projects: the 1982 publication of an updated glossary of osteopathic terminology; development of a core curriculum for osteopathic principles; and development of state-of-the-art textbook chapters highlighting the uses of palpatory diagnosis (use of touch) and manipulative treatment in multiple clinical disciplines.

Basic palpation and structural diagnosis and treatment skills are emphasized in preclinical American osteopathic education, and eight major manual medical methods are taught in osteopathic colleges. These eight methods are as follows:

1. Soft-tissue techniques that enhance muscle relaxation and circulation of body fluids.

2. Isometric and isotonic techniques (often referred to as muscle energy or post-isometric relaxation) that focus primarily on restoring physiological movements to altered joint mechanics.

3. Articulatory techniques (also called joint play and manipulation without impulse) that emphasize restoration of intrinsic joint mobility.

4. High-velocity, low-amplitude techniques (also called manipulation with impulse), designed to restore the symmetry of the movements associated with the vertebral joints.

5. Myofascial release techniques (also called fascial release techniques) that use combinations of so-called direct and indirect methods (see the glossary) to modify problems of individual and interactively related muscle groups and surrounding or covering (myofascial) tissues.

6. Functional techniques that emphasize treatment of restrictive patterns in joint, myofascial, and neural systems, using "ease," "bind," "sensing," and "motor" hands (see the glossary) as proprioceptive (see the glossary) diagnostic concepts.

7. Strain and counterstrain techniques, designed to locate sore places at specific sites on the body, tender points that relate to

specific patterns of abnormal joint movement. The points are "turned off" by moving the body or limb to a treatment position that quiets painful feedback. The position is held for 90 seconds. Reevaluation typically reveals improvement in movement and a decrease in local pain.

8. Cranial techniques (also called craniosacral techniques) that highlight the manual ability to assess and release tensions associated with subtle, reciprocating cranial (head) and sacral (tailbone) oscillations. These movements are thought to arise from a complex combination of dural (covering) and ligamentous (fibrous connecting tissue) relationships in the spinal network. Adams and Heisey have documented movement of cranial bones in studies using cats. They found cerebrospinal fluid waves having various frequencies and amplitudes (Adams et al., 1992; Heisey and Adams, 1993). Opportunities for research in this area abound.

A number of continuously evolving diagnostic and treatment systems that are osteopathically oriented and manually based incorporate various of these eight manual techniques. Some systems are meant to stand on their own, while others are integrated to a greater or lesser extent with medically (i.e., allopathically) oriented decision making.

Postdoctoral training, certification, and fellowship status in manual medicine are available to American osteopathic graduates, approximately 35 postdoctoral positions are available each year. Programs last 1 to 4 years. One-year fellowships are available for D.O.s and M.D.s who have finished a previously approved residency. Stand-alone 2-year programs leading to manual medicine certification are available in several colleges. Interdisciplinary 3- and 4-year programs that combine some of the many specialties and subspecialties are also available. The most popular are combinations of manual medicine with either family practice or physical medicine and rehabilitation.

Total patient care. Osteopathic physicians are involved in all aspects of total patient care (Northup, 1966), including structural diagnosis and manipulative treatment. Manipulative treatment is commonly used, especially by osteopathic family physicians, as adjunctive care for systemic illness and for various neuromusculoskeletal problems, such as low back, head, and neck pain. In this context, a wide variety of hands-on and—in some situations—"energy" applications are used in a range of disciplines, including family practice, pediatrics, geriatrics, physical medicine, surgery of all kinds, physical medicine and rehabilitation, neurology, rheumatology, pulmonology, and sometimes behavioral medicine and psychiatry. A few disciplines have conducted research using manual methods (Reynolds et al., 1993; Sleszynski and Kelso, 1993), but many questions remain.

Research base. Since its inception, the osteopathic profession has maintained and pursued active research in many areas. This work has usually been published in the Journal of the American Osteopathic Association, which until recently was not listed in Index Medicus. Present activities designing research tend to be directed toward evaluating (1) long-term effects of somatic dysfunctions and facilitated segments in disease states and (2) the outcome resulting from the use of manipulative treatment.

An extensive body of work supports a physiological basis for using osteopathic techniques in both musculoskeletal and nonmusculoskeletal problems. Of particular interest are studies dealing with

- interactions between internal body organs and neuromuscular structures.

- alterations in reflex thresholds,

- reliability of physician palpatory skills (interrater reliability studies), and

- effects of manipulative treatments on disease processes and a variety of physiological functions.

Early work performed by Louisa Burns demonstrated that spinal strain has adverse effects on both functional and motor neuron levels (Burns, 1917). Later work by Denslow and Korr demonstrated long-lasting, highly individual patterns of spinal hyperexcitability associated with neuromuscular and various visceral dysfunctions. This research led to the concept of the "facilitated segment" (fig. 29.1; also see "facilitation" in the glossary), which has been associated with a variety of clinical problems (Denslow et al., 1947; Korr, 1947, 1955). The concept of the facilitated segment is that repeated stimulation produces hyperactive responses, resulting in improper functioning of some body part.

By considering function along with structure, osteopathic theory has included conjecture on the role of the body's communication systems—nervous, circulatory, and endocrine—in initiating somatic dysfunction and causing additional responses in the body. Some early research (Northup, 1970) supports this supposition with regard to reflexes having a role in mediating both the origin of somatic dysfunctions and the effects of manipulative treatment. Osteopathic medicine needs continuing basic research on the role of the nervous system in establishing and maintaining somatic dysfunctions and effecting interactions with the rest of the body.

Figure 29.1 demonstrates potential effects of repeated facilitation; that is, inducing a hyperactive response, leading to somatic dysfunction. The term facilitation is usually used to describe enhancement or reinforcement of otherwise subthreshold neuronal activities that stimulate effector units to inappropriately carry out whatever action they are programmed to do. Examples of effector sites are muscle bundles, muscle groups, viscera, and other neural units and networks. Osteopathic treatment is designed to raise these stimulus thresholds so that the stimulatory event is less likely to occur.

More recent examples of osteopathic research include a preliminary assessment of the effectiveness of manipulative treatment for paresthesias (abnormal sensations) with peripheral nerve involvement (Larson et al., 1980) and thermographic studies of skin temperature in patients receiving manipulative treatment for peripheral nerve problems (Kappler and Kelso, 1984; Larson, 1984). Thermography was selected as a promising method to study segmental facilitation of sympathetic nerves without invading the body (as would be required if needle electrodes were used). Initial studies have been complicated, however, by the number of variables affecting skin-level circulation, including circulatory patterns, local influences, and local shunting. If methods can be developed to identify the effects of these variables, then thermography may prove useful for detecting changes in the sympathetic nervous system that affect skin-level circulation.

Other current clinical research projects that examine the effects of manual treatments have researched their effects on postoperative pulmonary flow rates (Sleszinski and Kelso, 1993), pain management (Zhu et al., 1993), and electromyographic changes associated with manual treatments. If vibration is applied to muscles near the spine or these paraspinal muscles contract voluntarily, weakened electrical potentials are observed in the cerebrum, the main part of the human brain. This finding suggests that muscle spindle receptors are responsible for providing signals that cause the early components of magnetically evoked brain potentials. The brain's evoked potentials return to normal amplitude (1) when the muscle spasm subsides after a period of time and (2) after spinal manipulative therapy is applied (Zhu et al., 1993).

Additional research on the interaction of visceral and somatic structures (Eble, 1960) has supported clinical findings that palpation of neuromuscular structures can help identify visceral disturbances (Johnston, 1992; Kelso et al., 1980) and that manual procedures can help restore both visceral and neuromuscular (somatic) functions (Buerger and Greenman, 1985; Korr, 1978; Northup, 1970). The latter include situations involving low back pain (Hoehler et al., 1981), neurological development in children (Frymann et al., 1992), carpal tunnel syndrome (Sucher, 1993), postoperative collapsed lung (Sleszynski and Kelso, 1993), and burning pain in an extremity (Levine, 1991). Moreover, in some preliminary observations with cadavers, Reynolds and Ward (Ward, 1994) found that palpatory diagnoses tended to correlate with radiographic and autopsy data.

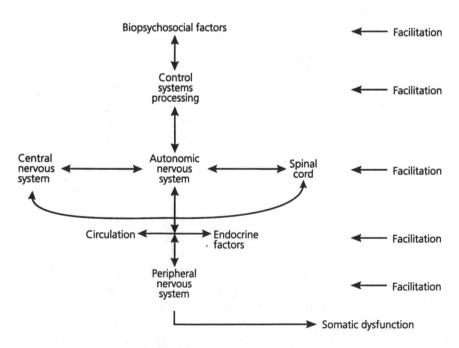

Figure 29.1. *Role of Facilitation in Somatic Dysfunction*

One example of the diagnostic potential of osteopathic palpation is the studies of Johnston and colleagues (Johnston et al., 1980, 1982b), comparing subjects with normal and high blood pressure. A significant number of the hypertensive patients were shown to have a stable pattern of musculoskeletal findings in the cervicothoracic spinal region. This finding suggests that osteopathic diagnoses could contribute to identifying internal difficulties.

Another issue that osteopathic researchers have addressed is the accuracy of their examinations of patients before and after manipulative treatment, including whether such observations are consistent among a group of osteopathic physicians. Several studies (Beal et al., 1980, 1982; Johnston, 1982a; Johnston et al., 1982a, 1982c, 1983; McConnell et al., 1980) have been conducted in which osteopathic physicians working independently have used a mutually agreed-upon test procedure. These studies of inter-rater reliability look for correlations in the observations of two or more independent raters. Results suggest that when there is prior training or agreement on which tests to use and what is clinically significant with respect to findings, inter-rater agreement can be achieved consistently. This ability to reach agreement becomes particularly important as the basis for establishing a method of setting up controlled clinical trials to determine the success of manipulative treatments.

Virtually all osteopathically oriented research has been funded from the private sector, mainly through the bureau of research of the American Osteopathic Association. The largest grant to date, $400,000, is for evaluating outcomes associated with the use of manipulation for back pain in a Chicago health maintenance organization population. This is a 3-year prospective study conducted by two osteopathic physicians specializing in musculoskeletal medicine. Patients having acute back pain with and without sciatica (pain radiating downward into the leg) are randomized into the project so that some receive manipulative care while others receive "standard" medical care. Clinical outcomes are evaluated by uninvolved clinicians. Preliminary data are expected in late 1994.

Barriers and key issues. Historically, Federal research initiatives relevant to osteopathic medicine (for example, from the National Institute of Neurological Disorders and Stroke at the National Institutes of Health (NIH) or from the Centers for Disease Control and Prevention) have been controlled by traditionally defined disciplines and their expert panels. Manual-methods research panels are not among them, and the result is a lack of genuine peer review capability.

This sociological fact of life has inhibited development and understanding of the manual medicine field, even though public acceptance has been and continues to be high throughout the world.

Some major issues to be considered in trying to improve osteopathic research opportunities are the following:

- Selecting appropriate patient populations in which to study the effects of manual manipulation.

- Arranging for knowledgeable peer review and research guidance, including (1) ensuring that persons with osteopathic experience serve on peer review panels and (2) determining appropriate procedures for measuring success of osteopathic treatments.

- Establishing whether previous inter-rater agreement studies support the use of the interrater agreement method in osteopathic and other kinds of research.

- Making previous osteopathic research more accessible (for example, the recent inclusion of the Journal of the American Osteopathic Association in Index Medicus), which could educate other investigators about osteopathic issues and possibly lead to collaborative research.

- Ensuring that osteopathic clinician-researchers are part of any research team so that persons inexperienced with osteopathic diagnosis and treatment do not conduct the work improperly. Additional training in planning, conducting, evaluating, and reporting clinical research should be made available to the osteopathic clinicians.

- Setting up a review process to integrate available information from outside the osteopathic profession with osteopathically based research on the structure-function relationship. Included would be research, for example, on homeostasis; short-, intermediate-, and long-term responses to different stressors; and adaptation to changes in internal and external environment. Useful new research questions are likely to result.

- Documenting anecdotal observations of patients and osteopathic clinicians who treat the somatic component of medical and health-related problems to tabulate patient benefits that include relief from stress and improvement in function and

410

well-being. Attention should be paid to all patient health outcomes, not just short-term benefits from manipulation; for example, reducing health risks, improving health maintenance,
and modifying adaptive responses would be included.

- Designing and conducting research to support or refute the use
  of palpatory examination and manipulative treatment for the
  somatic component of dysfunction and illness. Also researching
  the role of the somatic system; identifying the nature and effects of somatic dysfunctions and their incidence, prevalence,
  and effects on acute illness and long-term health; and any
  changes in those effects resulting from treatment.

- Developing alternative research designs for safety and efficacy
  studies that do not require blind controls for manual procedures. There are both practical and ethical reasons not to use
  blind controls for a hands-on procedure. One alternative is to
  use naive patients who lack any expectation that the treatment
  will be beneficial.

- Developing and integrating cost-benefit research that compares
  the use of palpatory examination and manipulative treatment
  with mainstream health care and disease management procedures. Common examples include headaches of all kinds, back
  pain, allergy, asthma, many orthopedic problems, postoperative
  and posttraumatic effects of all kinds, and various
  rheumatologic diseases.

Chiropractic

Chiropractic science is concerned with investigating the relationship between structure (primarily of the spine) and function (primarily of the nervous system) of the human body in order to restore and
preserve health. Chiropractic medicine addresses how to apply this
knowledge to diagnose and treat structural dysfunctions that affect
the nervous system.

Chiropractic philosophy and practice emphasize four major points:

- The human body has an innate self-healing ability and seeks to
  maintain homeostasis (see the glossary), or balance.

- The nervous system is highly developed in humans and influences all other systems in the body, thereby playing a significant role in health and disease.

411

- The presence of joint dysfunction and subluxation (see the glossary) may interfere with the ability of the neuromusculoskeletal system to act efficiently and may lead to or be a concomitant of disease.

- Treatment is based on the chiropractic physician's ability to diagnose and treat existing pathologies and dysfunctions by appropriate manual and physiological procedures.

The chiropractic physician relies heavily on hands-on procedures using touch (palpation) to determine both structural and functional joint "dysrelationships." These hands-on procedures are carried out alongside more traditional forms of diagnostic assessment. By training and by law, chiropractic physicians use manual procedures and interventions, not surgical or chemotherapeutic ones.

History and context. While manipulative medicine has been practiced for millennia, the chiropractic profession is only now preparing for its centennial. The profession was founded in the 1890s when Daniel David (D.D.) Palmer, a grocer and magnetic healer, applied his knowledge of the nervous system and manual therapies, thrusting on a thoracic vertebra to restore the hearing of Harvey Lillard, a local janitor. While Palmer was not the first to practice manual thrusting, he was the first to use the bony projections, or processes, of the vertebrae (specifically, the spinous and transverse processes) as levers for the manual contact.

Within 2 years of this initial discovery, Palmer had founded his Chiropractic School and Cure, while at the same time developing the concept of subluxation, a type of partial joint dislocation, as a causal factor in disease. For these reasons, D.D. Palmer is known as the Founder.

By 1902, Palmer's son Bartlett Joshua (B.J.) had enrolled in his father's school; he gained operational control by late 1904, and by 1906, D.D. Palmer was no longer associated with the college he had founded. The year 1906 also saw the development of the schism that still exists in the profession today; several faculty members, including John Howard, left Palmer College because of deep differences with B.J. Palmer (who came to be known as the Developer) over the role of subluxation in disease. By that time, B.J. was espousing subluxation as the cause of all disease; John Howard, however, saw a need for what he considered to be a more rational alternative to such thinking and focused his new National School of Chiropractic around a broad-based educational program incorporating basic and clinical sciences, laboratory work, dissection, and clinical care (Beideman, 1983).

From 1910 to 1920, many other chiropractic colleges came into existence; some followed the lead of B.J. Palmer in a "straight" form of chiropractic, while others followed the lead of Howard in developing "mixer" programs. The development of the profession could not have occurred without the missionary zeal of B.J. Palmer, who led his namesake college for 54 years. But others helped to advance the profession as well, including Carl Cleveland, Earl Homewood, Fred Illi, Joseph Janse, Herbert Lee, and Claude Watkins.

What these innovators did—in addition to all their educational and scientific advancements—was to place disease in a different context involving the concept of subluxation (Bergmann et al., 1993). Some factors are common to chiropractic and allopathic medicine. Both recognize the existence of bacteria and other "germs" and their role in creating disease; both mandate that a susceptible host be present along with the germ. Both also accept that the host's susceptibility depends on many factors. But only in the chiropractic model is the presence of subluxation stressed as an important factor; the contention of chiropractic is that since the subluxation can serve as a noxious irritant to the body, its removal becomes critical for restoring optimal health.

Chiropractors are responsible for the development and refinement of manual therapies, particularly those known as high velocity, short amplitude. Within the purview of these therapies, many systems have been developed concerning how to apply the various procedures. Examples include:

- *sacrooccipital technique*, originally developed by Major B. De Jarnette;

- *activator technique*, developed and advanced by Arlan Fuhr;

- *diversified technique*, which comes from many sources including manual medicine (physician John Mennell), and various chiropractors, including Arnold Hauser and Joseph Janse—and which was developed largely in the National College of Chiropractic;

- *Thompson terminal point technique*, developed by J. Clay Thompson;

- *flexion-distraction technique*, developed from original osteopathic concepts by James Cox (this is not a traditional thrusting procedure);

- *Gonstead technique*, developed by Clarence Gonstead; and

- *applied kinesiology*, developed by George Goodheart.

This list is by no means exhaustive; other innovators include L. John Fay, Henri Gillet, and John Grostic.

Today's common chiropractic procedures are refinements of systems developed during the past half-century, both in diagnosis (the motion palpation of Fay and Gillet, for example [Gillet and Liekens, 1984; Schaefer and Fay, 1989]) and in therapy.

Today chiropractic procedures are being examined by researchers from most of the chiropractic colleges, who also are receiving input from field-based chiropractors. Standards of care are being determined by coalitions of chiropractors, including practitioners, academics, researchers, and administrators. One group has already produced a set of guidelines called the Mercy Conference guidelines (Haldeman et al., 1992).

In reaching their decisions concerning practice parameters and standards of care, the various groups of chiropractors have been participating in consensus-development procedures (Hansen et al., 1992).

Demographics. In 1993 more than 45,000 licensed chiropractors were practicing in the United States alone. Licensing occurs in every State in the Union as well as in many foreign countries. Chiropractors provide various aspects of health care but cannot use surgery or drugs; they have several specialty areas, such as radiology, orthopedics, neurology, and sports medicine. Seventeen American chiropractic colleges graduate more than 2,000 chiropractors annually; colleges also exist in Canada, Australia, England, France, and Japan. Some other foreign countries are considering them (e.g., South Africa, Italy, and Germany). Chiropractors currently see 12 percent to 15 percent of the U.S. population, and most professionals practice in private office settings, usually solo.

Most chiropractic physicians incorporate structural diagnosis into their practice and use manual adjusting therapies as their main treatment mode. Today, most third-party payers accept chiropractic services, though they did not always. Increased chiropractic research has helped to allay the reluctance of insurance companies toward chiropractic, and the recent development of professional standards of care has opened new avenues for chiropractic coverage.

Chiropractic education. Today's chiropractic educational program is a 5-year curriculum that emphasizes chiropractic philosophy, basic and clinical science, and clinical care in outpatient settings. Standard forms of medical diagnosis are heavily detailed, with additional workloads in structural and functional diagnosis and chiropractic technique. All chiropractic colleges require at least 2 years of college education prior to matriculation, as well as a series of courses (e.g., chemistry, physics) meeting criteria set by the Council of Chiropractic Education (CCE).

Manual therapies include any procedure during which the hands are used to palpate, diagnose, mobilize, adjust, or manipulate the somatic or visceral structures of the body. There are two broad groups of joint manipulation procedures and soft-tissue manipulation procedures. Adjustments are the most commonly applied chiropractic therapy within either group. The most common forms of adjustment taught in chiropractic colleges are the diversified, Gonstead, activator, and sacrooccipital techniques.

Today CCE accredits chiropractic colleges on the professional level, while regional accreditation also occurs. All CCE-accredited colleges teach a comprehensive program that incorporates elements of basic science (physiology, anatomy, and biochemistry); clinical science (such as laboratory diagnosis, radiology, orthopedics, and nutrition); and clinical experience (e.g., patient management in the clinical setting). In addition, the profession offers postdoctoral training in a wide range of disciplines, with orthopedics and radiology the most popular. In this country, some hospital training has recently become available to chiropractic students and residents; such training has been available in Canada since 1975.

Research base. The chiropractic profession has performed rigorous research since its early days. However, at least in one sense, the research within the profession is still very much in its infancy, because the profession "lost" much of its early work for lack of an appropriate forum in which to publish it. Today the *Journal of Manipulative and Physiological Therapeutics* is the sole chiropractic research publication indexed in *Index Medicus*, Current Contents, BIOSIS, and Excerpta Medica. However, other journals such as Spine, which is indexed in the major medical data bases, do public chiropractic-related research.

Current chiropractic research interests include back and other pain, somatovisceral disorders, and reliability studies.

Back and other pain. Recent emphasis in research trials has been on manipulation and back pain, manipulation and various organic

415

disturbances, and reliability and validity. In 1984, Brunarski identified 50 trials of spinal manipulation (Brunarski, 1985); the number has increased since then. Studies by Bergquist-Ullman and Larsson (1977), Godfrey et al. (1984), Hadler et al. (1987), Mathews et al. (1987), and Waagen et al. (1986) were all important in establishing a definitive role for manipulation in the management of low back pain. The argument for including chiropractic in British National Health Service coverage was based on recent work by Meade et al. (1990), comparing chiropractic care to hospital outpatient care. The research of Koes (1992) served a similar role in the Netherlands. Further, the RAND report (cited in Haldeman et al., 1992), a recent and large undertaking examining all published literature on the use of manipulation for low back pain, made definitive comments regarding its use in specific situations.

The RAND report found that manipulation was effective in the following five situations: (1) acute low back pain without evidence of neurological involvement or sciatic nerve irritation; (2) acute low back pain with sciatic nerve irritation; (3) acute low back pain with minor neurological findings and sciatic nerve root irritation (although there was some conflicting evidence); (4) subacute low back pain with no evidence of neurological involvement or sciatic irritation; and (5) subacute low back pain with minor neurological findings and major neurological findings. In other situations, the literature was found to present too many conflicts to determine effectiveness of manipulation. Besides these trials, research has examined patient perceptual issues in the use of chiropractic care. Notable here is the research of Cherkin and MacCornack (1989), who reported that patients seeing chiropractors for low back pain were happier with the treatment they received than were similar patients seeing medical doctors for similar problems.

Studies examining manipulation for pain other than low back pain include work of Barker (1983) on thoracic pain; Molea et al. (1987) on post-exercise muscle soreness; Terrett and Vernon (1984) on paraspinal cutaneous pain tolerance; Vernon (1982) on headache; Jirout (1985) on C2-C3 vertebral dysfunction; and Parker et al. (1978) on migraine.

Somatovisceral disorders. One area that is gaining in research interest is the type O disorder (O for organic, as opposed to M for musculoskeletal). Much of the early impetus for studies of type O disorders came from osteopathic research examining somatic dysfunction. Examples of this work include studies by Johnston et al. (1985)

416

and Vorro and Johnston (1987) using kinematic and electromyographic instrumentation to investigate clinical signs of somatic dysfunction. Johnston developed a way to detect "mirror image asymmetries," a presumed indicator of the presence of somatic dysfunction (the osteopathic spinal lesion). He laid out palpatory procedures to look for these asymmetries and later refined his concepts in a series of three papers (Johnston, 1988a, 1988b, 1988c) discussing palpatory diagnosis.

Studies that have examined manipulation in treating hypertension include work of Fichera and Celander (1969), Morgan et al. (1985), and Plaugher and Bachman (1994). All of these studies demonstrated changes in blood pressure following spinal manipulation, but the changes were relatively transient. Kokjohn et al. (1992) examined manipulation to treat dysmenorrhea.

Reliability studies. Clinical trials are simply not possible unless their assessment procedures have themselves been tested and found reliable. A procedure is said to be reliable if it gives similar results when applied more than once to the same object it is measuring or when it gives similar results when applied to a series of objects with similar qualities. Reliability tests within chiropractic are commonly used to evaluate specific diagnostic procedures, such as motion palpation.

Motion palpation (examination for presence or absence of joint play) was first advanced by Gillet and Fay as a diagnostic procedure; it has since become a well-studied, common diagnostic procedure. Gonnella et al. (1982) used a seven-point scale to evaluate interexaminer and intraexaminer reliability, while Boline et al. (1988), Love and Brodeur (1987), Mior et al. (1985), Mootz et al. (1989), Nansel et al. (1989), and Wiles (1980) examined simple reproducibility. Beattie et al. (1987) studied the attraction method of measuring motion, and Lovell et al. (1989) used a flexible ruler to assess lumbar lordosis (spinal curvature, such as swayback).

Besides doing clinical studies of various chiropractic procedures, Haas (Haas, 1991; Haas et al., 1993) has made several important additions to reliability literature, even going so far as to study the reliability of reliability. Lawrence (1985) published a critique of reliability studies for measuring leg length, and Frymoyer et al. (1986) have looked at radiographic interpretation. (This list is by no means all-inclusive.)

The research described above has been accomplished largely without any Federal funding. The largest funding agency in the chiropractic profession is the Foundation for Chiropractic Education and Research, which generally has an annual research budget well below $1 million. Chiropractors have made an impressive addition to scientific knowledge despite the lack of encouragement and support by government agencies and medical personnel outside the chiropractic profession.

Barriers and key issues. Several barriers and key issues need to be addressed so that chiropractic research can progress:

- Lack of access to Federal funds has negatively affected the chiropractic research enterprise. Ways must be found to make funds available for chiropractic research through the various agencies. To date, no chiropractic research has been funded by NIH, although several approved studies later failed to meet funding cutoff guidelines. A Small Business Administration innovative research grant funded one study. One approach to alleviating this situation is through the workshops the Office of Alternative Medicine (OAM) is conducting on grant writing and research design. OAM's ability to fund small-scale projects is also a help. If research resources could be increased, much more could be accomplished.

- Lack of access to previous chiropractic research through indexing and databases also hampers research. As mentioned earlier, only a single solely chiropractic research publication is internationally indexed. (*The Journal of Manipulative and Physiological Therapeutics* is indexed in the former Soviet Union as well as in the Western publications previously cited.) Because other chiropractic research journals are unlikely to gain the status of indexing in a conventional database, it is necessary to consider including chiropractic research in an alternative medicine database. Meanwhile, the inclusion of CHIROLARS (Chiropractic Literature and Retrieval System) in BRS Colleague as a sub-database may help to make chiropractic literature more accessible.

- Philosophical differences (the straight-vs.-mixer controversy) continue to split the profession without any obvious solution. Unification is a goal that may still be years away.

- Inclusion of chiropractic in any of the proposed reforms of the health care system, such as those proposed by the Clinton administration, is not assured. It may be that the decision whether to include chiropractic in a national health care plan will be driven by congressional action. Major efforts are already under way to make contact with politicians regarding this issue, and chiropractic input was provided to the President's Health Care Task Force.

New avenues for the chiropractic profession have become available as a result of the decision against "biomedicine's" restraint of trade in the 1991 judgment rendered in Wilk et al. v. the American Medical Association (AMA). While it is likely to take many years to overcome the AMA's history of opposition to chiropractic, continuing quality research and patient care will negate this opposition. The current processes by which chiropractors are reviewing standards of care and chiropractic procedures should help solidify the public standing of this field.

Massage Therapy

Massage therapy is one of the oldest methods in the gallery of health care practices. References to massage are found in Chinese medical texts 4,000 years old. Massage has been advocated in Western health care practices in an almost unbroken line since the time of Hippocrates, the "father of medicine." In the 4th century B.C., Hippocrates wrote, "The physician must be acquainted with many things and assuredly with rubbing" (the ancient Greek and Roman term for massage).

Some of the greatest physicians in history advocated massage, including Celsus (25 B.C.-50 A.D.), who wrote *De Medicinia*, an encyclopedia of Roman medical knowledge that dealt extensively with prevention and therapeutics using massage; Galen (131-200), the most influential physician in the ancient, medieval, and Renaissance worlds, who addressed techniques and indications for massage in his book *De Sanitate Tuenda* (which is translated as The Hygiene, meaning prevention); and Avicenna (980-1037), a Persian physician who wrote extensively about massage in his *Canon of Medicine*, which was considered the authoritative medical text in Europe for several centuries. A sampling of other noted advocates includes Ambrose Pare, who wrote the first modern textbook of surgery; William Harvey, who demonstrated the circulation of the blood; and Herman Boerhaave, who introduced the clinical method of teaching medicine.

Modern, scientific massage therapy was introduced in the United States in the 1850s by two New York physicians, brothers George and

Charles Taylor, who had studied in Sweden. The first massage therapy clinics in this country were opened by two Swedes after the Civil War: Baron Nils Posse ran the Posse Institute in Boston, and Hartwig Nissen opened the Swedish Health Institute near the U.S. Capitol in Washington, D.C.. Several members of Congress and U.S. Presidents, including Benjamin Harrison and Ulysses S. Grant, were among the massage therapy clientele.

As the health care system in the United States became more influenced by biomedicine and technology in the early 1900s, physicians began assigning massage duties (which were also labor-intensive, requiring more time to be spent with patients) to assistants, nurses, and physical therapists. In turn, in the 1930s and 1940s, nurses and physical therapists lost interest in massage therapy, virtually abandoning it. However, a small number of massage therapists carried on until the 1970s, when a new surge of interest in massage therapy revitalized the field, albeit in the realm of alternative health care. That interest has continued to the present.

Basic approach. Massage therapy is the scientific manipulation of the soft tissues of the body to normalize those tissues. It consists of a group of manual techniques that include applying fixed or movable pressure, holding, and/or causing movement of or to the body, using primarily the hands but sometimes other areas such as forearms, elbows, or feet. These techniques affect the musculoskeletal, circulatory-lymphatic, nervous, and other systems of the body. The basic philosophy of massage therapy encompasses the concept of *vis medicatrix naturae*—that is, aiding the ability of the body to heal itself—and is aimed at achieving or increasing health and well-being.

Touch is the fundamental medium of massage therapy. While massage methods can be described in terms of a series of techniques to be performed, it is important to understand that touch is not used solely in a mechanistic way in massage therapy; there is also an artistic component. Because massage usually involves applying touch with some degree of pressure, the massage therapist must use touch with sensitivity to determine the optimal amount of pressure appropriate for each person. Touch used with sensitivity also allows the massage therapist to receive useful information about the body, such as locating areas of muscle tension and other soft-tissue problems. Because touch is also a form of communication, sensitive touch can convey a sense of caring—which is an essential element in the therapeutic relationship—to the person receiving massage. Using the wrong kind of touch—sometimes thought of as "toxic touch"—is counterproductive, tending to render a technique ineffective and to cause the body to defend or guard itself, which in turn introduces greater tension.

Demographics. The advancement of higher standards and the development of a system of professional credentials have paralleled the dynamic growth of the massage therapy profession. Massage therapists are currently licensed by 19 States and a number of localities; additional States are expected to adopt licensing acts in the near future. Most States require 500 or more hours of education from a recognized school program and a licensing examination. While some States require continuing education, most massage therapists voluntarily take additional courses and workshops on a regular basis during their careers.

The National Certification Exam, a professional certification program accredited by the National Commission for Certifying Agencies in December 1993 and currently administered by the Psychological Corporation, was inaugurated in June 1992. More than 9,000 people nationwide were certified as of July 1994. Six States have already adopted the exam as their licensing exam, and more States are expected to follow suit.

The Commission on Massage Training Accreditation/Approval, a national accreditation agency that was set up in accord with the guidelines of the U.S. Department of Education, currently recognizes 60 school programs. Curriculums must consist of 500 or more hours and include specified hours of anatomy, physiology, massage theory and practice, and ethics.

The primary sponsor of the national certification and accreditation programs is the American Massage Therapy Association (AMTA), the largest and oldest national professional membership association for massage professionals. AMTA currently has more than 20,000 members and publishes the Massage Therapy Journal. The association recently founded the public, charitable AMTA Foundation to fund projects for research, education, and outreach; the foundation awarded its first grants in June 1993.

Each of a number of other national nonprofit membership associations for massage professionals has between 200 and 1,500 members. These groups usually are formed for practitioners of specific methods. To alleviate the competition and infighting that are sometimes found among various professional groups, an innovative coalition known as the Federation of Therapeutic Massage and Bodywork Organizations was formed in 1991 by the AMTA, the American Oriental Bodywork Therapy Association, the American Polarity Therapy

Association, the Rolf Institute, and the Trager Institute. The federation fosters greater communication and cooperation among its members.

The number of massage therapists in the United States can only be estimated, because no formal census has been taken. Furthermore, a census or estimate would be affected by the criteria for inclusion, which would involve such variables as extent of training, number of hours worked, and whether methods used by an individual are considered forms of massage. It is estimated that there are approximately 50,000 qualified massage therapists in the United States, providing some 45 million 1-hour massage sessions per year. The number of massage therapists appears to be increasing rapidly along with a corresponding increase in use by the American public. An estimated 20 million Americans have received massage therapy. Indeed, in the study by Eisenberg and colleagues (1993)—which found that 34 percent of the American public used alternative health care-relaxation techniques, chiropractic, and massage were the most frequently used forms of alternative health care.

Methods. Some 80 different methods may be classified as massage therapy, and approximately 60 of them are less than 20 years old. There are several reasons why this is the case.

The period of the 1940s to the mid-1970s was relatively dormant for the massage therapy profession. Little standardization was established in the field. Then in the 1970s, stimulated by changes in society such as greater interest in fitness, healthier lifestyles, personal improvement, and alternative methods of health care to complement conventional medicine, interest in massage therapy increased. An influx of new practitioners brought with them a wave of new ideas and creativity regarding ways to use hands-on techniques. Since there was little standardization, these techniques sometimes developed into freestanding methods rather than being incorporated into an existing system of classification.

Another source of new techniques was the various forms of massage native to most cultures around the world but not previously described outside each culture. For example, many of the forms of massage that come from Asia are based on concepts of anatomy, physiology, and diagnosis that differ from Western concepts.

The proliferation of methods has slowed. It is expected—as has happened in the development of other professions—that as the development of standards and credentials continues, there will be some consolidation and integration of methods.

The forms of massage therapy described in this section are either among the most widely used or representative of a group of similar practices. Several forms that include additional techniques besides massage are listed briefly here and discussed in more detail in the following sections. In actual practice, many massage therapists use more than one method in their work and sometimes combine several.

Swedish massage uses a system of long gliding strokes, kneading and friction techniques on the more superficial layers of muscles, generally in the direction of blood flow toward the heart, sometimes combined with active and passive movements of the joints. This system is used to promote general relaxation, improve circulation and range of motion, and relieve muscle tension. Swedish massage is the most common form of massage.

Deep-tissue massage is used to release chronic patterns of muscular tension using slow strokes, direct pressure, or friction directed across the grain of the muscles with the fingers, thumbs, or elbows. It is applied with greater pressure and to deeper layers of muscle than Swedish massage.

Sports massage uses techniques that are similar to Swedish and deep-tissue massage but are specially adapted to deal with the needs of athletes and the effects of athletic performance on the body.

Neuromuscular massage is a form of deep massage that is applied specifically to individual muscles. It is used to increase blood flow, release trigger points (intense knots of muscle tension that refer pain to other parts of the body), and release pressure on nerves caused by soft tissues. It is often used to reduce pain. Trigger point massage and myotherapy are similar forms.

Manual lymph drainage improves the flow of lymph by using light, rhythmic strokes. It is primarily used for conditions related to poor lymph flow, such as edema, inflammation, and neuropathies.

The reflexology, zone therapy, tuina, acupressure, rolfing (structural integration), Trager, Feldenkrais, and Alexander methods are addressed in the following sections. The various methods of massage therapy can be divided into two major groupings:[2]

1. Traditional European methods based on traditional Western concepts of anatomy and physiology, using five basic categories of soft-tissue manipulation: effleurage (gliding strokes), petrissage (kneading), friction (rubbing), tapotement (percussion), and vibration. Swedish massage is the main example.

2. Contemporary Western methods based on modern Western concepts of human functioning, using a wide variety of manipulative techniques. These may include broad applications for personal growth; emotional release; and balance of the mind, body, and spirit in addition to traditional applications. These methods go beyond the original framework of Swedish massage and include neuromuscular, sports, and deep-tissue massage; and myofascial release, myotherapy, Bindegewebsmassage, Esalen, and manual Lymph Drainage.

In addition, there are structural, functional, and movement integration methods that organize and integrate the body in relationship to gravity through manipulating the soft tissues or through correcting inappropriate patterns of movement; methods that bring about a more balanced use of the nervous system through creating new, integrated possibilities of movement. Examples are Rolfing, Hellerwork, Aston patterning, Trager, Feldenkrais, and Alexander.

Current research. From 1873, when the term massage first entered the Anglo-American medical lexicon, through 1939, more than 600 journal articles appeared in mainline English language journals of medicine, including the *Journal of the American Medical Association, Archives of Surgery*, and the *British Medical Journal*. During the past 50 years, reports on nearly 100 clinical trials have been published in the medical and allied health literature. Many well-designed studies have documented the benefits of several methods of massage therapy for the treatment of acute and chronic pain; acute and chronic inflammation; chronic lymphedema; nausea; muscle spasm; various soft-tissue dysfunctions; grand mal epileptic seizures; anxiety; and depression, insomnia, and psychoemotional stress, which may aggravate significant mental illness. A larger number of studies also have been carried out in Europe, particularly in the former Soviet Union and East Germany. Unfortunately, the published reports on most of these have not been translated into English.

Research base. The following studies reflect the versatility of massage therapy and its broad and diverse range of applications.

Premature infants treated with daily massage therapy gain more weight and have shorter hospital stays than infants who are not massaged. A study of 40 babies with low birth weight found that the 20 massaged babies had 47-percent greater weight gain per day and stayed in the hospital an average of 6 fewer days than 20 similar infants who did not receive massage; the cost saving was approximately $3,000 per infant (Field et al., 1986). Cocaine-exposed preterm infants given massages three times daily for a 10-day period showed significant improvement. Results indicated that massaged infants had fewer postnatal complications and exhibited fewer stress behaviors during the 10-day period, had 28-percent greater daily weight gain, and demonstrated more mature motor behaviors at the end of the 10-day course of massage therapy (Field, 1993).

A study comparing 52 hospitalized depressed and adjustment-disorder children and adolescents with a control group that viewed relaxation videotapes found that the massage therapy subjects were less depressed and anxious and had lower saliva cortisol levels (an indicator of less depression) (Field et al., 1992).

Another study showed that massage therapy produced relaxation in 18 elderly subjects. This study demonstrated physiological signs of relaxation in measures such as decreased blood pressure and heart rate and increased skin temperature (Fakouri and Jones, 1987).

A combination of Swedish massage, shiatsu, and trigger point suppression in 52 subjects with traumatically induced spinal pain led to significant alleviations of acute and chronic pain and increased muscle flexibility and tone. This study also found massage therapy to be extremely cost-effective in comparison with other therapies, with savings ranging from 15 percent to 50 percent (Weintraub, 1992a, 1992b). Massage has also been shown to stimulate the body's ability to control pain naturally; in one study, massage stimulated the brain to produce endorphins, the neurochemicals that control pain (Kaarda and Tosteinbo, 1989). Fibromyalgia, a painful type of inflammation, is an example of a condition that may be favorably affected by this mechanism.

A pilot study of five subjects with symptoms of tension and anxiety found a significant response to massage therapy based on one or more psychophysiological parameters, including heart rate, frontalis and forearm extensor electromyograms, and skin resistance; these changes denote relaxation of muscle tension and reduced anxiety (McKechnie et al., 1983).

Another study found that massage therapy can have a powerful effect on psychoemotional distress in persons suffering from chronic inflammatory bowel disease. Stress can worsen the symptoms of ulcerative colitis and Crohn's disease (ileitis), which can cause great pain and bleeding and even lead to hospitalization or death. Massage therapy was effective in reducing the frequency of episodes of pain and disability in these patients (Joachim, 1983).

Lymph drainage massage has been shown to be more effective than mechanized methods or diuretic drugs to control lymphedema (a form of swelling) secondary to radical mastectomy (removal of breast tissues). It is expected that using massage to control lymphedema will significantly lower treatment costs (Zanolla et al., 1984).

Research opportunities. The pace of research in the United States involving massage therapy appears to be increasing, and the activities of OAM may play a supportive role. A list of studies (directed by Tiffany Field) under way at the Touch Research Institute of the University of Miami Medical School illustrates the range of possibilities for research:

- *Infant studies*—infants exposed to human immunodeficiency virus (HIV), depressed infants, infant colic, sleep disorders, and pediatric oncology.

- *Child studies*—asthma, autism, posttraumatic stress disorder following natural disasters, neglected and abused children in shelters, preschool behavior, pediatric skin disorders, diabetes, and juvenile rheumatoid arthritis.

- *Adolescent studies*—depressed adolescent mothers, adolescent mothers after childbirth, and eating disorders.

- *Adult studies*—job performance and stress, eating disorders, pregnancy and neonatal outcome, hypertension, HIV-positive adults, spinal cord injuries, fibromyalgia syndrome, rape and spouse abuse victims, and couples therapy.

- *Elderly studies*—volunteer foster grandparents giving and receiving massage, and arthritis.

Research recommendations. The preceding section indicates the diversity and breadth of applications of massage therapy and suggests the range of possibilities for future research.

General studies of the efficacy and effectiveness of massage therapy are still needed. Outcome studies are recommended that would allow massage therapists to work in a manner and setting that approximate actual working conditions as much as is possible. Cost-effectiveness studies also are needed. Several of the studies cited in this report have indicated that massage therapy provides substantial cost savings; this is a critical issue related to health care reform. To verify the savings, some of the more recent studies should be replicated as part of this approach.

There are numerous possibilities for studying effects of massage on many health conditions:

- Since massage therapy is especially effective with soft-tissue problems, studies involving muscle strains, sprains, tendinitis, problems related to acute and chronic muscle tension, and other such conditions would be useful, as would studies of the effect of massage on the tissue healing process.

- Because research offers mounting evidence that a significant percentage of health problems can be attributed to stress and that stress reduction can be a powerful means of preventing or treating such problems, studies of the stress-reduction effects of massage therapy would be valuable.

- Another question that needs to be addressed is whether massage can cause cancerous tumors to mestastisize.

- The various subject areas under investigation at the Touch Research Institute are also examples of areas that merit further study.

Barriers and key issues. Several barriers and key issues need to be addressed to make research on massage therapy more productive:

- *Study design.* A key issue related to research is the need for researchers to collaborate with massage therapists during the design stage of a study. Some previous studies used massage in an inappropriate or ineffective manner. For example, the duration of massage is an important factor; a common error is use of massage sessions that are too brief to be effective. Another error is the choice of techniques that are not effective.

- *Appropriate use of therapists.* Properly qualified and skilled massage therapists should be used in each study. Some studies have been carried out in which individuals who were untrained or undertrained applied massage; it then became impossible to discern whether any negative results meant that massage was ineffective or that it was not applied properly.

- *Collaborations.* Since few individuals are both doctorate-level researchers and massage therapists, it is recommended that NIH facilitate collaboration between researchers and massage therapists. Researchers would benefit by knowing more about interesting and promising possibilities for research, resources available from the massage therapy profession, and massage therapy itself. Massage therapists would benefit by being able to locate researchers with whom to collaborate (1) to pursue study ideas and (2) to have a better understanding of the needs of researchers and the research process itself.

- *Translations.* Because many studies are in foreign languages, translations of such studies are needed

- *Regulatory barriers.* Another key issue is the existence of barriers to practice that hinder massage therapists; these must be removed. In some States, regulatory boards use powers granted through licensing laws to limit the practice of legitimate massage therapy by qualified massage therapists. These barriers also restrict the ability to conduct research on massage therapy in traditional settings, such as clinics and hospitals, thereby hampering research efforts.

If regulatory, insurance payment, and research barriers are not removed, they will inhibit progress regarding massage therapy, along with other forms of alternative health care.

Pressure Point Therapies

Pressure point therapies use finger pressure on specific points—usually related to the oriental meridian points (see the glossary), but also other neurological release points—to reduce pain and treat various disease states. There are antecedents in Europe, Asia, and the United States. Adamus and A'tatis described a pressure system in 1582, and the sculptor Cellini (1500-71) wrote of using pressure points to relieve pain. In 1770 the Jesuit Amiat contributed to European understanding with an article on Chinese pressure point "massage." This article influenced the Swedish therapeutic massage pioneer Ling. In turn, Swedish therapeutic massage influenced traditional Japanese folk massage in the early 20th century, and this cross-fertilization became known as shiatsu. About 1913, Fitzgerald, an American, developed what came to be known as zone therapy. Fitzgerald had been influenced by Bressler in Europe. The use of pressure points has evolved under several systems, some of which are discussed below.

Reflexology. Fitzgerald's work with hand reflex points was developed and promoted by Ingram in the United States and Marquardt in Europe. Because in this system specific "zones" on the feet are related to specific organs, the system is often called zone therapy. There is a related system of hand zone therapy as well. The results reported for the process include relief of pain; release of kidney stones; and recovery from the effects of stroke, sinusitis, sciatica, and menstrual and other disorders (Marquardt, 1983).

Traditional Chinese massage. Traditional Chinese remedial massage methods were described in the texts of the Han period (202 B.C. to circa 220 A.D.). By the Tang Dynasty (618-907 A.D.), these systems were taught in special institutes. Both "tonification" (energizing) and "sedation" techniques are used to treat and relieve many medical conditions. Major techniques in use are

- *ma*, rubbing with palm or finger tips;
- *pai*, tapping with palm or finger tips;
- *tao*, strong pinching with thumb and fingertip;
- *an*, rapid and rhythmical pressing with thumb, palm, or back of the clenched hand;
- *nie*, twisting, with both thumbs and tips of the index fingers grasping and twisting the area being treated;
- *ning*, pinching and lifting in a stationary position;
- *na*, moving while performing ning; and
- *tui*, pushing, often with slight vibratory effect.

These techniques are usually used in combinations. Two prominent groupings of techniques are known as an-mo and tui-na.

Widely varying illnesses and conditions are treated with traditional Chinese massage, including the common cold, sleeplessness, leg cramps, painful menses, whooping cough, diarrhea, abdominal pains, headache, asthma, rheumatic pains, stiff neck, colic, bed-wetting, nasal bleeding, lumbago, and throat pains.

Acupressure systems. Currently, four systems in which the fingers manipulate the oriental meridian system are in widespread use in the United States. In all these systems, pressure is applied to meridian points (acupuncture points on the meridians; also called acupoints) to stimulate or sedate them. Amounts of pressure and length of application vary according to the system, the ailment, and the intent. All of these systems shiatsu, tsubo, jin shin jyutsu, and jin shin do—rely on traditional oriental medical theory (see the "Alternative Systems of Medical Practice" chapter), although their treatment methods vary considerably.

Shiatsu and tsubo rely largely on sequenced applications of pressure applied from one end of each meridian to the other. The patient reclines, usually lying on the back and then the front for approximately equal periods as the practitioner uses thumb pressure to stimulate the point through a combination of direct pressure and transference of qi (see the glossary) to the point from the practitioner's thumb. "Barefoot shiatsu" is a form that uses foot pressure to stimulate the meridian points. Sessions typically treat the meridians of the entire body in an attempt to bring relaxation, harmony, and balance to the patient. Shiatsu, which is traditional in Japan, has been used in the United States quite extensively for about 20 years. Therapy sessions have a strong focus on long-term health improvement. Procedures include specific treatments for a variety of functional disorders as well as postural, stress-related, and emotional problems. Conditions that have been improved include headache, asthma, bronchitis, diarrhea, depression, and circulatory problems (Namikoshi, 1969).

Jin shin jyutsu and jin shin do have developed sequences of meridian point pressure applications that are specific to the ailment being addressed. These systems are used more often than shiatsu and tsubo as alternative treatment approaches. Jin shin jyutsu, the "art of circulation awakening," was developed in Japan by Jiro Murai in the early 1900s and brought to the United States in the 1960s by Mary Iino Burmeister. It is the antecedent of jin shin do, which was developed in the United States by Iona Teeguarden in the 1980s. Sessions are primarily for treatment of specific problems. The approach is similar to that of acupuncture, as the meridian connections to the organs are understood and applied, but from somewhat different application perspectives. Pressure is applied to the meridian points, which are then held in specific patterns, to tonify or detonify (energize or enervate) the meridian qi. Conditions addressed include a wide range of organic dysfunctions (Teeguarden, 1987).

Postural Reeducation Therapies

Three prominent therapies in the United States use as their approach the reeducation of the body through movement and physical touch. In all three systems—Alexander, Feldenkrais, and Trager—patients are taught how to retrain their bodies to come into alignment to release and change postural faults, to improve coordination and balance, and to relieve structural and functional stress. A major principle underlying the three methods is that awareness has to be experienced rather than taught verbally. The awareness may then lead to more effective use of one's whole self.

Alexander technique. The Alexander method is a system of body dynamics, especially in respect to the head, neck, and shoulders. The technique was developed by the actor F.M. Alexander, who created the method after concluding that bad posture was responsible for his chronic periods of voice loss (Maisel, 1989). The technique includes simple movements that improve balance, posture, and coordination and relieve pain. During a session the client typically goes through a series of standing and seated exercises while the practitioner applies light pressure to points of contraction in the body. These pressures are intended to awaken kinesthetic response (sensitivity to motion by the muscles) and retrain the kinesthetic organs in the joints to their proper spatial relationship. The process is taught in many drama schools and is popular with performers. The techniques help clients learn how to use their bodies with less tension and more awareness and efficiency.

Alexander practitioners report success with neck and back pain, postural disorders, whiplash injury, breathing problems, myalgia, rheumatica, repetitive strain injury, hypertension, anxiety, stress, and other chronic conditions.

Feldenkrais method. The Feldenkrais method was developed by Moshe Feldenkrais, a Russian-born Israeli physicist, who turned his attention to the study of human functioning. His work integrated an understanding of the physics of the body's movement patterns with an awareness of the way people learn to move, behave, and interact

(Feldenkrais, 1949, 1972, 1981, 1985). He began teaching his method in North America in the early 1970s. The Feldenkrais method consists of two branches "awareness through movement" and "functional integration."

- *Awareness through movement.* This verbally directed form of the Feldenkrais method consists of gentle exploratory movement sequences organized around a specific human function (such as reaching, bending, or walking) with the intention of increasing awareness of multiple possibilities of action. A group of students may be standing, sitting, or lying on the floor. Thinking, sensory perception, and imagery are also involved in examining each function.

- *Functional integration.* This method involves the practitioner's use of words and gentle, non-invasive touch to guide an individual student to an awareness of existing and alternative movement patterns. The teacher communicates to the student—who may be lying, sitting, standing, kneeling, or in motion—how she or he organizes herself or himself and suggests additional choices for functional movement patterns. The use of touch is for communication, not correction, and there are no special techniques of pressing or stroking. Any changes in functioning result from the student's actions.

Practitioners report success with a variety of postural and functional disorders in such diverse applications as sports performance, equine training, physiotherapeutics, zoo animal rehabilitation, the performing arts, neurological and orthopedic physical therapy practice, pain management, and habilitation of developmentally impaired children.

Currently, the North American Feldenkrais Guild has approximately 1,000 members. As of January 1994, 31 training programs lasting 3 to 4 years were available around the world for Feldenkrais practitioners.

The method is a synthesis of modern ideas and basic research findings in perception, motor learning, neural plasticity, and sensory integration (Edelman, 1987; Georgopolus, 1986; Jacobson, 1964; Jenkins and Merzenic, 1987; Jenkins et al., 1990; Kaas, 1991; Kandel and Hawkins, 1992; Seitz and Wilson, 1987; and Sweigard, 1974). Only limited clinical research studies have been conducted to document the Feldenkrais method. Clinical successes have been cited in several review articles and clinical guidelines for physical therapy and pain management (DeRosa and Porterfield, 1992; Jackson, 1991; Lake, 1985; and Shenkman and Butler, 1989) and have included reports on exercise for the elderly and for persons recovering from spinal injury (Ginsberg, 1986; Gutman, 1977).

In one research study, Jackson-Wyatt and colleagues (1992) used video analysis to measure the kinetics of the change in motor ability in a vertical jump test in a subject who completed eight 5-day weeks of 6-hour training days in a Feldenkrais practitioner training program. Dramatic improvement in power, velocity, and movement efficiency were demonstrated.

Narula (1993) similarly examined the sit-to-stand movement, walking speed, and grip strength of four subjects with class 2 rheumatoid arthritis. After attending a twice-weekly 75-minute class for 6 weeks, all subjects showed decreased pain, improved walking performance, and improved kinetics of the sit-to-stand movement, but no improvement in grip strength. The results suggest that lessons in awareness through movement could be used by individuals to improve their functions despite long-term disabling medical conditions.

Ruth and Kegerries (1992) used a 25-minute, four-step process to test the flexion range of neck motion in college students before and after half the group received a 15-minute sequence from the awareness through movement methods. Compared with the control group, students experiencing this sequence showed measurably improved neck flexion motion and a decrease in the perceived effort to accomplish this motion.

Since Feldenkrais's functional integration method involves a highly individual interaction between practitioner and client, outcomes research should be long-term, using both subjective and objective measures. Such studies could establish whether various applications of the Feldenkrais method are useful both for medical care and in educational systems.

Trager psychophysical integration. The Trager method uses light, rhythmic rocking and shaking movements that loosen joints, ease movement, and release chronic patterns of tension. This method was developed by a Hawaiian physician, Milton Trager, on the basis of his experience as a trainer for the sport of boxing. The Trager practitioner uses his or her hands with the aim of influencing deep-seated psychophysiological patterns in the client's mind and interrupting the projection of those patterns into body tissues.

This method of movement reeducation is distinguished by compressions, elongations, and light bounces as well as rocking motions. These actions cause patients or clients to begin to experience freedom of movement of their body parts. Since practitioners believe they are affecting the inhibiting patterns at their source, it is expected that clients can experience long-lasting gains.

The goal of Trager work is general functional improvement, partly by creating a feeling of pleasure in being able to move body parts more freely. The process incorporates a meditative state called "hookup," which is intended to enhance sensory, kinesthetic, and other pleasurable experiences for the client.

Several case histories describe long-term improvement in movement function for persons with multiple sclerosis; in chest mobility with lung disease (Witt and MacKinnon, 1986); and in trunk mobility with childhood cerebral palsy (Witt and Parr, 1986). Other reports suggest success in treating chronic pain of various sorts, headaches, muscular dystrophy, muscle spasms, temporomandibular joint pain, recovery from stroke, spinal cord injuries, and polio.

The Trager method also includes Trager "mentastics," a system of mentally directed physical movements developed to maintain and enhance a sense of lightness, freedom, and flexibility. Mentastics is used by Trager practitioners and is taught to clients to enhance results.

There are now more than 800 certified Trager practitioners around the world. Training is available in the United States and several other countries.

Structural Integration (Rolfing)

Unlike most systems of body manipulation, which are concerned with the muscular system or the skeletal systems or both, structural integration focuses on the fascias, which are sheets of connective tissue. Ida Rolf, whose work was the foundation of the various systems of structural integration, noted that while bones support the body and muscles connect the bones. It is the enwrapping fascias that support and hold the muscle-bone combinations in place. Rolf's second precept was that the fascias would maintain not only the normal relationship of bone and muscle but also whatever postural misalignment the body might adopt. This misalignment could incorporate effects of trauma as well as poor posture.

Later theorists have used renowned architect and designer Buckminster Fuller's "tensegrity mast" as an explanatory model for

434

the relationship of the bones and fascias. In this structure, none of the solid elements are connected directly together but are held by tensioned wires. The structure becomes a model for the body if the solid segments are called the bones and the flexible wires are called the fascias (Robie, 1977).

When the body attempts to distribute the stress of an injury, the result is likely to be shortened and thickened fascias, which may in turn lead to symptoms somewhere other than the site of the original trauma. Structural integration is a system to "unwind" and stretch the distorted fascias back to their normal condition, thereby allowing the bones and muscles to come back to normal alignment and the body to return to normal functioning. Structural integration, or "Rolfing," involves stretching the fascia sheaths by applying sliding pressure to the affected area with fingers, thumbs, and occasionally elbows. In its early days, the process was known to be quite painful, but later refinements in technique have made Rolfing considerably more comfortable

Rolf postulated that the plasticity of the fascias in the body could offset the aging process (Rolf, 1973). Research in Rolfing has suggested beneficial results with cerebral palsy in children (Perry et al., 1981), state-trait anxiety (i.e., a person's current anxiety state or level is measured against his or her anxiety traits) (Weinberg and Hunt, 1979), the stress and symptoms of lower back pain and whiplash (Rolf, 1977), and changes in parasympathetic tone (degree of vigor and tension of muscles innervated by parasympathetic nerves) (Cottingham et al., 1988a, 1988b). Changes in psychological and physiological function have also been measured (Silverman et al., 1973).

The Rolf Institute, the first school to teach the principles of structural integration, offers a post-bachelor's degree training program requiring 28 weeks of classroom work. Today there are also three other schools based on Rolf's work and 1,500 practitioners who treat an estimated 150,000 individuals per year. Licensing requirements differ in various States.

Aston patterning, developed by Judith Aston, and Hellerwork, developed by Joseph Heller, are major offshoots of structural integration. Both incorporate movement reeducation training to bring the body into fuller activity and expression.

Bioenergetical Systems

Several therapeutic systems using manual healing are designed to release bodily held emotions through various combinations of activity

435

on the part of the client and applied pressure or holding on the part of the practitioner. These systems derive from Wilhelm Reich's original observations about bodily held emotions and his work with patients and clients to release emotion (Reich, 1973). In this work, the client assumes and holds one of several different postures, either seated or reclining. Simultaneously, the practitioner applies pressure to areas of abnormal stress that are revealed by the posture. The client may then be invited to breathe deeply into the stressed area. The combination of external, inwardly directed pressure and outwardly directed breath exaggerates holding patterns that have become so deeply imbedded that the client is no longer aware of them. Release of the emotion can be quite pronounced, resulting in spontaneously revealed insight, increased freedom of movement, and new social postures. Individual releases during the process may be accompanied by pronounced but brief periods characterized by increased body heat, tingles, and reported rushes of "energy."

Bioenergetics, core energetics, Lowenwork, neo-Reichian therapy, radix, and some other methods derive from Reich's basic approach.

Although some psychotherapists incorporate various forms of this work into their practices, there are constraints in some States because of ethical questions about touching the client. Discussions with various psychotherapists indicate that some would like to include these therapies but fear to do so at this time, when the legal and ethical considerations have not been resolved. Those who do the work operate in a dual capacity—as psychotherapist and bioenergetic body worker. However, they do not apply touch during straight psychotherapy sessions, and the straightforward touch used during the body work is clinically applied pressure and not sensually evocative.

Biofield Therapeutics

Overview

Biofield (see the glossary) therapeutics, often called energy healing or laying on of hands, is one of the oldest forms of healing known to humankind. Discovery, partial characterization, and use of the biofield have risen independently among peoples and cultures in every sector of the world (see table 29.1).

The earliest Eastern references are in the Huang Ti Nei Ching Su Wen (*The Yellow Emperor's Classic of Internal Medicine*), variously dated between 2,500 and 5,000 years ago (Veith, 1949). The earliest Western references are in hieroglyphics and in depictions of biofield healings dating from Egypt's Third Dynasty.[3] Hippocrates, a major figure in Western medicine, referred to the biofield as "the force which flows from many people's hands" (Schiegl, 1983). Franz von Mesmer, an Austrian physician who investigated and popularized this process in the late 18th century, referred to the biofield as "animal magnetism" to differentiate it from "metal magnetism," which he understood to be a similar but different medium (Mesmer, 1980). In the United States, use increased after Mesmer's "magnetic healing" became popular in the 1830s. (Among others, both Andrew Still (founder of osteopathy) and Daniel Palmer (founder of chiropractic) practiced for a time as magnetic healers (Gevitz, 1993)).

Historically, beliefs about causation in this type of healing have clustered around two views that remain active today. The first is that the "healing force" comes from a source other than the practitioner, such as God, the cosmos, or another supernatural entity. The second is that a human biofield, directed, modified, or amplified in some fashion by the practitioner, is the operative mechanism. Some of the terms presented in table 29.1 are devoid of religious or spiritual overtones, while others carry religious aspects common to the culture in which they were or are used.

Therapeutic application of the biofield is a process during which the practitioner places his or her hands either directly on or very near the physical body of the person being treated. In so doing, the practitioner engages the perceived biofield from his or her hands with the recipient's perceived biofield either to promote general health or to treat a specific dysfunction. The person being treated, who is usually clothed, reclines in some forms of the process but is seated in others.

The process is not instantaneous, as it is in "faith healing." (Faith is not a factor in the biofield process.) Treatment sessions may take from 20 minutes to an hour or more; a series of sessions is often needed to complete treatment of some disorders.

The ability to perform biofield healing appears to be universal, although most people seem unaware of possessing the talent. As with any innate talent, practice and learning appropriate techniques improve results.

There is consensus among practitioners that the biofield that permeates the physical body also extends outward from the body for several inches. Therefore, no real difference is seen between placing the hands directly on the body (either by direct skin contact or through clothing) or in close proximity to the body. In either case, the practitioner's biofield is understood to come into confluence with the

Table 29.1. Some Equivalent Terms for Biofield

Term	Source
Ankh	Ancient Egypt
Animal magnetism	Mesmer
Arunquiltha	Australian aborigine
Bioenergy	United States, United Kingdom
Biomagnetism	United States, United Kingdom
Gana	South America
Ki	Japan
Life force	General usage
Mana	Polynesia
Manitou	Algonquia
M'gbe	Hiru pygmy
Mulungu	Ghana
Mumia	Paracelsus
Ntoro	Ashanti
Ntu	Bantu
Oki	Huron
Orenda	Iroquois
Pneuma	Ancient Greece
Prana	India
Qi (chi)	China
Subtle energy	United States, United Kingdom
Sila	Inuit
Tane	Hawaii
Ton	Dakota
Wakan	Lakota

Source: Provided courtesy of the Biofield Research Institute.

recipient's biofield. There are advantages and disadvantages to each approach in clinical applications.[4]

Extension of the external portion of the biofield is considered variable and dependent on the person's emotional state and state of health. Practitioners describe the external portion, sometimes called the "aura," as tactilely detectable (see the "Biofield Diagnostics" section) and less dense than the portion permeating the physical body.

Biofield practitioners have a holistic focus, for most treatment sessions produce results that encompass more than one aspect of the person's health. Within that focus there is, however, a range of therapeutic intents:

- *General* (e.g., stress relief, improvement of general health and vitality).

- *Biologic* (e.g., reduction of inflammation, edema, chronic and acute pain; change in hematocrit and T-cell levels; and acceleration of wound healing and fracture repair).

- *Vegetative functions* (e.g., improvement of appetite, digestion, and sleep patterns).

- *Emotional states* (e.g., changes in anxiety, grief, depression, and feelings of self-worth).

- *Dysfunctions* often classified psychosomatic (e.g., treatment of eating disorders, irritable bowel syndrome, premenstrual syndrome, and posttraumatic stress disorder).

Some practitioners incorporate mental healing, or focused intent to heal, as part of their biofield treatments. This is also called psychic healing, distant healing, nonlocal healing, and absent healing. Mental healing can also be performed by itself at a considerable distance from the recipient. It is an active process on the practitioner's part, involving centered, focused concentration; it may include various imagery (visualization) techniques as well. (See the "Imagery" section and the "Prayer and Mental Healing" section in the "Mind-Body Interventions" chapter.)

A related mind effect sometimes used in biofield healing is described as the practitioner, by effort of will, extending the biofield (principally from the hands) into the recipient's body with increased force, sometimes from a distance of several feet. Chinese qigong masters are considered especially adept at this. The process appears to be draining; interviews with practitioners who do this procedure indicate they are limited in the number of treatments they can perform in a day.

Some practitioners meditate before giving a treatment in order to enter a so-called healing space; some others maintain a meditative state during treatment.

Biofield diagnostics. Detailed diagnostic methods have been developed to determine the condition of the patient's general health and present disorder by sensing, with touch, subtle perturbations in the biofield (clairsentience). Janet Quinn, researcher of the therapeutic touch method, writes that "assessment [of the external portion] focuses on perceiving the way this energy is flowing and is distributed in the patient" (Krieger, 1992). Patricia Heidt adds that areas of "accumulated tension" or "congested energy" are detected (Heidt 1981b). Barbara Brennan, developer of the healing science method, describes the use of "high sense perception," which includes other subtle perceptions of the external biofield (Brennan, 1987).

Biofield researcher Richard Pavek writes of similar subtle tactile cues detected when the hands are placed directly on the body during SHEN®[5] therapy as "changes in temperature . . . , tingles, prickles, 'electricity' (sensation of light static), pressure or 'magnetism' . . . sensations are usually different over an area of physical pain, inflammation, tension and/or when release of emotion occurs" (Pavek, 1987, p. 57).

Many practitioners develop their treatment plans entirely by interpreting these various tactile sensations. Others use biofield diagnostics to supplement conventional methods, such as nursing diagnostic forms or chronic pain evaluation forms.

Current status. Considerable interchange of technique occurs between Europe and the United States and some between the United States and Asia.

United States. The process of using biofields has been treated with a reflexive mixture of awe and disgust, reverence and fear, and belief and disbelief, but this situation appears to be changing as more and more people seriously investigate the process from a critically neutral perspective.

No formal census is available, but reasonable estimates suggest that some 50,000 practitioners in the United States provide about 120 million sessions annually (Pavek, 1994). Of these, about 30,000 have

440

trained in therapeutic touch (Benor, 1994). For some, it is a major part of their vocational activity; others use the process occasionally to help family and friends. Many practitioners have had no formal training in the process, and many have independently discovered biofield effects. Others learned rudimentary techniques from friends or trained in one of several schools that teach various forms of the process. Reviews of school enrollment records indicate that most practitioners are women.

Some practitioners, often those who have independently discovered the process, and some teachers ascribe to it a religious or spiritual basis.

A few link the process with specific religious activities.

No State has licensing requirements for biofield practitioners. Because legal constraints in many States prohibit the use of the terms patient and treatment, most practitioners use the terms receiver and session in describing their work.

Some, possibly because they fear being charged with practicing medicine without a license, have cloaked themselves by incorporating under the name of a healing church. They often deny attempting to treat biological disorders and describe their process as "healing the spirit," from which "healing of the physical" will follow.

In the past 20 years or so, formal training in the process has emerged in considerable strength in this country. At this time several teaching establishments with standardized training programs teach different forms of the process; most grant certificates. Schools differ considerably in curriculum, focus, length of training extent of internship, and certification requirements. Some schools are semistructured associations of instructors trained in a particular method; others are more centrally organized.

The major biofield therapies used in the United States are summarized in table 29.2.

At least four forms of biofield therapy—healing science, healing touch, SHEN® therapy, and therapeutic touch—have been taught in a number of medical establishments. Currently, student nurses are trained in one or another system in more than 90 colleges and universities around the world. Acupuncturists, massage practitioners, and nurses who pass these courses receive continuing education credit from several State bureaus for training in these four forms.

Most of the practitioners of this process work independent of conventional medical and health practitioners. The conventional practitioner may occasionally be aware that his or her patient-client is seeing a biofield practitioner collaterally, but most are not.

Table 29.2. Brief Features of the Major Biofield Therapies in the United States; continued on next page.

Therapy	Year originated	Developer	Theoretical basis	Diagnostic procedures	Certification	Placement of hands	Mental healing at a distance	Therapeutic intent
Healing science	1978	Barbara Brennan	Open system, incorporates chakras and psychic layers	High sense perception	Yes, after completion of advanced study	Both on and near the body	Yes	Treat the whole person and specific disorders
Healing touch	1981	American Holistic Nurses Association	Elements of therapeutic touch, healing science, and Brugh Joy's and other work	Tactile assessment	Yes	Both on and off the body	Yes	Whole person, specific disorders
Huna	Traditional Hawaiian		Involves mana (universal force) and aka (universal substance)	Various	No	Both on and near the body	Yes	Heal mind and body
Mari-el	1983	Ethel Lombardi	Vibrational energy is transmitted from a higher source through the practitioner to the patient, affecting cellular memory and the endocrine system	Tactile assessment	No	Usually off the body	Yes	Heal and harmonize the life of the individual
Natural healing	1974	Rosalyn Bruyere	Operates on a belief in a universal principle of energy	Tactile assessment	Graduates are ordained			Effect symptomatic relief, assists in proper use of energy
Qigong	Traditional Chinese		Qi flows through the body in meridians and other patterns; Qi is delivered with great force by many practitioners called qigong masters	Varies with practitioners	Not usually	At the meridian points or at a short distance from the body	Yes	Healing of biological disorders

Table 29.2. Brief Features of the Major Biofield Therapies in the United States; continued from previous page.

Therapy	Year originated	Developer	Theoretical basis	Diagnostic procedures	Certification	Placement of hands	Mental healing at a distance	Therapeutic intent
Reiki	Japan, 1800s; USA, 1936	Mikao Usui (introduced by Hawayo Takata)	Spiritual energy with innate intelligence, channeled through the practitioner; the spiritual body is healed, it in turn is expected to heal the physical; Uses rituals, symbols, spirit guides	Varies	Spiritual initiation (i.e., the power to heal is given after training)	A few standard hand placements (usually side by side; on the physical body)	Yes	
SHEN® therapy	1977	Richard Pavek	Biofield conforming to natural laws of physics, with a discernable flux pattern through the body	Conventional medical and psychotherapy instruments with questions designed to discover repressed emotional states	Yes, after internship. Practitioners meet requirements of U.S. Department of Labor Occupational Code 076.264-640.	Sequence of paired-hand placements, directly on the body, arranged according to flux patterns, usually with one on top and one underneath	No	Primarily emotional disorders and somatopsychic dysfunctions
Therapeutic touch	1972	Dora Kunz and Dolores Kreiger	Practitioner restores correct vibrational component to the patient's universal, unitary field	Tactile assessment	None	Generally near the body	Yes	Nonprescriptive healing of the whole person

Note: Polarity therapy was omitted from this table but is discussed in the "Combined Physical and Biofield Methods" section of this chapter.

443

However, while much of the current activity in this discipline can be considered separate and alternative, the process is beginning to seep upward into mainstream medical and health practices. It is likely that several thousand practitioners of conventional therapies currently combine one or another of the biofield therapy processes with their primary approaches. Among these are nurses, counselors, psychotherapists, chiropractors, and massage practitioners who at least occasionally use a form of biofield therapy as an adjunct.

At least three forms are currently in use in hospitals: healing touch and therapeutic touch are used for a variety of reasons in several hospitals (Quinn, 1981, 1993), and SHEN® therapy is used in alcohol abuse, drug abuse, and codependent recovery programs in a few hospitals (Sunshine and Wright, 1986).

Europe. The United States falls far behind other countries in legal recognition of biofield therapy. Currently, more than 8,500 registered healers in the United Kingdom (British Medical Association, 1993) "are permitted to 'give healing' (a term for the process in common usage in the United Kingdom) at the request of patients" (p. 92). Approval has been obtained to use the process at the 1,500 government hospitals. In some situations, biofield healers are paid under the U.K. National Health Service (Benor, 1993). Physicians receive postgraduate education credits for attending courses in the biofield process, and healers are able to purchase liability insurance policies similar to those covering physicians (Benor, 1992).

In Poland and Russia, biofield healing is being incorporated into conventional medical practice; some medical schools include instruction in the process in the curriculum. In Russia, the process is under investigation by the Academy of Science. In Bulgaria, a government-appointed scientific body assesses abilities and recommends licensing for those who pass rigorous examinations (Benor, 1992).

Asia. China leads the rest of the world in research on therapeutic application and methods of increasing biofield effects. Biofield healing is called wei qi liao fa, or "medical qigong" (chi kung), in China, where proficient practitioners are called "qigong masters." Qigong masters are described as having developed their qi (biofield) to a high degree through qigong exercises.[6] (A few qigong masters are reported to be able to anesthetize patients for surgery solely with this method [Houshen, 1988]). Reduction of secondary cancers by medical qigong masters is commonly reported; there are clinics for that purpose alone.

Departments of medical qigong research exist in every college of traditional Chinese medicine in China. Both national and regional governments sponsor periodic international conferences on medical qigong. American researchers are frequently invited to present papers at these conferences.

Explanatory models. No generally accepted theory accounts for the phenomena of biofields. As one might expect of a discipline often perceived as bordering between superstition and random process on the one hand and science and technique on the other, there are profound differences—both inside the discipline among practitioners and researchers, and outside among theoreticians—as to the exact nature of the phenomena. In many cases, the view of the biofield is not a clearly defined one; it often mixes concepts of physics and metaphysics, or ancient and modern wisdoms (see the glossary).

The current major hypotheses are that the biofield is:

- metaphysical (outside the four dimensions of space and time and untestable),

- an electromagnetic field effect, and

- a presently undefined but potentially quantifiable field effect in physics.

There are three metaphysical approaches:

- *Spiritual energy.* Practitioners of some methods believe that they are channeling a spiritual energy that has innate intelligence or logic and knows where and to what extent it is required (Baginski and Sharamon, 1988). Reiki and also "radiance," a form of reiki, are examples of this view (Ray, 1987). Reiki teaches that the practitioner is merely a conduit for spiritual energy. After training, the practitioner is initiated and given the power to heal; sacred symbols are often used to give added power to the process (Jarrell, 1992). Another system with a similar approach, mari-el, incorporates the use of angels or spiritual guides in the healing practice.

- *Interacting human and universal energy fields.* Heidt and others have postulated that both the healer and the healed are vibrating fields of energy (Heidt, 1981b) that interact with the environmental energy field around them for healing purposes.

445

Brennan describes a similar process as one of "harmonic induction" (Brennan, 1987).

• *Repatterning of resonant vibratory fields.* Going further, Quinn and nurse-theorist Rogers state that:

current assumptions (about Therapeutic Touch), which remain "untested" and "untestable," [are that] people are energy fields. We are not saying that people have energy fields in addition to what they are . . . [Instead they are] open systems engaged in continuous interaction with the environmental energy field. [Therefore] when a person is "sick" there is an imbalance in the person's energy field, [and] when a person uses his or her intent to help or heal a person, the energy field of the person may repattern towards greater wellness . . . The Therapeutic Touch practitioner knowingly participates in . . . "a healing meditation," facilitates repatterning of the recipient's energy field through a process of resonance, rather than "energy exchange or transfer" (Quinn, 1993).

The healing intervention is seen as a "purposive patterning of energy fields, a mutual process in which the nurse uses his or her hands as a mediating focus in the continuing patterning of the mutual patient-environment energy field process" (Rogers, 1990).

In addition, certain models in physics may offer some explanation of biofield phenomena. Although quantum physics, the branch of physics that treats atomic and subatomic particles, has been proposed to explain the effects of a related phenomenon, mental healing at a distance (see the "Mind-Body Interventions" chapter), it has not proved to be a useful model to explain biofield healing. For example, Brennan states, "I am quite unable to explain these experiences without using the old [classical physics] frameworks" (Brennan, 1987, p. 26).

Classical physics is a model that is applied with high precision to large-scale phenomena involving relatively slow motion, such as the flow of fluids, electromagnetic currents and waves, hydraulics, aerodynamics, and atmospheric physics. It appears to be a reasonable model to apply in studying biofield phenomena.

Indeed, much of the terminology used by biofield practitioners to describe their work— while somewhat imprecise and variable—clearly describes quantitative and qualitative factors similar to those in fields of classical physics. For example, qi appears to be equivalent to flux in electromagnetic fields, for it describes direction and quantity of field. Polarity between the hands and between different bodily regions appears to be equivalent to polar difference in electromagnetic fields and to pressure differential in hydrodynamics. Pavek describes the biofield as having "circulating [flux] patterns . . . similar in formation and function to magnetic fields or electrostatic fields" (Pavek, 1987, p. 61). (See table 29.3 for other analogies.)

Around 1850, Karl von Reichenbach (discoverer of kerosene and paraffin) demonstrated apparent biofield polarities and determined apparent velocity through a copper rod to be about 4 meters per second (von Reichenbach, 1851).[7] In 1947, L.E. Eeman demonstrated a polarity through the arms and hands and another through the spine with his device known as an Eeman screen (Eeman, 1947). (See fig. 29.2.)

In about 1950 Randolph Stone, developer of polarity therapy, determined that flux density showed polarities within the physical body (Stone, 1986).

In 1978, Pavek compared paired-hand placements and reversed paired-hand placements on patients by hundreds of trained and untrained practitioners; he noted that one arrangement consistently resulted in relaxation and feelings of well-being but that the other set consistently produced agitation and anxiety. From this he deduced normal (healthy) qi polarities and movement patterns in the body (Pavek, 1987). (See fig. 29.3.)

In 1985 Pavek expanded on these findings by demonstrating coherent linkages between qi patterns, emotional holding patterns, and autocontractile pain response while developing biofield treatments for disorders often classified as psychosomatic (Pavek, 1988b; Pavek and Daily, 1990) and correlating emotional holding patterns with Chinese five-phase theory (Pavek, 1988a).

In 1992, Isaacs conducted a double-blind study using Eeman screens, which confirmed polarity at the spine and arms (Isaacs, 1991).

It is unclear at this time whether the biofield is electromagnetic or some other presently unmeasured but potentially quantifiable medium. It is popularly hypothesized that the biofield is a form of bioelectricity, biomagnetism, or bioelectromagnetism.[8] This may well be the case but has yet to be established. Some researchers discount the possibility.[9]

Some Chinese researchers have conducted experiments indicating that when wei qi (the external biofield) is used in fa qi (healing), electro-magnetic radiation in the infrared range is produced; others found indications of infrasonic waves. However, both phenomena appear to be minor secondary effects (Shen, 1988; Xin et al., 1988).

Table 29.3. Rough Equivalencies in Applied Physics.

Atmospheric Physics	Biofield Physics[a]	Electromagnetics	Hydrodynamics
Air	Qi	Flux	Liquid
Density	Denseness	Charge	Viscosity
Wind	Flow	Current	Stream
High pressure	Sending hand[b]	Negative terminal	Source
Low pressure	Receiving hand[b]	Positive terminal	Slump
Friction	Resistance	Reluctance	Friction
System	Biofield	Field	Flow-field
Pressure	Force	Electromagnetic field	Pressure
Pressure gradient	Polarity	Polar difference	Pressure differential

Source: Provided courtesy of the Biofield Research Institute.

[a] Proposed category

[b] In some systems

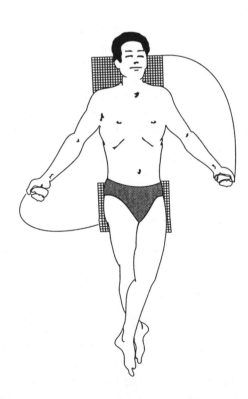

Figure 29.2. Arm and Spine Polarities

Research base. Rigorous research on biofield healing has been hindered by the belief, held by many, that nothing more than a placebo effect is the operative factor. This belief has affected funding, publishing, and status of researchers. Because funding organizations and scientific communities believed that any effects obtained were largely placebo effects, not real effects of biofields, research has been considered pointless. Moreover, many researchers have been unwilling to study biofield effects that they would otherwise be interested in, because they fear being ostracized by other researchers. Publication of research by the journals has been limited for similar reasons.

Notwithstanding these limitations, a number of studies have been implemented. In the United States, there are more than 17 published studies on biofield therapeutics.

Published U.S. studies. Because no comprehensive database of studies on biofield therapeutics exists, the following are considered to be only a sampling. In two controlled studies on therapeutic touch, Krieger found significant change in hemoglobin levels in hospitalized patients (Krieger, 1975, 1973). In a similar study, Wetzel found significant change in hematocrit and hemoglobin levels of 48 subjects receiving reiki, and no significant change with 10 controls (Wetzel, 1989).

Wirth found significant change in the healing rate of full-thickness skin wounds in a carefully controlled, double-blind study of therapeutic touch (Wirth, 1990), while Keller and Bzdek found highly significant decreases in pain scores recorded on the McGill-Melzak Pain Questionnaire by patients with tension headache in a controlled study of therapeutic touch (Keller, 1993; Keller and Bzdek, 1986).

Although Meehan found no significant difference on the Visual Analog Scale and Pain Intensity Descriptor Form between postoperative patients receiving therapeutic touch and controls, secondary analysis showed patients receiving therapeutic touch waited longer before requesting analgesia (Meehan, 1985, 1988). Similarly, Heidt found significant changes in anxiety levels of hospitalized cardiovascular patients receiving therapeutic touch versus controls as measured on the A-State Self-evaluation Questionnaire (Heidt, 1979, 1981a; Spielberger et al., 1983). Quinn (1983) found similar results in a study of therapeutic touch versus mimic therapeutic touch without centering and intention to assist.

In a replication study on patients before and after open heart surgery, using therapeutic touch versus mimic therapeutic touch and no-treatment groups, Quinn found no significant differences between the groups. Yet changes occurred in the expected direction, and there was a significant reduction in diastolic blood pressure among the therapeutic touch group that was not seen in the no-treatment group (Quinn, 1989). In another study of therapeutic touch versus mimic therapeutic touch, Parkes showed no significant differences among elderly hospitalized patients (Parkes, 1985).

Collins (1983), Fedoruk (1984), and Ferguson (1986) found significant relaxation effects of therapeutic touch with various subjects in different studies, and Quinn (1992), in a pilot study of four bereaved people, found significant reduction of suppressor T cells in all four after therapeutic touch. Moreover, Kramer found significant differences in stress reduction between treatment and control groups in a study of therapeutic touch with hospitalized children (Kramer, 1990).

Other U.S. studies. A number of pilot and case studies in fruitful areas have shown interesting results that are worthy of further investigation. These studies were conducted without controls, usually because of the severe limitations on funding.

In four uncontrolled cases, Pavek found that white cell decrease during chemotherapy reversed and rose significantly after single SHEN® therapy treatments at the thymus gland (Pavek, unpublished, 1984-85). In a pilot study on SHEN® therapy and premenstrual syndrome, Pavek noted significant long-term symptom relief and behavioral change with 11 of 13 subjects (Pavek, unpublished, 1986).

Beal, in an unpublished study of 12 hospitalized major depressives, found no statistical difference in time of release from the hospital between 6 subjects randomized to receive SHEN® therapy and 6 controls receiving sham SHEN®[9] therapy. However, in analyzing both subject and counselor reports, Pavek found significant change in dreaming, emotional expressiveness, and interpersonal contact with subjects receiving SHEN® therapy and much less change among controls (Beal and Pavek 1985).

Other therapeutic touch research with promising indications includes research on rehabilitation (Payne, 1989), helping patients to rest (Heidt, 1991), mental patients (Hill and Oliver, 1993), symptom control in acquired immunodeficiency syndrome (AIDS) (Newshan, 1989), and severe burn patients (Pavek, unpublished observations).

Promising research with SHEN®[9] therapy includes research with occupational therapy clients, third-trimester abdominal pain, reduction of pain during birthing without pain medication, irritable bowel syndrome, posttraumatic stress disorder, anorexia, bulimia, phobias, and chronic migraine.

International research. There has been considerable research on biofield therapeutics in other countries. In China, more than 30 controlled studies on effects of fa qi on both humans and animals were reported in the proceedings of just one meeting, the First World Conference for the Academic Exchange of Medical Qigong. At the same meeting, 32 studies were presented on effects on health of qigong exercises that raise qi (Proceedings, 1988).

In an overview report, Daniel Benor has compiled data on 151 healing studies from around the world (Benor, 1992). In many of these studies, mental healing efforts were combined with the biofield processes. However, 61 were controlled, published studies of biofield healing effects without the confounding factors of mental intent. These studies are shown in tables 29.4 and 29.5.

Table 29.4. Controlled Studies for Biofield Therapeutics With Humans

Subject	No. of studies	Significant results[a]
Anxiety	9	4 (+2)
Hemoglobin	4	4
Skin wounds	1	1
Asthma and bronchitis	1	0
Tension headache	1	1
Postoperative pain	1	0
Neck and back pain	1	$(?+1)^b$
Total	18	10 (2)
Percent of total		56% (11%)

Source: Benor, 1993.

[a]Significance $p<.01$; for values in parentheses, $p<.02-.05$.

[b]Possibly significant results, but faulty reporting or design prevented proper evaluation of the studies.

Research Recommendations

Promising clinical results. While technique, focus, and range of treatments attempted vary considerably, a number of results are common to all forms of the biofield process:

- Acceleration of wound healing.
- Reduction of the pain of thermal burns and acceleration of healing time.
- Reduction of sunburn pain and coloration.
- Reduction of acute and chronic pain.
- Reduction of anxiety.
- Release of pent-up grief.

In addition, practitioners of some forms of the process report consistently good results with:

- recurrent panic attacks;
- premenstrual syndrome;
- posttraumatic stress disorder;
- irritable bowel syndrome;
- nonbiological sexual dysfunction;
- drug, alcohol, and codependence recovery;
- migraine;
- anorexia and bulimia; and
- third-trimester pregnancy and birthing.

Characterization of the biofield. That the biofield has definable form, flux pattern, and polarities seems clear to practitioners from the wealth of empirical evidence available. However, characterization of the biofield is far from complete, and determining its nature is paramount to its further development among the healing arts.

Two hypotheses should be tested: first, that the biofield is a field in physics other than an already known field, and, second, that the biofield is bioelectromagnetism. One approach that would support the first hypothesis would be development of a device (transducer) that would react with the biofield so as to exclude the possibility of bioelectromagnetism. Research projects in China have shown that application of the biofield affects lithium fluoride thermoluminesence detectors, polarized light beams, Van de Graff generators, and silicone crystal plates (Proceedings, 1988). These preliminary experiments suggest possible approaches toward further characterization.

Research design considerations. The following should be considered in planning well-designed studies to evaluate potential effects of biofields on health:

- *Mental healing techniques.* Since mental healing techniques are often mixed with biofield techniques, care must be taken in all research designs to separate out the two factors. Unless this is done, unclear results will prevent reasonable analysis.

Table 29.5. Other Controlled Biofield Studies

Subject	No. of studies	Significant results[a]		
Enzymes	8	3	(+2)	(?+3)[b]
Fungus/yeast	6	4	(+1)	(?+1)[b]
Bacteria	2	?		
Red blood cells	1	1		
Cancer cells	3	1		(?+2)[b]
Snail pacemaker cells	4	4		
Plants	10	7		(?+2)[b]
Motility				
Flagellates	2	0		(?+1)[b]
Algae	2	1		
Moth larvae	1	1		
Mice				
Skin wounds	2	2		
Retardation of goiter growth	2	2		
Total	43	26	(3)	
Percent of total		61%	(7%)	

Source: Benor, 1993.

[a]Significance $p<.01$; for values in parentheses, $p<.02-.05$.

[b]Possibly significant results, but faulty reporting or design prevented proper evaluation of the studies.

- *Sham treatments.* Unlike placebo pills, biofield healing cannot be faked. According to the observations of practitioners, it is not possible to touch subjects in a clinical study in a purely physical way for any period of time without resulting in some effect from the practitioner's biofield. Nor is there a way to shield the biofield emitted by one person from another person's; this renders the notion of a "sham control" meaningless. This particular confounding factor has adversely affected results in several studies of biofield therapeutics (Beal and Pavek, 1985; Meehan, 1988; Parkes, 1985; Quinn, 1989). In these studies, controls were established by effecting a mimic, or sham, of the primary method. The practitioners' hands were brought into close proximity with the subject in a "sham treatment." In all such cases, some positive effect was obtained with the mimic or sham treatments that was greater than could be reasonably expected from no-treatment controls.

- *Double-blind studies.* Although it is not possible for a biofield healing practitioner to perform in a strict double-blind situation, it is possible to design studies in which the evaluators are blinded to the treatment method and subjects are blinded to the method and to the specific intended outcome.

- *Science and metaphysics.* Because the metaphysical model lies, by both definition and practice, outside the usual confines of science, research on metaphysical explanatory models will be difficult. However, outcome studies of clinical effect could be designed and executed.

- *Collaborations.* The process could be speeded up if experienced researchers sympathetic to energy healing work together with researchers experienced in developing appropriate criteria. These criteria must (1) provide the established medical and health communities with valid, reproducible data and (2) be constructed so as not to negate the operative treatment mechanism.

Barriers and Key Issues

Hindrances. For various reasons, biofield healing has been hindered from reaching its fullest potential. Principal among these reasons are the following:

- Until recently, few testable hypotheses.
- Few theoreticians who are also practitioners.

- The disdain of currently established scientists.
- Lack of a solid research base.
- Lack of an adequate outcomes database.
- Unsystematic accumulation of empirical evidence.
- Obscuring of the extent of efficacy by a plethora of conceptual confusions and conflicting claims as to causal factors, best methods, and procedures.

Placebo and efficacy. Some people have attributed any successful applications of biofield therapeutic to a high probability of placebo effect. This assumption has inhibited reviewers and editors from accepting as valid the usual, smaller pilot studies that would be acceptable for other types of therapy.

No studies that have been done, however, indicate that placebo factors are any higher with biofield therapies than with other healing methods. In fact, a number of situations in which placebo effects would have been highly unlikely cast doubt on the concern. Some such studies have had marked, positive results (Benor, 1992) with animals and with small children below the age of reason. There are also numerous anecdotal reports of children receiving treatments while asleep and awakening with marked change. Fevers have broken during such treatments, panic attacks have ceased, and comas have ended (Pavek, 1988).

Such evidence suggests that the reason why biofield treatments are effective is other than the placebo effect.

Peer review. At this time, there are no peer review groups that actually include "peers." True peers, who have a hands-on understanding of biofield therapeutics, should be included on review committees.

Recommendations

Because the stigma associated with "faith healing" has been attached to biofield therapy, it has not been seriously considered as a viable treatment method. Consequently, the discipline languishes in a research doldrum. The following steps are recommended:

1. The biofield should be characterized. Reasonable approaches exist, some of which have been described in this report.

2. Simple and appropriate instruments should be developed to begin the process systematically collecting clinical data. With

properly designed forms, individual case studies could be statistically sorted and grouped by disorder, treatment process, and results. This sorting would begin to establish relative efficacy in the various categories, suggesting productive avenues for future research. To implement this process, OAM should establish a small study group, including members familiar with intake and outcome forms and data collection and representative members of the discipline.

3. Studies should be undertaken to determine how much of biofield therapeutics is attributable to mental healing and how much is attributable to quantity and proper directional application of the biofield flows.

4. Appropriate review panels with actual peers should be established.

5. A number of open technical questions in the discipline should be resolved. OAM should invite the leaders of the various systems to a general meeting to discuss and compare techniques and methods and to begin resolving these questions. Resolving these differences will enhance the techniques of all biofield healing methods.

6. A number of clinical studies that have been done in Europe and in Asia could be replicated here. Replication is necessary to assure the American research community that the studies are valid and to point the way for further research here.

7. A wealth of serious study proposals are available. These should be reviewed, and the most promising should be implemented.

Conclusion

Biofield therapeutics and diagnostics have been struggling to cross the border from metaphysics to physics and gain mainstream acceptance for a long time. In spite of considerable difficulties, biofield methods are gaining acceptance from health professionals and the general public in two areas— (1) the medical clinic and (2) hospital and psychotherapeutic settings. In both, biofield treatments are reported to be of benefit for many people.

Biofield therapeutics are a low-cost, non-invasive, non-drug approach, and applications have been reported in many medical and health situations as alternatives or as complements to mainstream medicine. The potential reward-to-risk ratio is great, and relatively small amounts of money are needed to start a validation process, which should be done with dispatch.

Combined Physical and Biofield Methods

The following methods are described by their practitioners as combining physical and biofield aspects. The list, which is not all-inclusive, tends to be descriptive; little research is available as a basis for judging the usefulness of these methods. Most of them would benefit from research on their efficacy and their scientific bases.

Applied Kinesiology

Applied kinesiology, or "touch for health," consists of both a diagnostic method of determining dysfunctional states of the body and related therapeutics. Based on principles of physiology and the meridian system mentioned earlier, it was developed in the 1960s by George Goodheart. It uses both the meridian qi and the biofield qi in its diagnostics and therapeutics.

Neurolymphatic holding points, neurovascular holding points, meridian holding points, and the biofield external qi are all said to be incorporated in the process. A session starts with various "muscle testings" that are used to determine the state of qi flow through the meridians. Muscle testings give an indication of the area to be worked on and are a necessary part of the treatment.

A number of applied kinesiology practitioners use the process in conjunction with more established practices, such as chiropractic.

Network Chiropractic Spinal Analysis

Network chiropractic spinal analysis (NCSA) merges conventional chiropractic mechanical or structural approaches with biofield approaches to evaluate and correct anomalies of the spine and nervous system. At the clinical core of NCSA is the classification of spinal subluxations into two categories: (1) structural subluxation that involves mechanical dislocation of spinal sections and (2) soft-tissue subluxation that involves tension in the muscles and other soft tissue connected to the spinal sections. NCSA does not address structural subluxations until after a reduction of soft-tissue subluxations has occurred. (It has been noted that structural subluxations often

457

self-correct shortly after soft-tissue subluxations have been adjusted.) Application of the biofield is included for the soft-tissue adjustments and is applied first. Conventional chiropractic adjustments follow, as required, for structural adjustments.

The clinician uses a phased system to introduce order to the subluxated segments. Since the body often creates movement from a tense, restricted state, a spontaneous discharge of tension often occurs as the spinal distortions are resolved; this is a common occurrence. A wide range of responses is then observed with certain common elements. Among the unique individual responses typically seen is a period of deep and full respirations; other responses include periods of muscular movements and naturally occurring postures as the body and mind seek to purge mechanical tension or stored memories of traumatic experiences.

Polarity Therapy

Polarity therapy is a natural health system based on the idea of a "human energy field." Drawing from oriental and Indian sources, it asserts that well-being and health are conditions determined by the nature of the flow of this human energy field and that the flow can be affected by various natural methods. Polarity therapy incorporates a variety of strategies to enhance the flow of the energy field, including touch, diet, movement, and self-awareness. (Polarity practitioners generally believe that the energy field that they are enhancing is electromagnetic, but this point has not been established.)

The central concepts of polarity therapy are as follows:

- All phenomena have a fundamental structure involving charged particles in a relationship of expansion-contraction or attraction-repulsion. In East Asia this relationship is called the tao, or relationship of opposites (yin and yang).

- An "energy anatomy" precedes and creates physical anatomy, and this energy anatomy exists in several layers that are affected, and possibly distorted, by life experience.

- These distortions may be corrected by several methods, including touch, holding pressure points, and using the practitioner's hands to link various "polarities" in the client's body.

Commonly reported benefits of "polarity energy balancing" include relaxation, pain reduction, reduction of nervous conditions, heightened self-awareness, and improvement in range of motion.

Polarity therapy was developed in the 1950s by Randolph Stone, a chiropractor, osteopath, and naturopath. Today the American Polarity Therapy Association, which was founded in 1983, organizes and supports training and certification of practitioners; the association also is developing a research arm. At present there are more than 500 practitioners of polarity therapy, trained at several levels of proficiency.

Qigong Longevity Exercises

The qigong longevity or health exercises are a fairly recent addition to alternative health practices in the United States. Qigong exercises are similar in appearance to tijijuan (tai chi chuan), a rhythmical non-aerobic form of exercise; however, this appearance is only superficial. Qigong movement exercises do not flow from one position to another as in tai chi; they are done in shorter movement groups that are repeated many times. This, however, is not the essence of the practice, but only the visible form.

Qigong exercises combine repetitions of coordinated physical motions with mental concentration and directive efforts to move the qi in the body. During these exercises, which are based on slow, repetitive movements of the arms, legs, and torso, the exerciser's mind is focused on moving the qi (biofield flux) through the meridian pathways and non-meridian pathways that were developed by the ancient Taoist (Daoist) sages.

This mental effort is coordinated with specific movements; for example, qi may be directed up the back as the arms are raised and down the front as the arms are lowered. Large amounts of internal qi are said to be developed in the process. It is estimated that there are more than 100 different forms of qigong health exercises. There are considerable differences in the styles, but all consider the mental effort to be crucial. Qigong exercises are used daily for health improvement by several million Chinese, both in the People's Republic and in Chinese communities throughout Southeast Asia.

Qigong exercises are also used by qigong masters (see the "Biofield Therapeutics" section) to increase the quantity of qi available for healing; some use it in various forms of martial arts such as gongfu (kung fu).

In China, qigong exercises have been under study for their long-term effects on a number of medical conditions, such as cancer and arthritis, and for their effects on general health. More than 32 studies were recently presented at just one major conference on the effects on general and specific states of health of exercises enhancing qigong qi (Proceedings, 1988).

Several schools and organizations in this country focus entirely on these practices. The principal ones are China Advocates, the Chinese National Chi Kung Institute, the Qigong Academy, and the Qigong Institute. The practice of qigong is gaining in popularity in the United States both with Asians and non-Asians.

Craniosacral Therapy

Craniosacral therapy is a gentle, hands-on treatment method that focuses on alleviating restrictions to physiological motion of all the bones of the skull, including the face and mouth, as well as the vertebral column, sacrum, coccyx, and pelvis. Concurrently, the craniosacral therapist focuses as well on normalizing abnormal tensions and stresses in the meningeal membrane, with special attention to the outermost membrane, the dura mater, and its fascial connections. Attention is also paid to alleviating any obstacles to free movement by the cerebrospinal fluid within its membrane compartment and to normalizing and balancing perceived related energy fields. This approach is derived from experiments of John Upledger, an osteopathic physician and researcher (for example, see Upledger, 1977a and 1977b, which are discussed below).

As usually practiced, this therapy is a non-invasive treatment process that requires an uninterrupted treatment session of at least 30 minutes; often the session is extended beyond an hour. Practitioners indicate that successful treatment relies largely on the therapist's ability to facilitate the patient's own self-corrective processes within the craniosacral system. Postgraduate training in craniosacral therapy has been undertaken by a wide variety of physicians, dentists, and therapists. In the United States during 1993, 2,738 health care professionals completed the Upledger Institute's introductory-level workshop and seminar; 1,827 received training at the intermediate level, and 80 completed the advanced level. Training outside this country is available through the Upledger Institute Europe in the Netherlands and on a smaller scale in Japan, New Zealand, France, and Norway by American Upledger Institute teachers.

The most powerful effects of craniosacral therapy are considered to be on the function of the central nervous system, the immune system, the endocrine system, and the visceral organs via the autonomic nervous system. This therapy has been used with reported success in many cases of brain and spinal cord dysfunction. Although these successes have not been documented in formal studies, they have been observed subjectively or anecdotally by both patients and therapists. Most prominent among these success reports are cases of brain injury resulting in symptoms of spastic paralysis and seizure. Other areas of claimed success include cerebral palsy, learning disabilities, seizure disorders, depressive reactions, menstrual dysfunction, motor dysfunction, strabismus (a vision disorder), temporomandibular joint problems, various headaches, chronic pain problems, and chronic fatigue syndrome.

Research on tissues has documented the potential for movement between skull bones in adult humans, and pilot work with live primates has shown rhythmical movement of their skull bones. Interrater reliability studies, which look for correlations in the observations of two or more independent raters (see the "Osteopathic Medicine" section), have shown agreement between "blinded" therapists evaluating preschool-aged children ("blinding" means that the therapists making the observations did not know which children had received craniosacral therapy, nor did they know the history or problems of the children) (Upledger, 1977a). Controlled studies have shown high correlation between schoolchildren with various brain dysfunctions and specific dysfunctions of the craniosacral system; that is, the craniosacral exam scores correlated with recorded school teacher and psychologist opinions of "not normal," behavioral problems, motor coordination problems, learning disabilities, and obstetrical complications (Upledger, 1977b). Moreover, Upledger reports that a few pilot studies by dentists have demonstrated significant changes in the transverse dimension of the hard palate as well as in occlusion in response to craniosacral therapy.

At present, work is under way that appears to demonstrate fluctuations in what are called energy measurements in circuits between craniosacral therapists and patients. The circuits are established by attaching electrodes to the patient and the therapist with an ohmmeter and a voltmeter interposed in the circuits. In observations with 22 patients, measurements have ranged from more than 30 million ohms at the start of a treatment session to 448 ohms with a brain-injured child; voltages have fluctuated between 10 and 254 millivolts. Upledger's interpretation is that the elevation in resistances read with the ohmmeter correlate with the palpable resistances that craniosacral therapists feel with their hands and that the energy put into overcoming these resistances is reflected by elevations in the millivolt readings. On the basis of these preliminary studies, plans are under way to explore further whether the energetic changes measured in the circuits accompany specific landmarks in treatment processes.

Physical Therapy: An Example of Transition to Mainstream Health Care

Physical therapists are health care professionals who diagnose and treat problems related to physical function. While physical therapy is considered to be a part of mainstream medicine in this country, its practitioners frequently use manual healing methods that are categorized as alternative. Many of the methods identified in other sections of this chapter are part of the standard repertoire of physical therapy. The development of the profession and its transition into mainstream health care are discussed in this section. Some of the alternative procedures and the difficulties encountered in training for them are noted.

Background

Physical therapy is a relatively young profession in comparison with medicine and nursing, although its roots lie in ancient Rome and Greece. Its modern embodiment appeared at about the time of World War I, through the creation of the Women's Auxiliary Medical Aides, renamed Medical Aides and then again Reconstruction Aides, in the Office of the Surgeon General of the Army. Physical therapy training programs existed in France and England at this time under the name physiotherapy, a term that is still used in most Western nations outside the United States. It quickly became apparent that the United States also needed to train its own people in new ways to assist the war wounded. Few, if any, professionals who were trained in medicine or nursing at that time could deal with physical, vocational, and psychological problems associated with injuries sustained in war (Ramsden, 1978).

Educational preparation in 1917 consisted of 4-month sessions after graduation from high school but quickly moved to 12-month sessions that followed preparation in nursing or physical education. Since the 1920s, preparation for practice has shifted from an apprentice model to an academic model and from clinic-based education to universities. Currently, 50 percent of entry-level degrees are awarded at the master's degree level. Not included are master's degrees in physical therapy awarded to people already trained in the field. The professional doctorate—the D.P.T.—is available at three universities.

Adversity stimulated the growth of the profession, with major spurts during both world wars and during the polio epidemics in 1914, 1916, and the 1940s. Then a new creativity in prosthetics and orthotics in conjunction with physical therapy treatment evolved in response to the problems of thalidomide-affected babies after the belated recognition in 1961 that thalidomide was a teratogen (a substance affecting embryonic development). Thalidomide was given to pregnant women, primarily in Great Britain, to treat nausea, or "morning sickness."

The startling growth of physical therapy as a profession in the 1980s and l990s may be explained by many factors, including documented effectiveness of treatment of patients of all ages. The targets of treatment include virtually all problems affecting normal function resulting from trauma and illness as well as those resulting from genetically transmitted disease, trauma sustained in childbirth, developmental delay, and normal and abnormal consequences of aging.

The number of schools in the United States preparing men and women for the profession of physical therapy is now 140, with approximately 5,000 graduates each year (American Physical Therapy Association, 1993). There are additional schools at various stages in the accreditation process. Previously made up entirely of women from physical education and nursing, the professional ranks today include approximately 30 percent men. The curriculums draw applicants from a wide variety of academic backgrounds, including fine arts, basic science, humanities, behavioral sciences, engineering, and business. Membership in the American Physical Therapy Association is approximately 60,000, which is half the total number of practicing physical therapists in the United States.

The number of graduates from academic programs does not begin to meet society's need for physical therapy services. Because professional practice is relatively autonomous, physical therapists frequently work in private practice. Growing sophistication and autonomy have led to a nationwide effort by members of the profession to seek legislative changes in State practice acts to permit practice without referral. Twenty-eight States have enacted such legislation. Real shortages of physical therapists exist in many health care institutions; it is one of the professions having the greatest number of vacant positions in the Nation.

Current Practice

Physical therapists are licensed health care professionals. The therapist's normal scope of work for any given client involves evaluating the patient, identifying potential problems, and determining the diagnoses that are related to physical function; then the therapist establishes objectives or goals, provides treatment services, evaluates the effectiveness of treatment, and makes any modifications necessary to achieve the desired outcome.

Therapeutic interventions focus on posture, movement, strength, endurance, cardiopulmonary function, balance, coordination, joint mobility, flexibility, pain, healing and repair, and functional ability in daily living skills, including work.

Among the therapeutic activities included are therapeutic exercise; application of assistive devices; physical agents, such as heat and cold; ultrasound; electricity, such as electromyography and electrical muscle stimulation; manual procedures, such as joint and soft-tissue mobilization; neuromuscular reeducation; bronchopulmonary hygiene; and ambulation training with and without assistive devices.

This professional activity may take place in a wide variety of settings, including neonatal nurseries, intensive care units, bedside acute care, rehabilitation units, outpatient clinics, private offices, private homes, physical fitness or sports facilities, and schools. In addition to providing direct service, physical therapists are also involved in health maintenance programs and illness prevention programs, health policy development, administration, education, research, consultation, and other advisory services.

Physical therapists also apply many of the therapeutic interventions identified and discussed elsewhere in this chapter. Therapists using these procedures consider them fundamental tools in their repertoire. Among these procedures are acupressure, myofascial release, craniosacral therapy, massage techniques, Alexander technique, Feldenkrais method, and therapeutic touch.

Such procedures are rarely included in the academic preparation of physical therapy students. Rather, they may be learned through special programs with a select group of practitioners who conduct continuing education experiences throughout the country. Perhaps the inclusion of these procedures in the clinical practice of physical therapy is evidence of the belief by a growing segment in the profession that mind and body are connected, but we do not know or understand all the connections.

Several of these systems seem to share common threads. The therapy is aimed at restoring the homeostasis of a person's body-mind-spirit, using a comprehensive and holistic approach. The emphasis is on promotion of health, prevention of illness, and education approaches.

Philosophy

The philosophy of physical therapy is based on an educational model; the objective is to help individual patients help themselves to attain the maximum level of function they are capable of. The decisions about treatment—what to do, when to do it, and how much—are not made only on the basis of experience with what "works." A general understanding of the effects of an approach for a given condition is not adequate justification for applying that method.

The professional literature of physical therapy that appears in several refereed journals documents evidence of the efficacy, or lack thereof, of particular treatment interventions. Both quantitative and qualitative research methods are used with increasing sophistication. A major effort by physical therapists in academic and clinical leadership positions and by the professional association has contributed to the prominence of this kind of documentation for a wide variety of physical therapy interventions.

Current Research

Responding to a research mandate may be difficult for some physical therapists who are using procedures that are less well-known and not generally included in the traditional academic preparation (Hariharan, 1993). Research may be even more difficult for therapists whose work is entirely clinical and whose academic preparation did not include training in research methodology appropriate for clinical practice (Soderberg, 1991). Nevertheless, the research mandate for the profession today is clear: do it if it works, document carefully what has been done, develop careful research studies to determine the mechanisms involved, publish the results, and continue the research until everyone understands what is being done and why. As a corollary, a corresponding need has arisen for physical therapists to obtain training in research methodology.

Physical therapist researchers currently publish in major medical journals as well as the journal *Physical Therapy*. The research covers a wide range of subjects related to clinical practice and the underlying mechanisms of function (Bohannon, 1986). Recently published work on the following subjects illustrates the range: physical therapy treatment of peripheral vestibular dysfunction based on clinical case reports; impact of three posting methods on controlling abnormal subtalar pronation; a comparison of three different respiratory exercises in prevention of postoperative pulmonary complications after upper abdominal surgery; motor unit behavior in Parkinson's disease; a study of age and training on skeletal muscle physiology and on performance; a study of the factors associated with burnout of physical therapists working in a specific work environment; and a study of the discrete behaviors that differentiate the expert from the novice physical therapist.

Summary

Physical therapy began with a few women who trained briefly and learned on the job how to help care for seriously injured soldiers. The group grew dramatically, and the length of training increased as the scope of work became apparent and the amount of knowledge to impart expanded. With the knowledge and technology explosions, physical therapy became more sophisticated and moved into the mainstream of health care, contributing in significant ways to patient care and to the literature of research and practice.

Overall Recommendations

Research on manual healing methods is needed in four parallel and interactive directions:

- To determine the range of clinical benefits for the many common physical complaints and problems treated by therapists using these methods (e.g., back pain, headache, whiplash, and chronic fatigue syndrome).

- To determine the degree to which a general sense of well-being is enhanced by the various manual healing methods.

- To evaluate the effect of structural manipulation on body awareness (both visceral and external); regulation of motion; range of movement; ability to cope with stress; muscle tone and flexibility; growth, development, and aging; autonomic function (neural control systems); electrical patterns in muscles; immune system response; and cardiovascular and respiratory function.

- To determine the physiological and neurological mechanisms associated with specific manual healing methods.

[1]Robert Ward, an experienced osteopathic physician-researcher, estimated that 10 percent of osteopathic physicians use manual diagnosis and treatment a great deal and that some 60 percent use them in selected cases. Ward believes most patients receiving primary care from osteopaths probably receive a diagnostic workup involving manual diagnosis at some time, particularly if neuromusculoskeletal problems have been reported (Ward, 1994).

[2]The energetic and oriental manual techniques are categorized by some as massage techniques. However, in this chapter the energetic

techniques are addressed in the "Biofields Therapeutics" section and the "Combined Physical and Biofield Methods" section, and the oriental techniques are addressed in the remainder of the "Physical Healing Methods" section. The energetic methods are considered to affect the biofield—a field that is described as surrounding and infusing the human body—by pressure and/or manipulation of the physical body or by the passage or placement of the hands in, or through, that energetic field. These methods are based on traditional Ayurvedic, Eastern or Western esoteric, modern therapeutic, or other recognized and accepted systems of healing. Examples are polarity therapy and therapeutic touch. The oriental methods of treatment use pressure and manipulation based on traditional East Asian medical principles to assess and evaluate the energetic system (Jwing-Ming, 1992) or to provide actual treatment that affects and balances the energetic system. Examples are tuina (or tui-na), shiatsu, acupressure, an-mo, and jin shin do.

[3]These depictions can be seen in the Third Dynasty exhibit in the National Museum, Cairo, Egypt.

[4]The differences between direct and indirect contact are analogous to the two methods of illuminating a neon light. The first is to place the neon bulb in a strong electromagnetic field. This is the simpler way, as it requires no wiring or particular orientation; the bulb will glow wherever it is placed. However, a great deal of power is required for a given light output, and the light fluctuates sharply with small fluctuations in the field. The second method is to connect the neon bulb into an electric circuit. This method requires wires and knowledge of how to connect the bulb correctly; it produces much more light with far less power, but the light is less likely to fluctuate. Similarly, the biofield is described as having both external field and internal circuitry.

[5]SHEN® stands for Specific Human Energy Nexus. SHEN® therapy is described by Pavek as a biofield method of treating the so-called psychosomatic and related disorders by releasing repressed and suppressed debilitating emotions directly from the body.

[6]Quigong exercises are repetitive physical motions coordinated with breath and mental efforts to move the qi through meridians and other "channels." They are gaining popularity in the United States. (See the "Combined Physical and Biofield Methods" section.)

[7]Flow is much slower through human tissue and varies with the person's health and emotional state.

[8]An erroneous report, "New Technologies Detect Effects of Healing Hands, in *Brain/Mind Bulletin*, vol. 10, no. 16, contributed to this supposition when it stated that one researcher, John Zimmerman, had measured electromagnetic effects of healers' hands during healing with a SQUID (superconducting quantum interference device); actually, he made his measurements at the healers' heads while measuring very low amplitude electromagnetic brainwave activity.

[9]No one has yet been able to detect either current flow or electromagnetic flux emanating from the hands of a practitioner. Dry skin electrical impedance at the hands is quite high, 210 megohms (10 million ohms). Silver/silver chloride electrodes, as used in biofeedback, measure skin conduction, not flux emanations.

Chapter 30

Massage

Massage is a manual technique which uses a variety of strokes to move the muscles and soft tissue of the body. The movements break up the fibrous tissue, loosen stiff joints and clear them of acids and deposits. The massage strokes can also affect the blood, lymph and nervous system.

Massage aims to alleviate pain and then to rebalance and strengthen the affected area.

When giving a massage the room and the therapist's hands should be warm, and only parts of the body being worked on are exposed. A pure oil can be used for the massage and, if appropriate additional training has been undertaken, essential oils can be added.

A massage should be a pleasant experience, but there are therapists who believe that some pain may be necessary in order to release tensions in the body. People who are having a massage should feel able to discuss how much pain they are able to accept and to indicate how vigorous a massage they prefer. A whole-body massage usually takes about one hour. There are many different types of therapeutic massage, each of which place a different emphasis on different elements of the therapy. Intuitive massage, for example, emphasizes the importance of 'getting in touch' with the client's tensions and emotional state. Holistic massage, however, places the treatment within a broader framework of the client's life.

Some of the most commonly used massage strokes are illustrated here.

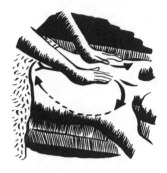

Figure 30.1. Effleurage

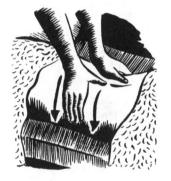

Figure 30.2. Deeper pressure strokes (such as petrissage)

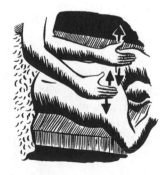

Figure 30.3. Tapotement (such as hacking or cupping)

Giving a Simple Hand Massage

This technique can safely be used, among friends and colleagues, but should not be offered to patients.

Make your friend or colleague comfortable and ensure his or her hands are easily accessible. This sequence can be done with or without oil, but if oil is used, make sure the receiver's clothes will not become stained: roll up his or her sleeves and place a towel under his or her hands. Gently take one hand and massage gently around the wrist with your thumbs. Hold the receiver's hand palm up and stroke the palm with the heel of your other hand. Then turn the hand over and support it with the fingers of both your hands while you stroke the back of the receiver's hand with your thumbs. Next wring and stretch each finger in turn, and complete the massage by gently stroking the receiver's arms and hands.

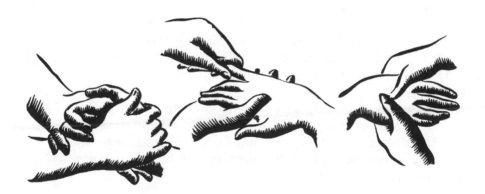

Figure 30.4. Simple Hand Massage

Historical Background

Massage as a therapy is known to have been used by the Chinese as far back as 3000 years BC, and there are references to massage in the *Ayur Veda*, an Indian text written in 1800 BC.

In the West, the value of massage was first described by Hippocrates. Other ancient Greek converts to massage included Homer, Plato and Socrates.

The Roman physician Celsus used to recommend massage for a variety of conditions and Pliny had regular massage for his asthma. In the second century AD Galen was recommending massage to the gladiators of Pergamum, before and after exercise, something we now know helps prevent sports injuries by warming and loosening the muscles.

Massage decreased in popularity in the Middle Ages but by the Renaissance it was popular again. For example, Ambroise Pare (1517-1590), physician to four French monarchs, was a keen exponent of the art.

In the 19th century a Swedish doctor, Per Hendrik Ling (1776-1839), developed a scientific system of massage, the Swedish movement treatment, which became popular with the medical profession. The techniques he described have been incorporated within most forms of massage offered today. As technology improved, however, the power of touch became neglected and it was not until the recent boom in complementary therapies that therapeutic massage again became popular.

Claims

As massage is associated with relieving stress by relaxing the muscles and hence the whole of the body, it is thought to be helpful in treating stress-related problems such as insomnia, headaches and backache.

Therapists also claim that massage can help with problems such as high blood pressure, arthritic and rheumatic pain, asthma, colds, constipation, depression, muscular strain and sciatica. Massage is strongly associated with health promotion inducing, as it can, a sense of well-being and relaxation.

Contraindications

Massage should not be undertaken in the following situations:

- If the client has eaten within two hours, has an infectious disease, high fever or acute inflammation

- If the client has a serious health problem such as heart disease or cancer, or has recently undergone surgery (unless consent from the appropriate consultant has been given)

- If the client is in the first three months of pregnancy. During the remaining six months, only gentle massage should be offered, avoiding the ankles, lower back and pelvic area.

472

Scar tissue, varicose veins, bruising, tender or inflammed areas, and sites of recent fractures should not be massaged directly. Clients should not drink alcohol or take non-prescription drugs before or straight after a massage.

If there is any doubt about the appropriateness of offering massage to a client, expert advice should be sought.

Research

As with many complementary (alternative) therapies, there is still a dearth of good research into the therapeutic value of massage. The following list of studies is not comprehensive, but aims to give the reader an idea of the range of research that has been undertaken.

- Premature babies given three 15-minute massages during three consecutive hours per day for 10 days averaged a 21 percent weight gain per day (34 versus 28) and were discharged five days earlier than babies assigned to the control group.

  Scafidi, F.S., Field, T.M., Schanberg, S.M. et al. Massage stimulates growth in pre-term infants: a replication. *Infant Behaviour and Development* 1990; 13: 167-188.

- In a study of 52 hospitalized, depressed children and adolescents with adjustment disorders, those who received a daily 30-minute back massage over a five-day period were found to be less depressed and anxious and had lower saliva cortisol levels than the control group who simply viewed videotapes.

  Nurses also reported that night-time sleep improved among the massage group, and the urinary cortisol and norepinephrine levels decreased among the depressed patients who received massage.

  Field, T., Morrow, C., Vaideon, C. et al. Massage reduces anxiety in child and adolescent psychiatric patients. *Journal of the American Academy of Childhood and Adolescent Psychiatry* 1992; 31: 1,125-131.

- Twenty-one elderly people who were residents in a home were randomly allocated to three groups: those who received back massage with normal conversation, those who received conversation only and those who received no intervention.

473

There was a statistically insignificant decrease in mean scores of anxiety levels, electromyographic recordings and systolic blood pressure in the back massage group.

There was a statistically significant difference in the mean anxiety scores between the back massage group and the no-intervention group. The difference in anxiety scores between the back massage group and the conversation-only group approached statistical significance.

Fraser, J.. Kerr, J.R. Psychophysiological effects of back massage on elderly institutionalized patients. *Journal of Advanced Nursing* 1993; 18: 238-245.

- Other research studies conducted over recent years include:

Avakyan, G.N. Pressure and massage therapy to relieve fatigue. *Advanced Clinical Care* 1990; 5: 5, 10-11.

Kampschroeder, F. Trigger point and transfictional massage: a care report. *Chiropractic* 1990; 6: 2, 40-42.

Li, Y. Facial cosmetic massage. *Journal of Traditional Chinese Medicine* 1990; 10: 3, 219-221.

Puustjarvi, K. The effects of massage in patients with chronic tension headache. *Acupuncture and Electrotherapy Research* 1990; 15:2,159-162.

Shao, X. Effect of massage and temperature on the permeability of initial lymphatics. *Lymphology* 1990; 23: 1,48-50.

Implications for Nursing

Massage is already being used to benefit patients in a variety of health-care settings —either by nurses, midwives or health visitors who have undertaken training, or by professional massage therapists.

It is also a therapy that can be beneficial to health-care staff—a five-minute neck-and-shoulder massage may release tension and pains which were making a shift seem twice as long.

If you want to begin incorporating massage into the care you give to your patients, however, a thorough training is necessary.

Examples of the use of massage in the health service include:

In intensive care:

Caroline Stevenson, an intensive care sister at the Middlesex Hospital in London has introduced massage in her unit with good results and helps train nurses from the health authority in massage techniques.

Stevenson, C. Holistic power. *Nursing Times* 1992;88:38,68-70.

In the care of the dying:

As a staff nurse at Mount Edgcumbe Hospice in St Austell, Rosemary Byass offers massage to patients. She believes it is a "beneficial, holistic and harmless means of helping patients 'live until they die,' and it only requires empathy and a pair of hands."

Byass, R. Soothing body and soul. *Nursing Times* 1988; 84:24, 39-41.

In health visiting:

Gill Thornton is a health visitor working in Wickham. After training at the London College of Massage she offers massage privately and takes patients referred to her by the GP. She also teaches baby massage at antenatal classes.

In general practice:

Jackie Pietroni is a nurse tutor. After training at the Clare Maxwell Hudson School of Massage she has held regular massage clinics at her husband's GP surgery in Ealing since 1991. The clinics are part of the surgery's health promotion initiatives and are very popular.

Pietroni, J. NHS funds GP massage clinic. *Massage* 1991, 3:1.

—by Joanna Trevelyan

Joanna Trevelyan is deputy editor, *Nursing Times*

Chapter 31

Rolfing:
Realigning Body and Mind

For Bren Jacobsen, pain was the mother of inspiration.

A director of a meditation center in Buffalo, N.Y., in 1970, Mr. Jacobsen was injured in a car accident that resulted in constant neck and shoulder pain. He sought relief from acupuncturists, chiropractors and physical therapists.

Then he got Rolfed—and his pain vanished. Duly impressed, he became a Rolfer himself.

"Rolfing works where nothing else does, and the results last," Mr. Jacobsen, 55, says in his Annapolis office.

Rolfing employs deep-tissue manipulation to improve a person's posture and well-being. Named after its developer, American biochemist Ida Rolf, the method was invented in the 1940s with the aim of treating the whole person, not just certain symptoms. The technique involves deep-tissue manipulation and alignment that straighten and balances the body and bring it in balance with the person's mind.

Today scores of celebrities and sports figures swear by its effectiveness:

- Olympic skaters Brian Orser, Michelle Kwan and Elvis Stojko say it gives them an edge in their performances.

- Pianist Leon Fleisher, who suffered from repetitive motion syndrome for 22 years, now plays with both hands.

- Operatic soprano Patricia Johnson noticed that her voice "opened up" after a few Rolfing sessions.

"It is amazing how the body responds, how your body continues to unravel after the treatment" says Jean Canale, 39, of Annapolis. She was Rolfed by Mr. Jacobsen two years ago for a neck and shoulder ache.

Rolfing involves straightening and balancing the body, helping it to adjust properly to gravity, Mr. Jacobsen says, adding that the treatment links body and mind, improves physical performance and fosters a balanced psyche.

"By straightening the person, the body will have support from gravity instead of fighting it, which causes pain," says the advanced Rolfer, who uses his hands to manipulate deep tissue, lengthen and loosen muscles, and bring the body into alignment.

Mr. Jacobsen studied the practice at the Rolf Institute in Boulder, Colo., where he received his practitioner certificate in 1977.

Since then, he has Rolfed and talked about Rolfing all over the world. One of 39 active Rolfers in Maryland, Virginia and the District, he is scheduled next month to address the Washington Ethical Society on the topic.

(The United States has 847 Rolfers, according to the Rolf Institute and the Guild for Structural Integration.)

Some New Age adherents have ascribed almost mystical attributes to Rolfing, saying it releases the physical "memory" of negative emotions and events residing deep in muscle tissue, thus creating happier humans.

But Mr. Jacobsen says Rolfing is just a good physical experience.

"Some results of Rolfing are that people get rid of their pain, get more energy, are better able to cope with stress and anxiety, look better and take care of themselves better since they become more aware of what's happening in their body," he says.

A Rolfing treatment is done in 10 sessions of 90 minutes each, with a fee of $95 per session.

Kim Weiss, 28, of Annapolis says she has a strong back from her work as a nurse, but she felt her pelvis was out of alignment after two pregnancies. She is halfway through her treatment with Mr. Jacobsen.

"I have noticed a big improvement. I exercise a lot, and I can jog better now. Rolfing is good for runners since it improves alignment and flexibility," says Miss Weiss, who is trying to make a career as a model.

Mr. Jacobsen notes the different reasons that clients seek his services. Some "people come to get Rolfed because it makes them look better," he says. "You look taller and slimmer when aligned, and will move more gracefully since you are better balanced and grounded"

David Canale, 39, says he has been Rolfed to cope better with all the stress from his work as a lawyer.

"At least 70 percent of everything doctors see people for is stress-related problems," Mr. Jacobsen says. "Rolfing is tremendously anti-stress."

Dr. Jacob Teitelbaum, a board-certified internist, says Rolfing can be helpful in relieving headaches, back pains, even fibromyalgia—the mysterious symptoms of exhaustion and body aches often associated with chronic fatigue syndrome.

"The work [Mr. Jacobsen] does is superb," says Dr. Teitelbaum, who heads a fibromyalgia research clinic in Annapolis. "People who have suffered from chronic pain for 20 years will be amazed at how their pain goes away."

The 46-year-old physician has specialized in chronic pain and sought Mr. Jacobsen's services for his own bout with fibromyalgia.

"Rolfing is a very powerful tool, and a very important tool for me to have for my patients, and I know I feel better," Dr. Teitelbaum says, adding that the treatment even cured his snoring.

—by Elin Walfridsson

Chapter 32

Chiropractic

Chiropractic (from the Greek *cheiro* and *praktikos*, meaning done by hand) is a manipulative therapy that seeks to diagnose and correct disorders of function associated with joints and the tissues of which they are comprised. Most treatment centers on the spine, which, because of its close relationship with the nervous system, is believed to be intimately connected with a whole range of health problems, should there be any misalignment.

Chiropractors claim to be practitioners of holistic medicine in that they treat the whole person, not simply the presenting problem.

Historical Background

Spinal manipulation as a therapy has existed since at least Hippocrates' time, and possibly much earlier[1]; variations, such as the native American practice of "backwalking," have been noted in many cultures[2]. During the Middle Ages, there arose a group of healers in Europe known as "bone-setters," who practiced manipulation of joints for a range of ailments, and they flourished in Britain until the early years of the 20th century[3]. In the last quarter of the 19th century, in the USA a form of spinal manipulation called "osteopathy" appeared, which was to win many adherents.

Chiropractic was the invention of Canadian Daniel David Palmer, who had a special interest in the spine and developed a theory that misalignments of the vertebrae could be at the root of many medical conditions.

In 1895, 21 years after the principles of osteopathy were first described, Palmer performed his first documented chiropractic treatment. A man who said he had been deaf for 17 years following an accident when he hurt his neck lifting received three manipulations, and his hearing allegedly returned.

Palmer set up a school to teach his method and was imprisoned for practicing medicine without a license. His son, B.J. Palmer, developed the theory further, but different schools of thought led to schisms within the fledgling profession.

The first US state license was granted by Kansas in 1913; now all US states recognize chiropractic as a valid therapy, as do Australia, Canada, New Zealand and several other countries. In Europe, Denmark, Sweden, Switzerland, Norway, Liechtenstein and, until its split, the former Yugoslavia have chiropractic legislation.

The British Chiropractors' Association, forerunner of the British Chiropractic Association (BCA) was formed in 1925, and the therapy enjoyed some success until the founding of the NHS in 1948 saw the end of the Approved Health Insurance Societies, many of which had been willing to pay for chiropractic treatment. Under the new rules, only treatment provided within the NHS was free to users. An application by the BCA to join the NHS in 1974 was rejected, but the profession received a boost three years later when the General Medical Council ruled that, providing doctors retained ultimate clinical responsibility, they could officially refer their patients to a chiropractor when appropriate

A major survey of the use of "nonorthodox" therapies, undertaken by public health researchers at Sheffield University and published in the British Medical Journal in 1991[5], found that over three-quarters of the people seeking help from complementary therapies did so for musculoskeletal problems; this suggests that there is considerable demand for the kind of therapy that chiropractors offer.

How it Works

The theory behind chiropractic is, on the surface, quite simple: if there is any malfunction of the vertebrae leading to restricted, excessive or in any way abnormal movement within the spinal column, then the result will be a bodily malfunction. The spine, chiropractors point out provides protection for a large part of the central nervous system—the spinal cord—and although the link is not always completely understood, problems with vertebral alignment can manifest themselves in a whole range of sensory, organic, vascular and muscular problems. Chiropractic involves manipulation of joints, with the aim of restoring function, and a teacher of the technique suggests that this works on three levels[6]:

- Mechanical/anatomical: restoring movement by improving anatomical relationships and functions through a variety of spinal manipulation and joint mobilization techniques

- Neurological/reflexive: specific soft and hard tissue (joint muscles and fascia) manipulations that change nerve signalling patterns and therefore physiological functioning

- Mental/emotional: the healing aspects of human contact, its hands-on methodology and its effects on the mind and motivation of a patient.

Chiropractors use the term "biomechanics" in explaining their techniques. This implies that mechanical function (or dysfunction) in the body is intimately related to biological function, both in health and illness.

The aim of treatment is to identify any areas of the spine where movement is in any way abnormal, establish the reason or reasons for this abnormality and if manipulation is an appropriate treatment, to attempt to restore normal movement.

What it Claims to Do

About half of all chiropractic consultations are made because of low back pain, including hip problems, and around 40 percent deal with head, neck and chest pain, including cervical spondylosis and migraines. The remainder is made up of people seeking treatment for problems with wrist, ankle, knee and elbow problems and health problems that do not, at first sight, appear to have much connection with joints, such as asthma, dysmenorrhoea and disorders of the gastrointestinal tract[4,7]; chiropractors believe that such conditions can result from restricted joint movement.

Contraindications

Because of the damage that can be caused by spinal manipulation, qualified practitioners are very careful about what conditions they treat.

Inflammation in and infections of the spine, and any neoplastic disease in the area, are absolute contraindications. Osteoporosis, ligament damage and fractures call for the avoidance of certain techniques, and circulatory problems such as the presence of an aneurysm or advanced arteriosclerotic disease, also impose a requirement for extra caution in treatment.

Technique

The first two steps in treatment are the collection of a detailed history, including as much information as possible about the person's lifestyle, and a series of general observations of posture and gait. After this, the principal diagnostic tools are, unsurprisingly, the practitioner's hands, but X-rays are also widely used. Qualified chiropractors are extremely cautious about inappropriate treatment and may well, at this stage, refer the patient to a doctor if the condition is not one amenable to chiropractic. Once diagnosis has been reached, a treatment regime can begin. This may include:

Mobilization. The person is asked to move the joint as far as they can until they reach the end of their range of active movement. Mobilization involves the chiropractor exerting enough force to take the joint a little further until the end of the range of passive movement is reached.

Manipulation. When a joint has been passively moved as far as it will go, the resistance encountered can be overcome by manipulation, in which further force is applied until the joint surfaces are moved apart This may be accompanied by a sound like that made by people "cracking their knuckles," when carbon dioxide is freed from the synovial fluid that bathes the joint.

Manipulation, or "adjustment," as it is called, is a precise skill, as a very slight over-exertion of force could damage the joint.

There are 36 different adjustments but the two most used are classed as dynamic (high-velocity thrust) or recoil. A chiropractor describes the difference in the following way. In a recoil adjustment, the patient lies in a neutral and relaxed position, often face down on the treatment table.

The chiropractor makes contact with the edge of her palm on a specific joint to be adjusted and removes any slack from the skin. This thrust has a high speed but a low amplitude or depth in order to avoid any damage to the structures in the area.

With the dynamic or high-velocity thrust adjustment, the part of the body being adjusted has to be positioned so that the joint is at the limit of its active range of motion.

For the lower back, this requires the patient to lie on one side with the upper body twisted in the opposite direction to the pelvis to introduce an element of rotation and lateral flexion to the spine. This in turn brings the spinal joints to the limit of their active range of movement. By causing a counter-rotation on the spine, achieved by varying the extent to which the hips and knees are bent, a point of tension can be obtained at which the chiropractor makes a specific contact with her hand on the area to be adjusted.

She then carefully turns the patient's body so that the joint is taken through its range of movement to the elastic barrier of resistance (the point at which manipulation needs to be applied, if further movement is to be effected).

The chiropractor applies a small thrust, again of high speed but short amplitude. The thrust is given in a specific direction in order to restore normal spinal and joint mechanics and function and integrity. It may be necessary to repeat this action at more than one level in the lumbar spine and first on one side and then the other.

Note: although the chiropractor is referred to as "she" in this example, approximately two-thirds of practitioners are male.

What the chiropractor is treating is a perceived alteration in the normal function of a motor unit (a joint and all its associated structures); this is sometimes called a fixation. This does not mean that the joint is actually "fixed" or immobile; rather, that there is some degree of restriction on normal movement, that which in turn can have effects on tissues at some distance from it. Fixations can be divided into three types:

1. **Static motor unit fixations**—the joint is fixed in flexion, extension, lateral flexion or rotation.

2. **Kinetic motor unit fixations**—the joint cannot move freely—it is hypomobile—and to compensate other motor units become hypermobile.

3. **Structural alterations**—as the term implies, the fixation results from an alteration in the spine's normal shape (for example, kyphosis or "dowager's hump," in which the thoracic spine curves outward) or scoliosis, where the spine curves sideways. Postural problems may also be implicated.

Chiropractors believe that the causes of fixations fall into three groups:

1. **Mechanical**—for example, trauma or the use of badly designed chairs and beds;

2. **Chemical**—this includes allergic reactions and nutritional problems;

3. **Psychological**—the chief of these being stress.

Establishing the cause of the presenting problem is a priority in the chiropractor's initial assessment; with this grouping of causes it can be seen that the history-taking has to be very wide-ranging to elicit all relevant information.

Research

In 1963, the American Medical Association formed a "Committee on Quackery" and its final verdict on chiropractic was that it was "an unscientific cult." As one author notes, "the hostility of the medical establishment forced chiropractic to get its scientific act together"[2]

Palmer established a research center in 1935 in the USA, and although his work lacked the hallmarks of scientific rigor expected today, "the seeds of research planted by him . . . were reaped in the 1970s and 1980s when a small band of researchers applied scientific principles to the examination of chiropractic theories, this time to dramatic and positive effect."[4]

In 1974 the Canadian Memorial Chiropractic College in Toronto established the Chiropractic Research Abstracts Collection, which forms an index of international research; a 1985 publication listed 120 books available in English[8], and in 1986 *The Chiropractic Theories: A Synopsis of Scientific Research* was published[9].

Chiropractors acknowledge the need for properly conducted clinical evaluation of their therapy[7], and all students undertaking the BCA-recognized training at the Anglo-European College of Chiropractic undertake research as a course requirement[10].

Other Research

Perhaps the most complete recent research project carried out in Britain was one carried out by Medical Research Council epidemiologists and a rheumatologist, whose results were published in the British Medical Journal in 1990.

In a randomized, controlled, multicenter trial, 741 patients, aged between 18 and 65, all having severe lower back pain of mechanical origin, received either chiropractic (from BCA-registered practitioners) or hospital outpatient treatment. The chiropractors were to give no more than 10 treatments, preferably within a three-month period, but they could spread them over a year if necessary; the paper does not give details of any constraints on the hospital teams.

Progress was measured using the results of the Oswestry pain disability questionnaire (a recognized and validated research tool) and tests of straight leg raising and lumbar flexion exercises. Follow-up was initially planned to last for two years.

The results showed that with the Oswestry scores only one hospital department (out of 11) appeared to get better results than chiropractors, and results were equivocal in two more, leaving eight centers where chiropractic was significantly more effective.

With leg raising and lumbar flexion, patients treated by chiropractors did better than those treated as hospital outpatients.

The comparative benefits of chiropractic became more marked at six months into the follow-up period and, as a result, the researchers extended this by another year. The improvements—including a decreased chance of the patient needing further treatment—were maintained.

The authors concluded: "For patients with low back pain in whom manipulation is not contraindicated, chiropractic almost certainly confers worthwhile, long-term benefit in comparison with hospital outpatient management. The benefit is mainly seen in those with chronic or severe pain. Introducing chiropractic into NHS practice should be considered."

Meade, T.W., Dyer, S., Browne, W. et al. Low back pain of mechanical origin: randomized comparison of chiropractic and hospital outpatient treatment. *British Medical Journal* 1990; 300: 6737, 1431-1437.

The principal author published another paper, summarizing its findings but containing the additional idea of training physiotherapists in chiropractic technique.

Meade, T.W. Chiropractic treatment of low back pain. *MRC News* 1990; 48: 23-24.

Implications for Nursing

Chiropractic is a very highly skilled therapy for which a training period equivalent to five years' full-time study (six years from September 1993) is needed and, as with all manual skills, continuous practice is necessary.

However, no chiropractic technique should ever be attempted by nurses who have not received the necessary training.

References

1. Stanway, A. *Alternative Medicine*. London: Bloomsbury Books, 1992.

2. Olsen, K. *The Encyclopaedia of Alternative Medicine*. London: Piatkus, 1991.

3. Inglis, B. *Natural Medicine*. London: Collins, 1979.

4. Copland-Griffiths, M. *Dynamic Chiropractic Today*. Wellingborough: Thorsons, 1991.

5. Thomas, K.J., Carr, J., Westlake, L. et al. Use of non-orthodox and conventional health care in Great Britain. *British Medical Journal* 199 1; 302: 6770,207-210.

6. Meeker, W. *The Encyclopaedia of Alternative Medicine*. London: Piatkus, 1991.

7. Moore, S. *A Guide to Chiropractic*. London: Hamlyn, 1988.

8. West, R., Trevelyan, J.E. *Alternative Medicine: A Bibliography of books in English*. London: Mansell, 1985.

9. Leach, R.A. *The Chiropractic Theories: A Synopsis of Scientific Research*. Baltimore, Md: Williams and Wilkins, 1986.

10. Howitt Wilson, M.B. *Chiropractic*. Wellingborough: Thorsons, 1991.

11. Moore, S. *Chiropractic*. London: Macdonald Optima, 1988.

12. King's Fund. *Report on Chiropractic*. London: King's Fund, 1993.

—by Brian Booth

Brian Booth is assistant clinical editor, Nursing Times

Chapter 33

The Gentle Power of Acupressure

When I was first introduced to acupressure 15 years ago, I was more than a little skeptical. At the time, I was still totally committed to the Western medicine mind set and there was no rational place for acupressure within that framework. Little did I realize that this ancient healing art would one day become a major part of my practice.

Acupressure developed in China thousands of years ago; it's even older than acupuncture. Scholars believe prehistoric humans found that holding the part of the body that hurt brought relief and comfort. Over the centuries, the technique was refined, taking into account rivers of energy flowing throughout the body—what we've come to call meridians. This body energy, also called Qi, exists internally as well as externally, like the fields of energy that run through and surround a magnet.[1]

According to acupressure theorists, disease signifies an imbalance of the flow of Qi along the river-like meridians. Stimulating certain points on the skin along these meridians, however, can release muscle tension, increase circulation, and allow Qi to flow evenly and become balanced, thus healing disease.[1,2]

As traditional Chinese medicine has evolved, acupressure has developed into a complex healing art that uses 12 meridians and eight regulatory channels. The 12 meridians correspond approximately to 12 major organs—including the heart, kidneys, liver, lungs, colon, spleen, and bladder—and pressure along them is used to treat specific

---

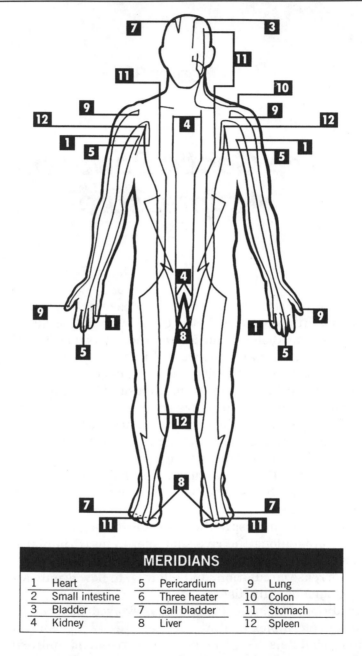

MERIDIANS					
1	Heart	5	Pericardium	9	Lung
2	Small intestine	6	Three heater	10	Colon
3	Bladder	7	Gall bladder	11	Stomach
4	Kidney	8	Liver	12	Spleen

Figure 33.1. *Acupressure meridians: Numerous pressure points exist along each of the 12 meridians used in Chinese medicine. Meridians 2 and 6 are not shown in the drawing because they run along the side and back of the body.*

disorders, depending on where pressure is exerted. The regulatory channels, on the other hand, function to gently restore balance to the entire body. There are a number of pressure points along each channel, too.[1]

Overcoming My Skepticism

Modern researchers are slowly beginning to find scientific evidence to support the existence of these meridians. One has developed a machine that is supposed to be able to measure electronic impulses in the skin that run along the acupressure meridians.[3]

This kind of evidence alone wasn't enough to convince me that acupressure worked. Not until I had met people who were using the technique as part of their nursing practice and seen the outstanding results their patients were getting, did my mindset begin to change.

As I began using some simple acupressure skills in my practice, I also began to see positive results in my patients. So I enrolled in an acupressure certification program. There I quickly began to appreciate that the art of laying on of hands can have a profound relaxing and healing effect on patients, demonstrating a type of caring that can't be communicated by mere words.

Of course, learning the more complex principles of the acupressure meridians and their relation to specific organs was much more of a challenge. But with the greater challenge came greater rewards. The more knowledge I gained, the easier it was to select the most effective treatment combination. And the results were sometimes dramatic.

My Patients Made Me a Firm Believer

Take Sarah Collins, for instance, a 76-year-old woman who had been suffering for four months with malaise, muscle weakness, occasional dizziness, mild anorexia, and weight loss. After many trips to her internist and a number of antibiotics, she was referred to an ear specialist. He could find nothing specific but told her she probably had a viral infection. Eventually she was given lorazepam (Ativan) to help her cope with the anxiety of dealing with the situation.

Having once been a student in my stress management class, Mrs. Collins decided to see if acupressure could help alleviate her condition. During our first session, I used a treatment pattern that incorporated pressure points along the Bridge regulatory channel. Stimulating this channel can often gently restore energy balance in older patients suffering from dizziness. Because her physician also suspected a viral infection, I also used points along the lung and large intestine meridians to stimulate the body's immune response.

In acupressure, you use your fingertips to create gentle but firm pressure. In areas where there's a blockage of energy, certain points may be very sensitive, so you must rely on patient feedback to determine how much pressure to apply. You never press down so strongly that it's uncomfortably painful.

The other important precaution to remember when using acupressure involves the pregnant patient—obviously not one of Mrs. Collins' concerns. One commonly used pressure point is called the Hoku point, located in the web between the thumb and the index finger. It's helpful in relieving headache, gastrointestinal problems, insomnia, and depression but, because it stimulates the lower abdomen, overuse may bring on premature labor.[4]

As a general rule, I'll hold down on a pressure point for two to five minutes. After holding a point for awhile, an experienced practitioner can usually feel a slight pulse. This pulse is the energy that flows along the body. When you feel it, it means that the Qi was blocked and is once again flowing.

During the process of holding and releasing the various pressure points—a single session can last up to an hour—the patient usually becomes very calm as the body secretes endorphins and enkephalins, relaxation hormones that help the body heal itself.[5]

Mrs. Collins responded very well to her first session. In fact, she was amazed that she could feel the strength returning to her arms and legs so quickly. Six follow-up sessions brought continuing improvement. Now she's committed to maintaining her health by doing self-acupressure, using points I demonstrated for her.

Lorraine Amico saw similar benefits from her acupressure sessions. Originally she came to see me seeking relief from severe shoulder tension and pain. After three sessions she was so delighted by her response that she asked if acupressure might help her ear problem. A year earlier she'd developed inner ear congestion during an airplane flight. Her ears buzzed often but her doctor had told her she'd have to live with it.

For Ms. Amico's ear problem, I used a point on the small intestine meridian that's located in front of the ear, a point that's specific for tinnitus.[4] Not only did the buzzing go away, but when she went on a recent flight, she was able to use acupressure to prevent an attack. Her tinnitus has not returned.

As a healing art, acupressure blends beautifully with nursing practice. It's easy to learn the basic skills and it can be used to treat a wide variety of symptoms, in a wide variety of patient care settings.[6] It's also easy to teach patients how to use the pressure points themselves so they can participate in their own healing.

The skeptic in me is gone, replaced by a sense of awe that something so simple, gentle, and respectful can be such a potent therapeutic tool.

For More Information

Additional information on acupressure, including a list of courses for health professionals, can be obtained by contacting: Acupressure Institute 1533 Shattuck Avenue Berkeley, CA 94709 (800) 442-2232 (510) 845-1059 (In California)

References

1. Hin, K. (1994). *Chinese massage and acupressure* (5th ed.). New York: Bergh.

2. Teeguarden, 1. (1978). *Acupressure way of health: Jin shin do*. New York: Japan Publications.

3. Hover-Kramer, D. (1996). *Healing touch: A resource for health care professionals*. New York: Delmar.

4. Gach, M. (1984). *Intermediate and advanced acupressure course booklet*. Berkeley, CA: The Acupressure Institute.

5. Locke, S., & Colligan, D. (1967). *The healer within: The new medicine of mind and body*. New York: E.P. Dutton.

6. Calbert, J., Gach, M., & Wilder, M. (1990). *Acupressure for health professionals*. Berkeley, CA: The Acupressure Institute.

—by Jan Maxwell, RN, BA

The author is a health counselor and educator in private practice in Castro Valley, California

Chapter 34

Shiatsu

Shiatsu is a Japanese word which translates as "finger pressure". The Japanese Ministry of Health and Welfare defines shiatsu therapy as "a form of manipulation administered by the thumbs, fingers and palms, without the use of any instrument, mechanical or otherwise " to apply pressure to the human skin, to correct internal malfunctioning, promote and maintain health and treat specific diseases".

The theory behind shiatsu is very closely related to traditional Chinese medicine (TCM). A fuller discussion can be found in the chapter on traditional Oriental medicine and acupuncture, but a much abbreviated summary follows:

Ki (the Japanese word for *Qi*, a fundamental concept in TCM) is energy, in the widest sense: everything in the universe is a manifestation of it. *Ki* is never static, which means that everything is in a constant state of change.

Ki has two qualities: yin and yang, which are opposites, but neither can exist without the other. Everyone has a tendency to be more yin or yang in their nature, but a balance is usually maintained. If one becomes too predominant, though, the imbalance may be manifested as signs and symptoms: too much yin is associated with bodily coolness and lethargy, while excessive yang causes restlessness and fevers.

Ki is believed to circulate throughout the body, but there are several meridians, or channels, where its flow is most concentrated.

Where the meridians pass near the surface, acupressure can be applied; these areas are called acupoints, or tsubo. When a channel or tsubo is judged to be "full", the term used is jitsu; if it is "empty", the term is kyo. Jitsu and kyo correspond to yin and yang, but "fullness" and "emptiness" are relative, not absolute terms. The meridians connect organs, but these are not seen in the same way by TCM and Western medicine. For example, a problem with the heart meridian may be associated with emotional disturbances, an association that is hard to explain in physiological terms.

The reason for this is apparently straightforward; in Oriental medicine, the organ referred to does not mean only the physical structure but also relates to a whole series of perceived related functions. So, when the heart is referred to, the practitioner is not talking only about cardiac function, as a Western medical practitioner would understand it, but also a whole range of emotional activity (which, interestingly, corresponds almost exactly to lay understanding of "matters of the heart").

To avoid confusion, many texts have adopted the convention of capitalising the first letter of an organ's name—for example, Heart—when referring to it in this extended, almost metaphorical, sense.

There are two additional "organs": the "Heart Governor", and the "Triple Heater". The first of these is also referred to as the Pericardium, using the capital letter convention, or Heart Protector, and is considered to be concerned with the physical actions of the heart as a pump. The Triple Heater refers to three central energy centers, or *chakras*, found at the levels of, respectively, the heart, the solar plexus and the *tanden* (an area three fingers' width below the umbilicus). Each Heater is connected with the organs in its vicinity and, as a whole, acts as the body's temperature regulator.

Disturbances in the flow of *Ki* come from a disturbance in the balance of yin and yang, and the result is ill health. In shiatsu, the presumed causes of imbalance are the same as in other branches of Oriental medicine: internal, external or "other". Internal causes are linked with emotions; external causes include climate, which is thought to have an effect upon the body's health; while "other causes" include just about every other possible reason for the appearance of symptoms, including stress, level of physical activity, trauma, toxic substances (both natural, such as bee stings, and synthetic, such as pharmaceutical products) and "constitution", which may be used as shorthand for an expression of how much *Ki* an individual has in reserve.

A typical treatment session might last up to an hour. The first one is taken up with a health assessment, in which the practitioner uses visual and verbal clues and information gained from the client about past and present health, lifestyle, family history, and so on, to build up an overall picture of the person he or she will be treating.

A physical assessment is then carried out, in which the shiatsu practitioner "feels" the quality of *Ki* within the person by touching areas of the torso. By its very nature, it is quite subjective.

One practitioner explains this: "Where too much *Ki* causes a blockage along a channel, the blocked *Ki* feels like a swelling from which *Ki* is trying to break out. It feels "active" and "hard" in the same way as an over-inflated balloon feels hard; the more you press it, the more it resists. It may not present as an actual swelling, but will definitely feel energetically confined and under pressure. As with a balloon, you would not want to press it too hard for fear of an explosion. An explosion of pain accompanies pressure which is too direct and heavy upon the blocked area . . . Insufficient *Ki* in an area makes that area feel empty, lifeless and devoid of zest. It . . . may well feel soft, lacking resilience. It may also feel hard, but not the hardness of an inflated balloon or car tire—this is the hardness of inert matter such as the dried-out crust on top of a stale loaf of bread. Contrast this with a loaf of bread just out of the oven, which has the *Ki* of freshness and warmth to give it some bounce."[2]

There are two areas on the torso which the shiatsu practitioner can use as an aid in formulating a diagnosis. One is the *hara*, on the abdomen and another is an area that covers most of the back. Information can also be gathered by feeling pulses at six positions on each wrist, while the tongue and face also have diagnostic potential.

Diagnostic touch is always carried out through a layer of clothing, preferably a single one of natural fibre. The assessment can be carried out in a sitting position, but treatment is likely to be carried out with the client lying down. There are three basic techniques: tonification, dispersal and calming.

Techniques

Tonification. This is sustained pressure, delivered at right angles to the body, which is intended to increase the circulation of both blood and energy in an area.

Dispersal. There are several techniques included under "dispersal", all of which involve active movement, such as stretching and squeezing. As the name suggests, the aim is to break up a blockage of blood or energy.

Calming. There is little or no pressure in "calming", which can consist of a simple holding or gentle rocking movement. This is intended to counteract agitated energy.

The key to successful treatment is efficient use of the therapist's bodyweight and position, and should be almost effortless.

Claims

As shiatsu is believed to be a potent reliever of stress, it may be of value to any person at an time, but especially when a health problem could be stress-related.

Disorders of the gastrointestinal tract, including diarrhoea, constipation, indigestion and stomach cramp, are all conditions that practitioners feel they can alleviate, while a whole range of muscular problems may benefit from the therapy.

One well-documented area is the treatment of nausea, whether caused by motion, pregnancy or drugs; this is discussed under "Research."

Contraindications

Shiatsu practitioners have lists of conditions that their treatment would not help, ones where treatment is impractical and others where matters could possibly be worsened. In the first group, acute fevers and burns are listed; in the second, contagious diseases are an obvious category.

A primary aim of the therapy is increasing the blood flow within the body, so where there is a risk of hemorrhage, or where thrombosis is expected, shiatsu should probably be avoided. For the same reason, some practitioners recommend extreme caution when there may be a tumor in the area to be treated.

Because a degree of pressure is used, the same cautions observed in massage apply;[3] when the person has osteoporosis, or if there has been any recent tissue damage, inflammation or bone fractures, particular care must be taken before applying pressure to any part of the body that has been affected.

If a person has high blood pressure or epilepsy, some points on the skull should be avoided.

Pregnancy is another difficult area, for although mothers to be may enjoy the relaxation engendered by shiatsu there are some pressure points on the leg which practitioners say can, if manipulated, increase the chance of miscarriage.

There is another group of conditions that shiatsu has no direct part in treating, but the experience of touch alone might be beneficial for the patient—particularly in neoplasm and AIDS.

Research

There is very little published research on shiatsu.

One related area which has received a lot of attention is the use of acupressure bands in the treatment of nausea. The theory is that there is a point on the Pericardium meridian, found on the inside of the wrist—Pericardium 6, also referred to as P6 or nei kuan—which, if pressed, will directly suppress nausea. The acupressure bands are elasticated, and a small stud on the inner surface is thus held above the P6 point. If nausea is felt, pressure can be applied. Several studies have been carried out to see whether the effect is real or not, and the results have tended to be positive:

- The incidence of morning sickness was greatly reduced in 350 pregnant women in a Belfast hospital, when pressure was applied to P6.

  Dundee, J., Ghaley, G., Bell, F.F. et al. P6 acupressure reduces morning sickness. *Journal of the Royal Society of Medicine* 1988; 81:456-458.

- A trial carried out in the USA found acupressure bands relieved morning sickness in 12 out of the 16 pregnant women studied, and improved mental well-being was reported during the periods they were worn.

  Hyde, E. Acupressure therapy for morning sickness. *Journal of Nurse-Midwifery* 1989; 34:4, 171-177.

- Forty female patients, admitted to a Buckinghamshire hospital for major gynecological surgery, were paired with controls for age, sex and surgical procedure. Members of each pair were randomized to either wear acupressure bands and to be given anti-emetics as necessary, or anti-emetics alone.

Full data were available on 28 index patients and their controls. The study showed that patients wearing the bands needed about 15.5 percent fewer doses of anti-emetics, having a significantly reduced level of nausea and vomiting.

Phillips, K., Gill, L. A point of pressure. *Nursing Times* 1993; 89: 45, 44-45.

- A Hampshire study of 38 patients receiving chemotherapy, where half the group wore the bands on the ankle, found a significant decrease in nausea and improvements in mood in those who wore the bands in the correct position.

  Price, H., Lewith, G., Williams, C. Acupressure as an anti-emetic in cancer chemotherapy. *Complementary Medical Research* 1991; 5: 2, 3-94.

- In 1991 and 1992, a small pilot study was carried out by a shiatsu practitioner in Oxford. Thirteen people with thalamic pain were approached and asked if they would participate in some research; seven consented, but only two went through with it. Three other people were already receiving shiatsu for thalamic pain.

Of these five, three felt that shiatsu had helped, while two felt worse; as the researcher points out, thalamic pain can be worsened by touch. Further details about this study can be obtained from the Shiatsu Society.

Implications for Nursing

Training in shiatsu takes several years, part time, but the basics are reasonably simple, and it can be practiced on oneself without too much trouble, providing the cautions given above are heeded.

Before embarking on administering shiatsu, nurses should have attended some form of practical study course, run by a member of the register of the Shiatsu Society. The risks may be small, but they are no less real for that.

As with massage therapy, shiatsu calls for a closer degree of physical contact than many people might find comfortable, and this must always be borne in mind.

It seems that nurses who have undergone a recognized training course in this therapy might have a lot to offer patients in their care, as it is relatively safe and offers relief from a number of conditions. Unfortunately it appears that to date no nurses have published anything about the use of shiatsu in their practice.

References

1. Trevelyan, J. Acupuncture. *Nursing Times* 1993; 89:28,26-28.

2. Jarmey, C. *Thorson's Introductory Guide to Shiatsu*. London: Thorsons, 1992.

3. Trevelyan, J. Massage. *Nursing Times* 1993; 89: 19,45-47.

When therapeutic techniques are described, it is purely for illustration and not intended to act as a guide to practice. No therapeutic interventions should ever be carried out by nurses, midwives or health visitors who have not undergone the appropriate training

— *by Brian Booth, RGN, is clinical editor, Nursing Times*

Recommended Reading

Jarmey, C., Mojay, G. *Shiatsu: The Complete Guide*. London: Thorsons, 1991.

Jarmey, C. Thorsons. *Introductory Guide to Shiatsu*. London: Thorsons, 1992.

Liechti, E. *Shiatsu: Japanese Massage for Health and Fitness*. Shaftesbury: Element, 1992.

Lundberg, P. *The Book of Shiatsu*. London: Goia, 1992.

Sofroniou, P. Shiatsu: The practitioner's story. In: Booth, B. *Complementary Therapy*. London: Nursing Times/Macmillan, 1993.

Resources

Training and Regulation

There are several different types of shiatsu, which lay emphasis on different areas. They include Namikoshi-style, which is rooted in a Western-style approach to physiology; Zen shiatsu, which proposes a more complex network of meridians than that taught in the "traditional"schools, and, Tsubo Therapy, which is more closely-related to acupuncture in its concentration on specific points on the body. There are other variants, but the aims of each are the same: to revitalize the body and mind through the use of finger pressure on the body. Unlike some therapies, though, it is not considered a disadvantage to be familiar with more than one of these variants—the Shiatsu Society, in fact, encourages it.

It is possible to attend classes that give a basic grounding in shiatsu for use on oneself, but, as might be expected, training as a practitioner is a more lengthy procedure.

Chapter 35

Acupuncture

National Institutes of Health Consensus Development Conference Statement Acupuncture November 3-5, 1997

NIH Consensus Statements are prepared by a nonadvocate, non-Federal panel of experts, based on (1) presentations by investigators working in areas relevant to the consensus questions during a 2-day public session; (2) questions and statements from conference attendees during open discussion periods that are part of the public session; and (3) closed deliberations by the panel during the remainder of the second day and morning of the third. This statement is an independent report of the panel and is not a policy statement of the NIH or the Federal Government.

Introduction

Acupuncture is a component of the health care system of China that can be traced back for at least 2,500 years, The general theory of acupuncture is based on the premise that there are patterns of energy flow (Qi) through the body that are essential for health. Disruptions of this flow are believed to be responsible for disease. The acupuncturist can correct imbalances of flow at identifiable points close to the skin. The practice of acupuncture to treat identifiable

NIH Consensus Statement, November 3-5, 1997.

pathophysiological conditions in American medicine was rare until the visit of President Nixon to China in 1972. Since that time, there has been an explosion of interest in the United States and Europe in the application of the technique of acupuncture to Western medicine.

Acupuncture describes a family of procedures involving stimulation of anatomical locations on the skin by a variety of techniques. The most studied mechanism of stimulation of acupuncture points employs penetration of the skin by thin, solid, metallic needles, which are manipulated manually or by electrical stimulation. The majority of comments in this report are based on data that came from such studies. Stimulation of these areas by moxibustion, pressure, heat, and lasers is used in acupuncture practice, but due to the paucity of studies, these techniques are more difficult to evaluate. Thus, there are a variety of approaches to diagnosis and treatment in American acupuncture that incorporate medical traditions from China, Japan, Korea, and other countries.

Acupuncture has been used by millions of American patients and performed by thousands of physicians, dentists, acupuncturists, and other practitioners for relief or prevention of pain and for a variety of health conditions. After reviewing the existing body of knowledge, the U.S. Food and Drug Administration recently removed acupuncture needles from the category of "experimental medical devices" and now regulates them just as it does other devices, such as surgical scalpels and hypodermic syringes, under good manufacturing practices and single-use standards of sterility.

Over the years, the National Institute of Health (NIH) has funded a variety of research projects on acupuncture, including studies on the mechanisms by which acupuncture may have its effects, as well as clinical trials and other studies. There is also a considerable body of international literature on the risks and benefits of acupuncture, and the World Health Organization lists a variety of medical conditions that may benefit from the use of acupuncture or moxibustion.

Such applications include prevention and treatment of nausea and vomiting; treatment of pain and addictions to alcohol, tobacco, and other drugs; treatment of pulmonary problems such as asthma and bronchitis; and rehabilitation from neurological damage such as that caused by stroke.

To address important issues regarding acupuncture, the NIH Office of Alternative Medicine and the NIH Office of Medical Applications of Research organized a 2 1/2-day conference to evaluate the scientific and medical data on the uses, risks, and benefits of acupuncture procedures for a variety of conditions. Cosponsors of the conference

504

were the National Cancer Institute, the National Heart Lung, and Blood Institute, the National Institute of Allergy and Infectious Diseases, the National Institute of Arthritis and Musculoskeletal and Skin Diseases, the National Institute of Dental Research, the National Institute on Drug Abuse, and the Office of Research on Women's Health of the NIH. The conference brought together national and international experts in the fields of acupuncture, pain, psychology, psychiatry, physical medicine and rehabilitation, drug abuse, family practice, internal medicine, health policy, epidemiology, statistics, physiology, and biophysics, as well as representatives from the public.

After 1 1/2 days of available presentations and audience discussion, an independent, non-Federal consensus panel weighed the scientific evidence and wrote a draft statement that was presented to the audience on the third day. The consensus statement addressed the following key questions:

- What is the efficacy of acupuncture, compared with placebo or sham acupuncture, in the conditions for which sufficient data are available to evaluate?

- What is the place of acupuncture in the treatment of various conditions for which sufficient data are available, in comparison or in combination with other interventions (including no intervention)?

- What is known about the biological effects of acupuncture that helps us understand how it works?

- What issues need to be addressed so that acupuncture can be appropriately incorporated into today's health care system?

- What are the directions for future research?

Question 1: What is the efficacy of acupuncture, compared with placebo or sham acupuncture, in conditions for which sufficient data are available to evaluate?

Acupuncture is a complex intervention that may vary for different patients with similar chief complaints. The number and length of treatments and the specific points used may vary among individuals and during the course of treatment. Given this reality, it is perhaps encouraging that there exist a number of studies of sufficient quality to assess the efficacy of acupuncture for certain conditions.

According to contemporary research standards, there is a paucity of high-quality research assessing efficacy of acupuncture compared with placebo or sham acupuncture. The vast majority of papers studying acupuncture in the biomedical literature consist of case reports, case series, or intervention studies with designs inadequate to assess efficacy.

This discussion of efficacy refers to needle acupuncture (manual or electroacupuncture) because the published research is primarily on needle acupuncture and often does not encompass the full breadth of acupuncture techniques and practices. The controlled trials usually have only involved adults and did not involve long-term (i.e., years) acupuncture treatment

Efficacy of a treatment assesses the differential effect of a treatment when compared with placebo or another treatment modality using a double-blind controlled trial and a rigidly defined protocol, Papers should describe enrollment procedures, eligibility criteria, description of the clinical characteristics of the subjects, methods for diagnosis, and a description of the protocol (i.e., randomization method, specific definition of treatment, and control conditions, including length of treatment, and number of acupuncture sessions). Optimal trials should also use standardized outcomes and appropriate statistical analyses. This assessment of efficacy focuses on high-quality trials comparing acupuncture with sham acupuncture or placebo.

Response Rate. As with other interventions, some individuals are poor responders to specific acupuncture protocols. Both animal and human laboratory and clinical experience suggest that the majority of subjects respond to acupuncture, with a minority not responding. Some of the clinical research outcomes, however, suggest that a larger percentage may not respond. The reason for this paradox is unclear and may reflect the current state of the research.

Efficacy for Specific Disorders. There is clear evidence that needle acupuncture is efficacious for adult post-operative and chemotherapy nausea and vomiting and probably for the nausea of pregnancy.

Much of the research is on various pain problems. There is evidence of efficacy for postoperative dental pain. There are reasonable studies (although sometimes only single studies) showing relief of pain with acupuncture on diverse pain conditions such as menstrual cramps, tennis elbow, and fibromyalgia. This suggests that acupuncture may have a more general effect on pain. However, there are also studies that do not find efficacy for acupuncture in pain

There is evidence that acupuncture does not demonstrate efficacy for cessation of smoking and may not be efficacious for some other conditions.

While many other conditions have received some attention in the literature and, in fact, the research suggests some exciting potential areas for the use of acupuncture, the quality or quantity of the research evidence is not sufficient to provide firm evidence of efficacy at this time.

Sham Acupuncture. A commonly used control group is sham acupuncture, using techniques that are not intended to stimulate known acupuncture points. However, there is disagreement on correct needle placement. Also, particularly in the studies on pain, sham acupuncture often seems to have either intermediate effects between the placebo and "real" acupuncture points or effects similar to those of the "real" acupuncture points. Placement of a needle in any position elicits a biological response that complicates the interpretation of studies involving sham acupuncture. Thus, there is substantial controversy over the use of sham acupuncture as control groups. This may be less of a problem in studies not involving pain.

Question 2: What is the place of acupuncture in the treatment of various conditions which sufficient data are available, in comparison with or in combination with other interventions (including no intervention)?

Assessing the usefulness of a medical intervention in practice differs from assessing formal efficacy. In conventional practice, clinicians make decisions based on the characteristics of the patient, clinical experience, potential for harm, and information from colleagues and the medical literature. In addition, when more than one treatment is possible, the clinician may make the choice taking into account the patient's preferences. While it is often thought that there is substantial research evidence to support conventional medical practices; this is frequently not that case. This does not mean that these treatments are ineffective. The data in support of acupuncture are as strong as those for many accepted Western medical therapies.

One of the advantages of acupuncture is that the incidence of adverse effects is substantially lower than that of many drugs or other accepted medical procedures used for the same conditions. As an example, musculoskeletal conditions, such as fibromyalgia, myofascial pain, and "tennis elbow," or epicondylitis, are conditions for which acupuncture may be beneficial. These painful conditions are often treated with, among other things, anti-inflammatory medications (aspirin, ibuprofen, etc.) or with steroid injections. Both medical interventions have a potential for deleterious side effects, but are still widely used, and are considered acceptable treatment. The evidence supporting these therapies is no better than that for acupuncture.

In addition, ample clinical experience, supported by some research data, suggests that acupuncture may be a reasonable option for a number of clinical conditions. Examples are postoperative pain and myofascial and low back pain. Examples of disorders for which the research evidence is less convincing but for which there are some positive clinical reports include addiction, stroke rehabilitation, carpal tunnel syndrome, osteoarthritis, and headache. Acupuncture treatment for many conditions such as asthma, addiction, or smoking cessation should be part of a comprehensive management program.

Many other conditions have been treated by acupuncture; the World Health Organization, for example, has listed more than 40 for which the technique may be indicated.

Question 3: What is known about the biological effects of acupuncture that helps us understand how it works?

Many studies in animals and humans have demonstrated that acupuncture can cause multiple biological responses. These responses can occur locally, i.e., at or close to the site of application, or at a distance, mediated mainly by sensory neurons to many structures within the central nervous system. This can lead to activation of pathways affecting various physiological systems in the brain as well as in the periphery. A focus of attention has been the role of endogenous opioids in acupuncture analgesia. Considerable evidence supports the claim that opioid peptides are released during acupuncture and that the analgesic effects of acupuncture are at least partially explained by their actions. That opioid antagonists such as naloxone reverse the analgesic effects of acupuncture further strengthens this hypothesis. Stimulation by acupuncture may also activate the hypothalamus and the pituitary gland, resulting in a broad spectrum of systemic effects. Alteration in the secretion of neurotransmitters and neurohormones and changes in the regulation of blood flow, both centrally and peripherally, have been documented. There is also evidence that there are alterations in immune functions produced by acupuncture. Which of these and other physiological changes mediate clinical effects is at present unclear.

Despite considerable efforts to understand the anatomy and physiology of the "acupuncture points," the definition and characterization of these points remains controversial. Even more elusive is the scientific basis of some of the key traditional Eastern medical concepts such as the circulation of Qi, the meridian system, and the five phases theory, which are difficult to reconcile with contemporary biomedical information but continue to play an important role in the evaluation of patients and the formulation of treatment in acupuncture,

Some of the biological effects of acupuncture have also been observed when "sham" acupuncture points are stimulated, highlighting the importance of defining appropriate control groups in assessing biological changes purported to be due to acupuncture. Such findings raise questions regarding the specificity of these biological changes. In addition, similar biological alterations including the release of endogenous opioids and changes in blood pressure have been observed after painful stimuli, vigorous exercise, and/or relaxation training: it is at present unclear to what extent acupuncture shares similar biological mechanisms.

It should be noted also that for any therapeutic intervention, including acupuncture, the so-called "non-specific" effects account for a substantial proportion of its effectiveness, and thus should not be casually discounted. Many factors may profoundly determine therapeutic outcome including the quality of the relationship between the clinician and the patient, the degree of trust, the expectations of the patient, the compatibility of the backgrounds and belief systems of the clinician and the patient, as well as a myriad of factors that together define the therapeutic milieu.

Although much remains unknown regarding the mechanism(s) that might mediate the therapeutic effect of acupuncture, the panel is encouraged that a number of significant acupuncture-related biological changes can be identified and carefully delineated. Further research in this direction not only is important for elucidating the phenomena associated with acupuncture, but also has the potential for exploring new pathways in human physiology not previously examined in a systematic manner.

Question 4: What issues need to be addressed so that acupuncture can be appropriately incorporated into today's health care system?

The integration of acupuncture into today's health care system will be facilitated by a better understanding among providers of the language and practices of both the Eastern and Western health care communities. Acupuncture focuses on a holistic, energy-based approach to the patient rather than a disease-oriented diagnostic and treatment model.

An important factor for the integration of acupuncture into the health care system is the training and credentialing of acupuncture practitioners by the appropriate state agencies. This is necessary to allow the public and other health practitioners to identify qualified acupuncture practitioners. The acupuncture educational community has made substantial progress in this area and is encouraged to continue along this path. Educational standards have been established for training of physician and non-physician acupuncturists. Many acupuncture educational programs are accredited by an agency that is recognized by the U.S. Department of Education. A national credentialing agency exists that is recognized by some of the major professional acupuncture organizations and provide examinations for entry-level competency in the field.

A majority of States provide licensure or registration for acupuncture practitioners. Because some acupuncture practitioners have limited English proficiency, credentialing and licensing examinations should be provided in languages other than English where necessary. There is variation in the titles that are conferred through these processes and the requirements to obtain licensure vary widely. The scope of practice allowed under these State requirements varies as well. While States have the individual prerogative to set standards for licensing professions, harmonization in these areas will provide greater confidence in the qualifications of acupuncture practitioners. For example, not all States recognize the same credentialing examination, thus making reciprocity difficult.

The occurrence of adverse events in the practice of acupuncture has been documented to be extremely low. However, these events have occurred in rare occasions, some of which are life threatening (e.g., pneumothorax). Therefore, appropriate safeguards for the protection of patients and consumers need to be in place. Patients should be fully informed of their treatment options, expected prognosis, relative risk, and safety practices to minimize these risks prior to their receipt of acupuncture. This information must be provided in a manner that is linguistically and culturally appropriate to the patient. Use of acupuncture needles should always follow FDA regulations, including use of sterile, single-use needles. It is noted that these practices are already being done by many acupuncture practitioners; however, the practices should be uniform. Recourse for patient grievance and professional censure are provided through credentialing and licensing procedures and are available through appropriate State jurisdictions.

It has been reported that more than 1 million Americans currently receive acupuncture each year. Continued access to qualified acupuncture professionals for appropriate conditions should be ensured. Because many individuals seek health care treatment from both acupuncturists and physicians, communication between these providers should be strengthened and improved. If a patient is under the care of an acupuncturist and a physician, both practitioners should be informed. Care should be taken so that important medical problems are not overlooked. Patients and providers have a responsibility to facilitate this communication.

There is evidence that some patients have limited access to acupuncture services because of inability to pay. Insurance companies can decrease or remove financial barriers to access depending on their willingness to provide coverage for appropriate acupuncture services. An increasing number of insurance companies are either considering this possibility or now provide coverage for acupuncture services. Where there are State health insurance plans, and for populations served by Medicare or Medicaid, expansion of coverage to include appropriate acupuncture services would also help remove financial barriers to access.

As acupuncture is incorporated into today's health care system, and further research clarifies the role of acupuncture for various health conditions, it is expected that dissemination of this information to health care practitioners, insurance providers, policymakers, and the general public will lead to more informed decisions in regard to the appropriate use of acupuncture.

Question 5. What are the directions for future research?

The incorporation of any new clinical intervention into accepted practice faces more scrutiny now than ever before. The demands of evidence-based medicine, outcomes research, managed care systems of health care delivery, and a plethora of therapeutic choices makes the acceptance of new treatments an arduous process. The difficulties are accentuated when the treatment is based on theories unfamiliar to Western medicine and its practitioners. It is important, therefore, that the evaluation of acupuncture for the treatment of specific conditions be carried out carefully, using designs which can withstand rigorous scrutiny. In order to further the evaluation of the role of acupuncture in the management of various conditions, the following general areas for future research are suggested.

What are the demographics and patterns of use of acupuncture in the U. S. and other countries?

There is currently limited information on basic questions such as who uses acupuncture, for what indications is acupuncture most commonly sought, what variations in experience and techniques used exist among acupuncture practitioners, and whether there are differences in these patterns by geography or ethnic group. Descriptive epidemiologic studies can provide insight into these and other questions. This information can in turn be used to guide future research and to identify areas of greatest public health concern.

Can the efficacy of acupuncture for various conditions for which it is used or for which it shows promise be demonstrated?

Relatively few high-quality, randomized, controlled trials have been published on the effects of acupuncture. Such studies should be designed in a rigorous manner to allow evaluation of the effectiveness of acupuncture. Such studies should include experienced acupuncture practitioners in order to design and deliver appropriate interventions. Emphasis should be placed on studies that examine acupuncture as used in clinical practice, and that respect the theoretical basis for acupuncture therapy.

Although randomized controlled trials provide a strong basis for inferring causality, other study designs such as used in clinical epidemiology or outcomes research can also provide important insights regarding the usefulness of acupuncture for various conditions. The have been few such studies in the acupuncture literature.

Do different theoretical bases for acupuncture result in different treatment outcomes?

Competing theoretical orientations (e.g., Chinese, Japanese, French) currently exist that might predict divergent therapeutic approaches (i.e., the use of different acupuncture points). Research projects should be designed to assure the relative merit of these divergent approaches, as well to compare these systems with treatment programs using fixed acupuncture points.

In order to fully assess the efficacy of acupuncture, studies should be designed to examine not only fixed acupuncture points, but also the Eastern medical systems that provide the foundation for acupuncture therapy, including the choice of points. In addition to assessing the effect of acupuncture in context, this would also provide the opportunity to determine if Eastern medical theories predict more effective acupuncture points, as well as to examine the relative utility of competing systems (e.g., Chinese vs. Japanese vs. French) for such purposes.

What areas of public policy research can provide guidance for the integration of acupuncture into today's health care system?

The incorporation of acupuncture as a treatment raises numerous questions of public policy. These include issues of access, cost-effectiveness, reimbursement by state, federal, and private payors, and training, licensure, and accreditation. These public policy issues must be founded on quality epidemiologic and demographic dam and effectiveness research.

Can further insight into the biological basis for acupuncture be gained?

Mechanisms which provide a Western scientific explanation for some of the effects of acupuncture are beginning to emerge. This is encouraging, and may provide novel insights into neural, endocrine and other physiological processes. Research should be supported to provide a better understanding of the mechanisms involved, and such research may lead to improvements in treatment

Does an organized energetic system exist in the human body that has clinical applications?

Although biochemical and physiologic studies have provided insight into some of the biologic effects of acupuncture, acupuncture practice is based on a very different model of energy balance. This theory may provide new insights to medical research that may further elucidate the basis for acupuncture.

How do the approaches and answers to these questions differ among populations that have used acupuncture as a part of its healing tradition for centuries, compared to populations that have only recently begun to incorporate acupuncture into health care?

Conclusions

Acupuncture as a therapeutic intervention is widely practiced in the United States. There have been many studies of its potential usefulness. However, many of these studies provide equivocal results because of design, sample size, and other factors. The issue is further complicated by inherent difficulties in the use of appropriate controls, such as placebo and sham acupuncture groups.

However, promising results have emerged, for example, efficacy of acupuncture in adult postoperative and chemotherapy nausea and vomiting and in post-operative dental pain. There are other situations such as addiction, stroke rehabilitation, headache, menstrual cramps, tennis elbow, fibromyalgia myofascial pain, osteoarthritis, low back pain, carpal tunnel syndrome, and asthma where acupuncture may be useful as an adjunct treatment or an acceptable alternative or be included in a comprehensive management program. Further research is likely to uncover additional areas where acupuncture interventions will be useful.

Findings from basic research have begun to elucidate the mechanisms of action of acupuncture, including the release of opioids and other peptides in the central nervous system and the periphery and changes in neuroendocrine function. Although much needs to be accomplished, the emergence of plausible mechanisms for the therapeutic effects of acupuncture is encouraging.

The introduction of acupuncture into the choice of treatment modalities that are readily available to the public is in its early stages. Issues of training, licensure, and reimbursement remain to be clarified. There is sufficient evidence, however, of its potential value to conventional medicine to encourage further studies.

There is sufficient evidence of acupuncture's value to expand its use into correctional medicine and to encourage further studies of its physiology and clinical value.

Part Seven

Mind/Body Control

Chapter 36

Mind-Body Medical Interventions:

Psychotherapy, Support Groups, Meditation, Imagery, Hypnosis, Biofeedback, Yoga, Dance Therapy, Music/Sound Therapy, Art Therapy, and Prayer and Faith Healing

Introduction

Most traditional medical systems appreciate and make use of the extraordinary interconnectedness of the mind and the body and power of each to affect the other. In contrast, modern Western medicine has regarded these connections as of secondary importance.

The separation between mind and body was established during the 17th century. Originally it permitted medical science the freedom to explore and experiment on the body while preserving for the church the domain of the mind. In the succeeding three centuries, the medicine that evolved from this focus on the body and its processes has yielded extraordinary discoveries about the nature and treatment of disease states.

However, this narrow focus has also tended to obscure the importance of the interactions between mind and body and to overshadow the possible importance of the mind in producing and alleviating disease. The focus of medical research has been on the biology of the body and of the brain, which is part of the body. Concern with the mind has been left to non-biologically oriented psychiatrists, other mental health professionals, philosophers, and theologians. Psychosomatic medicine, the discipline that has addressed mind-body connections, is a subspecialty within the specialty of psychiatry.

Extracted from NIH Publication No. 94-066. December 1994. Due to space considerations, bibliographic data have not been reprinted in this chapter. However, the in-text references have been retained.

During the past 30 years, there has been a powerful scientific movement to explore the mind's capacity to affect the body and to rediscover the ways in which it permeates and is affected by all of the body's functions. This movement has received its impetus from several sources. It has been spurred by the rise in incidence of chronic illnesses—including heart disease, cancer, depression, arthritis, and asthma—which appear to be related to environmental and emotional stresses. The prevalence, destructiveness, and cost of these illnesses have set the stage for the exploration of therapies that can help individuals appreciate the sources of their stress and reduce that stress by quieting the mind and using it to mobilize the body to heal itself.

During the same time, medical researchers have discovered other cultures' healing systems, such as meditation, yoga, and tai chi, which are grounded in an understanding of the power of mind and body to affect one another; developed techniques such as biofeedback and visual imagery, which are capable of facilitating the mind's capacity to affect the body; and examined some of the specific links between mental processes and autonomic, immune, and nervous system functioning—most dramatically illustrated by the growth of a new discipline, psychoneuroimmunology.

The clinical aspect of the enterprise that explores, appreciates, and makes use of mind-body interactions has come to be called mind-body medicine. The techniques that its practitioners use are mind-body interventions. The chapter discusses the evidence that supports the mind-body approach, describes some of these techniques, and summarizes the results of some of the most effective interventions.

This approach is not only producing dramatic results in specific arenas, it is forming the basis for a new perspective on medicine and healing. From this perspective it is becoming clear that every interaction between doctors and patients—between those who give help and those who receive it—may affect the mind and in turn the body of the patient. From this perspective all of medicine, indeed all of health care, is grounded in the mind-body approach. And all interventions, alternative or conventional, can be enhanced by it.

Meaning of Mind-Body

Any discussion of mind-body interventions brings the old questions back to life: What are mind and consciousness?[1] How and where do they originate? How are they related to the physical body? In approaching the field of mind-body interventions, it is important that the mind not be viewed as if it were dualistically isolated from the body, as if it were doing something to the body. Mind-body relations are always mutual and bidirectional—the body affects the mind and is affected by it. Mind and body are so integrally related that, in practice, it makes little sense to refer to therapies as solely "mental" or "physical." For example, activities that appear overwhelmingly "physical," such as aerobic exercise, yoga, and dance, can have healthful effects not only on the body but also on such "mental" problems as depression and anxiety; and "mental" approaches such as imagery and meditation can benefit physical problems such as hypertension and hypercholesterolemia as well as have salutary psychological effects. Even the use of drugs and surgery has its psychological side. The use of these methods often requires placebo-controlled, double-blind studies to estimate and factor out the physical effects of patients' beliefs and expectations.

When the term mind-body is used in this report, therefore, there is no implication that an object or thing—the mind—is somehow acting on a separate entity—the body. Rather, "mind-body" could perhaps best be regarded as an overall process that is not easily dissected into separate and distinct components or parts. This point of view, which was put forward a century ago by William James, the father of American psychology, has recently been reaffirmed by brain researchers Francis Crick and Christof Koch (1992).

Timeless Factors in Healing

Throughout history the value of "human" factors in healing has been recognized. These factors include closeness, caring, compassion, and empathy between therapist and patient. Though these factors are theoretically acknowledged by contemporary medicine, they are largely ignored in current practice, partly because they are hard to define and measure and cannot be easily taught. In many mind-body interventions, however, their relevance is obvious. A research agenda for the future should include an investigation of the impact of these qualities on healing—not only on alternative, mind-body interventions but on orthodox therapies as well.

Healing and Curing

Mind-body interventions frequently lead patients to new ways of experiencing and expressing their illness. For example, although healing usually denotes an objective improvement in health, patients commonly state that they feel "healed" but not "cured"—that is, they experience a profound sense of psychological or spiritual well-being and wholeness although the actual disease remains. Distinctions between curing (the actual eradication of a disease) and healing (a sense of wholeness and completeness) have little place in contemporary medical practice but are important to patients. A place should be made for these distinctions. Acknowledging that "healing without curing" is both permissible and honorable requires the recognition of spiritual elements in illness.[2] It also requires honoring the wishes of individuals in deciding what is best in the course of their disease process. Sometimes, zealous attempts to cure may have disastrous effects on patients' quality of life for the years they have left.

Evidence of Mind-Body Effects in Contemporary Medical Science

Social Isolation

Biological scientists have long been aware of the importance of social relationships on health. As the evolutionary biologist George Gaylord Simpson observed, "No animal or plant lives alone or is self-sustaining. All live in communities including other members of their own species and also a number, usually a large variety, of other sorts of animals and plants. *The quest to be alone is indeed a futile one, never successfully followed in the history of life*" (emphasis added) (Simpson, 1953, p. 53).

This observation is nowhere truer than in the human domain, where perceptions of social isolation and aloneness may set in motion mind-body events of life-or-death importance. This point has been demonstrated in research on many dimensions of human experience, among them the following:

- **Bereavement.** The idea that a person can die of being separated suddenly from a loved one is rooted in history and spans all cultures—the "broken heart" syndrome. In the United States, 700,000 people aged 50 or older lose their spouses annually. Of these, 35,000 die during the first year after the spouse's death. Researcher Steven Schleifer of Mount Sinai Hospital, New York, calculates that 20 percent, or 7,000, of these deaths are directly caused by the loss of the spouse. The physiological processes responsible for increased mortality during bereavement have been the subject of extensive investigations and include profound alterations in cardiovascular and immunological responses. In study after study, the mortality of the surviving spouse during the first year of bereavement has been found to be 2 to 12 times that of married people the same age (Dimsdale, 1977; Engel, 1971; Holmes and Rahe, 1967; Lown et al., 1980; Lynch, 1977; Schleifer et al.,1983; Stoddard and Henry, 1985). These studies have far-reaching therapeutic implications as well. Individual and group support can—and have been shown to—help mitigate the devastating effects of loss.

- **Poor education and illiteracy.** A more general and pervasive form of isolation results from poor education and illiteracy, which are in turn associated with increased incidence of disease and death. As Thomas B. Graboys of Harvard Medical School has stated, poor education is "an Orwellian recipe in which the estranged worker, besieged from above and below, mixes internal rage and incessant frustration into a fatal brew" (Graboys, 1984).

Many believe that the common factor in poor education, poor health, and higher mortality is simply that the poorly educated take worse care of themselves. However, research shows that smoking, exercise, diet, and accessibility to health care, while important, do not explain the poorer health and earlier death of these people; the influence of social isolation and poor education is more powerful. Moreover, poor education appears to be only a stand-in or proxy for stress and loneliness—that is, low education actually does its damage through the stress and social isolation to which it leads (Berkman and Syme, 1982; House et al., 1982, 1988; Ruberman et al., 1984; Sagan, 1987).

The underlying pathophysiological processes by which social isolation may bring about poor health have been illuminated by studies of primates in the wild. Low-ranking baboons, whose entire life is spent in constant danger with little control, demonstrate high circulating levels of hydrocortisone, which remain elevated even when the stressful event has passed. In addition, chronic psychological stress and isolation have been associated with decreased concentrations of high-density lipoproteins, which protect against heart disease, and weaker immune systems with fewer circulating disease-fighting lymphocytes (Sapolsky, 1990).

Work Status

Attitude toward work and work status may also be intimately related to health and well-being. Several lines of evidence point to these correlations:

- When researcher Peter L. Schnall and his colleagues examined the relationship between "job strain," blood pressure, and the mass of the heart's left ventricle, they found—after adjusting for age, race, body-mass index, type A behavior, alcohol intake, smoking, the nature of the work site, sodium excretion, education, and the physical demand level of the job—that job strain was significantly related to hypertension. They concluded that "job strain may be a risk factor for both hypertension and structural changes of the heart in working men" (Schnall et al., 1990; Williams, 1990).

- Epidemiologist C. David Jenkins demonstrated in 1971 that most people in the United States who experience their first heart attack when they are under the age of 50 have no major risk factors. Although Jenkins's findings must be tempered by the more recent redefinition of what constitutes "normal" cholesterol and blood pressure, the point remains: a purely physical approach may be inadequate for understanding the origins of coronary artery disease in our culture (Jenkins, 1971).

- In a 1973 survey in Massachusetts, a special Department of Health, Education, and Welfare task force reported that the best predictor for heart attack was none of the classic risk factors, but the level of one's job dissatisfaction (*Work in America: Report of a Special Task Force to the Secretary of Health, Education, and Welfare,* 1973). It is possible that this finding may be related to the observation that heart attacks in the United States, as well as in other Western industrialized nations, cluster on Monday mornings from 8 to 9 a.m., the beginning of the work week (Kolata, 1986; Muller et al., 1987; Rabkin et al., 1980; Thompson et al., 1992).

- Robert A. Karasek and colleagues have shown that the job characteristics of high demand and low decision latitude have predictive value for myocardial infarction. Occupational groups embodying these personality traits—waiters in busy restaurants, assembly line workers, and gas station attendants, for example—are at increased risk for heart attack. Their hypothesis is that increasing job demands are harmful when environmental constraints prevent optimal coping or when coping does not increase possibilities for personal and professional growth and development (Bergrugge, 1982; Bruhn et al., 1974; Karasek et al., 1982, 1988; Palmore, 1969; Sales and House, 1971; Syme, 1991).

- Psychologist Suzanne C. Kobasa and colleagues have identified job qualities that offer protection against cardiovascular morbidity and mortality, even in psychologically stressful job settings. They refer to the "three Cs": (1) control—a sense of personal decision making; (2) challenge—the sense of personal growth and wisdom; becoming a better person; and (3) commitment to life on and off the job—to work, community, family, and self. Persons experiencing these qualities are said to possess "hardiness" and are relatively immune to job-induced illness or death (Kobasa et al., 1982).

Perceived Meaning and Health

Perceived meaning—how one perceives an event or issue, what something symbolizes or represents in one's mind—has direct consequences to health.[3] The annals of medicine are replete with anecdotes illustrating the power of perceived meaning—for example, accounts of sudden death after receiving bad news. Moreover, perceived meanings affect not just health, they also influence the types of therapies that are chosen. For example, if "body" means "machine," as it has tended to for people since the Industrial Revolution, illness is likely to be seen as a breakdown or malfunction, and the tendency is to prefer mechanically oriented approaches to treating illness.

Therapies, therefore, are likely to be designed to repair the machine when it malfunctions—surgery, drugs, irradiation, and so on. Or, if illness symbolizes an attack from the outside by "invading" pathogens or foreign substances, as it does to many people, people are apt to look for magic bullets in the form of antibiotics or other substances to protect them from these threats. Society may even declare counterattacks, such as the "wars" on acquired immunodeficiency syndrome (AIDS), heart disease, cancer, high blood pressure, or cholesterol. Perceived meanings, therefore, can be translated into the body as potent influences, and they can strongly influence the design of medical interventions.

More recently, careful studies have indicated the pivotal role of perceived meaning in health. Sociologists Ellen Idler of Rutgers University and Stanislav Kasl of the Department of Epidemiology and Public Health at Yale Medical School studied the impact of people's opinions on their health—what their health meant to them. The study involved more than 2,800 men and women, and the findings were consistent with the results of five other large studies involving more than 23,000 people. All these studies lead to the same conclusion: One's own opinion about his or her state of health is a better predictor than objective factors, such as physical symptoms, extensive exams, and laboratory tests, or behaviors such as cigarette smoking. For instance, people who smoked were twice as likely to die during the next 12 years as people who did not, whereas those who said their health was "poor" were seven times more likely to die than those who said their health was "excellent" (Idler and Kasl, 1991).

Placebo Response

Dorland's *Illustrated Medical Dictionary*, twenty-fifth edition, defines the word placebo (in Latin, "I will please") as an inactive substance or preparation given to satisfy the patient's symbolic need for drug therapy and used in controlled studies to determine the efficacy of medicinal substances. It is also a procedure with no intrinsic therapeutic value, performed for such purposes. Although the placebo response is perhaps the most widely known example of mind-body interaction in contemporary scientific medicine,[4] it is at the same time one of the most undervalued and neglected assets in today's medical practice (Benson and Epstein, 1975). Even the definition from the medical dictionary suggests the term's uselessness apart from its narrow role in testing drugs. However, throughout most of medical history—in the centuries before antibiotics and other "wonder drugs"—the placebo effect was the central treatment physicians offered their patients (Benson and Epstein, 1975). Doctors hoped that their reassuring attention and their belief in their treatments would mobilize powers within their patients to fight their illnesses.

Today the placebo response is considered primarily a way of testing new drugs: if patients who have been given a placebo improve as much as those who took the new medication, the drug is dismissed as ineffective and with it the placebo. "Since a beneficial effect is the desired result," say cardiologist Herbert Benson and psychiatrist Mark Epstein, "should not the placebo effect be further investigated so that we might better explain its worthwhile consequences?" (Benson and Epstein, 1975).

The placebo response relies heavily on the interrelationship between doctor and patient. Patients bring with them to the doctor's office their attitudes, expectations, hopes, and fears. Doctors, in turn, have their own biases, attitudes, expectations, and methods of communication, which have a profound effect on patients. Doctors who believe in the efficacy of their treatment communicate that enthusiasm to their patients; those who have strong expectations of specific effects and are self-confident and attentive are the most successful at eliciting a positive placebo response (Wheatley, 1967). It is the interrelationship between the doctor and patient and the congruence of their expectations that bring about a positive placebo response. If the congruence is lacking, a favorable response rarely occurs (Hankoff et al., 1960).

The placebo response says a great deal about the importance of the doctor-patient relationship and the need to pay greater attention to it—and to provide further medical training on how that relationship can be heightened. It is particularly important in this highly technological era of medicine, when doctor-patient contacts are diminishing.

Although the literature of mind-body interaction documenting the placebo response is too vast to be reviewed here, several additional mind-body issues raised by this research deserve emphasis:

- The placebo response is almost ubiquitous. Studies show that in virtually any disease, roughly one-third of all symptoms improve when patients are given a placebo treatment without drugs (Goleman and Gurin, 1993).

- Placebo responses can be extraordinarily dramatic and offer valuable insights into the extent of the "powers of the mind" (Levoy, 1989).

- The nocebo response, a toxic or negative placebo event, raises serious questions about what is meant by "the natural course" or "the inherent biology" of any particular disease and suggests the great degree to which attitudes and expectations can affect one's state of health and the course of an illness.

- Nocebo effects can also be dramatic, are very common, and should be more widely acknowledged. Even anaphylactoid reactions (Wolf and Pinsky, 1954) and addictions to placebos (Rhein, 1980)—reactions not commonly thought to be "mental" in origin—have been reported, along with a variety of other noxious reactions. In one controlled study by the British Stomach Cancer Group, 30 percent of the control (placebo-treated) group lost their hair, and 56 percent of the same group had "drug-related" nausea or vomiting (Fielding et al., 1983).

Spirituality, Religion, and Health

"Spirituality" is, generally speaking, one's inward sense of something greater than the individual self or the meaning one perceives that transcends the immediate circumstances. "Religion" may be described as the outward, concrete expression of such feelings.

The therapeutic potential of spirituality and religion have generally been neglected in the teaching and practice of medicine. However, epidemiologists Jeffrey S. Levin and Harold Y. Vanderpool have assembled what they term an "epidemiology of religion"—a large body of empirical findings "lying forgotten at the margins of medical research . . . specifically . . . nearly 250 published studies dating back over 150 years which [present] the results of epidemiologic, sociomedical, and biomedical investigations into the effects of religion. Nearly all of these investigations were large-scale studies" (Levin, 1989; Levin and Schiller, 1987; Levin and Vanderpool, 1991; Vanderpool and Levin, 1990).

Reviewing this immense database, Schiller and Levin found significant associations with variables such as religious attendance and subjective religiosity for a wide assortment of health outcomes, including cardiovascular disease, hypertension and stroke, uterine and other cancers, colitis and enteritis, general mortality, and overall health status (Schiller and Levin, 1988). These data are so consistent that Levin and Vanderpool suggest that infrequent religious attendance or observance should be regarded as a consistent risk factor for morbidity and mortality of various types (Levin and Vanderpool, 1987).

These findings are consistent with those of David B. Larson and Susan S. Larson who surveyed 12 years of issues of the *American Journal of Psychiatry* and the *Archives of General Psychiatry*. They found that 92 percent of the studies that measured participation in religious ceremony, social support, prayer, and relationship with God showed benefit for mental health, whereas 4 percent were neutral, and 4 percent showed harm (Larson and Larson, 1991). Craigie and colleagues, in a 1990 review of 10 years of issues of the *Journal of Family Practice*, reported similar findings: 83 percent of studies showed benefit for physical health, 17 percent were neutral, and 0 percent showed harm (Craigie et al., 1990).

Matthews, Larson, and Barry made a major contribution in bringing together the research in this field—a two-volume report that compiles hundreds of studies, titled T*he Faith Factor: An Annotated Bibliography of Clinical Research on Spiritual Subjects* (Matthews et al., 1993). Because research indicates that religious and spiritual meanings are correlated with increased physical and mental health and a lower incidence of a variety of diseases, and because religious and spiritual issues also affect profoundly how physicians regard death and treat the elderly, the quarantine against bringing up these matters in the doctor-patient relationship must be lifted. Becoming sensitive to these delicate issues does not require physicians to advocate any particular religious point of view. It does imply, however, that they should honor the salutary effects of spiritual meanings in their patients' lives, and inquire about spiritual and religious issues as assiduously as any physical factor.[5]

Spontaneous Remission of Cancer

The belief that life-threatening diseases such as cancer may disappear suddenly and completely is universal. This idea is usually coupled with the conviction that radical healing is somehow connected with one's state of mind.

Opinions vary as to how often cancer regresses spontaneously, leaving the person healthy. In their 1966 book on spontaneous regression of cancer, Everson and Cole collected 176 case reports from various countries around the world and concluded that spontaneous regression occurs in one of 100,000 cases of cancer. Other authorities believe the incidence may be much higher. Everson and Cole found that almost any therapy to induce remission seems to work some of the time. Regression of cancer follows such diverse measures as intercessory prayer, conversion to Christian Science, mud packs, vitamin therapy, and force-feeding. They found that spontaneous regression occurs after both insulin and electroshock treatments. Since almost any treatment seems to work occasionally but not consistently, many have concluded that these measures are equally worthless and that spontaneous regression of cancer is purely a random event (Everson and Cole, 1966).

This point of view is a historical oddity. Prior to the 20th century, both physicians and patients believed the mind was a major factor in the development and course of cancer. In the years since Everson and Cole's review, this perspective has been recovered and reexamined. Many investigators—including psychologist Lawrence LeShan (1977) of New York and psychiatrist Steven Greer (1985) of King's College Hospital, London—have produced studies that suggest that emotions, attitudes, and personality traits may affect the onset of cancer as well as its course and outcome.

The Institute of Noetic Sciences has just published the most comprehensive investigation of spontaneous remission ever done—*Spontaneous Remission: An Annotated Bibliography* (O'Regan and Hirshberg, 1993).[6] This 15-year project was the work of biochemist Caryle Hirshberg and researcher Brendan O'Regan, who combed

3,500 references from more than 800 journals in 20 languages. The report deals not only with cancer but also with the spontaneous remission of a wide spectrum of diseases. It is the largest database of medically reported cases of spontaneous remission in the world. Key findings are as follows:

- Remission is a widely documented phenomenon, almost certainly more common than generally believed.

- Remission is an extremely promising area of research. Studying the psychobiological processes involved may provide important clues to understanding the body's self-regulatory processes and the breakdowns that precede the onset of many diseases.

- Data on remissions can have an important influence on how patients are treated and handled when diagnosed with a terminal illness. Restoring hope may help instill a "fighting spirit," an important factor in recovery from illness.

This interest in the possible role of the mind in the causation and course of cancer has been significantly stimulated by the discovery of the complex interactions among the mind and the neurological and immune systems, the subject of the rapidly expanding discipline of psychoneuroimmunology.

The relationship between psychological strategies and the regression of cancer is immensely complex and cannot be fully reviewed here. Two salient points should be made, however, that contradict popular belief and illustrate the complexity of these events: (1) Although an aggressive, fighting stance is generally advocated in stimulating spontaneous regression of cancer, University of California-Los Angeles psychologist Shelley E. Taylor has shown that (a) psychological denial following the diagnosis of breast cancer and (b) openly facing the disease and its implications are associated with near-equal survival statistics (Taylor, 1989). (2) Sometimes a mode of psychological acceptance, not aggressiveness, toward the diagnosis seems to set the stage for spontaneous remission. This point is particularly obvious in a series of spontaneous cancer remissions reported from Japan by Y. Ikemi and colleagues (Ikemi et al., 1975).

The profound differences in the psychological stances taken by people who survive cancer suggest that not only is there extreme variation between cultures, there are profound differences in the psychology of cancer survivors within cultures as well. Because the causal mechanisms involved are not known, and in view of the sheer variety of the psychological states that are apparently involved in spontaneous regression of cancer, physicians are currently unjustified in recommending uniformly that patients with cancer adopt a specific psychological stance in hopes of getting well. Still, spontaneous remission of cancer is a fact. Far more knowledge is needed about when and why it happens and what can be done to promote it.

Specific Therapies

The Panel on Mind-Body Interventions has selected the following therapies in an attempt to illustrate the diversity of this field and to illustrate some of the scientific work that has been done. The panel has not attempted to be exhaustive in this review, nor does it believe an exhaustive approach is possible in this document. Space does not allow discussion of many alternative therapies in which mind-body interactions are obviously prominent, such as anthroposophically extended medicine (see the "Alternative Systems of Medical Practice" chapter), Christian Science, and many others. Even though the sampling of specific therapies is necessarily restricted, the panel hopes this limited discussion will contribute to the development of a larger dialog in which all perspective mind-body interventions can eventually be considered.

Psychotherapy

It may be an error to focus on psychotherapy as an adjunctive therapy. Only from a perspective that views doctors as mechanics does psychotherapy become simply a technique. In fact, psychotherapy is the medium and basis of all care. It influences to some degree the efficacy of all health interventions, even those thought to be purely physical in nature.

Derived from Greek words meaning "healing of the soul," psychotherapy means treatment of emotional and mental health, which is in turn closely interwoven with physical health. Psychotherapy encompasses a wide range of specific treatments, including combining medication with discussion, listening to the patient's concerns, and using more active behavioral and emotive approaches. It also should be understood more generally as the matrix of interaction in which all the helping professions operate.

The number of health care professionals in the United States with some level of training in psychiatric and psychological counseling is immense. Currently, the American Psychiatric Association registers approximately 37,000 members; the American Psychological Association, 54,562 (approximately 60 percent clinical and 40 percent research and academic). The Department of Labor estimates that there are between 380,000 and 400,000 social workers; the American Medical Association lists 615,000 physicians, and the American Nurses Association lists 2,000,000 nurses. All of these people, as well as alternative health care practitioners, make conscious or unconscious use of psychotherapeutic interventions in their contacts with patients.

Conventional psychotherapy is conducted primarily by means of psychological methods such as suggestion, persuasion, psychoanalysis, and reeducation. It can be divided into the following six general categories. All of the following therapies can be undertaken either individually or in groups.

1. Psychodynamic therapy is derived from psychoanalysis. Current emotional reactions are related to past experiences, usually those of early childhood. It is generally directed toward changing fundamental personality patterns.

2. Behavior therapy emphasizes making specific behavior changes, such as learning not to be afraid of public speaking.

3. Cognitive therapy facilitates changing specific behaviors but focuses on habitual thoughts that affect behavior.

4. Systems therapy emphasizes relationship patterns and may involve all family members in therapy sessions.

5. Supportive therapy concentrates on helping people in major emotional crises, and treatment may include drug therapy.

6. Body-oriented therapy hypothesizes that emotions are encoded in and may be expressed as tension and restriction in any part of the physical body. Therapy uses breathing techniques, movement, and manual pressure and probing to help people release emotions that are believed to have been located in their tissues.

Any and all of these approaches may be used, but if a patient has a physical illness, the therapist focuses on short-term treatment dealing with any emotional state directly related to the physical condition. For example, depression and anxiety are common effects of any serious illness and may make it worse. Psychotherapy helps patients acknowledge the presence of these emotions and diminish their effects, thus enhancing recovery. According to a study by James J. Strain (1993), an average of "one of every five people in the United States has a psychological disorder every six months—most commonly anxiety, depression, substance abuse, or acute confusion." At present, approximately three-fifths of patients with psychological problems are seen only by primary care physicians, many of whom are not well trained in psychotherapy and do not have adequate time to spend with each patient. Thus, despite the enormous need for psychological care, most people with medical illnesses do not receive screening or treatment for their psychiatric symptoms.

Clinical applications. Studies have shown that psychotherapy has had beneficial effects with medical crises and somatic illness

Medical crises. Research indicates that psychotherapeutic treatment can hasten a recovery from a medical crisis and is in some cases the best treatment for it. According to Strain, brief psychotherapy reduced the hospital stay of elderly patients with broken hips by an average of 2 days. These patients had fewer rehospitalizations and spent fewer days in rehabilitation (Strain, 1993). Other studies show that psychotherapy is most effective when begun soon after a patient is admitted to a hospital. Currently, however, most psychological problems associated with physical illnesses remain undiagnosed or are not identified until near the end of a hospital stay.

In-hospital psychotherapy helps people cope with fears about their medical state by providing them with a supportive atmosphere in which to verbalize feelings. This atmosphere may give them a sense that their concerns are understood. It may also, by altering mood and attitude, be a significant factor in improving outcome. At the University of Minnesota, 100 patients preparing to go through bone marrow transplant for leukemia were examined for depression. Of the 13 patients diagnosed with major depression, all but one died in the following year; but all of the other 87 patients were still alive 2 years later.

Somatic illness. Somatic illnesses, in which physical symptoms appear to have no medical cause, are often improved markedly with psychotherapy. The emotional mechanism triggering somatic illness is presumed to be a problem that is not acceptable to the person and is transformed into a physical ailment. Studies measuring rates of return visits to a health maintenance organization after receiving a brief interval of psychotherapy are very positive. Another study demonstrated a reduction in visits following group support and psychotherapeutic treatment. A physician who recognizes this condition can save time and money and alleviate the physical suffering of the patient.

Cost-effectiveness. Psychotherapy has been shown to speed patients' recovery time from illness. Faster recovery in turn leads to smaller medical bills and fewer return visits to medical practitioners. In a study by Nicholas Cummings (Cummings and Bragman, 1988), patients who frequently visited medical clinics were offered short-term psychotherapy, and "these patients showed significant declines in their visits to doctors, days spent in the hospital, emergency room visits, diagnostic procedures, and drug prescriptions." The overall health care costs decreased by 10 to 20 percent in the years following brief psychotherapy.

A more specific example of cost-effectiveness was demonstrated in a study by Margaret Caudill and colleagues (1991), in which 10 group sessions of 90 minutes of psychotherapy and relaxation techniques significantly reduced the severity of pain. In a study of clinic use by chronic pain patients, patients who participated in the outpatient behavioral medicine program used 36 percent fewer clinic visits than those who did not. Cost savings were estimated at more than $100 per patient per year (Caudill et al., 1991).

Support groups. Social, cultural, and environmental contexts, which have a powerful impact on bringing about both psychological and physiological change, should be more fully investigated. The literature on support groups demonstrates that in a wide variety of physical illnesses, such as heart disease, cancer, asthma, and strokes, a support group can have a powerful positive effect.

Consider the potential role of group support and psychological counseling in cancer and heart disease, the two major causes of death in the United States. One recent, well-publicized example of this ubiquitous effect is David Spiegel's study on women with metastatic breast cancer. Women who took part in a support group lived an average of 18 months longer (a doubling of the survival time following diagnosis) than those who did not participate. In addition, all the long-term survivors belonged to the therapy group (Spiegel et al., 1989).

In a well-known study of patients with established coronary artery disease, group support, and psychological counseling were combined with diet and exercise. Symptoms such as angina pectoris rapidly diminished or disappeared altogether, and after 1 year the coronary artery obstructions were demonstrated to be smaller. This strongly suggests that coronary artery disease, the Nation's most deadly and expensive health care problem, is reversible through a complementary, non-invasive, diet and behavioral modification approach that emphasizes group psychotherapy (Ornish, 1990). (See the "Diet and Nutrition" chapter for more details on this approach.)

Support groups have two other major benefits: (1) they help members form bonds with one another, an experience that may empower members for the rest of their lives; and (2) they are inexpensive or even free (e.g., Alcoholics Anonymous).

Research needs and opportunities. Future opportunities for research on the interconnectedness of mind and body include the following:

- Studies should be directed toward devising methods for integrating psychotherapy into all aspects of health care and evaluating its efficacy in all treatments.

- Researchers should try to understand better how small shifts in behavior, thoughts, and attitudes can help change a person's entire physical and psychological state.

- Whether behavioral intervention can delay or prevent the onset of illness should be assessed.

- How support groups work should be explored. What types of groups are best? Leaderless or directed groups? Participants with single or mixed diagnoses? With time-limited or open-ended sessions? What type of personality is most likely to find them useful? Are they harmful to certain types of individuals? If so, what types?

- The role of psychotherapy in treating serious illness should be emphasized. Unfortunately, many people, including health care professionals and academicians, consider psychotherapeutic intervention in physical illness a luxury or frill. However, the studies cited above suggest that psychological intervention works best when used early and may actually make the difference between life and death in certain illnesses.

- Research should be undertaken on just how the body records and expresses emotions and on the possible effectiveness of body-oriented therapies in releasing physical tensions and resolving emotional problems.

- Mental health researchers should direct more attention to certain anomalous and unexplained mind-body events that have long existed on the periphery of medicine and that are generally ignored. Examples include the falling off of warts with suggestion; psychological profiles of extremely long-lived people; and the spontaneous and unanticipated remission of "fatal" cancer. If explained, these events could yield major gains in understanding the mind and its relationship to the body and could yield valuable new approaches to health.

- Mental health departments in teaching institutions should be bolder in entertaining novel explanations of mind and consciousness and the relationship between mind and brain. Currently, almost all academic institutions teach models of consciousness that largely equate mind and consciousness with the physical brain. This perspective is incomplete; it entirely ignores the considerable data implying that a nonlocal concept of consciousness may be a more encompassing explanation for the manifestations of consciousness. (See Dossey, 1989, 1992; Jahn, 1981; and Josephson and Ramachandran, 1980.) For patients, a physically based view of illness is restrictive, expensive, and often harmful. As long as mind is equated with brain, the routine tendency to employ physical interventions such as drugs for mental disturbances will continue to overshadow other methods that conceivably might be safer, more effective, and less costly.

- Mental health professionals should explore other areas of science areas usually considered "off base" and "irrelevant"—for perspectives that might be enriching. Quantum mechanics, dissipative structure theory, chaos theory, and nonlinear dynamics are only a few areas of science that have great potential relevance for understanding the mind and consciousness.[7]

- The concept of what constitutes appropriate areas for psychiatric intervention should be enlarged. Impressive evidence exists that "disorders of meaning" (a person's sense that his or her life lacks meaning) are epidemic in society and that these disorders can have life-and-death consequences. Mental health professionals should deal more effectively with issues involving meanings and values, which are usually shunted aside by medical professionals. Some of these problems are spiritual and require a reexamination of the traditional distinctions psychiatrists have made between psychiatry and religion, and between "science" and "spirit."[8]

- The cost-effectiveness of psychiatric intervention in physical illness deserves to be better known and should be more widely publicized. In an era of continued escalation of health care costs, these interventions offer a very real opportunity to improve health and limit costs simultaneously.

Meditation

Meditation is a self-directed practice for relaxing the body and calming the mind. The meditator makes a concentrated effort to focus on a single thought—peace, for instance; or a physical experience, such as breathing; or a sound (repeating a word or mantra, such as "one" or a Sanskrit word such as "kirim"). The aim is to still the mind's "busyness"—its inclination to mull over the thousand demands and details of daily life.

Most meditative techniques have come to the West from Eastern religious practices—particularly those of India, China, and Japan—but they can be found in all cultures of the world. Christian contemplation—saying the rosary or repeating the "Hail Mary"—brings similar effects and can be said to be akin to meditation. Michael Murphy, the cofounder of Esalen Institute, claims that the concentration used in Western sports is itself a form of meditation. While most meditators in the United States practice sedentary meditation, there are also many moving meditations, such as the Chinese martial art tai chi, the Japanese martial art aikido, and walking meditation in Zen Buddhism. Yoga can also be said to be a meditation.

Until recently, the primary purpose of meditation has been religious, although its health benefits have long been recognized. During the past 15 years, it has been explored as a way of reducing stress on both mind and body. Cardiologists, in particular, often recommend it as a way of reducing high blood pressure.

There are many forms of meditation—with many different names—ranging in complexity from strict, regulated practices to general recommendations, but all appear to produce similar physical and psychological changes (Benson, 1975; Chopra, 1991; Goleman, 1977; Mahesh Yosti, 1963).

If practiced regularly, meditation develops habitual, unconscious microbehaviors that produce widespread positive effects on physical and psychological functioning. Meditating even for 15 minutes twice a day seems to bring beneficial results.

While many individuals and groups have examined the effects of meditation, two major meditation programs have extensive bodies of research: transcendental meditation and the relaxation response.

Transcendental meditation. Transcendental meditation (TM) was developed by the Indian leader Maharishi Mahesh Yogi, who eliminated from yoga certain elements he considered nonessential. In the 1960s he left India and came to the United States, bringing with him this reformed yoga, which he felt could be grasped and practiced more easily by westerners. His new method did not require the often difficult physical or mental exercises required by yoga and could be easily taught in one training session. TM was soon embraced by some celebrities of that day, such as the Beatles, and can now probably claim well over 2 million practitioners.

TM is simple. To prevent distracting thoughts a student is given a mantra (a word or sound) to repeat silently over and over again while sitting in a comfortable position. Students are instructed to be passive and, if thoughts other than the mantra come to mind, to notice them and return to the mantra. A TM student is asked to practice for 20 minutes in the morning and again in the evening.

In 1968, Harvard cardiologist Herbert Benson was asked by TM practitioners to test them on their ability to lower their own blood pressures. At first, Benson refused this suggestion as "too far out" but later was persuaded to do so. Benson's studies and an independent investigation at the University of California at Los Angeles were followed by much additional research on TM at Maharishi International University in Fairfield, IA, and at other research centers. Published results from these studies report that the use of TM is discretely associated with:

- reduced health care use;

- increased longevity and quality of life;

- reduction of chronic pain (Kabat-Zinn et al., 1986);

- reduced anxiety;

- reduction of high blood pressure (Cooper and Aygen, 1978):

- reduction of serum cholesterol level (Cooper and Aygen, 1978);

- reduction of substance abuse (Sharma et al., 1991);

- longitudinal increase in intelligence-related measures (Cranson et al., 1991);

- treatment of posttraumatic stress syndrome in Vietnam veterans (Brooks and Scarano, 1985);

- blood pressure reduction in African-American persons (Schneider et al., 1992); and

- lowered blood cortisol levels initially brought on by stress (MacLean et al., 1992).

Relaxation response. Convinced that meditation was a possible treatment for high blood pressure, Benson later pursued his investigation at the Mind-Body Medical Institute at Harvard Medical School. He identified what he calls "the relaxation response," a constellation of psychological and physiological effects that appear common to many practices: meditation, prayer, progressive relaxation, autogenic training, and the presuggestion phase of hypnosis and yoga (Benson, 1975). He published his method in a book of the same name.

Over a period of 25 years, Benson and colleagues have developed a large body of research. During this time, meditation in general and the relaxation response specifically have slowly moved from alternative to mainstream medicine, although they are still overlooked by many conventional doctors. Benson's research has demonstrated a wide range of effects from meditation (or the relaxation response) on bodily functions: oxygen consumption and carbon dioxide and lactate production, adrenocorticotropic hormone excretion, blood elements such as platelets and lymphocytes, cell membranes, norepinephrine receptors, brain wave activity, and utilization of medical resources.

In addition, one study by Benson's group indicated that chronic pain patients who meditated had a net reduction in general health care costs, suggesting that this approach is cost-effective (Caudill et al., 1991).[9]

Although the positive effects of meditation clearly outnumber and outweigh the negative effects, the latter have also been studied (Blackmore, 1991). Potential adverse effects include adverse psychological feelings (e.g., feelings of negativity, disorientation) in a small percentage of meditators after meditation retreats; and elicitation of acute episodes of psychosis by intensive meditation in schizophrenics.

Despite the breadth and clarity of the research[10] indicating that meditation is a useful, low-cost intervention, it continues to be regarded as unconventional and is still ignored by most medical professionals. The report of the National Research Council (NRC) on meditation, which drew heavily on a negative review by Holmes (1984), emphasized concerns about weak experimental design's failure to discriminate meditation from other sources of effects, and conceptual issues such as the lack of an underlying mechanism. A critique of the NRC report by Orme-Johnson and Alexander responded to these criticisms using quantitative reviews which they claimed provided strong arguments for taking a deeper look at meditation (Orme-Johnson and Alexander, 1992).

Current clinical use. In September 1987, science writer Daniel Goleman reported in the *New York Times Magazine* that some 400 universities offered some level of training in behavioral medicine, including meditation, and "thousands of hospitals, clinics, and individual practitioners offer the treatments." Harvard Medical School's Mind-Body Medical Institute has several thousand patient visits per year in its clinical arm and maintains an active research program as well as training programs for doctors, nurses, social workers, and psychologists, in conjunction with the school's continuing education program (Benson and Stuart, 1992). Other hospitals want clinics of this kind, and dissemination is proceeding. The first affiliate is at Mercy Hospital in Chicago. Others sites being negotiated are Morristown, NJ; Columbus, OH; Charlottesville, VA; and Houston, TX. Many other independent clinics employ meditation techniques, such as the Cambridge Hospital behavioral medicine program and the University of Massachusetts Medical School program.

Meditation and healing. In addition to being used by individuals, meditation is also an important part of the unconventional healing approaches used by mental, spiritual, and psychic healers. Almost all healers consider some form of meditation or quiet prayer fundamental to their practice. (Mental healing is discussed in the "Prayer and Mental Healing" section.) Indeed, the state of focused attention and exclusive concern that some doctors demonstrate in orthodox medicine can be thought of as a form of meditation. In addition, meditation is often practiced by some physicians for their own benefit, even though they do not use it in treating their patients.

Cost-effectiveness and potential economic impact. Insurance statistics for a group of 2,000 meditators compared with 600,000 nonmeditators show that the use of medical care was 30 percent to 87 percent less for meditators in all but one of 18 categories (childbirth)

(McSherry, 1990; Orme-Johnson, 1987). In another study at the Harvard Community Health Plan, patients who attended a 6-week behavioral medicine group that included meditation made significantly fewer visits to physicians during the 6 months that followed; the savings were estimated at $171 per patient.

If the definition of meditation is expanded to include more or less formal religious practices that emphasize quiet prayer, the number of people using some form of meditation becomes enormous and the potential health benefits correspondingly large. In the United States, TM has been taught to well over a million people, and it is estimated that most continue the practice regularly. Benson's Mind-Body Medical Institute currently has 7,000 patient visits per year and has trained thousands of health professionals in applying the relaxation response.

Theory and rationale. How and why does meditation work? There are several related theories about the underlying mechanism. Ken Walton, director of the Neurochemistry Laboratory, Maharishi International University, states:

> The frequently striking results of [studies of TM] have not been widely discussed in the medical literature, purportedly because "there is no reasonable mechanism" which could explain such a spectrum of health effects from a simple mental technology . . . Only in the last year has the stress connection emerged with the degree of clarity it now has. The . . . bottom line is the proposed vicious circle linking chronic stress, serotonin metabolism, and hippocampal regulation of the hypothalamic-pituitary-adrenocortical (HPA) axis (Nelson, 1992).

Similarly, Everly and Benson have proposed that meditation is effective in a wide variety of disorders that may be called "disorders of arousal," in which the limbic system of the brain has become over-stimulated. Relaxation and meditation training serve to "retune" the nervous system by damping the production of adrenergic catecholamines, which stimulate limbic activity. Everly and Benson (1989) suggest also that excessive limbic activity may inhibit immune function—a possibility that may account for the association of chronic stress and increased susceptibility to infection.

Research needs and opportunities. The following points may be made about research needs in the area of meditation:

- More than 30 years of research, as well as the experiences of a large and growing number of individuals and health care providers, suggest that meditation and similar forms of relaxation can lead to better health, higher quality of life, and lowered health care costs. This research should be collected and critically evaluated, and its results should be widely disseminated to health professionals.

- Some of the research needs to be replicated and the physiological and biochemical dimensions more fully investigated to facilitate education, application, and acceptance into mainstream medicine.

- Research is needed into the commonalities and differences of meditation and other forms of self-regulation such as hypnosis, relaxation, and guided imagery.

- The nature and purpose of meditation need to be made more explicit by its advocates. In most traditions, meditation was originally considered primarily a technique for changing consciousness and achieving spiritual understanding; improvements in health were considered only byproducts. Today, meditation seems to be popularly regarded as utilitarian, as simply as a tool for improving physical health. Future research should compare the health benefits that result when meditation is undertaken for explicit health reasons versus for its own sake.

- Most meditation research has involved young or middle-aged Americans who have practiced meditation for several months to several years. Understanding would be enhanced by more studies of advanced, expert meditators who have spent a lifetime of meditation in a variety of traditions and cultures. This approach would be more likely to shed light on the maximal health benefits possible from meditation.

- Many different schools of meditation exist, advocating a variety of techniques. Prospective studies should investigate whether any particular school offers special health benefits.

- To ameliorate the objections of many Christian religious groups to meditation, cross-disciplinary dialog and communication should be encouraged that would examine (1) the commonalities

between Christian prayer and contemplation and Eastern meditation, and (2) the extraordinary similarities in the esoteric
mystical traditions of East and West.

Most important, meditation techniques offer the potential of learning how to live in an increasingly complex and stressful society while
helping to preserve health in the process. Given their low cost and
demonstrated health benefits, these simple mental technologies may
be some of the best candidates among the alternative therapies for
widespread inclusion in medical practice and for investment of medical resources.

Imagery

Imagery is both a mental process (as in imagining) and a wide
variety of procedures used in therapy to encourage changes in attitudes, behavior, or physiological reactions. As a mental process, it is
often defined as "any thought representing a sensory quality"
(Horowitz, 1983). It includes, as well as the visual, all the senses—
aural, tactile, olfactory, proprioceptive, and kinesthetic. Imagery is
often used synonymously with visualization; this use is misleading,
because the latter refers only to seeing something in the mind's eye,
whereas imagery can mean imagining through any sense, as through
hearing or smell.

Imagery is a common ingredient in many behavioral therapies not
specifically labeled imagery. Since it often involves directed concentration, it can also be thought of as a form of meditation (see the
"Meditation" section). Imagery can be taught either individually or
in groups, and the therapist often uses it to affect a particular result,
such as quitting smoking or bolstering the immune system to attack
cancer cells.

Practices that have a component of imagery are almost ubiquitous.
They include, among many others, biofeedback, desensitization and
counterconditioning, psychosynthesis, neurolinguistic programming,
gestalt therapy, rational emotive therapy, and hypnosis (see the "Hypnosis" section). Any therapy that relies on imagery or fantasy to motivate, communicate, solve problems, or evoke heightened awareness
and sensitivity could be described as a form of imagery. Forms of
meditation that involve repeating a sound or mantra (e.g., TM) or
focusing attention on an object that has no concurrent external ref-
erent (such as a whale in the ocean) could also be developed as aspects of imagery. Likewise, relaxation techniques that involve

instruction (e.g., "Your hands are heavy"), such as autogenic training, have an imagery component.

Whether imagery differs from hypnosis in terms of purpose and state of consciousness is currently debated. Hypnotherapists, particularly those who train clients in methods of self-hypnosis, are often indistinguishable from practitioners of imagery. What has been agreed on is that there is a correlation between the ability to image and the capacity to enter into an altered state of consciousness, including the hypnotic state (Barber, 1984; Hilgard, 1974; Lynn and Rhue, 1987).

Numerous studies indicate that mental imagery can bring about significant physiological and biochemical changes. These findings, which have encouraged the development of imagery as a health care tool, include its capacity to affect the following: oxygen supply in tissues (Olness and Conroy, 1985); cardiovascular changes (Barber, 1969); vascular or thermal change (Green and Green, 1977); the pupil and the cochlear reflex (Luria, 1968); heart rate and galvanic skin response (Jordan and Lenington, 1979); salivation (Barber et al., 1964; White, 1978); gastrointestinal activity (Barber, 1978); increase in breast size (Barber, 1984); the Mantoux reaction (Black et al., 1963); and blood glucose levels (Stevens, 1983). Several hundred studies using biofeedback, which Green and Green (1977) refer to as an "imagery trainer," expand the list considerably, running the gamut from effects on the firing of single motorneurons (Basmajian, 1963) to brain wave alterations (Brown, 1977).

Some of these findings are from well-controlled studies, but the vast majority represent reports of single cases or small studies that have not been replicated. Nevertheless, the overriding conclusion is that there is a relationship between imagery of bodily change and actual bodily change. Without question, imagery calls for further and more precise investigation.

Clinical applications. Procedures for imagery fall into at least three major categories: (1) evaluation or diagnostic imagery, (2) mental rehearsal, and (3) therapeutic intervention.

Techniques used in evaluation or diagnostic imagery involve asking the person to describe his or her condition in sensory terms. The therapist gathers information regarding the disease, the effect of treatment, and any natural inner healing resources the person might be sensing. The patient is asked, literally, "How do you feel?" In psychotherapy settings, dreams or fantasies might be used in this way, as a means to gaining insight or control over a situation.

Evaluation imagery is usually done early in a therapy session and serves as a format for designing both mental rehearsal and therapeutic intervention strategies. It also is an indicator of the person's understanding of the mechanisms of health and disease and provides opportunity for patient education.[ll]

Typically, a relaxation strategy is taught, then the treatment and recovery period are described in sensory terms as the patient is taken on a guided imagery "trip." Care is taken to be factual without using emotion-laden or fear-provoking words, and the medical procedure is reframed in a positive way whenever possible. The patient is taught coping techniques such as distraction, mental dissociation, muscle relaxation, and abdominal breathing.

Published results with mental rehearsals (or sensory education) are almost uniformly positive and often dramatic. Effects include reduced pain and anxiety; decreased length of hospital stay; the use of fewer pain medicines, barbiturates, tranquilizers, and other medications; and reduced treatment side effects. Mental rehearsal is a cornerstone of certain natural childbirth practices. It has also been tested in burn debridement (Kenner and Achterberg, 1983) and as a preparation for spinal surgery (Lawlis et al., 1985), cholecystectomy, pelvic examination, cast removal, and endoscopy (Johnson et al., 1978). In each of these instances, rehearsal through imagery has been found to diminish pain and discomfort and to reduce side effects.

Imagery as a therapeutic intervention is based on the idea that the images have either a direct or an indirect effect on health. Therefore, either the patients are shown how to use their own flow of images about the healing process or, alternatively, they are guided through a series of images that are intended to soothe and distract them, reduce any sympathetic nervous system arousal, or generally enhance their relaxation. The practitioner may also use "end state" types of imagery, having patients imaging themselves in a state of perfect health, well-being, or successfully achieved goals.

A major and serious criticism of imagery literature (as well as hypnosis literature) is that clinic protocols are seldom provided. Therefore, it is impossible to know what type of therapeutic strategy was used, and of course it cannot be replicated.

Some practitioners even regard their protocols as trade secrets and refuse to divulge them.

Whether imagery is merely an antidote to feelings of helplessness or whether the image itself has the capacity to induce the desired physical effect is still unclear. Existing research suggests both conclusions are justified, depending on the situation in question.

Imagery has been successfully tested as a strategy for alleviating nausea and vomiting associated with chemotherapy in cancer patients (Frank, 1985; Scott et al., 1986), to relieve stress (Donovan, 1980), and to facilitate weight gain in cancer patients (Dixon, 1984). It has been successfully used and tested for pain control in a variety of settings; as adjunctive therapy for several diseases, including diabetes (Stevens, 1983); and with geriatric patients to enhance immunity (Kiecolt-Glaser et al., 1985).

Imagery is usually combined with other behavioral approaches. It is best known in the treatment of cancer as a means to help patients mobilize their immune systems (Borysenko, 1987; Siegel, 1986; Simonton et al., 1978), but it also is used as part of a multidisciplinary approach to cardiac rehabilitation (Ornish, 1990; Ornish et al., 1983) and in many settings that specialize in treating chronic pain.

In a survey of alternative techniques used by cancer patients (Cassileth et al., 1984), imagery was cited as the fourth most frequently used. And 46 percent of the respondents listed "self" as practitioner, indicating that imagery is often used as a self-help tool.

Imagery assessment tools. The measurement of imagery as a mental process is fraught with the same problems faced in measuring any other so-called hypothetical construct, including learning, motivation, and perception. So far, psychology has risen to the occasion and developed reliable and meaningful measurement strategies.

A number of instruments with varying purposes, degrees of validity, and reliability are currently in use for measuring imagery. Sheikh and Jordan (1983) have reviewed the imagery test used for psychological diagnosis. Imagery of cancer, diabetes, and spinal pain have been specifically analyzed by Achterberg and Lawlis, using a protocol to elicit sensory information on healing mechanisms, treatment, and the disease itself (Achterberg and Lawlis, 1984). These tests have been found to be accurate predictors of treatment outcome in a number of clinics and rehabilitation facilities.

Research accomplishments. Recent studies suggest a direct impact or correlation between imagery (both as a mental process and a set of procedures) and immunology. These findings include the following:

- Correlations between various types of leukocytes and components of cancer patients' images of their disease, treatment, and immune system (Achterberg and Lawlis, 1984).

- Increased phagocytic activity following biofeedback-assisted relaxation (Peavey et al., 1985).

- Enhanced natural killer cell function following a relaxation and imagery training procedure with geriatric patients (Kiecolt-Glaser et al., 1985) and in adult cancer patients with metastatic disease (Gruber et al., 1988).

- Changes in lymphocyte reactivity following hypnotic procedures (Hall, 1982-83) and instruction in relaxation and imagery in adult cancer patients with metastatic disease.

- Altered neutrophil adherence or margination, as well as white blood cell count, following an imagery procedure (Schneider et al., 1983).

- Increased secretory immunoglobulin A (IgA) (significantly higher than control group) following training in location, activity, and morphology of IgA and 6 weeks of daily imaging.

- The specificity of imagery training was suggested by a study on training patients in cell-specific imagery of either T lymphocytes or neutrophils. The effects of training, which were assessed after 6 weeks, were statistically associated with the type of imagery procedure employed (Achterberg and Rider, 1989).

Research issues. Although this early research is very promising, further investigations are badly needed. Longitudinal studies are virtually nonexistent. Consequently, the major question remains: Will the physiological-biochemical changes noted in imagery studies have an ultimate impact on health or on the course of the disease?

Distinguishing clinical from statistical significance is critical. Relying on statistical significance alone may obscure much valuable information, such as the few outstanding cases in which the methods were remarkably successful.

For complex clinical research, innovative research paradigms and statistical treatments are needed. Traditional research methodology is based on the idea of a univariate, linear model, which is rare (if not completely absent) in the real world. The spirit of discovery is not served by clinging to models that obscure much of the richness of the human condition. Furthermore, there are a number of complex variables that need to be accounted for in developing a research design. The following are examples:

545

- The randomized control group design is often impossible, impractical, and unnecessary. Its general efficacy and the ethics of its application are now being seriously challenged (Rider et al., 1990). Other designs should be considered.

- Participant and therapist-researcher motivation and belief are critical and significant variables to consider in this type of behavioral research and should serve as factors in group selection and measurement.

- Studies should be designed to maximize the possibility of good outcome on health and well-being.

- Research into the relationship between imagery and biological parameters—particularly those related to immunology—is hindered by the state of the art in that area. For instance, normative data are often absent, and reliability of assay procedures is questionable. Clinical significance of any changes may or may not be known. The specific impact of diet, season, environment, age, mood, or even the time of day on many of the immune assays is not well studied.

Research needs and opportunities. Existing data suggest at least two major research directions:

1. The impact of imagery as part of a multimodal treatment with conditions such as cancer, AIDS, or autoimmune disorders. The research should include repeat immunologic testing and follow up. Specific studies could be embedded within the overall design; for example, studies on the effect of imagery specifically designed to enhance medical treatment, the relationship between imagery and outcome of disease, types of patients who respond to imagery, and so on.

2. Replication and expansion of earlier intriguing—but small or poorly controlled—studies that indicated a direct effect of imagery on biologic function.

Hypnosis

Hypnosis, derived from the Greek word hypnos (sleep), and hypnotic suggestion have been a part of healing since ancient times. The induction of trance states and the use of therapeutic suggestion were a central feature of the early Greek healing temples, and variations of these techniques were practiced throughout the ancient world.

Modern hypnosis began in the 18th century with Franz Anton Mesmer, who used what he called "magnetic healing" to treat a variety of psychological and psychophysiological disorders, such as hysterical blindness, paralysis, headaches, and joint pains. Since then, the fortunes of hypnosis have ebbed and flowed. The famous Austrian neurologist Sigmund Freud at first found hypnosis extremely effective in treating hysteria and then, troubled by the sudden emergence of powerful emotions in his patients and his own difficulty with its use, abandoned it.

In the past 50 years, however, hypnosis has experienced a resurgence, first with physicians and dentists and more recently with psychologists and other mental health professionals. Today it is widely used for addictions, such as smoking and drug use, for pain control, and for phobias, such as the fear of flying.

Hypnosis is a state of attentive and focused concentration in which people can be relatively unaware of, but not completely blind to, their surroundings. If something demands attention—such as a fire in the wastebasket—hypnotized people easily rouse themselves to react to the situation. In this state of concentration, people are highly responsive to suggestion. But, contrary to popular folklore, people cannot be hypnotized involuntarily or follow suggestions against their wishes. They must be willing to concentrate their thoughts and to follow the suggestions offered. In the end, all hypnotherapy is self-hypnosis. Some people usually those with a vivid fantasy life-are better hypnotic subjects than others.

Hypnosis has three major components: absorption (in the words or images presented by the hypnotherapist); dissociation (from one's ordinary critical faculties); and responsiveness. A hypnotherapist either leads a client through relaxation, mental images, and suggestions or teaches clients to do this for themselves. Many hypnotherapists provide guided audiotapes for their clients so they can practice the therapy at home. The images presented are specifically tailored to the particular client's problems and may employ one or all of the senses.

Physiologically, hypnosis resembles other forms of deep relaxation: a generalized decrease in sympathetic nervous system activity, a decrease in oxygen consumption and carbon dioxide eliminations, a lowering of blood pressure and heart rate, and an increase in certain kinds of brain wave activity (Spiegel et al., 1989).

The most prominent organization of clinical professionals in the field is the American Society for Clinical Hypnosis, which numbers approximately 3,000 members (M.D.s and Ph.D.s). In addition, there are probably thousands of others who use hypnotherapy as part of their practice (e.g., R.N.s, M.S.W.s, marriage and family counselors, and lay therapists).

Clinical applications. One of the most dramatic uses of hypnosis is the treatment of congenital ichthyosis (fish skin disease), a genetic skin disorder that covers the surface of the skin with grotesque hard, wartlike, layered crust. Dermatologists thought ichthyosis was incurable until an anesthesiologist, Arthur Mason, in the mid-1950s used hypnosis by chance to effectively treat a patient he thought had warts. After Mason used hypnosis on the patient (a 16-year-old boy), the boy's scales fell off, and within 10 days, normal pink skin replaced it. Since that time, hypnosis has been used to treat ichthyosis—not always resulting in complete cure but often resulting in dramatic improvement (Goldberg, 1985).

Hypnosis is, however, most frequently used in more common ailments, either independently or in concert with other treatment. The following are a few examples:

- **Pain management.** Pain increases with heightened fear and anxiety. Because hypnotherapy helps a person gain control over fear and anxiety, pain is also reduced. Hypnotic suggestion (one may suggest that a part of the body become numb) can be used instead of or together with an anesthetic. Twelve controlled studies have demonstrated that hypnosis is a superior way to reduce migraine attacks in children and teenagers. In one experiment, schoolchildren were randomly assigned a placebo or propranolol, a blood-pressure lowering agent, or taught self-hypnosis; only the children using self-hypnosis had a significant drop in severity and frequency of headaches (Olness et al., 1989). Another pain study of patients who were chronically ill reports a 113-percent increase in pain tolerance among highly hypnotizable subjects versus a control group who did not receive hypnosis (Debenedittis et al., 1989).

- **Dentistry.** Some people have learned how to tolerate dental work with hypnotherapy as the only anesthetic. Even when an anesthetic is used, hypnotherapy can also be employed to reduce fear and anxiety, control bleeding and salivation, and reduce postoperative discomfort.

- **Pregnancy and delivery.** Women who have hypnosis prior to delivery have shorter labors and more comfortable deliveries. Women have also used self-hypnosis to control pain during delivery (Rossi, 1986).

- **Anxiety.** Hypnosis can be used to establish a new reaction to specific anxiety-causing activities such as stage fright, plane flights, and other phobias.

- **Immune system function.** Hypnotherapy can have a positive effect on the immune system. One study has shown that hypnosis can raise immunoglobulin levels of healthy children (Olness et al., 1989). Another study reported that self-hypnosis led to an increase in white blood cell activity (Hall, 1982-83).

Other studies in the past 40 years have shown that hypnosis can affect a wide variety of physical responses, including reduction of bleeding in hemophiliacs (Lucas, 1965), reduction in severity of attacks of hay fever and asthma (Mason and Black, 1958), increased breast size (Honiotest, 1977; LeCron, 1969; Staib and Logan, 1977; Willard, 1977; Williams, 1973), the cure of warts (Ahser, 1956; Sinclair-Geiben and Chalmers, 1959; Surman et al., 1973; Ullman and Dudek, 1960), the production of skin blisters and bruises (Bellis, 1966; Johnson and Barber, 1976), and control of reaction to allergens such as poison ivy and certain foods (Ikemi, 1967; Ikemi and Nakagawa, 1962; Platonov, 1959).

No one knows exactly how such bodily changes are brought about by hypnosis, but they clearly occur because of the connections between mind and body. It is also clear that suggestions have the capacity to affect all systems and organs of the body in a variety of ways.

To flow naturally in and out of hypnotic states is common; it happens to people watching television, for instance. We are also likely to move into a trance state in situations of extreme stress. When a person in a position of power yells, the yelling may have effects that become as strong as posthypnotic suggestions. When physicians or other health care providers make predictions about an illness, they may have a similar effect. It is particularly important that physicians understand this state and the potential power of the positive and negative suggestions they use with their patients.

Research needs and opportunities. The following needs exist in the area of hypnosis:

- Because of the profound influence of hypnosis, an understanding of how to apply it in all therapeutic settings is needed. Future study must be directed toward influencing and maximizing the beneficial capacity of trance states occurring in doctors' offices and on operating tables as well as minimizing the destructive effects of negative or offhand remarks made in these places. And of course, further research is needed on explicit, hypnotic treatment for specific illnesses.

- The cases in which hypnosis has resulted in dramatic improvements of severely disfiguring genetic diseases such as ichthyosis deserves further scientific attention. They raise fundamental questions about the extent and limits of the mind's powers and suggest that such limits may be very wide indeed.

- Hypnosis is often reserved as a "backup" therapy to be used when conventional treatments fail. However, the examples above show the broad spectrum of its usefulness and suggest that in some conditions hypnosis may be appropriately considered as a first-line therapy instead of a last resort.

Biofeedback

Originating in the late 1960s, biofeedback is a treatment method that uses monitoring instruments to feed back to patients physiological information of which they are normally unaware. By watching the monitoring device, patients can learn by trial and error to adjust their thinking and other mental processes in order to control bodily processes heretofore thought to be involuntary, such as blood pressure, temperature, gastrointestinal functioning, and brain wave activity.

Biofeedback can be used to treat a wide variety of conditions and diseases ranging from stress, alcohol and other addictions, sleep disorders, epilepsy, respiratory problems, and fecal and urinary incontinence to muscle spasms, partial paralysis or muscle dysfunction caused by injury, migraine headaches, hypertension, and a variety of vascular disorders. More applications are being developed yearly.

In a normal session, electrodes are attached to the area being monitored (the involved muscles for muscle therapy, the head for brain wave activity); these electrodes feed the information to a small monitoring box that registers the results by a sound tone that varies in pitch or on a visual meter that varies in brightness as the function being monitored decreases or increases. A biofeedback therapist leads the patient in mental exercises to help the patient reach the desired result (e.g., muscle relaxation or contraction, or more alpha and theta brain waves). Through trial and error, patients gradually train themselves to control the inner mechanism involved. Training for some disorders requires 8 to 10 sessions. Patients with long-term or severe disorders may require longer therapy. Obviously, the aim of the treatment is to teach patients to regulate their own inner mental and bodily processes without help from the machine. In its simplest form, biofeedback therapy always involves a therapist, a patient, and a monitoring device capable of providing accurate physiological information.

A major reason why many patients like biofeedback training is that, like behavioral approaches in general, it puts them in charge, giving them a sense of mastery and self-reliance over their illnesses and health. Such an attitude may play a crucial role in the lower health care costs seen in patients after learning biofeedback skills.

Background. In 1961, experimental psychologist Neal Miller proposed that the autonomic, or visceral, nervous system was entirely trainable. Miller's suggestion ran contrary to prevailing orthodoxy, which held that all autonomic responses—heart rate, blood pressure, regional blood flow, gastrointestinal activity, and so on—were beyond voluntary control. In a remarkable series of experiments he showed that instrumental learning and control of such processes were indeed possible. One result of his work was the creation of biofeedback therapy.

In the succeeding three decades, Miller's work has been expanded by scores of researchers. Approximately 3,000 articles and 100 books have been published to date describing biofeedback and its applications. There are currently about 10,000 practitioners in the United States. Two organizations certify biofeedback professionals and paraprofessionals, and more than 2,000 individuals have received national certification.

Biofeedback does not belong to any particular field of health care but is used in many disciplines, including internal medicine, dentistry, physical therapy and rehabilitation, psychology and psychiatry, pain management, and more.

The most common forms of biofeedback involve the measurement of muscle tension (electromyographic, or EMG, feedback), skin temperature (thermal feedback), electrical conductance or resistance of the skin (electrodermal feedback), brain waves (electroencephalographic, or EEG, feedback), and respiration. More recently, increasingly sophisticated measurement devices have expanded biofeedback possibilities. Sensors can now measure and feed back the activity of the internal and external rectal sphincters (for the treatment of fecal incontinence), the activity of the detrusor muscle of the urinary bladder (for the treatment of urinary incontinence), esophageal motility, and stomach acidity (pH). Currently there are approximately 150 applications for biofeedback. Medical awareness of biofeedback is increasing, and referrals to biofeedback clinics continue to climb. Some treatments are already widely accepted. The American Medical Association, for example, has endorsed EMG biofeedback training for treating muscle contraction headaches.

Research accomplishments and clinical applications. Substantial research exists demonstrating the effectiveness of biofeedback in a number of conditions, including bronchial asthma, drug and alcohol abuse, anxiety, tension and migraine headaches, cardiac arrhythmias, essential hypertension, Raynaud's disease/syndrome, fecal and urinary incontinence, irritable bowel (spastic colon) syndrome, muscle reeducation (strengthening weak muscles, relaxing overactive ones), hyperactivity and attention deficit disorder, epilepsy, menopausal hot flashes, chronic pain syndromes, and anticipatory nausea and vomiting associated with chemotherapy (Basmajian, 1989).

Like all other forms of therapy, biofeedback is more useful for some clinical problems than for others. For example, biofeedback is the preferred treatment in Raynaud's disease/syndrome (a painful and potentially dangerous spasm of the small arteries) and certain types of fecal and urinary incontinence. However, it is one of several preferred treatments for muscle contraction (tension) headaches, migraine headaches, irritable bowel (spastic colon) syndrome, hypertension, asthma, and a variety of neuromuscular disorders, especially during rehabilitation. EEG biofeedback therapy is one of several preferred treatments for certain patients with epilepsy or attention deficit disorder.

Cost-effectiveness. Biofeedback-assisted relaxation training has been shown to be associated with decrease in medical care costs to patients, decrease in number of claims and costs to insurers in claims payments, reduction of medication and physician usage, reduction in hospital stays and rehospitalization, reduction of mortality and morbidity, and enhanced quality of life (Schneider, 1987).

Efforts are being made to further increase the cost-effectiveness of biofeedback therapy through the use of group and classroom instruction, reduced therapist contact, and home-based training. No studies have yet been made that discuss cost-benefit issues for the non-relaxation-based biofeedback therapies, such as neuromuscular education and seizure reduction training.

Research needs and opportunities. The following are some of the research questions about biofeedback that need answering:

- What is actually learned during biofeedback? An awareness of some internal response or an awareness of associations between stimuli and responses?

- What variables influence learning in the biofeedback setting? How do they exert their effects? For example, what are the effects of the quality and quantity of reinforcements used to promote learning?

- What is the full range of bodily responses that can be modified by instrumental training procedures? Are the influences of biofeedback large enough to make a clinical difference? Or, are they laboratory curiosities?

- Which physiological responses are best to modify with respect to a specific disorder? For example, is lowering of blood pressure best achieved by feedback of blood pressure, or is feedback of muscle tension or skin temperature more effective?

- To what extent does transfer of training take place from the laboratory to real life? Can an individual self-regulate a physiological response at home as well as in a clinic? How long does the learning last?

- How do motivation and expectancy relate to the successful learning of biofeedback skills? What criteria predict who will be a successful biofeedback subject?

- How does biofeedback compare with other approaches (e.g., meditation, relaxation, suggestion, hypnosis) in altering physiological processes?

- How can biofeedback's effects be separated from other treatment variables such as the therapist's attention, verbal exchanges, suggestion, patient expectation, the clinical atmosphere, or participation in a self-help program?

- In which situations can biofeedback-assisted learning be used in lieu of pharmacological or surgical therapies, and in which situations as an adjunct to these approaches?

- For what conditions might group instruction in biofeedback skills be as effective as individual teaching? How can subjects be identified as more suitable for group teaching or individual instruction?

- How can biofeedback teaching procedures be more widely applied to the medical problems of children? Might the widespread teaching of biofeedback skills to children emphasizing self-care and self-responsibility at a young age counteract the widespread dependence and reliance on the medical system demonstrated by adults?

- What innovations in chip and microprocessor technology are needed to open up new areas of experimental and clinical research in biofeedback? How might miniaturization provide opportunities for patients to wear portable devices in real-life situations, thus expanding biofeedback learning?

Progress in this field, as in many other alternative and orthodox therapies, will entail three general steps or phases:

I. Pilot studies to determine whether there are any promising effects worthy of investigation and to detect any negative side effects or practical difficulties. These may be anecdotal case reports, systematic case studies or uncontrolled single-group studies.

II. Controlled comparisons with the best available other techniques or with placebo treatments, using larger groups of patients, double-blind procedures, and adequate follow up.

III. Broad clinical trials on large patient populations under ordinary conditions, to determine the effectiveness of the treatment in conditions other than unusually favorable ones with especially talented therapists.

Most clinical research in biofeedback has been done in Phase I, although some studies have appeared in Phase II. Phase III studies are needed and can be expected if funding becomes available.

Yoga

In India, where it has been practiced for thousands of years, yoga is a way of life that includes ethical precepts, dietary prescriptions, and physical exercise. Its practitioners have long known that their discipline has the capacity to alter mental and bodily responses normally thought to be far beyond a person's ability to modulate. During the past 80 years, health professionals in India and the West have begun to investigate the therapeutic potential of yoga. To date, thousands of research studies have shown that with the practice of yoga a person can indeed learn to control such physiological parameters as blood pressure, heart rate, respiratory function, metabolic rate, skin resistance, brain waves, body temperature, and many other bodily functions (see also the "Ayurvedic Medicine" section in the "Alternative Systems of Medical Practice" chapter).

As the practice of yoga has gradually moved into the West, it has been used most often as part of an integral program of health enhancement as well as for the treatment of chronic diseases. A prime example of the latter application is Dr. Dean Ornish's use of yoga in conjunction with dietary changes, moderate aerobic exercise, meditation, and group support to reverse coronary artery disease (Ornish, 1990) (see the "Diet and Nutrition" chapter).

For the most part, the West has adopted three aspects of entirely different yoga practices: the postures (or asanas) of hatha yoga, the breathing techniques of pranayama yoga, and meditation. Studies of meditation were discussed previously in this section. Here, the focus is on the therapeutic utility of programs that combine hatha yoga and pranayama yoga.

A typical yoga session as practiced in the United States lasts 20 minutes to an hour. Some people practice daily at home, while others practice one to three times a week in a class. A session usually begins with gentle postures to relax tension in the muscles and joints, then moves to more difficult postures. Every movement should be made gently and slowly, and practitioners are urged not to stretch beyond what is comfortable for them. Rather, practice should be "easeful." Emphasis is placed on breathing slowly from deep in the abdomen. Specific pranayama breathing exercises also are an important part of the practice. Guided (or self-guided) relaxation, meditation, and sometimes visualization follow the asanas. The session frequently ends with chanting, such as a repeating Om shanti ("Let there be peace"), to bring the body and mind into a deeper state of relaxation.

The physical and psychological benefits of yoga reportedly include massage of muscles and internal organs; increased blood circulation; rebalancing of the sympathetic and parasympathetic nervous systems; increase in brain endorphins, enkephalins, and serotonin; deeper breathing; increased lymph circulation; countering of the effects of gravity on the body; increasing nutrient supply to the tissues; and augmenting alpha and theta brain wave activity, which reflects a greater degree of relaxation.

Research. Since it began in the 1920s, scientific research on yoga has been enormous. Some 1,600 studies are listed by Monroe and colleagues (1989), and many more have been undertaken since that bibliography was published in 1989. Following are a few examples of those studies:

- Rats who were placed in headstands for an hour a day and then subjected to a variety of shocks adapted more rapidly to stressful situations than the control group (Udupa, 1978).

- Human beings doing postures such as the shoulder stand daily became more "stress hardy" (Gaertner et al., 1965).

- People practicing yogic meditation showed a 200-percent increase in skin resistance (less stress) within 10 minutes after beginning to meditate. The anxiety level remained altered (reduced) for long periods after the meditation training session ended (Benson, 1972).

- With the practice of yoga, the heart works more efficiently (Ornish et al., 1983), and the respiratory rate decreases (Bakker, 1976).

- Blood pressure is lowered, accumulated carbon dioxide diminishes, and the brain waves reflect a more relaxed state (Anand and Chhina, 1961; Blacknell et al., 1975; Fenwick et al., 1977).

- EEG synchronicity, a unique change in brain waves found only in deep meditation, reflects improved communication between the right and left brain with regular yoga practice (Banquet, 1972).

- Physical fitness (as measured by the Fleishman Battery of Physical Fitness) is improved (Therrien, 1968).

- With yoga training in conjunction with dietary changes, cholesterol levels have been shown to drop an average of 14 points in 3 weeks (Ornish et al., 1983).

- Yoga brings increased chest expansion, better breath-holding abilities, and increased vital capacity and tidal volume (Maris and Maris, 1979; Shivarpita, 1981).

- Blood sugar levels improve and diabetes is better controlled after regular yoga practice (Monroe and Fitzgerald, 1986).

- Yoga, because of its psychological benefits, has been used successfully for drug treatment among prisoners, to help people stop smoking (Benson, 1969), and to improve job satisfaction (Maris and Maris.1979)

- Yoga can be used successfully as an adjunctive therapy for asthma (Gore, 1982), high blood pressure (Blacknell et al., 1975), drug addiction (Benson, 1969), heart disease (Ornish et al., 1983), migraine headaches (Benson et al., 1977), and cancer (Frank, 1975).

- Yoga has been used successfully with arthritis and the arthritic symptoms of lupus (Coudron and Coudron, 1987).

Research needs and opportunities. Although many possibilities to further research can be considered, two areas are of primary importance—surgery and cancer. Yoga should be studied as a form of pain relief for surgical patients. Use of yoga both before and after surgery should be studied and evaluated in terms of the number of days of recuperation and the level of pain experienced. Studies also should be done with cancer patients who practice 1 hour of yoga a day for a year together with specific, ongoing lifestyle changes: a low-fat, high-fiber diet and weekly group support meetings.

Dance Therapy

Because dance is a direct expression of the mind and body, it is an intimate and powerful medium for therapy. Throughout the world, people have always danced to celebrate major events, to bond communities, to share sentiments, and to heal the sick and the alienated.

Applications. The use of dance as a medical therapy in the United States began in 1942 through the pioneering efforts of Marian Chace. Psychiatrists in Washington, D.C., found that their patients were deriving therapeutic benefits from attending Chace's dance classes. As a result, Chace was asked to work on the back wards of St.

Elizabeth's Hospital with patients who had been considered too disturbed to participate in group activities. At about the same time, Trudi Schoop, a dancer and mime, volunteered to work with patients at Camarillo State Hospital in California. A group approach for nonverbal and noncommunicative patients was needed, and dance/movement therapy (DMT) met that need.

In 1956, dance therapists from across the country founded the American Dance Therapy Association, which has now grown to more than 1,100 members.[12] It publishes a journal, the *American Journal of Dance Therapy*; fosters research; monitors standards for professional practice; and develops guidelines for graduate education. It also maintains a registry for therapists: the certification registered dance therapist (D.T.R.) is granted to individuals with a master's degree and 700 hours of supervised clinical internship; the certification "Academy of Dance Therapists Registered" (A.D.T.R.) is awarded after therapists have completed 3,640 hours of supervised clinical work, which qualifies an individual to teach, supervise, and engage in private practice.

Dance/movement therapists are employed in a wide range of facilities, work with diverse populations, and address the needs of a broad spectrum of specific disorders and disabilities. Typically, dance/movement therapists work with individuals who have social, emotional, cognitive, or physical problems. Evolving specializations include using DMT as a disease prevention and health promotion service with healthy people and as a method of reducing the stress of caregivers and of patients with cancer, AIDS, and Alzheimer's disease.

Therapy goals vary according to the population served: for the emotionally disturbed, goals are to express feelings, gain insight, and develop attachments; for the physically disabled, to increase movement and self-esteem, have fun, and heighten creativity; for the elderly, to maintain a healthy body, enhance vitality, develop relationships, and express fear and grief; and for the mentally retarded, to motivate learning, increase body awareness, and develop social skills.

The underlying assumption in DMT is that visible movement behavior is analogous to personality. Thus, the process of changing how one moves (e.g., from fragmented to integrated or graceful) can effect total functioning. Specific aspects in DMT—such as music, rhythm, and synchronous movement—promote the healing processes by altering mood states, reawakening stored memories and feelings, organizing thoughts and actions, reducing isolation, and establishing rapport. Dancing in a group creates the emotional intensity necessary for behavioral change, and physical activity increases the endorphin level, inducing a state of well-being. Total body movement stimulates functioning of body systems (circulatory, respiratory, skeletal, and neuromuscular). Activating muscles and joints reduces body tension and body armoring. Unspeakable events, expressed in dance, can then be verbalized.

DMT has been demonstrated to be clinically effective in developing body image, improving self-concept, increasing self-esteem, facilitating attention, ameliorating depression, decreasing fears and anxieties, expressing anger, decreasing isolation, increasing communication skills, fostering solidarity, decreasing bodily tension, reducing chronic pain, enhancing circulatory and respiratory functions, reducing suicidal ideas, increasing feelings of well-being, promoting healing, and increasing verbalization (Fisher and Stark, 1992).

Research needs and opportunities. Although the efficacy of DMT has been demonstrated since the 1940s through extensive clinical practice, the following kinds of research should be done:

- Experimental studies to establish cause-effect relationships between specific approaches and patient outcomes. For example, what is the effect of daily DMT on depressed teenagers and drug abusers? What are the effects of psychotropic drugs on the ability of patients to respond to DMT? What are the effects of DMT on the ability of autistic children to communicate (Holtz, 1990)?

- Reression studies to isolate the independent and interactive effect of DMT. In many settings DMT is but one of several treatment modalities. Studies addressing the question of how much of the variation in patient change is accounted for by DMT alone and by DMT in combination with other therapies would yield useful information (Holtz, 1990).

- Studies about how specific elements of dance—such as exuberance, vitality, social contact, and bonding—promote healing, longevity, and health-enhancement. Can the effects of these different components be dissected and quantified?

- If dance is engaged in for a specific purpose, is its therapeutic effect diminished? That is, to what extent does the effect of dance depend on spontaneity?

- Studies indicate that DMT is an aid to recovery after illness. However, few studies exist on the use of dance therapy for prevention of illness. Studies could be done to evaluate the adjunctive use of dance in blood pressure control or in reduction of blood lipids.

Music Therapy

Throughout history, music has been used to facilitate healing. Aristotle believed the flute in particular was powerful. Pythagoras taught his students to change emotions of worry, fear, sorrow, and anger through the daily practice of singing and playing a musical instrument. The first accounts of the influence of music on breathing, blood pressure, digestion, and muscular activity were documented during the Renaissance (Munro and Mount.1978).

Music, more than the spoken word, "lends itself as a therapy because it meets with little or no intellectual resistance, and does not need to appeal to logic to initiate its action . . . [and] is more subtle and primitive, and therefore its appeal is wider and greater" (Altshuler, 1948). This wide appeal, as well as the considerable research base, suggests music may be used more and more both by itself and in conjunction with other treatments to ameliorate certain illnesses

Music therapy began as a profession in the 1940s, when the Veterans Administration Hospital incorporated music into rehabilitation programs for disabled soldiers returning from World War II. The National Association for Music Therapy, Inc. (NAMT), was established in the United States in 1950. At the same time, degree programs were developing to educate and train professional music therapists. Since then, the organization has established curricular programs in music therapy, which include both clinical practice and internships at sites in a wide variety of medical and community settings; organized an impressive scientific database for the profession; developed standards of practice and a code of ethics; and fostered the development of a theoretical rationale for music's beneficial effect on the mind and body.

There are more than 5,000 registered music therapists (R.M.T.s) in the United States, and more than 80 undergraduate and graduate degree programs. In addition, there are 165 clinical internship training sites. A baccalaureate degree in music therapy requires course work in music therapy; psychology; music; biological, social, and behavioral sciences; disabling conditions; and general studies. It includes field work in community facilities or on-campus clinics serving individuals with special needs. After graduation, a student must serve a 6-month internship in an approved facility to be eligible to take the exams to become a board-certified therapist.

Two refereed journals are sponsored by NAMT: the *Journal of Music Therapy* and *Music Therapy Perspectives*. Three published indexes in music therapy exist with more than 6,000 citations of periodical articles published between 1960 and 1980 (Eagle, 1976, 1978; Eagle and Minter, 1984). An electronic database of medical music therapy (Computer-Assisted Information Retrieval Service System, CAIRSS) has been established with citations from more than 1,000 journals including empirical studies, case reports, and program reviews.

Music therapy is used in psychiatric hospitals, rehabilitation facilities, general hospitals, outpatient clinics, day care treatment centers, residences for people with developmental disabilities, community mental health centers, drug and alcohol programs, senior centers, nursing homes, hospice programs, correctional facilities, halfway houses, schools, and private practice.

Music therapy is used to address physical, psychological, cognitive, and social needs of individuals with disabilities and illnesses. After assessing the strengths and needs of each client, a qualified music therapist provides the appropriate treatment, which can include creating music, singing, moving to music, or just listening to it. Music therapy can be used to meet medical goals in many areas, including the following:

- Physical and emotional stimulation for those with chronic pain or impaired movement. Music evokes a wide range of emotional responses. It can be a sedative to promote relaxation, or it can be a stimulant to promote movement to other physical activity (Coyle, 1987; Kerkvliet, 1990; Zimmerman et al., 1989).

- Communication for those with autism or communication disorders. Music is a unique form of communication. Using music with people who are nonverbal or who have difficulty communicating facilitates their social interaction and may increase their functioning (Grimm and Pefley, 1990; Street and Cappella, 1989).

- Emotional expression for those with mental health problems. Music can be used to express a wide variety of emotions, ranging from anger and frustration to affection and tenderness.

561

These feelings often take the form of vocalizations that may or may not employ words (Jochims, 1990; Schmettermayer, 1983).

- Associations with music for those with Alzheimer's disease and other dementias. Selecting music from an individual's past may evoke memories of times, places, and persons. These memories can contribute additional information to the treatment of the individual (Clair and Bernstein, 1990; Gibbons, 1988; Hanser, 1990).

Research accomplishments. Thousands of specific research studies have been undertaken in the clinical uses of music in medical and dental treatment, and many others are currently in process. Among those clinical uses are the following:

- **As an analgesic.** As early as 1914, Kane investigated using a phonograph in the operating room for calming patients prior to anesthesia. Music as an analgesic for dental procedures was one of the earliest and most thoroughly investigated areas. It also has been used successfully during childbirth and with obstetric patients. A 1985 study using music as an anxiolytic showed suppressed stress hormone levels in orthopedic, gynecologic, and urologic surgery patients (Bonny and McCarron.1984: Frandsen.1989).

- **As a relaxant and anxiety reducer for infants and children.** Many studies have dealt with music's effect on hospitalized infants and pediatric patients. Lullabies in the neonatal nursery increased the weight gain and movements of newborns; music activities reduced fear, distress, and anxiety in hospitalized infants, toddlers, and their families and promoted "wellness" attributes in very ill children (Aldridge, 1993; Armatas, 1964; Atterbury, 1974; Chetta, 1981; Crago, 1980; Daub and Kirschner-Hermanns, 1988; Fagen, 1982; Kamin et al., 1982; Locsin, 1981; MacClelland, 1979; Mullooly et al., 1988; Oyama et al., 1983; Sanderson, 1986; Tanioka et al., 1985).

- **With burn patients.** Burn patients experienced alleviation of aesthetic sterility and distraction from constant pain.

- **With terminally ill individuals.** Cancer patients, using music therapy, increased their ability to discuss their feelings and talk about the trauma of the disease (Fagen, 1982; Frampton, 1986: Gilbert.1977: Walter 1983).

- **With persons with cerebral palsy.** As early as 1950, music therapy together with physical therapy was shown to reduce the neurological problems of children with cerebral palsy.

- **With individuals who have had strokes or have Parkinson's disease.** Federal funding from the Administration on Aging is currently being used for research into the effects of music therapy and physical therapy on people with strokes or Parkinson's disease.

- **With persons who have sensory impairments or AIDS.** Many studies have explored the applications of music therapy to individuals who have sensory impairments (visual and hearing), mental retardation, or AIDS.

- **With elderly persons.** In 1991 the U.S. Senate Special Committee on Aging convened a hearing on the therapeutic benefits of music for elderly persons, which included neurologist Dr. Oliver Sacks, singer Theodore Bikel, rock musician Mickey Hart, music therapists, and clients. The hearing record documents in detail the benefits of music therapy to the elderly (Special Committee on Aging, 1991). After the hearing, Senator Harry Reid (D-NV) introduced the Music Therapy for Older Americans Act, which was later folded into the Older Americans Act Amendments of 1992. This act lists music therapy as both a supportive and a preventive health service. The new Title IV initiative creates research and demonstration projects and education and training initiatives, for which Congress appropriated nearly $1 million. In 1993, six nationwide music therapy projects were funded (Renner, 1986).

- **With persons with brain injuries.** In 1993, the Office of Alternative Medicine awarded one of its first 30 grants "to investigate any beneficial effects of a specific music therapy intervention on empirical measures of self-perception, empathy, social perception, depression, and emotional expression in persons with brain injuries." This research is now under way (Lehmann and Kirchner, 1986; Lucia, 1987).

Research needs and opportunities. In areas where it has not been done, systematic review and metaanalysis should be performed to assess the quality and outcomes of the research. In addition, further research is needed in the following areas:

- Neurological functioning, communication skills, and physical rehabilitation.

- Perception of pain, need for medication, and length of hospital stay.

- Cognitive, emotional, and social functioning in those with cognitive impairments.

- Emotional and social well-being of caregivers and families of those with disabilities.

- Clinical depression and other mental disorders.

- Disease prevention and health promotion of persons with disabilities.

Art Therapy

Art therapy is a means for patients to reconcile emotional conflicts, foster self-awareness, and express unspoken and frequently unconscious concerns about their disease. In addition to its use in treatment, it can be used to assess individuals, couples, families, and groups. It is particularly valuable with children, who often cannot talk about their most pressing and painful concerns.

The connection between art and mental health began to be recognized with the advent of mental institutions in the late 1800s and the early 1900s. Prinzhorn's book *Artistry of the Mentally Ill,* published in 1922, with stunning art made by institutionalized adults, helped ignite inquiries into the spontaneous graphic outpouring of disturbed patients. In addition to the interest in the artistic or diagnostic value of the patients' productions, there was the realization that the production of art was valuable in rehabilitating a patient's mental health.

In the 1940s, Margaret Naumberg blended ideas about psychoanalytic interpretive techniques and art to develop art as a tool to help release "the unconscious by means of spontaneous art expression . . . and on the encouragement of free association . . . The images produced . . . constitute symbolic speech" (Naumberg, 1958). A decade later, Edith Kramer began her own exploration into the use of art. She focused her approach on the art-making process itself. In her brand of therapy, a therapist is able to bring "unconscious material closer to the surface by providing an area of symbolic experience wherein changes may be tried out, gains deepened and cemented. The art therapist must be at once artist, therapist, and teacher . . . "

(Kramer, 1958). Then, in 1958, Hana Kwiatkowska translated what she knew as an artist into the field of family work and introduced specific evaluation and treatment techniques at the National Institute of Mental Health.

Art therapy was formalized in the founding of the American Art Therapy Association in 1969.[13] Along with the Art Therapy Credentials Board, the 4,000-member organization sets standards for the profession, strives to educate the public about the field, has a code of ethics and a system of approving educational programs and registering art therapists, and will soon certify art therapists. Registered art therapists (A.T.R.s) must have graduate degree training and a strong foundation in the studio arts as well as in therapy techniques and must complete a supervised internship with work experience. Currently, 2,250 art therapists are registered by the association. They practice in psychiatric centers, drug and alcohol rehabilitation programs, prisons, day care treatment programs, schools for the mentally retarded, residences for the developmentally delayed, geriatric centers, and hospices. Two journals are available: *Journal of Art Therapy* and *Art Therapy Journal*.

Art therapy differs from regular art classes such as painting, sculpture, and drawing, in that the therapist is trained both in diagnosis and in helping patients with specific health problems. In their art, for instance, patients may focus on parts of their bodies that unconsciously concern them but which they have never mentioned to their physicians or nurses. Such revelation can lead to further investigation and additional diagnosis. In helping patients express their feelings about a disease—such as cancer, for instance—therapists may lead them to draw images of themselves with cancer. These images may reveal a great deal about their feelings about their cancer, its severity, and its effect on their health and well being.

Research accomplishments. Research on art therapy has been conducted in clinical, educational, physiological, forensic, and sociological arenas. Studies on art therapy have been conducted in many areas.

- Burn recovery in adolescent and young patients (Appleton, 1990).

- Eating disorders.

- Emotional impairment in young children (Bowker, 1990)

- Reading performance (Catchings, 1981).

- Chemical addiction (Chickerneo, 1993).

- As a prognostic aid in childhood cancer.

- As an aid in assessing ego development and psychological defensiveness in young children (Kaplan, 1986; Levick, 1983).

- Childhood bereavement (Zambelli et al., 1989).

- As a modifier of locus of control in behavior-disordered students.

- Sexual abuse in adolescents.

- Deafness, aphasia, autism, emotional disturbance, physical handicap, and brain injury in children (Silver, 1966).

Research needs and opportunities. Among the areas for further research are the following:

- Test the effect of art therapy on anxiety levels of patients subjected to invasive medical procedures.

- Determine whether art therapy enhances recovery and diminishes hospital stays for hospitalized patients.

- Examine whether art enhances relaxation art in guided imagery and relaxation training.

- Develop specific art interventions for children with communication problems and test the impact on their academic and social performance.

- Determine whether clients' choice of art materials and quality of art affects their psychophysical state.

- Assess group therapy as a tool to improve corporate working relationships.

- Assess self-portraits as a prognostic indicator for clients with eating disorders.

- Examine use of art therapy with juvenile offenders to assess moral development—and modify impact of peer pressure.

- Investigate art therapy as an avenue to pain control.

- Test whether art therapy increases acceptance of physical and psychological changes in the elderly.

- Assess the utility of art therapy as a coping technique with survivors of natural disasters.

Prayer and Mental Healing

The use of prayer in healing began in human prehistory and continues to this day. Contemporary surveys reveal that most Americans pray and that they pray frequently, and almost always when they or their loved ones are ill.

The terms mental healing and spiritual healing are frequently used interchangeably. What does "spiritual" mean in this context? For many healers, spiritual healing is an integral part of their personal religion (e.g., healing comes from Jesus, Mary, a particular saint, God, and so on). Yet this cannot be the whole story, because spiritual and prayer-based healing is universal. It cannot be attributed to any particular religious point of view; it occurs in non-theistic traditions such as Buddhism just as it does in the theistic traditions of the West and in animistic societies as well. What is the unifying principle in mental-spiritual healing that seemingly transcends personal religious views? Is mental-spiritual healing a direct effect of mind or consciousness? Are personal religious interpretations irrelevant? What is the most fundamental, basic requirement for mental-spiritual healing, without which it cannot occur?

Techniques vary widely from culture to culture and are too diverse to be reviewed here. Overall patterns can nonetheless be discerned among mental-spiritual healers practicing in the United States.

One of the most thorough and innovative evaluations of this field is by psychologist Lawrence LeShan, a pioneer in investigating the relationship between psychological states and cancer (LeShan, 1966). LeShan found that mental-spiritual healing methods are of two main types. In type 1 healing, which LeShan considered the most important and prevalent kind, the healer enters a prayerful, altered state of consciousness in which he views himself and the patient as a single entity. There need be no physical contact and there is no attempt to "do anything" or "give something" to the person in need, only the desire to unite and "become one" with him or her and with the Universe, God, or Cosmos.

Type 1 healers uniformly emphasize the importance of empathy, love, and caring in this process. When healing takes place, it does so in the context of an enveloping sense of unity, compassion, and love. These healers state that this type of healing is a natural process that does not violate the laws of innate bodily function but rather speeds up ordinary healing—a very rapid self-repair or self-recuperation.

LeShan's type 2 healers, on the other hand, do touch the patient and describe some "flow of energy" through their hands to the patient's area of pathology. Feelings of heat are common in both healer and patient. In this mode, unlike type 1, the healer tries to heal. Some type 2 healers see themselves as originators of this healing power; others describe themselves as transmitters of it.

Type 1 healers do not have to be close to the patient to facilitate healing; for them, the degree of spatial separation from the person in need is irrelevant. Type 2 healers work on site in the presence of the patient.

These healing techniques are offered only as generalities. Some healers use both methodologies, even in the same healing session, and other healing methods could be described.

Rationale. How does this type of healing occur? There is no explanation within contemporary medical science, particularly for type 1, nonlocal healing.

The absence of an underlying "mechanism" is the greatest impediment to progress in this field, if such a word is even applicable. The lack of an explanation for these events prompts many people to dismiss them without investigating the evidence: since they cannot occur, they do not occur. Proponents of this foregone conclusion regard any "evidence" for mental healing as illusory, nothing more than artifacts of poor experimentation or data processing, or chance results of complex random processes.

The absence of a known mechanism, however, does not necessarily mean that mental healing does not or cannot occur, or that the research supporting it is necessarily flawed. Until the turn of this century, scientists had no explanation for a very common event: sunshine. An understanding of why the sun shines had to await the development of modern nuclear physics. Of course, the ignorance of scientists did not annul sunlight. Likewise, although the evidence is not so immediate, mental healing may be valid in the absence of a validating theory.

What might a future model of the mind that permits mental-spiritual healing look like? Such a model will almost certainly be nonlocal.

The idea prevalent in contemporary science is that the mind and consciousness are entirely local phenomena—that is, they are localized to the brain and body and confined to the present moment. From this point of view, distant healing cannot occur in principle, since the mind cannot stray outside the "here and now" to cause a remote event. Studies in distant mental influence and mental healing, however, challenge these assumptions. Dozens of laboratory experiments suggest that the mind can bring about changes in faraway physical bodies, even when the distant person or organism is shielded from all known sensory and electromagnetic influences. They imply that mind and consciousness may not always be localized or confined to points in space, such as brains or bodies, or in time, such as the present moment (Braud, 1992; Braud and Schlitz, 1991; Jahn and Dunne, 1987).

For medicine, the implications of a nonlocal concept of the mind may be profound. Among them are the following:

- Nonlocal models of the mind may be helpful in understanding the actual dynamics of healing. They may help explain instances in which a cure appears suddenly, radically, and unexpectedly; or when healing appears to be influenced by events occurring at a distance from the patient and outside his or her awareness.

- Nonlocal manifestations of consciousness may complicate traditional experimental designs and require innovative research methods because they suggest, among other things, that the mental state or expectation of the experimenter may influence the experiment's outcome, even under "blind" conditions (Solfvin, 1984).

At the same time, however, nonlocal manifestations suggest unmistakable spiritual qualities of the psyche, including the possibility that a nonlocal consciousness might survive the death of the local brain. The temporal barrier may also be violated: information apparently may be received by a distant person, at global distances, before it is mentally transmitted by the sender (Radin and Nelson, 1989). These events, replicated by careful observers under laboratory conditions, suggest that there is some aspect of the psyche that is unconfinable to points in space or to points in time. In sum, these events point toward a nonlocal model of consciousness, which at the very least allows for the possibility of distant healing information exchange and perhaps distant healing influences.

A nonlocal model of consciousness implies that at some level of the psyche there are no fundamental spatio-temporal separations between individual minds. If so, at some level and in some sense there may be unity and oneness of all minds—what Nobel physicist Erwin Schroedinger called the One Mind.[14]

In a nonlocal model of consciousness, therefore, distance is not fundamental but is completely overcome—in which case the mind of the healer and the patient are not genuinely separate but in some sense united. "Distant" healing thus becomes a misnomer, and because of the unification of consciousness, the patient may be said to be healing himself or herself.

Offering nonlocality as the bedrock of mental healing merely shifts the question: instead of asking how mental healing occurs, now one must ask how nonlocality happens. Currently no one knows, not even the physicists whose many experiments have established it as a solid part of modern physics. The saying comes to mind, "Physicists never really understand a new theory, they just get used to it." Perhaps the same may be said of physicians and their attempts to understand mental healing. Nonlocal mental models imply "action at a distance," which has been an abhorrent concept to most scientists since Galileo. But that situation may be changing. Physicists have repeatedly documented that nonlocal phenomena occur in the subatomic, quantum domain, wherein information can seemingly be "transferred" between distant sites by processes that are "immediate, unmitigated, and unmediated."[15] Whether quantum nonlocality is a possible explanation or rationale for biological or mental nonlocality is a question for future research. Nobel prize-winning physicist Brian D. Josephson of Cambridge University has suggested that nonlocal events occur in the biological world as well as the quantum domain. He proposes that human ways of knowing, particularly the human capacity to perceive patterns and meaning, make possible "direct interconnections between spatially separated objects." Josephson suggests that these interconnections permit the operation of "psi functioning" between humans, currently held by biomedical science as impossible (Josephson and Pallikara-Viras, 1991). In any case, the fact that nonlocal events are now studied by physicists in the microworld suggests a greater permissiveness and freedom to examine phenomena in the biological and mental domains—such as mental healing—that may possibly be analogous.

Research accomplishments and major reviews. Anecdotal accounts of the power of prayer in "mental," "spiritual," "psychic," "distant," or "absent" healing are both legendary and legion. Countless books on these subjects are available, but this literature contains little scientific value.

Scientific attempts to assess the effects of prayer and spiritual practices on health began in the 19th century with Sir Francis

Galton's treatise entitled "Statistical Inquiries into the Efficacy of Prayer" (Galton, 1872). Galton assessed the longevity of people frequently prayed for, such as clergy, monarchs, and heads of state. He concluded that there was no demonstrable effect of prayer on longevity. Judged by modern research standards, Galton's study contains many flaws, but he succeeded in advancing the idea that healing methods involving prayer and similar spiritual practices could be subjected to empirical scrutiny.

Since Galton's time, a sizable body of scientific evidence has accumulated in the field of spiritual healing showing positive results. This information is little known to the scientific community. Psychologist William G. Braud, a leading researcher in this field, summarizes this research in a recent review:

> There exist many published reports of experiments in which persons were able to influence a variety of cellular and other biological systems through mental means. The target systems for these investigations have included bacteria, yeast, fungi, mobile algae, plants, protozoa, larvae, insects, chicks, mice, rats, gerbils, cats, and dogs, as well as cellular preparations (blood cells, neurons, cancer cells) and enzyme activities. In human "target persons," eye movements, muscular movements, electrodermal activity, plethysmographic activity, respiration, and brain rhythms have been affected through direct mental influence (Braud, 1992; Braud and Schlitz, 1991).

These studies in general assess the ability of humans to affect physiological functions of a variety of living systems at a distance, including studies in which the "receiver" or "target" is unaware that such an effort is being made. The fact that these studies commonly involve nonhuman targets is important; lower organisms are presumably not subject to suggestion and placebo effects, a frequent criticism when human subjects are involved.

Many of these studies do not describe the psychological strategy of the influencer as actual "prayer," in which one directs entreaties to a Supreme Being, a Universal Power, or God. But almost all of them involve a state of prayerfulness—a feeling of genuine caring, compassion, love, or empathy with the target system, or a feeling that the influencer is one with the target.

In addition to the review by Braud, two other major reviews of this field have been published in the past decade by researchers Jerry Solfvin and Daniel J. Benor (Benor, 1990, 1993; Solfvin, 1984). These reviews examine the results of more than 130 controlled studies of distant mental effects, approximately half of which show statistically significant results. *The Future of the Body: Explorations Into the Further Evolution of Human Nature*, a scholarly, encyclopedic work by Michael Murphy, cofounder of the Esalen Institute, reviews the major research accomplishments in the field of mental healing and related fields and is a valuable guide (Murphy, 1992). The potential relevance of this area for medical practice has been examined by Larry Dossey (1993).

Experiments in distant hypnosis deserve in tense scientific scrutiny. In such studies a subject is hypnotized remotely, is unaware when the hypnosis is taking place, and has no sensory contact with the hypnotist. Several such experiments were performed in France in the late 1800s by Janet and Gilbert and were repeated with greater refinement in 260 laboratory experiments in 1933 and 1934 by Vasiliev and colleagues in Leningrad (Vasiliev, 1976). These studies offer tantalizing suggestions that the human mind may display nonlocal characteristics (see the next section). For reasons to be discussed there, exploring this possibility scientifically should be given high priority. Extent of the nonlocal perspective. The nonlocal manifestations of consciousness are not limited to prayer. Consciousness appears to manifest nonlocally in secular laboratory settings as freely as in a church, implying that prayer is only one of the possible avenues for the expression of these events. If nonlocal mental events are indeed ubiquitous, they may pervade all healing endeavors to some degree, even those that appear overwhelmingly mechanical, such as pharmacological and surgical therapies. Therefore it is unclear whether any therapy can be considered totally mechanical or "objective" (Braud, 1992). Nonlocal mental events may affect all therapies to some degree, and the nonlocal perspective may have to be considered when any therapy is assessed.

Research needs and opportunities. In addition to demonstrating whether there is a distant healing effect of the mind, future research should examine the following questions:

- How robust, reliable, and dependable is the mental healing effect?

- What qualities in the praying person and the recipient facilitate and retard distant healing effects?

- How can talented or potential healers be identified?[16]

- Is healing a "gift," or can individuals be trained to heal?[17]

- Do some prayers work better than others in mental-spiritual healing?[18]

- Why does the ability to heal fluctuate? Why is it not constant? Are mental healers like talented athletes, who can be either "hot" or "cold"? Since healing abilities seem to fluctuate, how can experimental protocols allow for this variation? Is it justifiable to apply the same experimental designs to healers as to penicillin, which presumably does not have an "off" day?

- How can mental healing be integrated with orthodox medical approaches, particularly in hospital environments? Can medical and surgical approaches be used simultaneously with mental healing, or are these methods incompatible?

- Can mental healing be tested in the same way as a new drug or surgical procedure? Is the randomized, prospective, double-blind methodology equally appropriate for physically and for mentally-spiritually based therapies?

- How can the public be protected from fraudulent or misguided mental "healers"? Is it possible to establish a requirement akin to board certification for healers in an attempt to ensure efficacy and protect consumers from worthless "healers" and predatory quacks?[19]

- What about more general ethical considerations? Is a mental healer justified in attempting to heal people without their knowledge and consent?

- Is it possible to harm distant organisms and aid them through distant mental influences?[20]

There are two related but separate directions of research in the field of nonlocal therapy: (1) the need to develop actual healing methods, and (2) the need to shed light on the fundamental nature of human consciousness. The first goal obviously requires the use of some type of living organisms as the recipient, but the second need not. In fact, the effects of consciousness can be studied in certain laboratory settings that offer greater precision and control than is offered by the usual experiments that involve living organisms as recipients. An example is the sophisticated studies in remote human-machine interactions that have been done for a decade at the Princeton Engineering Anomalies Research laboratory by Robert G. Jahn, former dean of engineering of Princeton University, and his colleagues Jahn and Dunne, (1987).

Conclusions. Appallingly little is known about the origins of consciousness and how it relates to the physical brain. Although hypotheses purporting to explain consciousness abound, there simply is no consensus among expert neuroscientists, psychologists, artificial intelligence researchers, and philosophers as to its nature. Perhaps the lack of knowledge is not surprising; in medical research, scientists usually consign consciousness to last-place status and opt for "practical" research areas—the development of new drugs, surgical therapies, vaccines, and so forth.

Research in this area is analogous to basic investigations in other exotic areas of science such as particle physics, which have no immediate, bottom-line value. There is a need to know more about the basic, fundamental nature of consciousness—its spatial and temporal characteristics and its precise relationship with matter, including the brain. Without this basic understanding, progress in all forms of therapy, alternative and traditional, will be hampered, because the effects of consciousness are to some degree involved in all of them.

Summary

The mind-body interventions described in this chapter are part of a neglected dimension in health care. They offer what people are hungry for—a medicine that addresses more than the body. In addition to preventing or curing illnesses, these therapies by and large provide people with the chance to be involved in their own care, to make vital decisions about their own health, to be touched at deep emotional levels, and to be changed psychologically in the process.

There is nothing inherent in many alternative medical therapies that necessarily sets them apart from the way contemporary drugs and surgery are used. Because they are, after all, things, it is possible to use diets, herbs, homeopathic remedies, and most other alternative treatments with the same impersonal, remote objectivity that prompts people today to say, "My doctor doesn't care about me!" It is possible to convert any alternative technique into the "new penicillin" or the "latest surgery"—something given or done to a body without regard for the person involved. The mind-body approach outlined here is potentially a corrective to this tendency, a reminder of the

574

importance of human connection and the power of patients acting on their own behalf. Caring and compassion are not enough, and "putting the patient back into health care" is not sufficient. Alternative therapies, including the mind-body approaches that have been described, must be proved to work, must be safe, and must be cost-effective. While more work needs to be done, evidence also is already substantial that many of these mind-body therapies, if appropriately selected and wisely applied, meet these demands.

Recommendations

To further the development of alternative medical practices and mind-body interventions, the Panel on Mind-Body Interventions recommends the following:

- Development of educational materials, models, and programs in each of the mind-body areas discussed in this chapter, and dissemination to faculty and students in medical and other schools of health education.

- Development of comprehensive reviews of the literature in the various areas of the mind-body field. Such reviews would document the enormous body of work already done and specify directions for future research, thus facilitating the most efficient use of resources. Five areas should receive focus in a comprehensive review:

  1. The theoretical foundations, research accomplishments, and clinical applications of mind-body interventions as well as the commonalities and differences among various self-regulation strategies.

  2. The dynamics of the therapeutic relationship between providers and patients. What qualities, for example, allow therapists and patients to work well together? What factors distinguish "technicians" from "healers"? How do beliefs and attitudes of both patients and physicians affect health care and treatment outcomes?

  3. The influence of social context on health and illness, including the impact of family, work, education, economic status, and culture.

  4. The effects of belief, values, and meaning on health and illness.

5. The influence of nonlocal phenomena on health and illness.

- Development of a clearinghouse for information dealing with mind-body approaches to health and illness, including the publication of a journal on mind-body medicine.

- Evaluation of the legal, regulatory, and economic barriers to the integration of the mind-body perspective and techniques into the health care system.

- Institution of studies dealing with integration of mind-body techniques already shown to be effective (e.g., biofeedback plus hypnosis plus imagery), with attention to possible increases in cost-effectiveness when these approaches are used integrally rather than singly.

- Comparison of the long- and short-term effects of various self-regulation strategies.

- Basic investigations of the nonlocal effects of consciousness. These studies would involve human-machine as well as human-human interactions and would employ degrees of spatial separation of global or greater distances. Such research is vital in laying a theoretical foundation for understanding the role of consciousness in health in general and for progress in the mind-body field.

- Research addressing mind-body factors in chronic illness in poor and minority communities.

- Development of stress reduction techniques and non-pharmacological health education programs in elementary and secondary schools. Such programs would emphasize the role of self-responsibility in young children as well as the impact of attitudes, beliefs, and emotions in health.

- Development of drug rehabilitation and recidivism-reduction programs that emphasize mind-body techniques.

- A project to investigate how patient education affects the outcome of research studies. If the findings so justify, research designs should be developed that inform patients fully of the nature of the protocol in which they are participating and that provide immediate feedback of results.

- Funding and support of small pilot programs in the mind-body field.

- A study of the psychosocial characteristics of people who experience spontaneous remissions of cancer and chronic disease.

- Development of research methods that include subjective ways of knowing and "state-specific" observations.

- The beginning of a systematic study of what it means to be healthy.

- A task force on the nature of consciousness to be formed within the Office of Alternative Medicine. This task force would be composed of representatives from various disciplines whose work deals with the nature of consciousness, including psychologists, neurophysiologists, artificial intelligence experts, physicists, physicians, and philosophers. The mission of this group would be to formulate a model of consciousness that, as completely as possible, would account for the manifestations of consciousness that surface in mind-body research. Such a model would be of significant value in legitimizing the area of mind-body interventions and in stimulating progress in this field.

Notes

1. In this report, mind and consciousness are used interchangeably, and the following definition is accepted: "Our use of the term consciousness is intended to subsume all categories of human experience, including those commonly termed 'conscious,' 'subconscious,' 'superconscious,' or 'unconscious,' without presumption of specific psychological or physiological mechanisms" (Jahn and Dunne, 1987).

2. "Spiritual elements are those capacities that enable a human being to rise above or transcend any experience at hand. They are characterized by the capacity to seek meaning and purpose, to have faith, to love, to forgive, to pray, to meditate, to worship, and to see beyond present circumstances" (Clifford Kuhn, a quoted in Aldridge, D. 1993. Is there evidence for spiritual healing? *Advances* 9:445). "The spiritual dimension . . . is that aspect of the person concerned with meaning and the search for absolute reality that underlies the world of the

senses and the mind and, as such, is distinct from adherence to a religious system" (J. Hiatt. 1986. Spirituality, medicine, and healing. *Southern Medical Journal* 79:736-74.3).

3. For a review of the impact of perceived meaning on health, see Dossey, 1991.

4. T.J. Silber, for example, writing in the *Journal of the American Medical Association* in 1979, found 1,500 articles on the subject of placebos in English, German, and Spanish.

5. Larson and Larson assembled a teaching module that physicians could fruitfully follow in dealing with these delicate issues with patients without appearing to advocate any particular religious tradition or point of view (Larson and Larson, 1991). In the study, physicians who were not religious seemed to achieve better results with the inquiry than physicians who were.

6. This publication can be obtained from the Institute of Noetic Sciences, Box 909, Sausalito. CA 94966-0909.

7. As an example of the cross-fertilization that might occur between the disciplines of psychiatry and modern physics, see Zohar, 1990. See also Jahn, 1981; and Josephson and Ramachandran, 1980.

8. See Ravindra, 1991. Ravindra is both an academic physicist and a theologian at Dalhousie University. See also the "Spirituality, Religion, and Health" section of this chapter.

9. Although TM and the relaxation response have been most intensively studied, other investigators (including Jon Kabat-Zinn, Ilan Kutz, and Joan Borysenko) have demonstrated the effectiveness of South Asian vipassana, or mindfulness meditation, in the reduction of chronic pain and as an adjunct to psychotherapy (Kabat-Zinn et al., 2985; Kutz et al., 1985).

10. The most comprehensive review of meditation research is a set of five volumes compiled by Maharishi International University (Orme-Johnson and Farrow, 1977) (a sixth is in preparation), containing more than 500 original research, review, and theoretical papers by some 360 researchers at 200 universities and a meta-analysis. Comparing various techniques for reducing trait anxiety, researchers found the largest overall

effect was produced by TM (Eppley et al., 1989). Murphy and Donovan surveyed more than 600 studies of physiological and psychological effects of meditation (Murphy, 1992; Murphy and Donovan, 1989). Schneider addressed the search for an optimal behavioral treatment for hypertension (Schneider et al., 1992). Walsh and Vaughan provide a compact and readable summary of the state of the art in meditation research as a chapter in a new book (Walsh and Vaughan, in press).

11. Many evaluation formats appear in the nursing literature. For a comprehensive presentation of this information as it relates to nursing practice and assessment, see Dossey et al., 1992, and Zahourek, 1988. General health evaluation tools. as well as those specific to certain diseases, have been published by Achterberg and Lawlis (1980, 1984). Mental rehearsal is an imagery technique used before medical techniques, usually in an attempt to relieve anxiety, pain, and side effects, which are exacerbated by heightened emotional reactions. Surgery or a difficult treatment is rehearsed before the event so that the patient is prepared and is rid of any unrealistic fantasies.

12. The American Dance Therapy Association is located at 2000 Century Plaza, Suite 108, Columbia, MD 21044-3363, telephone 410-9974040.

13. References documenting work in art therapy in addition to those cited in this report can be obtained from the American Art Therapy Association. Inc., 1202 Allanson Road, Mundelein, IL 60060, telephone 708-949-6064, fax 708-566-4580.

14. For a discussion of Schroedinger's views on the nonlocal, unitary nature of human consciousness, see L. Dossey, "Erwin Schroedinger," in *Recovering the Soul* (Dossey, 1989, pp. 129139). Nonlocality, furthermore, implies infinitude in space and time, because a limited nonlocality is a contradiction in terms. A nonlocal model of the mind, therefore, suggests that some component of the psyche is omnipresent, eternal, and immortal. For elaboration, see Recovering the Soul.

15. For a review of the current status of nonlocality in contemporary physics, see physicist Nick Herbert's *Quantum Reality* (Herbert, 1987).

579

16.   Efforts to identify potential spiritual healers and encourage or accelerate their development are being made by the National Federation of Spiritual Healers of America, Inc., P.O. Box 2022, Mt. Pleasant, SC 29465.

17.   An exemplary training program for spiritual healers is the Consciousness Research and Training Project, Inc., 315 East 68th Street, Box 9G, New York, NY 10021-5692. The director is Joyce Goodrich, Ph.D. This organization developed from the research of psychologist Lawrence LeShan, a pioneer in the scientific study of spiritual healing, and it advocates his general philosophy in this area.

18.   This question has also been investigated extensively by Spindrift, Inc., of Lansdale, PA (see next footnote). These researchers have repeatedly demonstrated in quantitative experiments that although both approaches work, an open-ended "Thy will be done" prayer strategy is more effective than a specific, goal-directed request in bringing about healing. These results may depend, however, on innate personality characteristics of the praying person, a possibility that Spindrift has not addressed.

19.   Spindrift researchers have developed a laboratory test they believe can prove which healers are talented and which are not. They have shown that healers differ widely in their abilities. Spindrift's suggestion that all so-called healers "take the test" evoked bitter criticism and hostility from the Christian Science Church ("It is heresy to bring God into the laboratory!"). See L. Dossey, "How Should We Pray? The Spindrift Experiments," in *Recovering the Soul* (New York. Bantam, 1989), 55-62.

20.   This possibility is suggested by many anthropological accounts such as the "death prayer," used at a distance by Kahuna shamans of Hawaii. These phenomena are unlike hexing and voodoo, which are local in nature, mediated through sensory exchanges between perpetrator and recipient.

Chapter 37

Alexander Technique

The principal aim of the Alexander technique is to help people learn how to "use" themselves better. It is a method of psycho-physical education which is claimed to work at a fundamental level—affecting how we think, react, support our bodies and move.

Proponents of the technique claim that learning it allows an individual to become more poised and balanced in attitude and movement—more elastic, fluid and graceful—as potentially self-damaging, awkward, stiff, jerky, overhasty or over-tense movements are gradually eliminated from an individual's repertoire.

According to the Society for Teachers of the Alexander Technique, "from Alexander's own observations, since confirmed by scientific research, it has become apparent that there are natural postural reflexes to organize this support and balance for us without great effort, provided that we have the necessary understanding and degree of 'relaxation in activity' to allow these to work freely."

Practitioners of the technique call themselves teachers rather than therapists because they see their task as one of education, not therapy.

Their clients are referred to as pupils or students since they work with the teacher rather than passively receive a treatment.

The technique is usually taught on a one-to-one basis, although group sessions are offered as a useful introduction. A "lesson" generally lasts about 30 minutes, during which time a teacher will work with his or her pupil in a variety of ways.

Lessons start with the pupil being asked to quieten and calm themselves.

During a lesson, a teacher may ask the pupil to sit on a chair and spend some time gently guiding the pupil in and out of the chair. In this way the pupil is gradually made aware of his or her poor posture and begins to learn new ways of sitting, standing and moving.

The teacher may also use other ways of moving, such as crawling or walking, with the aim of facilitating the release of over-tight muscles and restore normal curvature of the spine.

Kathleen Ballard, chairwoman of the Society of Teachers of the Alexander Technique, summarizes the dynamics of a lesson thus: "By words and subtle informed touch pupils are taught how to allow the neck to be free, the head to be released forward and up and the back to lengthen and widen. They learn how to promote this lengthening and freedom when moving from standing to sitting and vice versa. The teacher's touch and advice helps the pupils become aware of habitual misuse and enables them to make changes."

Teachers of the technique generally agree that between 20 and 30 lessons are needed in order to learn the technique properly.

Historical Background

The Alexander technique owes its existence to an Australian actor and recitationist called Frederick Matthias Alexander(1869-1955).

Alexander had been having trouble with his voice, which became strained and hoarse during performances, on occasion disappearing completely. When the doctors failed to identify the cause of the problem, Alexander decided to find out what was wrong himself.

Using mirrors he watched himself perform—reasoning that the cause of his problem must lie in the way that he performed. Through a process of detailed observation Alexander established a set of principles of good and bad "use" of the body, and overcame his voice problem. He felt his general health also improved.

Alexander went on to teach the technique he had developed and, in time, doctors began to refer patients to him. Later he travelled to London and began teaching there. He soon became popular, particularly with theater people, including George Bernard Shaw and Aldous Huxley.

During the First World War, Alexander went to America and established the technique over there—work that was continued by his brother when Alexander returned to the UK in 1931.

Back in London, Alexander set up a training course for teachers of his technique and continued to work and teach until his death in 1955.

Indications

The most common reasons for seeking lessons in the Alexander technique are back or neck problems, although some people simply want to improve their posture. After a lesson pupils often report greater ease in physical mobility and feeling re-energized. There may also be physical changes such as the disappearance of a stoop, less back pain or fewer leg cramps at night.

While teachers generally do not claim to be able to "treat" problems, learning the technique has been found to be helpful with stress-related conditions such as migraines. One Alexander technique teacher, Wilfred Barlow, has even claimed to help people with rheumatic disorders, epilepsy and problems during pregnancy. The Alexander technique is, however, fundamentally, a self-help technique for learning to acquire good "use." Since many health problems arise because of poor "use," they will often disappear once the technique has been mastered.

Contraindications

There are no age restrictions to learning the technique, but it may not be suitable for individuals with learning disabilities or mental illness.

Research

The observations made by Alexander are in sympathy with what we now know about anatomy and physiology. Research into the technique itself, however, did not begin until after the Second World War.

- Wilfred Barlow, for example, conducted many studies. In one he gave lessons to a group of students from the Royal College of Music in London—photographing them before and after the course of lessons. Their "use" improved dramatically.

  As a control group in this study, students from the Central School of Speech and Drama in London were given exercises aimed at improving posture, rather than receiving Alexander technique lessons. Their use deteriorated rather than improved.

Stevens, C. *The Alexander Technique*. London: Macdonald Optima, 1987.

- In the 1950s, Professor Frank Pierce-Jones of the Institute for Applied Experimental Psychology at Tufts University demonstrated the effect of the technique on patterns of movement using multiple-image photography. Pierce-Jones, F. *Body Awareness in Action*. New York: Schocken Books, 1976.

  Chris Stevens and Professor Finn Boyson-Moller of the University of Copenhagen used electrical recordings of muscle activity and found that a guided movement required less force, less muscle activity and was smoother than the habitual movement.

  Stevens, C. *The Alexander Technique*. London: Macdonald, Optima, 1987.

- John Austin, professor of clinical radiology at the Department of Radiology, Columbia University, New York, investigated the effects of Alexander technique on respiratory function in adults. He found that Alexander lessons increased peak expiratory flow, maximal voluntary ventilation and maximal inspiratory mouth pressure.

  Austin, J.H.M., Ausubel, P. Enhanced respiratory muscular function in normal adults after lessons in propriceptive musculoskeletal education without exercise. *Chest* 1992; 102:2, 486-490.

Implications for Nursing

To become an Alexander technique teacher takes three years of full-time study, so few nurses are likely to incorporate this technique within their practice. However, teachers do recommend the technique to nurses themselves to counteract the stress of the physical nature of their work.[1]

The Alexander technique is, however, being used within the NHS. According to the Society of Teachers of the Alexander Technique, General Practicioners are referring patients to teachers, and a report by the National Association of Health Authorities and Trusts[2] notes that one family health services authority has given approval for a health promotion clinic offering the Alexander technique. Certainly nurses, midwives and health visitors should be aware of the benefits of the

Alexander technique in order to answer patients' questions and to be able to suggest it to patients as appropriate.

References

1. Maitland, J., Goodliffe, H. The Alexander technique. *Nursing Times* 1989; 85:42,55-57.

2. National Association of Health Authorities and Trusts. *Complementary Therapies in the NHS*. London: NAHAT, 1993.

—by Joanna Trevelyan

Joanna Trevelyan is deputy editor, *Nursing Times*

When therapeutic techniques are described, it is purely for illustration and not intended to act as a guide to practice. No therapeutic interventions should ever be carried out by nurses, midwives or health visitors who have not undergone the appropriate training

Recommended Reading

Alexander, F.M. *Use of the Self*. London: VictorGollancz, 1985.

Barlow, W. *The Alexander Principle*. London: VictorGollancz, 1990.

Brennan, R. *The Alexander Workbook*. Shaftesbury: Element Books, 1992.

Gelb, M. *Body Learning*. London: Aurum Press, 1987.

Gray, J. *Your Guide to the Alexander Technique*. London: VictorGollancz, 1990.

Steven, G. *Alexander Technique*. London: Macdonald Optima, 1991.

Chapter 38

Chronotherapy Tunes in to the Body's Rhythms

How our bodies marshal defenses against disease depends on many factors, such as age, gender and genetics. Recently, the role of our bodies' biological rhythms in fighting disease has come under study by some in the medical community.

Our bodies' rhythms, also known as our biological clocks, take their cue from the environment and the rhythms of the solar system that change night to day and lead one season into another. Our internal clocks are also dictated by our genetic makeup. These clocks influence how our bodies change throughout the day, affecting blood pressure, blood coagulation, blood flow, and other functions.

Some of the rhythms that affect our bodies include:

- **ultradian**, which are cycles shorter than a day (for example, the milliseconds it takes for a neuron to fire, or a 90-minute sleep cycle)

- **circadian**, which last about 24 hours (such as sleeping and waking patterns)

- **infradian**, referring to cycles longer than 24 hours (for example monthly menstruation)

- **seasonal**, such as seasonal affective disorder (SAD), which causes depression in susceptible people during the short days of winter.

FDA Consumer magazine (April 1997). web version http://www.fda.gov/fdac/features/1997/397/_chrono.html.

"The biology of human beings is not constant throughout the day, the menstrual cycle, and the year," says Michael Smolensky, Ph.D., director of the Chronobiology Center at the University of Texas. "Instead, it varies predictably in time."

Coordinating biological rhythms (chronobiology) with medical treatment is called chronotherapy. It considers a person's biological rhythms in determining the timing—and sometimes the amount—of medication to optimize a drug's desired effects and minimize the undesired ones.

According to Smolensky, patients are more likely to follow schedules for taking their medications when those medications are formulated as chronotherapies because of better medical results and fewer adverse side effects. "With better compliance, the disease can be better contained, which means fewer doctor visits and potential trips to the hospital because of acute flare-ups," he says.

The area in which chronotherapy is most advanced—drug chronotherapy—for the most part does not involve new medicines but using old ones differently. Revising the dosing schedule, reformulating a drug so its release into the bloodstream is delayed, or using programmable pumps that deliver medicine at precise intervals are some of the simple changes that may reap enormous benefits. Drugs that are reformulated as chronotherapeutics are regulated by the Food and Drug Administration.

Here's a look at how chronotherapy is being used or studied for various diseases.

Asthma

Normal lung function undergoes circadian changes and reaches a low point in the early morning hours. This dip is particularly pronounced in people with asthma.

Chronotherapy for asthma is aimed at getting maximal effect from bronchodilator medications during the early morning hours. One example is the bronchodilator Uniphyl, a long-acting theophylline preparation manufactured by Purdue Frederick Co. of Norwalk, Conn., and approved by FDA in 1989. Taken once a day in the evening, Uniphyl causes theophylline blood levels to reach their peak and improve lung function during the difficult early morning hours. There are other bronchodilators that act similarly to address the early morning dip in lung function, but the manufacturers have not sought or received FDA approval for chronotherapeutic labeling.

Writing in the April 15, 1996, issue of *Hospital Practice,* Richard Martin, M.D., who directs the division of pulmonary medicine at the

National Jewish Center for Immunology and Respiratory Medicine in Denver, stated his belief that "the key to managing [asthma] cases is chronotherapy. I have found that unless treatment improves night-time asthma, it is hard to improve its daytime manifestations." For people with severe asthma who wake up several times a night gasping for breath, a good night's sleep can be a dream come true.

Arthritis

Chronobiological patterns have been observed with arthritis pain. People with osteoarthritis, the most common form of the disease, tend to have less pain in the morning and more at night. But for people with rheumatoid arthritis, the pain usually peaks in the morning and decreases as the day wears on. Recent animal studies showing that joint inflammation in rats fluctuates over a 24-hour period support these observations by both patients and physicians.

Chronotherapy for all forms of arthritis uses standard treatment, nonsteroidal anti-inflammatory drugs and corticosteroids; however, the dosages are timed to ensure that the highest blood levels of the drug coincide with peak pain.

For osteoarthritis sufferers, the optimal time for a nonsteroidal anti-inflammatory drug such as ibuprofen would be around noon or mid-afternoon. The same drug would be more effective for people with rheumatoid arthritis when taken after the evening meal. The exact dose would depend on the severity of the patient's pain and his or her individual physiology.

Cancer

Animal studies suggest that chemotherapy may be more effective and less toxic if cancer drugs are administered at carefully selected times.

"The data in animals are very compelling," says Gerald Sokol, M.D., an oncologist with the division of oncology in FDA's Center for Drug Evaluation and Research. However, he says, additional studies in humans are needed.

"There really aren't any controlled trials demonstrating that chronotherapy for cancer is important," says Robert Justice, M.D., deputy director of the division. "I'm not saying it can't be. I just don't think it's been demonstrated."

The studies so far suggest that there may be different chrono-biological cycles for normal cells and tumor cells. If this is true, the goal would be to time the administration of cancer drugs to the chronobiological cycles of tumor cells, making them more effective against the cancer and less toxic to normal tissues, Sokol explains.

Before chronotherapy could become part of standard cancer treatment, Sokol adds, it would have to be determined whether there is an optimal time to give a drug.

Also to be determined would be how to handle the logistics of giving drugs at scattered times throughout the day and night. "Chronotherapy means we can't bring in all our cancer patients in the morning to receive their drug therapies," says Sokol, who also has a hospital practice in Tampa, Fla. "Some patients may be better served by getting their drugs late in the afternoon or even at night."

Portable infusion pumps may hold the answer. "The patient can be sent home with an implantable pump that will automatically distribute the drug at the appropriate time," he explains.

Cancer Surgery

The optimal timing of cancer surgery, particularly breast cancer, has also come under study. Some researchers believe that in premenopausal women, surgical cure of breast cancer is more likely if surgery is performed in the middle of a woman's menstrual cycle in the week or so following ovulation.

At the May 1996 International Conference on Breast Diseases in Houston, Umberto Veronesi, M.D., of the European Institute of Oncology in Milan, Italy, presented 20 years of follow-up data on nearly 1,200 premenopausal women who underwent surgery for breast cancer. Of patients who had surgery in the week following ovulation, 76 percent were tumor-free after five years, compared with 63 percent in patients who had surgery earlier in their menstrual cycle.

Many experts believe that any improved outcome is hormone-related. In the first half of the menstrual cycle, estrogen levels are high, and progesterone is not produced. In the second half, progesterone rises and estrogen falls. It is believed that progesterone may inhibit the production of some enzymes that help cancer spread.

However, some experts dispute the need to time breast cancer surgery according to the menstrual cycle. G.M. Clark, M.D., of the University of Texas Health Science Center at San Antonio, reported at the conference that retrospective analyses from at least 23 studies involving more than 6,000 patients failed to find any significant impact of the menstrual cycle division on breast cancer prognosis.

Regulatory Implications

Chronotherapeutics present new challenges to regulators and scientists alike. For example, according to FDA's Sokol, chronotherapeutic clinical studies need to consider additional parameters not usually required of other clinical trials. Among additional factors that must be considered, he says, are:

- time of day a drug is administered

- time-related biological factors, such as seasonal disorders (for example, seasonal affective disorder)

- patients' normal routines (for example, eating times and sleep patterns).

Making chronotherapy the focus of more clinical trials would be welcome news to many in the medical community, according to a 1996 American Medical Association survey. The study found that about 75 percent of the doctors surveyed said they would like more treatment options to match a patient's circadian, or daily, rhythms.

But chronotherapy has a way to go, considering that only 5 percent of the doctors surveyed said they were "very familiar" with the subject.

"Chronotherapy is not well recognized in the medical community," Sokol says, "but awareness is increasing. The implications are broad in every area of medicine."

—by Isadora Stehlin

Isadora Stehlin is a member of FDA's public affairs staff.

Chapter 39

Aura (Kirlian) Photography: Mundane Physics or Diagnostic Tool?

Abstract

Kirlian photography is often associated with the paranormal. Many people believe it records the auras of living objects and that it can be used as a diagnostic tool. This paper argues against these beliefs and maintains that there is a simple, scientific explanation of the Kirlian effect.

It is claimed that the Kirlian effect, captured on photographic film, is a complex paranormal phenomenon and that it shows the aura of human objects such as fingertips and hands.

Singer claims the photographs record "information about the physiological, psychological and psychic state of the individual and for plant and animal parts, [and] that the aura carries information about their 'lifeforce,' 'life-energy' or 'bioplasma.'"[1]

The phenomenon has also been the subject of discussion in *Nursing Times* as part of an examination of complementary medicine.[2] It was stated that if it is assumed there is no trickery involved, Kirlian photographs have shown something unusual which conventional science cannot explain away as electrical disturbance of photographic emulsion.

Actually the opposite is the case. Science provides a perfectly adequate explanation of the processes that produce the Kirlian effect recorded on photographic film. Claims about links to the paranormal are simply the result of a misunderstanding of the physical processes involved.[3]

Scientific studies of the Kirlian effect have shown that what is responsible is a rather mundane physical process—an electrically excited (energized) gas re-emitting energy (radiation) in the form of photons (light) which is recorded on photographic film.

All gases are made up of atoms, either alone or bonded together as molecules. According to the nuclear model, atoms contain a central nucleus of neutral neutrons and positively charged protons, surrounded by a swarm of orbiting, but strongly held, negatively charged electrons.

In order to strip the strongly held electrons from their atoms, the atoms must be subjected to a high-intensity electric field. This is done by running a current between two conductors or electrodes. One electrode is given a strong positive charge and the other given a strong negative charge. In the electric field between the two conductors, a negatively charged electron will be attracted towards the positive electrode and will be stripped from its atom.

If ambient air is introduced between the electrodes, the stripped electrons will flow as a current through the air, colliding with, and therefore giving energy to, other atoms and molecules. These in turn give off energy in the form of photons of light, creating a visible glow.' This is the essence of the process that produces the aura inherent to corona discharge or Kirlian photography.

A Kirlian apparatus consists of an electrical circuit which has at one end an object such as a leaf, the palm of a hand or a fingertip, acting as an electrode. They are then placed on a photographic plate, which is in turn placed on a glass sheet.

Atoms and molecules in the electric field surrounding the surface of the hand or leaf, in contact with the photographic plate, have their electrons stripped from them. These electrons energize other atoms in the air which in turn discharge that energy as light, or a corona discharge, above the photographic film. This process decreases further away from the surface of the object and therefore the luminous discharge is confined to a small area around the object's surface.

Two additional points are worth mentioning here. First, the amount of positive or negative charge in a given area is greatest where there is sharp curvature, such as at the fingertips or the prominences of a leaf, and so the corona discharge is greatest around these points.

Second, if the process is conducted in a vacuum, no image is recorded on the photographic plate. These two observations are precisely predictable if the phenomenon is an ordinary corona discharge, but not if it is an "energy body."[1] Further, Watkins and Bickel observed that the corona discharge or aura also appears from mechanical or lifeless objects, such as coins. Since the aura appears from both organic and inorganic objects, it cannot be the result of "life-energy."[3]

Armed with this background information, we can now critically evaluate some of the assertions and interpretations placed on specific characteristics of the aura patterns that result from corona discharge photography.

There are many claims about Kirlian photography,—but only a few can be dealt with here. The first claim is that the "auras" change according to the subject's mood. This change has been well documented and carefully researched.[4]

Moisture, passed onto the photographic plate and into the air immediately in the vicinity of the object to be photographed, has been found to be responsible for the modification of the corona's shape. Moisture is also responsible for the corona's size and brightness and for the reduction in density of the 'needles' of light that are produced from the object's sharply curved contact points, such as fingertips or the prominences of a leaf.[1,4]

Further investigations have found that various factors which induce an emotional response, such as pain and sudden noise, modified the corona or aura's appearance. These changes are also connected to the amount of moisture in the person's skin.[1,4]

Another parameter, also linked to emotional response, which influences human electricity conductivity is the electrical skin resistance. Changes in this are known as the psychogalvanic skin reaction. Ellison says electrical skin resistance can be changed by heavy breathing and altered radically by deep relaxation, the skin's resistance increases greatly in a state of trance.[5]

Another claim involves what is known as "the phantom leaf effect." Two sets of Kirlian photographs are taken of a rose leaf before and after a section of the leaf is cut away. The second photograph shows the aura persisting around the space left by excision. In their experiments examining the phantom leaf effect, Watkins and Bickel placed torn and broken leaves, keeping the pieces separate on the photographic plate.[3]

When several of the experimental results showed a phantom leaf effect, further investigation revealed that the cause was easily explained. When the leaves were photographed using the conducting pressure plate placed on top of them, moisture and leaf fluids were excreted onto the photographic plate, together with adhering dust particles. After the leaf was removed and the metal plate carefully repositioned in its original position, the faint imprint provided an aura photograph of the entire missing leaf.[3] When there was no imprint there was no "phantom-leaf effect."

The final claim is that Kirlian photography can be used as a diagnostic tool, by using information from the various patterns created by an aura and relating it to the state of the individual. But to make such a claim the Kirlian practitioner, or indeed any medical practitioner, must be able to provide scientific evidence that the person's condition caused any of the effects seen in the aura.

According to Watkins and Bickel, however, "there is no evidence as yet that any feature, character or property of the aura pattern is related to the physiological, psychological or psychic condition of the sample."[3]

Although certain physiological and psychological problems are outwardly observable and measurable, there is no scientific evidence to warrant the claim that the Kirlian technique is a "direct or meaningful link" to such problems.

Kirlian photography is dependent on many variables that, if not properly controlled, can affect the process. Singer, referring to a Kirlian photograph of a fingertip, claims such factors include: position and pressure of the finger on the photographic plate; air temperature; skin resistance; moisture extruded from the skin; and photograph interpretation.[1]

Further factors that have been identified are the electrical properties of the circuit, photographic plate properties (such as the types of emulsion), electrode and insulator characteristics.[1,3,4]

Pehek, Kyler and Faust also noticed that when two consecutive photographs of a fingertip were taken within a short time of each other, the first corona affected the second, which appeared much denser. This phenomenon suggests "the effect is either a dehydration of the stratum corneum or sweat duct emptying, accompanied by depolarization of the sweat duct neurons by the electric field."[4]

As Watkins and Bickel point out, the challenge is now to "control the parameters and demonstrate in several specific cases that the aura produces information inaccessible to, or better than, other techniques."[3]

As with other fringe therapies, what is required is rigorous scientific research into the efficacy of Kirlian photography. If that is carried out, paying customers who entrust their health, safety and welfare to practitioners of the technique will be reassured that the methods used are demonstrably safe and effective.[6]

References

1. Singer, B. Kirlian Photography. In: Abell, G. and Singer B. (eds) *Science and the Paranormal* London: Junction Books, 1981.

2. Booth, B. Iridology, radionics, Kirlian photography. *Nursing Times* 1995; 91:11,29-31.

3. Watkins, A.J., Bickel, W.S. A study of the Kirlian effect. *The Skeptical Inquirer* 1986; 10: 3, 244-257.

4. Pehek, J.O., Kyler, H.J. and Faust, D.L. Image modulation in corona discharge photography. *Science* 1976; 194:263-270.

5. Ellison, A.J. A crack in Kirlian's halo. *The Unexplained*. 32, 630-633

6. Brewin, T. What's wrong with alternative medicine? *The Skeptic* 1995;8:6,6-9.

—by Michael Stanwick

Michael Stanwick, BA, is a qualified teacher and a science student.

Chapter 40

Music's Surprising Power to Heal

Marianne Strebely, severely injured in an auto accident, lay in the operating room of St. Luke's Hospital in Cleveland, awaiting anesthesia. Surrounded by a surgical team, Strebely was hooked up to a computer that monitored her heart rate and brain waves. She was also hooked up, by earphones, to a tape recorder playing Vivaldi's The Four Seasons.

During the operation, the surgical team listened to Mozart and Brahm's from another tape recorder. "Music reduces staff tension in the operating room," says Dr. Clyde L. Nash, Jr., Strebely's surgeon, "and also helps relax the patient."

"The music was better than medication," Strebely claims, comparing this surgery with a previous one. "I remained calm before the operation and didn't need as much sedation." At home, convalescing to music, Strebely was even able to forgo her prescribed painkillers.

Nash is one of many physicians around the country who are finding that music, used with conventional therapies, can help heal the sick. Adds Dr. Mathew H. M. Lee, acting director of the Rusk Rehabilitation Institute at New York University Medical Center, "We've seen confirmation of music's benefits in helping to avoid serious complications during illness, enhancing patients' well-being and shortening hospital stays."

- At California State University in Fresno, psychologist Janet Lapp studied 30 migraine-headache sufferers for five weeks.

Some of the 30 listened to their favorite music; others used bio-feedback and relaxation techniques; a control group did neither. All three groups received similar medication. Music proved the most effective supplemental therapy, especially over the long term. A year later, the patients who had continued to listen to music reported one-sixth as many headaches as before; these were also less severe and ended more quickly.

- Clinical researchers at the U.C.L.A. School of Nursing in Los Angeles, and at Georgia Baptist Medical Center in Atlanta, found that premature babies gained weight faster and were able to use oxygen more efficiently when they listened to soothing music mixed with voices or womb sounds. At Talla-hassee (Fla.) Memorial Regional Medical Center, premature and low-birth-weight infants exposed to an hour and a half of soothing vocal music each day averaged only 11 days in the Newborn Intensive Care Unit, compared with 16 days for a con-trol group.

- At Baltimore's St. Agnes Hospital, classical music was provided in the critical-care units. "Half an hour of music produced the same effect as ten milligrams of Valium," says Dr. Raymond Bahr, head of the coronary-care unit. "Some patients who had been awake for three or four straight days were able to go into a deep sleep."

How does music help? Some studies show it can lower blood pressure, basal-metabolism and respiration rates, thus lessening physiological responses to stress. Other studies suggest music may help increase production of endorphins (natural pain relievers) and S-IGA (salivary immunoglobulin A). S-IGA speeds healing, reduces the danger of infection and controls heart rate.

Music therapy is proving especially effective in three key medical areas:

1. Pain, anxiety and depression. "When I had my first baby," says Susan Koletsky of Shaker Heights, Ohio, "I was in difficult labor for two days. The second time around, I wanted to avoid the pain." Relaxing jazz calmed her in the delivery room; Bach and Beethoven paced her during contractions; finally, the closing movement of Brahms's Symphony No. 1 energized her for the last phase of delivery. "The music produced a much easier experience," she claims.

600

Cancer patients often brood in their hospital rooms, refusing to talk with doctors and nurses. "The music therapist can give them a positive outlook," says Dr. Nathan A. Berger, director of the Ireland Cancer Center at University Hospitals of Cleveland. "That makes it easier to communicate and encourages them to cooperate more in their treatment."

A 17-year-old patient at the center, with extensive skin damage from cancer treatments, was withdrawn and silent. When music therapist Deforia Lane saw her, the teenager was wrapped in gauze, sitting in a wheelchair.

Lane gave her a quick lesson in the omnichord, a small music synthesizer; then they played and sang together for 45 minutes. After the session, the patient's mother told Lane in a voice choked with emotion, "This is the first time Ginny has shown any happiness since she walked into this hospital."

2. Mental, emotional and physical handicaps. The Ivymount School in Rockville, Md., helps youngsters with developmental problems ranging from emotional disturbances to mental retardation, autism and severe to moderate learning disabilities. Ruthlee Adler, a music therapist for more than 20 years, uses song and dance to help the children learn—and cope. "While the seriously handicapped may ignore other kinds of stimulation, they respond to music," she says.

One five-year-old lacked fine muscular skills, didn't know left from right, and was so shy he refused to sing. The boy became fascinated with the xylophone, however, and through this interest Adler taught him numbers, left from right, and the concept of sharing. Eventually he learned to read music and play the piano, and he even led the group in singing.

At Colorado State University's Center for Biomedical Research in Music, ten stroke victims were hooked up to sensors that measured muscle activity in their legs and the timing of their strides as they walked to a rhythmic dance piece. Over four weeks, the patients were tested first without, then with, the music. Significant improvement in stride symmetry was seen when the patients walked to musical accompaniment. "In almost every case," says Michael Thaut, director of the center, "the timing of the stride improved with music."

3. Neurological disorders. Dr. Oliver Sacks, whose work with sleeping-sickness victims led to the book and movie Awakenings, reports that patients suffering neurological disorders who cannot talk or move are often able to sing, and sometimes even dance, to music. "The power of music is remarkable in such people," Sacks observes.

Studies indicate both hemispheres of the brain are involved in processing music. Dr. Sacks explains, "The neurological basis of musical responses is robust and may even survive damage to both hemispheres."

In a group session for elderly patients at Beth Abraham Hospital in New York City, a 70-year-old stroke victim sat by himself, never speaking. One day, when therapist Connie Tomaino played an old Jewish folk song on her accordion, the man hummed. Tomaino played the tune regularly after that. Finally, the man sang some of the words. "Before you knew it," says Tomaino, "he was talking."

Music's therapeutic benefits, of course, aren't confined to those who are ill. "Apart from the simple enjoyment that music provides, we're learning how much it can also help us in our daily personal lives," says Ireland Cancer Center's Dr. Berger. To "psyche up" for important presentations and meetings, Berger hums the theme music from the movie Rocky or the triumphal march from the opera Aida. "Music can also act as a tension—or pain—reliever for something as routine as going to the dentist," he says, "or it can simply give expression to our moods."

To gain the full benefit of music, you need to work it into your daily schedule. During his lunch hour, Jeffrey Scheffel closes his office door at the Mayo Clinic in Rochester, Minn., slips on a pair of earphones and, leaning back in his desk chair, tunes in some light jazz or Mozart, depending on the mood he wants to build. "It rejuvenates me," explains Scheffel, research administrator at the famed medical center. "It gives my brain a break, lets me focus on something else for a few minutes, and helps me get through the rest of the day."

Dana Gentry of Las Vegas recently discovered the added power that music can have when we share it with others. One of Gentry's earliest memories is of her grandmother holding her in her arms, singing their favorite song, "True Love." Now Gentry's grandmother is in a nursing home, her mind lost to Alzheimer's disease.

One day Gentry knelt beside the woman's wheelchair and sang "their" song. "At first," Gentry says, "I noticed a glimmer of recognition on her face. Then she joined in and sang the entire song in harmony. As tears rolled down my cheeks, she cried, too, as if realizing what she had accomplished. We sing our song every visit now. It turns a sad time into a happy time."

Few people understand the therapeutic powers of music better than Cleveland music therapist Deforia Lane. Ten years ago, during her own bout with cancer, singing helped her relax and take her mind off the disease. Since then, she has used that experience to help others. "Music is not magic," says the 44-year-old therapist with the warm smile and rich soprano voice. "But in a hospital or at home, for young people or older ones, it can be a potent medicine that helps us all."

— by David M. Maize

Chapter 41

Prayer as Therapy

Worth a Prayer?

Is prayer really an effective therapeutic tool for seriously ill individuals who worship God?

The answer, says a southern California internist who studied nearly 400 heart patients over a 10-month period, would seem to be Amen!—but not without some reservations.

The idea of someone praying for the well-being of someone else is hardly new; nevertheless, very little serious scientific research has been done on prayer's effectiveness with hospital patients, and the few studies that have been attempted are inconclusive. To describe and evaluate the effects, if any, of intercessory prayer on a patient's condition and recovery while in the hospital, Dr. Randolph C. Byrd picked at random 393 heart patients admitted to the cardiac care unit of the San Francisco General Hospital Medical Center between August 1982 and May 1983. The patients had agreed to be placed into two groups. Byrd assigned Roman Catholic and Protestant individuals outside the hospital to pray daily to the western world's most-worshipped deity, the Judeo-Christian God, for the well-being and recovery of 192 patients in one group; the remaining 201 patients in the other group were left without assigned persons to pray for them.

Byrd found no significant differences between the two groups at first; however, follow-up studies on all patients revealed slightly fewer

Medical Education and Research Foundation 1989. *Medical Update*, March 1989 v12 n9 p2(2). Reprinted with permission.

medical complications among the first group. Of the various conditions measured, congestive heart failure, cardiopulmonary arrest, and pneumonia were seen less frequently in the prayer group. This same group also used fewer diuretics, antibiotics, and intubation/ventilation procedures than the second, non-prayer group.

Finally, Byrd rated 85 percent of the prayer group as having a good medical course after entry (i.e., no new diagnoses, problems or therapies were recorded during these patients' stays), compared with 73 percent of the non-prayer group. A bad hospital course (high morbidity and risk of death, or death itself) was observed in 14 percent of the prayer group, in contrast with 22 percent of the non-prayer group.

Byrd points to several references in the Bible (Genesis 20:17, 18; Numbers 12:13; Acts 28:8) where intercessory prayer was used as a healing mechanism. However, Byrd admits it is possible that the study's intercessors might have prayed for those in the non-prayer group, even though they were expressly told not to. Also, there was no attempt to limit the amount of prayer by the intercessors, nor was anyone hired to check up on the praying individuals to make sure they were doing their jobs. Byrd even allows for the possibility that others not assigned to the study might have been praying alongside the assigned intercessors; then, too, he says, it is impossible to accurately assess just exactly what the Judeo-Christian God actually did and if he did anything because, or in spite of, the prayers of the individuals considered by the researcher to be "born-again" Christians as defined in the Biblical verse John 3:3.

Nevertheless, Dr. John Thomison, editor of the Southern Medical Journal, says he would like to read of further studies exploring this topic more thoroughly. Prayer, believes Thomison, is "about as benign a form of treatment as there is. There is no danger whatsoever." Byrd likewise presumes the effect of prayer to be "beneficial," based on the data presented in the study, as well as the general consensus of almost all the study's patients that "prayer probably helped and certainly could not hurt."

Part Eight

Pharmacological and Biological Treatments

Chapter 42

Pharmacological and Biological Interventions:

Antineoplastons, Cartilage Products, EDTA Chelation Therapy, Ozone, Immunoaugmentative Therapy, 714-X, Hoxsey Method, Essiac, Coley's Toxins, MTH-68, Neural Therapy, Apitherapy, Iscador/Mistletoe, and Rivici's Guided Chemotherapy

Overview

The alternative pharmacological and biological treatments discussed in this chapter are an assortment of drugs and vaccines that have not yet been accepted by mainstream medicine. If and when they are accepted, many of these drugs and vaccines will fit into conventional medicine as it is practiced today. Thus, these treatments differ from other alternative health measures in this report because, by and large, they do not represent an entirely new theory or unified approach to health and disease.

Despite their diversity, the alternative pharmacological approaches share some or all of the following themes:

- Unlike many mainstream drugs, most unconventional substances are believed to be nontoxic.

- Many are directed not toward eradicating a specific disease entity but toward stimulating the patient's immune system to fight the onslaught of a pathological condition or organism. Frequently, these methods may have to be tailored to individual patients to be effective.

- For other approaches, practitioners may postulate an entirely new defense system altogether.

Extracted from NIH Publication No. 94-066. December 1994. Due to space considerations, bibliographic data have not been reprinted in this chapter. However, the in-text references have been retained.

- Other alternative substances are derived from old Native American herbal remedies or are turn-of-the-century remedies that were cast aside during the rapid advance of biomedicine.

Hundreds of alternative drugs and vaccines could have been included in this report. The ones that are included were chosen because they met one or more of the following criteria:

- **Therapeutic promise.** Available evidence suggests that they may be effective.

- **Wide use.** Because they are now used by many people, public health considerations indicate that they should be investigated. If any of these products prove harmful, that news needs to be spread quickly; if any prove effective, this should be officially recognized and they should be put to further use. An up-to-date example is the use of cartilage products for acquired immune deficiency syndrome (AIDS), cancer, and arthritis. Since a "60 Minutes" television program about them in late February 1993, some 50,000 Americans are currently reported to be taking shark cartilage even though properly designed trials have not yet been conducted. (Another consideration besides safety and effectiveness for the users is that demand for these products entails destroying many sharks.) Ozone is another example of a substance now being used widely—particularly as a self-medication in the AIDS community—without solid evidence of its usefulness.

- **Subject of controversy.** Some other pharmacological or biological products have been the subject of long-standing controversies that need to be resolved. This point is particularly true for certain medicines derived from Native American remedies, such as the Hoxsey method and Essiac.

- **Former use or use elsewhere.** Some products have been tested and well documented in the scientific literature but for various reasons have fallen by the wayside. An example is Coley's toxins, an immunotherapy for cancer that was developed at the turn of the century by a New York bone surgeon and which is currently being used in China and Germany. Similarly MTH-68, a nontoxic, biological vaccine, is reported to buttress the immune system against cancer. Another example is the use of a local anesthetic (often novocaine) for neural therapy to combat

610

chronic pain, allergies, and other problems; this approach is in wide use in Europe.

A major impediment to full investigation of alternative pharmacological treatments is the high expense of conducting the trials necessary to meet Food and Drug Administration (FDA) approval. Nearly every one of the few drugs that FDA approves each year is marketed by one of the major pharmaceutical companies. Nevertheless, even well-capitalized biotechnology firms have sometimes been driven out of the marketplace by the difficulty in meeting FDA requirements.

Another problem for many alternative materials such as herbs, nutrients, and common chemicals is their lack of sponsorship. Because they are in the public domain and therefore inexpensive and not patentable, drug companies understandably lack interest in investing the enormous sums required for full trials. Therefore, most such alternatives lack both sponsors and funding for clinical trials of their safety and effectiveness.

Marketing most of the substances discussed in this chapter is not allowed by FDA on the basis of its interpretation of Title 21, article 355, of the U.S. Code, which states that unless a developer has presented "substantial evidence" of a drug's safety and efficacy, the FDA can deny approval for marketing that substance. "Substantial evidence" is defined as "adequate and well-controlled investigations, including clinical investigations, by experts qualified by scientific training and experience to evaluate the effectiveness of the drug involved."

Many alternative medical practitioners have attempted to market new drugs or vaccines under this statute, but few have succeeded. The failure often occurs because "qualified experts" are defined as those who adhere to mainstream medical practices. To be an alternative practitioner has, until now, been reason enough to disqualify a person to evaluate the usefulness of the drug in question.

Moreover, "clinical investigations" are generally interpreted to mean randomized, double-blind, placebo-controlled studies (see the "Research Methodologies" chapter) of the kind that only pharmaceutical companies and major medical centers can afford to conduct. This is true despite a declaration by Jay Moskowitz, former deputy director of the National Institutes of Health in September 1992, that "not all alternative medical practices are amenable to traditional scientific evaluation, and some may require development of new methods to evaluate their efficacy and safety." Thus, the reluctance of conventional medicine to accept for examination and possible use the materials assessed here appears to be tied to measuring them with the wrong yardstick.

The remaining sections of this chapter deal with the existing research base for 14 specific treatments, future research opportunities for these 14 treatments, and key issues and recommendations that are relevant to all such biological and pharmacological treatments. Each treatment fits one or more of the criteria cited earlier—such as wide use, controversy, and therapeutic promise and may require selection or development of appropriate methodologies for proper evaluation.

Research Base for Specific Treatments

Hundreds of potentially useful alternative drugs or vaccines are supported by data indicating that they may be useful in the treatment of such diseases as cancer, AIDS, heart disease, hepatitis, and other major health problems. What follows is only a sampling of the many products available for study.

Antineoplastons

Antineoplastons are peptide fractions originally derived from normal human blood and urine, although a method for synthesizing them was subsequently developed by Dr. Stanislaw Burzynski. Burzynski has named some of these peptides A2, A5, A10, and AS2-1. He first discovered antineoplastons as a graduate student in Poland in 1967 (Moss, 1989) when he compared normal urine and urine from people with cancer and noted an anomalous streak on electrophoresis of the normal urine that was not present in the urine of cancer patients. He then chemically defined these antineoplastons at Baylor College of Medicine in Houston (Burzynski, 1973, 1976, 1986; Burzynski and Kubove, 1986a, 1986b; Moss, 1992). He depicts these substances as a newly discovered, natural form of anticancer protection, apart from the lymphocyte system.

Burzynski reported that the antineoplaston peptides are essentially nontoxic (Burzynski, 1986) and that preliminary clinical results indicated tumor responses (shrinkages) in a number of difficult cases, most of which involved subjects who had exhausted conventional treatments (Burzynski, 1986; Moss, 1992). He also reported at the 1992 International Conference on AIDS that some patients infected with human immunodeficiency virus (HIV) responded to antineoplastons by a marked increase in certain white blood cells (CD4+ lymphocytes);

other observations included increases of energy and weight and a decrease of opportunistic infections.

Although antineoplastons have been employed against a wide variety of tumors, the greatest interest has been generated by using them with otherwise incurable brain cancers. Burzynski reports that he has been most successful treating prostate cancer and brain cancer (specifically, several forms of childhood glioma) and has had good results with (in descending order) non-Hodgkins lymphomas and pancreatic cancers, breast cancer, lung cancer, and colon cancer. Burzynski has published scores of medical articles in peer-reviewed journals, mostly in Europe (Bertelli, 1990; Bertelli and Mathe, 1985, 1987; Kuemmerle, 1988). At the 18th International Congress of Chemotherapy in Stockholm on July 1, 1993, more than a dozen papers were presented by researchers from Brazil, Holland, Japan, Poland, and the United States in a special session on antineoplastons.

In the late 1970s, controversy began swirling around Burzynski when he left a position at Baylor College of Medicine during a disagreement about an interdepartmental transfer, research freedom, research funding, and maintenance of a private medical practice. Since then, Burzynski has worked independently, paying for his research from patients' fees. Some research physicians are fascinated by his work, but many others have attacked it. On one hand, after conducting a review of a "best case series," including a site visit in October 1991, the National Cancer Institute (NCI) concluded that antitumor activity by antineoplastons may have been demonstrated by Burzynski in seven cases of incurable brain cancer (confirmation by NCI communication, 1994). Consequently, NCI agreed that conducting confirmatory trials would be a worthwhile effort. On the other hand, Saul Green, formerly a researcher at Memorial Sloan-Kettering Cancer Research Center, attacked treatments with antineoplastons in the *Journal of the American Medical Association* (Green, 1992).

The trials that NCI proposed are Phase II studies (that is, small-scale clinical trials), in which researchers examine the effectiveness of a potential treatment in some 25 to 40 subjects. The Office of Alternative Medicine (OAM) has contributed to the funding of these trials; Burzynski has participated in the planning steps and provided a supply of synthetic antineoplastons A10 and AS2-1. (He informed NCI that he no longer uses urine-derived products.) In late 1993 and early 1994, three sites opened enrollment for these trials: Memorial Sloan-Kettering in New York, the Mayo Clinic in Minnesota, and the Clinical Pharmacology Branch of NCI in Maryland. The subjects to receive antineoplastons are patients with two types of brain tumors, gliomas and astrocytomas. They are required to have a particularly small tumor, at Burzynski's request.

Because of the possible promise of some of Burzynski's products and the controversy surrounding them, further research should be conducted.

Cartilage Products

Investigations of cartilage to improve health began with a graduate student wondering whether cartilage could assist wound healing. Physician-researcher John Prudden decided to find out, using a powdered and washed cartilage product. There is now a long list of reported effects of cartilage preparations, including accelerating wound healing, possessing topical anti-inflammatory capability, alleviating autoimmune diseases, relieving osteoarthritic pain, alleviating scleroderma (a disease in which the skin hardens), easing skin symptoms of herpesvirus infections, alleviating psoriasis (a chronic, scaly skin disease), and inhibiting a wide spectrum of cancers (Prudden, 1985). A recent report adds relieving swollen and tender joints of patients with rheumatoid arthritis (Trentham et al.; 1993). This study bolsters previous anecdotal reports that cartilage products can palliate the painful effects of rheumatoid arthritis.

The various cartilage products under study or reported on anecdotally derive from cattle, sheep, sharks, and chicken cartilage; some products, such as Prudden's "Catrix," are a form of repeatedly powdered and cleaned cartilage; others are relatively pure substances, such as the type II collagen used by Trentham et al. (1993) in a randomized double-blind trial.

The popularity of cartilage products increased dramatically after the television program "60 Minutes" produced a segment on the possible benefits of shark cartilage in late February 1993, citing a 16-week clinical trial in Cuba with some allegedly positive results. Medical centers have since been inundated with calls about the effectiveness of shark cartilage in treating AIDS, cancer, and arthritis. Since the show, this product has been aggressively marketed in the United States, and some 50,000 Americans are said to be currently taking shark cartilage at an individual cost of approximately $7,000 or more per year.

The numbers of persons and amount of money they are spending are together sufficient reason to undertake an evaluation of the safety and effectiveness of shark cartilage treatments.

As for one or more scientific bases, a scientific hypothesis for the effectiveness of cartilage products as anticancer agents relates to their effects on blood vessel formation. A substance present in very small amounts in cartilage is believed to act by inhibiting angiogenesis, or interfering with the ability of a tumor to create a network of new blood vessels. It has been shown that if a tumor cannot establish a new blood network, it cannot grow any larger than the point of a pencil (Brem and Folkman, 1975; Folkman, 1976; Langer et al., 1976). Thus it has been proposed that cartilage, and appropriate substances purified from cartilage, may act against cancer through angiogenesis-inhibiting effects.

A researcher at NCI has proposed another anticancer mechanism involving a class of protein that are produced in normal tissues such as cartilage and bone (Liotta, 1992). These proteins are called tissue inhibitors of metalloproteinases (TIMPs); TIMPs appear to block the action of certain metal-containing enzymes (the metalloproteinases) that help tumor cells to invade surrounding tissue.

A detailed explanation for the successful treatment of rheumatoid arthritis with type II collagen (Trentham et al., 1993) is still being sought. A working hypothesis is that the large amount of collagen taken by mouth (in daily doses in orange juice) suppresses autoimmune reactions; this observation was made in previous studies with animal models of autoimmune diseases and in small pilot human studies of patients with multiple sclerosis and with rheumatoid arthritis. Possibly the collagen stimulates certain immune system cells to produce anti-inflammatory cytokines.

In reviewing the scientific literature on cartilage, Prudden (1985) described other health-promoting activities studied by other researchers. Wound-healing activity is attributed to a polymer of N-acetyl glucosamine. Inhibition of cell division and inflammation appear to be attributable to a different "fraction" of cartilage. Although practitioners of alternative medicine tend to prefer dealing with natural substances, such as cartilage, the more conventional academic view is that such mixtures must be separated into identifiable, pure products. The most recent work with cartilage itself, rather than purified products, is probably the anticancer shark cartilage studies. NCI informally reviewed the results of the 16-week Cuban study that "60 Minutes" cited when the chief Cuban investigator presented a seminar in the United States. Staffers from NCI's Cancer Treatment Effectiveness Program noted the uncertainty of accurate drug delivery by enemas (apparently enemas had to be used because the preparation's taste was so bad that subjects would not eat it) and what they called the lack of any clear benefits in the cases described. Nevertheless, the NCI staff indicated that it would be willing to reconsider this product if additional data should prove positive

Charles Simone—an oncologist from Lawrenceville, NJ, who has NCI research experience—examined the results of the Cuban study for "60 Minutes" and was guardedly optimistic. In his own practice, he has treated some patients who initiated self-medication with cartilage. He has said that some of his patients experienced dramatic improvement, including the clearing of liver metastases and rapid reduction in certain prostate antigens in prostate cancer (Simone, 1993). Simone provided OAM with a copy of a protocol (study plan) and has begun a prospective study on shark cartilage. In early 1994, he received IND (investigational new drug) approval from FDA for shark cartilage.

Most previous studies with cartilage have used bovine cartilage. Catrix, a trade-named product derived from the tracheal rings of cattle, was developed by John Prudden, who holds a patent on the use of all cartilage products (including shark) and an FDA IND permit to conduct research studies. Prudden was formerly a surgeon at Columbia-Presbyterian Hospital in New York and associate professor of clinical surgery at Columbia University. He has published more than 60 papers on the use of cartilage, mostly to accelerate wound healing but also to treat psoriasis, cancer, and rheumatoid arthritis. In 1985, Prudden reported on results of a study in which 31 cancer patients were treated continually with Catrix. The overall response rate, measured as a greater than 50-percent reduction in tumor size, was reported as an unusually high 90 percent; 61 percent had complete disappearance of tumors.[1] Both oral and injectable forms of Catrix were used, and Prudden concluded that the oral route was superior.

Clinical trials using Catrix in kidney (renal cell) cancer patients are currently under way at Westchester Medical Center in Valhalla, NY, and Royal Victoria Hospital in Montreal. Renal cell cancer is an intractable tumor, resistant to cure, relief, and control; response rates with Catrix are said to be about 25 percent (Prudden, 1993).

The proposed usefulness of cartilage for AIDS patients would be for treatment of AIDS-related cancers such as Kaposi's sarcoma and AIDS-related lymphoma and for opportunistic infections caused by viruses other than HIV. Although cartilage is reported to have activity against herpes infections, it does not directly affect herpesviruses (Prudden, 1993). Prudden proposes that the antiviral effects result from stimulation of patients' immune systems; this point should be explored in more detail.

EDTA Chelation Therapy

Chelation is the major form of alternative therapy for cardiovascular disease and one of the most popular alternative pharmacological treatments. Chelation employs ethylene diamine tetraacetic acid (EDTA), a material that readily binds to metallic ions. EDTA is used in standard medicine as the preferred treatment for lead poisoning as well as for removing more than a dozen other toxic metals ranging from cadmium to zinc (Berkow, 1992).

Since shortly after EDTA was synthesized in the 1950s, its use has been suggested to treat heart disease and circulatory problems, including atherosclerosis (Clarke et al., 1955), high blood pressure (Schroeder and Perry, 1955), angina pectoris (Clarke et al., 1956), occlusive vascular disease (Clarke, 1960), and porphyria (Peters, 1960). Chelation has also been suggested as a potential treatment for rheumatoid arthritis (Boyle et al., 1963) and even as a preventive for cancer (Blumer and Cranton, 1989).

Several mechanisms have been proposed for the therapeutic action of EDTA. Since the molecule is known to be able to incorporate a metal ion into its own ring structure, it may maintain cellular health by removing those ions that cause harmful peroxidation of lipids (fatty materials). EDTA is also believed to remove calcium particles deposited in the arterial wall-various kinds of plaques by analogy to its standard use in heavy-metal poisoning. But it may also lower the ionized calcium levels by blocking the slow calcium currents in the arterial wall, thus functioning as a kind of "calcium-blocking agent," a category of drugs known to have potent coronary vasodilating effects (Casdorph, 1981). EDTA has also been identified as acting to increase the concentration of vasodilator (Cranton and Frackelton, 1989).

Most recently, the various mechanisms proposed for EDTA's therapeutic action have been brought together under a unified but controversial theory that they all involve protective effects against detrimental actions of free radicals (Cranton and Frackelton, 1989). This protection may lead indirectly to such activities as removing deposits from the walls of arteries or dilating blocked arteries.

Various peer-reviewed articles support the use of EDTA chelation in heart disease because of the observed effects on the health of patients, but clear demonstration of physiological change has been possible only in the past few years. In the early 1980s, the problem was how to directly measure arterial effects of EDTA, because measurements of the size (diameter) of arteries were accurate within only 25 percent (Cranton and Frackelton, 1982); yet dilations of 10 to 15

617

percent may have significant (doubling) effects on blood flow (Cranton, 1985; Olszewer and Carter, 1989). One 1982 study did report decreased blockage of arteries in 88 percent of 57 patients by means of a non-invasive analysis (McDonagh et al., 1982) that relies on a technique developed by Langham and To'mey (1978). Later research involving some of the same investigators (Rudolph et al., 1991) using ultrasound showed a decrease in blockage of carotid arteries using chelation therapy that was statistically significant in both males and females and was an average of 21 percent lower than initial values. The investigators calculated large improvements in blood flow as a result of the decreased blockage. Furthermore, a large retrospective study of 2,870 patients in Brazil showed that 89 percent of the patients treated with EDTA had marked or good improvement (Olszewer and Carter, 1989). Olszewer et al. (1990) followed the retrospective study with a small, randomized, double-blind clinical trial of EDTA treatments for 10 men with peripheral vascular disease. After 10 of 20 intended EDTA treatments, it was clear that some patients were showing dramatic improvements. When the code that identified which patients were receiving medication was broken, the group that had improved were all identified as persons who received EDTA. All patients were then placed on EDTA treatment, and the ones previously receiving placebo showed improvement comparable to that of the first EDTA group. The group continuing on EDTA showed additional improvements as well, although later progress was not as dramatic as the initial changes.

Chelation is currently available in nearly every State of the United States as well as many foreign countries. In the United States, the four major organizations promoting acceptance of chelation therapy are the American Board of Chelation Therapy, the American College for Advancement in Medicine, the Great Lakes Association of Clinical Medicine, and the International Bioxidative Medicine Association. Chelation therapy is administered as an outpatient treatment, costing $75 to $120 per visit; the average cost for a course of 20 to 30 treatments is approximately $3,000. Since 1960, 500,000 patients have received chelation in more than five million treatments.

The toxicity of EDTA is a matter of some dispute. Advocates claim that it is essentially nontoxic, with approximately the same "danger" as that of normal doses of aspirin. They explain that early adverse effects, especially on the kidney, resulted from preexisting kidney disease or from using greater doses and rates of administration than those now recommended (the protocol available from the American College for Advancement in Medicine for use of intravenous EDTA also includes dietary supplements with multivitamins and trace elements). Although some reports claimed EDTA-related deaths, proponents state that these claims were erroneous, explaining, for example, that some deaths resulted from heavy-metal toxicity. See Cranton and Frackelton (1989) for references reviewing the field.

Hundreds of physicians are convinced that EDTA chelation therapy is of greater benefit to their patients than conventional treatments that are more dangerous and costly, such as bypass operations or toxic cardiotonic drugs such as digoxin. For example, Cranton (1985) compared 4,000 deaths from bypass surgery over a 30-year period with fewer than 20 associated with EDTA treatment (both procedures had approximately 300,000 patients during that time). Proponents also note that in issuing an IND permit to the American College for Advancement in Medicine to study EDTA to treat peripheral vascular disease, FDA officials indicated that "safety is not an issue" (Olszewer and Carter, 1989).

A double-blind, placebo-controlled study that might have settled the question of the usefulness of EDTA treatment was begun at three military hospitals in the 1980s under the FDA-approved IND application cited in the preceding paragraph. This study was dropped in November 1991, reportedly because of the exigencies of Operation Desert Storm in the Persian Gulf. At that time, 31 patients had completed their dosages, but the double-blind code was not broken.

At present, it is estimated that the study could be resumed by an interested sponsor at a cost of $3.75 million for the remaining 150 patients, or $25,000 per patient. Since EDTA is an unpatented drug in the public domain, no drug company is likely to sponsor this research or develop it for sale. Proponents of alternative medicine believe that EDTA could and should be evaluated in less costly ways.

Ozone

Anecdotal claims abound for ozone therapy among persons infected with HIV (the virus causing AIDS). Yet there have been only a few test tube (in vitro) and clinical evaluations of ozone as an antiviral therapy.

One such study (Wells et al., 1991) showed that ozone caused test tube inactivation of HIV by inhibiting an enzyme called reverse transcriptase and by disrupting viral particles and viral attachment to target cells. Ozone in nontoxic concentrations (4.0 g/mL) was also shown to inactivate this virus in both serum (Freeburg and Carpendale, 1988) and whole blood (Wagner et al., 1988). These test tube results appeared promising, but that was true for a number of other proposed AIDS treatments that were not subsequently successful for treating human beings.

More recently, two small sets of clinical trials using ozone-treated blood have been described in published reports (Garber et al., 1991; Hooker and Gazzard, 1992) and one clinical study using rectal administration of ozone (Carpendale et al., 1993). Garber and colleagues reported on withdrawing blood from patients infected with HIV, treating the blood with ozone, and returning the blood to the patient. Their hypothesis was that this technique would return killed HIV to patients that could then stimulate their immune systems.[2] In a Phase I study, which examines safety of the treatment in a small number of subjects, ozone therapy was reported to be safe and also possibly effective; the latter was suggested because three of ten patients showed some improvement in various measurements associated with HIV infection. (Study participants were HIV-infected persons who either refused or could not tolerate zidovudine [AZT] treatments.) Next, a Phase II randomized, double-blind study was initiated to look for signs of effective treatment in 14 subjects. On the basis of this 12-week study and blood, biochemical, and clinical laboratory tests, the authors reported that ozone had no significant effect.

Although a suggestion has been made that different dosing or other procedural variations might have produced positive results, the work of Hooker and Gazzard corroborates the negative results discussed above. Hooker and Gazzard conducted an open study of nine patients, using a procedure like that of Garber and colleagues and following the participants for 12 weeks. These researchers concluded, "We agree with Garber et al. that there is no evidence to support a belief that ozone, used by this method, is beneficial during HIV infection."

Nevertheless, persons applying or receiving ozone therapy tend to rely on the test tube results concerning ozone killing HIV and stimulating interferon, and on anecdotal information such as the following: To obtain additional information on ozone therapy in actual practice, the Research Department of Bastyr College of Natural Health Sciences in Seattle collected anecdotal data in 1993 from three physicians who used ozone in the treatment of their HIV and AIDS patients. In examining the case records of nine cases of HIV-positive patients treated with ozone by a physician in Washington State, Bastyr scientists concluded that some patients with CD4 counts above 500 showed increased counts of these cells after several weeks of treatment.[3] Patients with CD4 counts of 200 and below (more critical levels) did not seem to respond, although the doctor reported anecdotally that these patients were doing well clinically. Bastyr's researchers expressed interest in conducting a clinical trial.

A physician with a 5-year history of interest in ozone therapy, John Pittman, recently announced plans to open the North Carolina Bio-Oxidative Health Center in August 1994 and provide there a holistic treatment approach that includes ozone therapy. Previously, Pittman had closed his office to comply with an order from the State board of medical examiners, which considered ozone use nonconventional. North Carolina subsequently passed a "freedom of medicine law" that allows physicians choice among therapies so long as they have not been proved ineffective or dangerous. Pittman has indicated that the center will collect data on the effectiveness of its treatments.

A different approach to ozone use by AIDS patients appears to deserve further exploration. This application is not for attacking HIV, but for treating a debilitating and deleterious symptom-diarrhea. Carpendale et al. (1993) treated five patients with AIDS-related, in-tractable diarrhea using rectal administration of ozone gas daily for three to four weeks. This choice of treatment was based on reports from the 1930s that ozone was effective for three kinds of diarrhea. Diarrhea in three of the five patients was resolved, and one other patient improved as well. The ozone had no toxic effects. The authors suggest that further investigation is warranted, that longer treatment periods and different doses be studied, and that attention be paid to whether good results depend on the initial immunological state of the patients.

The fact that many people are receiving some kind of ozone treat-ment and that some practitioners continue to regularly apply such treatments is sufficient reason to recommend that definitive studies be undertaken to determine whether these treatments have any util-ity. Possibly, Pittman's new center will be able to provide this infor-mation.

Immunoaugmentative Therapy

Immunoaugmentative therapy, which was developed by Lawrence Burton, is "one of the most widely used unconventional cancer treat-ments," according to the Office of Technology Assessment (OTA)(Office of Technology Assessment, 1990). It has also been one of the most bit-terly contested. The process is patented, and some details of it appear to have been kept secret, although this situation may change since Burton's death in early 1993. The attempt to achieve a fair evalua-tion of immunoaugmentative therapy led some of its proponents, such as Frank Wiewel of People Against Cancer, to work for the establishment of OAM (Mason, 1992).

Essentially, immunoaugmentative therapy is an experimental form of cancer immunotherapy consisting of daily injections of processed blood products. Several blood fractions recovered by means of centrifugation are used in an attempt to restore normal immune function to the person with cancer. These fractions are said to include the following substances: (1) deblocking protein—an alpha-2 macroglobulin derived from the pooled blood serum of health donors; (2) tumor antibody 1 (TA1)—a combination of alpha-2 macroglobulin with other immune proteins (IgG and IgA) derived from the pooled blood serum of healthy donors; and (3) tumor antibody 2 (TA2) also derived from healthy blood serum but differing in potency (and possibly in composition) from TA1.

Proponents of immunoaugmentative therapy hypothesize that the tumor antibodies attack the tumors and that the deblocking proteins remove a "blocking factor" that prevents the patient's immune system from detecting the cancer.

Originally a New Yorker with a clinic in Great Neck, Long Island, Burton established a new base in Freeport, the Bahamas, in the late 1970s after he failed to obtain FDA approval for his blood fraction medications. This move followed nearly 20 years of work with tumor-inducing and tumor-inhibiting factors at various institutions. During the 1960s and 1970s, Burton and a colleague, Frank Friedman, reported discovering cancer-inhibiting factors in mice (Friedman et al., 1962). In one experiment, daily administration of these factors was said to eliminate palpable disease in 26 of 50 mice with leukemia. The treated animals appeared to survive significantly longer than the controls. In another experiment, Burton reported that 37 of 68 experimental animals survived for an average of 131 days without any evidence of leukemia, versus a 12-day average survival of untreated mice (Office of Technology Assessment, 1990). Burton concluded that the study of the biological action and interaction of these components in mice suggests the existence of an inhibitory system involved in the genesis of tumors and capable of causing specific tumor cell breakdown.

In July 1985, Burton's Freeport clinic was suddenly closed by the Bahamian health authorities and the Pan American Health Organization on charges of contamination with HIV (then called HTLV-III) and hepatitis virus. Despite alarming stories in the media, no patient has yet been found who became HIV positive or succumbed to AIDS because of Burton's treatment. Investigations by the Immunoaugmentative Therapy Patients Association (now People Against Cancer) suggest that there may never have been any HIV contamination (Moss, 1989). Some 500 patients were receiving 8 to 10 injections per day; during the year after the clinic was closed, several hundred all tested negative for HIV (Wiewel, 1994). Additional standard HIV tests of serum and blood supply used to prepare the treatment were all negative as well.

The Freeport clinic, which reopened in January 1986 through the actions of Burton's patients and some members of the U.S. Congress, remains open at present despite Burton's death. More than 5,000 patients have received immunoaugmentative therapy in Freeport.

In spite of the many patients treated and the stories of remissions, extensions of life, and improvements in the quality of life, very little documentation exists of either the methods or the results of Burton's therapy. After the hostile reaction by the cancer establishment in the 1970s, Burton retaliated by withdrawing from his former colleagues and ignoring the basic requirements of scientific documentation. A standoff resulted, which OTA was unable to resolve. It is possible that the Freeport clinic, now led by R.J. Clement, and the other existing clinic in Germany will be more willing to cooperate in concrete studies and that serious investigations of immunoaugmentative therapy can now be launched.

714-X

The ideas of French-born Gaston Naessens are a controversial area on the fringe of modern medicine. Naessens, a microbiologist whose formal education was interrupted by World War II before he could earn an advanced degree, has proposed a theory that cancer cells are deficient in nitrogen and can become normal cells if they receive it. Naessens' treatment to provide the nitrogen is a mixture of camphor and nitrogen called 714-X. The camphor is present reputedly to help deliver the nitrogen when 714-X is injected into the lymph system in the region of the abdomen. Naessens also uses the treatment for AIDS. To find out whether the 714-X treatment is working, Naessens uses a special microscope that he invented, called a somatoscope. The somatoscope has been described as an altered dark-field microscope. Naessens claims it can visualize living things at magnifications unattainable through the ordinary light microscope. He monitors improvement in his patients by the status of their "somatids," variable particles that he has described in his viewings with the somatosocope.

In the 1980s in Quebec, Naessens was prosecuted for health fraud and threatened with life imprisonment. He was acquitted, however, after many people testified not only to his character, but also to beneficial results from using 714-X. Some of the individuals claiming cures for cancer and AIDS are quoted in *Galileo of the Microscope* (Bird, 1989).

Many Americans, including former congressman Berkley Bedell (Bedell, 1993), have used 714-X as an unconventional treatment for cancer.[4] It has penetrated a number of alternative clinics that concentrate on other treatments. Stories are circulating of dramatic improvements or, with AIDS, of conversion from HIV positive to HIV negative. However, Naessens has not published in peer-reviewed literature. Without impartial scientific evaluation, it is difficult to reach conclusions on his work.

Hoxsey Method

The Hoxsey treatments are among the oldest U.S. alternative therapies for cancer and have been some of the most controversial. Like Essiac (see next section), they use a mixture of powerful herbs. These mixtures were probably derived from early Native American Indian medicines, although that connection is not as well established as with Essiac. Some of the same herbs are included in the formulas for both methods.

In the early part of the century Harry Hoxsey, an uncredentialed layman, marketed several cancer treatments in his clinics across the South. He claimed his remedies had been passed down to him by his father and grandfather, and he kept the ingredients secret until 1950. Eventually U.S. authorities shut down Hoxsey's clinics, but the treatment is still available at the Bio-Medical Center in Tijuana, Mexico, which is headed by Mildred Nelson, Hoxsey's former nurse assistant. Hoxsey indicated that some of his herbal components were present to necrotize tumors and others, as purgatives, to carry away the waste.

Hoxsey's remedies basically consist of an external salve and an herbal potion. The external medicine is an escharotic—a kind of burning paste—composed of zinc chloride, antimony, trisulfide, and bloodroot; its purpose is to corrode cancers. The paste is used principally for skin cancer (usually basal cell carcinomas), and many ambitious claims have been made for it. However, few reports on its efficacy (or lack thereof) exist in peer-reviewed literature. Moh's micrographic surgery, an orthodox procedure that bears some relationship to the Hoxsey treatment, is cited (Swanson, 1983): Moh's method consists of the use of zinc chloride paste to "fix" the tumor in place; the tumor is then removed in a series of steps.

The internal medication, which is the primary concern here, is made up of various herbs added to a base of potassium iodide and cascara, which is a bark preparation. The principal herbs are pokeweed root, burdock root, barberry (Berberis), buckthorn bark, stillingia root, and prickly ash. As Patricia Spain Ward noted in a contract report to OTA for its Unorthodox Cancer Treatments project, many of these roots and barks are now known to have anticancer and immunostimulatory effects.[5] The following items discuss several:

- **Pokeweed.** Pokeweed root (*Phytolacca americana*) has several effects on the immune system including stimulation of the production of two cytokines (see the glossary), interleukin 1 (IL-1) and tumor necrosis factor (TNF) (Bodger et al., 1979a, 1979b). Boosting the immune system is generally thought to help the body fight cancer.[6] Although pokeweed root is poisonous, it apparently has been used without serious toxicity problems since the mid-18th century.

- **Burdock root.** Burdock root (*Arctium lappa*) contains what Japanese scientists have called the "burdock factor" (Morita et al., 1984), which is reputed to act as a desmutagen, that is, a substance that reduces mutations. Burdock also has been shown to inhibit HIV, according to the World Health Organization (1989). In Japanese and macrobiotic diets young burdock roots are eaten as a vegetable called "gobo."

- **Buckthorn.** Buckthorn contains emodin, which has shown antileukemic activity in the laboratory (Kupchan and Karim, 1976).

It is noteworthy that, despite intense opposition, the Hoxsey formula has persisted as a cancer treatment for almost 100 years (Chowka, 1985). Among numerous anecdotal accounts of its effectiveness. some are hard to dismiss out of hand; it therefore warrants investigation. Despite decades of controversy, no clinical trials have ever been performed by either supporters or detractors of the Hoxsey therapies.[7] But since the Hoxsey formula contains the poisonous substance pokeweed, testing the formula is also a public health concern.

Essiac

Like Hoxsey therapy, Essiac is an herbal treatment. Reported to be of Native American (Ojibwa) origin, it was first brought to public attention in 1922 by an Ontario nurse named Renee Caisse (Essiac is Caisse spelled backward). Caisse was impressed by the case of a local woman who claimed to have been cured of breast cancer by a local Native American healer. Caisse set up a clinic in Bainbridge and treated thousands of patients before being shut down by the Canadian medical authorities in 1942. One problem was that Caisse never made the formula public during her lifetime (1888-1978).

In 1982 a Canadian government report concluded, "No clinical evidence exists to support the claims that Essiac is an effective treatment for cancer." Nevertheless, the relevant government agency, Health and Welfare Canada (equivalent to FDA in the United States), agreed to make this medication legally available to advanced cancer patients under Canada's Emergency Drug Regulations. It is currently produced as a trademarked product in Canada. This and other versions of Essiac are also widely available through the "cancer underground" in the United States.

There are several different Essiac products, each of which claims to be the one and only authentic Caisse formula. According to author Gary L. Glum, a Los Angeles chiropractor, authentic Essiac contains four ingredients: (1) sheep sorrel (Rumex acetosella); (2) burdock (*Arctium lappa*); (3) slippery elm inner bark (*Ulmus fulva*); and (4) Turkey rhubarb (*Rheum palmatum*) (Glum, 1988).

- **Sheep sorrel.** The main ingredient, sheep sorrel—not to be confused with the more readily available vegetable garden sorrel, also known as "sour grass"—contains vitamins, minerals, carotenoids, and chlorophyll, all of which supposedly have anti-cancer effects either directly or through immunological or anti-mutagenic activity (Moss, 1992). Sorrel was the basis of a celebrated cancer "cure" in Virginia in the 1740s, and as jiwisi it was a noted remedy of the Algonquin Ojibwa (Snow, 1993). In folk tradition it is reputed to have many other medicinal qualities as well.

   Sorrel also contains generous amounts of oxalic acid as well as emodin, which has been shown to have "significant antileukemia activity" (see discussion of buckthorn in the "Hoxsey Method" section).

- **Burdock.** (See also the "Hoxsey Method" section.) That the two long standing remedies of Hoxsey and Caisse have burdock in common is suggestive, although both formulas were long held in secret, and it is unlikely that Hoxsey and Caisse communicated or even knew of each other's existence. Burdock has been shown to be bioactive in a number of experiments (Dombradi and Foldeak, 1966; Foldeak and Dombradi, 1964; Morita et al., 1984; World Health Organization, 1989).

- **Slippery elm inner bark.** Slippery elm inner bark was tested by NCI without producing any sign of anticancer activity. Slippery elm lozenges, powdered bark, and slippery elm extracts are often available in health food stores and catalogs, with a wide range of curative and restorative claims listed for them.

- **Rhubarb.** Rhubarb has been used in Chinese medicine since at least 220 BC It is believed to exert a beneficial effect on the liver and gastrointestinal tract. Rhubarb extract showed anticancer activity in the sarcoma 37 test system (Belkin and Fitzgerald, 1952). It contains rhein, an anthraquinone, which has been shown to have antitumor effects (Office of Technology Assessment, 1990).

Essiac is widely used throughout North America, although, unlike use of Hoxsey's formula, use of Essiac is not associated with any particular clinic (Snow, 1993).

Coley's Toxin

Like many of the other pharmacological and biological treatments, Coley's toxins have attracted considerable medical and political controversy. More than 100 years ago, a New York bone surgeon at Memorial Hospital, William B. Coley, was investigating new approaches to curing cancer after his surgery failed to save a 19-year-old cancer patient. Coley chose to buttress a patient's immune system by giving him a bacterial infection that would cause a high fever and potently mobilize the patient's immune system to fight the cancer cells. Today, Coley is widely recognized as the first pioneer of immunotherapy— an approach that was virtually unknown in the 1890s.

The preparations that Coley developed were a mixture of killed cultures of bacteria from *Streptococcus pyogenes* and *Serratia marcescens*. Although not all patients responded to Coley's toxins, his treatment is reported to have shown dramatic curative effects on various cancers for many patients (Coley, 1894). These results were documented by Coley's daughter, Helen Coley Nauts, in a series of articles and monographs (Nauts, 1976, 1982, 1989.) Helen Nauts also founded the Cancer Research Institute in New York in 1953; this institute devotes itself to "the immunological approaches to the diagnosis, treatment, and prevention of cancer."

Nauts's monographs outline remarkable cures from the use of Coley's methods. Lloyd Old, an immunologist at Memorial Sloan-Kettering Cancer Research Center and a colleague, wrote, "Those who have scrutinized Dr. Coley's records have little doubt that the bacterial products that came to be known as Coley's toxins were in some instances highly effective" (Old and Boyse, 1973).

Over the years, Coley's work led to other discoveries. For instance, in the course of work on Coley's toxins in the 1940s, M.J. Shear of NCI discovered lipopolysaccharide (LPS), a component of bacterial cell walls. By injecting LPS into mice previously treated with bacillus Calmette-Guerin, Old discovered TNF (Old, 1987, 1988; Oettgen, 1980).

The original Coley formulas are no longer being used, even experimentally, in the United States. Until the 1980s, they were being tested at Temple University, Pennsylvania (Havas et al., 1958; Havas et al., 1990). In his 1990 paper, Havas pointed out that using purified LPS to evoke immune reactions is problematic because of its toxicity and proposed returning to a cruder mixture, a mixed bacterial vaccine similar to Coley's toxins. The research reported in that paper showed the mixed bacterial vaccine to have anticancer and immunostimulatory properties at nontoxic levels in animals with tumors. The authors concluded that the vaccine "compares favorably with other biological response modifiers."

Outside the United States, Coley's toxins are being used in Beijing Children's Hospital, the People's Republic of China, and Germany (Kolmel et al., 1991).

MTH-68

The MTH-68 vaccine is a form of immunotherapy that employs a little-known biological product against viral diseases and various kinds of cancer. Developed by Laszlo K. Csatáry, a Hungarian-American physician who currently resides in Ft. Lauderdale, FL, MTH-68 therapy is based on the idea that certain nonpathogenic viruses can be used to interfere with the growth of cancer in humans and the activity of harmful viruses.

MTH-68 is a modified attenuated strain of the Newcastle disease virus of chickens (paramyxovirus). In poultry, it causes an acute, fever-causing, generally fatal disease. In humans, however, the worst it does is trigger an acute but transient conjunctivitis (pinkeye), but this side effect is rare (Moss, 1992).

While Csatáry was searching for a virus that would be harmless to humans but would attack cancer viruses, it came to his attention that a chicken farmer in Hungary with advanced metastatic gastric carcinoma had undergone a complete regression of his cancer after his flock experienced an epidemic of Newcastle disease. Csatáry published his early observation in the British medical journal *Lancet* (Csatáry, 1971). In 1982, 1984, and 1985 he published study results and a general article on interference between pathogenic and non-pathogenic viruses (Csatáry et al., 1982, 1984, 1985).

Researchers in Hungary—under the direction of Sandor Eckhardt, the 1990-94 president of the International Union Against Cancer and the director of the Institute of Oncology—completed a multicenter, Phase II, double-blind, placebo-controlled clinical trial with terminal cancer patients (Csatáry et al., 1990; Moss, 1992). According to the statistical analysis in internal reports on the Phase II study, "the number of cases with stabilization or regression was significantly higher in the MTH-68/N group; favorable response in subjective parameters, such as pain relief, occurred in a significantly higher percentage in the MTH-68/N group; and performance status improved in the MTH-68/N group and significantly deteriorated in the placebo group."

Patients in Phase II received MTH-68/N by nasal drops or by inhalation (MTH-68/N is a live virus vaccine derived from the attenuated strain). The researchers say that the treatment has proved to be nontoxic and devoid of side effects. Currently, the Hungarian research team is still waiting for financial arrangements for Phase III trials.

A recently published report provides more details concerning the Phase II study (Csatáry et al., 1993). The study subjects had advanced cancers with multiple and widely distributed metastases. The duration of the protocol was 6 months, but those patients who had reacted favorably to treatment were continued on therapy. Further evaluation about survival was done after 1 and 2 years.

There were 59 patients in the study-33 in the MTH-68/N group and 26 in the placebo group. Their tumor types included lung, pancreas, kidney, sigmoid colon, and stomach cancer. In the MTH-68/N group, 2 patients experienced complete remissions, 5 experienced partial remission, 1 had moderate remission, and 10 had stabilization, for a total of 18 positive responses. Median survival time was significantly extended beyond that of the placebo group, which had only 2 stabilizations.

In addition, 26 subjects in the MTH-68/N group versus only 7 in the placebo group had either unchanged or increased weight. In the MTH-68/N group, 15 subjects had a sense of better well-being, 13 reported increased appetite, and 11 reported decreased pain; no one in the placebo group reported these effects (Csatáry et al., 1993).

Csatáry is currently negotiating with an American biotechnology company to speed development in the United States, and he has expressed willingness to have OAM conduct clinical trials of his product. He does not treat patients in the United States. Csatáry's explanation of how MTH-68 works is based on his belief that many human cancers are of viral origin.

Three possible mechanisms of antitumor action by the nonpathogenic avian viruses include direct cytolysis (cell killing), tumor-specific immune enhancement, and cytokine (see the glossary) stimulation. Thus, the avian viruses may modify tumor cells and enhance tumor-specific immunity (Schirrmacher et al., 1986). Or they may selectively kill cancer cells. Or they may stimulate a wide variety of cytokines (Csatáry, 1986, 1989), such as TNF (Lorence et al., 1988), interferons (Wheelock, 1966), and interleukins (Van Damme et al., 1989).

Neural Therapy

Neural therapy is a healing technique for attempting to deal with chronic pain and other longstanding illnesses and conditions. It involves injecting local anesthetics into autonomic ganglia (nerve cell bodies), peripheral nerves, scars, glands, acupuncture points, trigger points (points that produce a sharp pain when pressed), and other tissues and anatomical sites. Though unfamiliar to most American practitioners—and therefore part of alternative medicine neural therapy is apparently quite widely used in Europe, especially for the treatment of chronic pain. According to its advocates, such as the American Academy of Neural Therapy, this "gentle healing technique" can instantly and lastingly resolve chronic problems when correctly applied (Klinghardt, 1991).

The history of neural therapy began with the discovery of local anesthetics in the late 19th century. In 1883, the Russian physiologist Ivan Petrov (1849-1936) laid the basis for the entire field when he hypothesized that the nervous system exercises a coordinating influence over all organic functions. Before he developed psychoanalysis, Sigmund Freud (1856-1939) discovered the anesthetic effect of cocaine on mucous membranes. In 1890, abdominal surgery was first performed using a 0.2-percent solution of cocaine. In 1903, a French surgeon first employed cocaine as an epidural anesthetic.

One obvious problem with cocaine, however, was its potential to be addictive. In 1904, Alfred Einhorn discovered procaine (novocaine), still widely used in medicine. In 1906, G. Spiess observed that wounds and inflammations subsided with fewer complications if they were first injected with novocaine. In 1925, a French surgeon, Rene Leriche, used this compound for treating chronic intractable arm pain. He called novocaine "the surgeon's bloodless knife." In the same year, two German physicians described another local effect, claiming that an intravenous injection of novocaine could abolish migraine headaches (Dorman and Raven, 1991; Dosch, 1984).

A key development came in 1940, when Ferdinand Huneke discovered an instant healing reaction—what is now called the "lightning reaction" or the "Huneke phenomenon." First, Huneke injected novocaine into the shoulder joint of a woman with a severely painful, frozen right shoulder, but without any beneficial local effect. Instead, unexpectedly, the woman developed severe itching in a seemingly unrelated and relatively distant scar on her lower left leg. On a hunch, Huneke then injected novocaine into the itching scar, and within seconds the woman obtained full and painless range of motion in her right shoulder. The woman's scar dated from an operation on an infected tibia (shin bone). Although the leg operation was a "success," the woman soon afterward developed the frozen shoulder on the opposite side of her body. The initial scar had become, in neural therapy terminology, an interference field (Huneke, F., 1950; Huneke, W., 1952).

By combining the use of local anesthetics with the treatment of such (inferred) interference fields, Huneke and colleagues created an entirely new healing system they called neural therapy (Dosch, 1985). Neural therapy is said to be widely used for pain control in Europe, Russia, and Latin America and by 35 percent of all Western German physicians.

At first sight, it seems improbable that a scar on the left leg could cause a pain in the right shoulder or be resolved by an injection of local anesthetic into a scar at a site so distant from the shoulder. Dietrich Klinghardt offers several possible explanations for this phenomenon (Klinghardt, 1991), including one that he calls the "nervous system theory." Klinghardt's teacher, A. Fleckenstein, demonstrated that normal body cells and cells in scar tissue have a different electric potential across the cell membrane. In cells that have lost normal potential, the ion flux across the membrane stops (Fleckenstein, 1950). This means that toxic substances and abnormal minerals build up inside the cell. In turn, the cell becomes unable to heal itself and resume normal functioning. Treatment with local anesthetic may help restore ion flux for 1 to 2 hours, which could be enough time for the cell to partially repair itself and resume normal activity.

Another theory is that scar tissue can become, in effect, a "battery" of about 1.5 volts in the body. This scar "battery" sends forth abnormal electrical signals that disturb the autonomic nerve fibers (which lack the protective myelin coating possessed by most other nerve cells in the body). This electrical abnormality can disturb the overall autonomic nervous system, leading to systemic, and often severe, bodily dysfunction.

Also proposed is what Klinghardt calls the "fascial continuity theory." According to this theory, the fascia, or sheaths of connective tissues, are all interconnected. If scar tissue is present anywhere in this system, fascial movement can become impaired. Klinghardt claims that back pain, for instance, can sometimes be completely resolved by injecting a local anesthetic (novocaine or lidocaine without epinephrine) into a scar, such as that from an appendectomy or gallbladder operation.

In addition to its anti-pain functions, neural therapy has been used to treat allergies, chronic bowel problems, kidney disease, prostate and female urogenital problems, infertility, and tinnitus (Brand, 1983), as well as other problems (Pischinger, 1991). Klinghardt contends that although many diseases and conditions can be successfully treated by a variety of healing techniques, some conditions can be treated successfully only with neural therapy.

If it is an effective method, why is neural therapy not more widely accepted in the United States? One explanation may be that it does not lend itself to a double-blind study. According to Klinghardt, "each patient with low back pain needs to be treated in a different way." In addition, neural therapy also requires a meticulous injection technique and detailed history taking, both of which are time-consuming.

Apitherapy

Apitherapy is the medicinal use of various products of *Apis mellifera*—the common honeybee— including raw honey, pollen, royal jelly, wax, propolis (bee glue), and venom. Various studies attribute antifungal, antibacterial, anti-inflammatory, antiproliferative, and cancer-drug-potentiating properties to honey (Science News, 1993). In China, for example, raw honey is applied to burns as an antiseptic and a painkiller. Recently, propolis (the bee product that cements a hive together) has been identified as containing substances called caffeic esters that inhibit the development of precancerous changes in the colon of rats given a known carcinogen (Rao et al., 1993). Preparations from pieces of honeycomb containing pollen are reported to be successful for treating allergies, and bee pollen is touted as an excellent food. This section focuses on bee venom to treat chronic inflammatory illness because of the popularity of this treatment and the availability of related research material.

That forms of apitherapy have been used since ancient times is not remarkable, because bees formed an important part of many early economies. Ancient writers as diverse as Hesiod (ca. 800 BC), Aristophanes (ca. 450-ca. 388 BC), Varro (166-27 BC), and Columella (1st century AD) all wrote on the cultivation of the hive, and Charlemagne (742-814 AD) is said to have had himself treated with beestings. The Koran (XVI: 71) refers to bee products in the following terms: "There proceeded from their bellies a liquor wherein is a medicine for men" (Kim, 1986). For apiculture and the scientific understanding of bees, real progress began about 100 years ago when physician Phillip Terc of Austria advocated the deliberate use of beestings in his 1888 work, Report about a Peculiar Connection Between the Beestings and Rheumatism.

Today's proponents of apitherapy cite the benefits of bee venom for alleviating chronic pain and for treating many ailments including various rheumatic diseases involving inflammation and degeneration of connective tissue (e.g., several types of arthritis), neurological disease (e.g., multiple sclerosis, low back pain, migraine), and dermatological conditions (e.g., eczema, psoriasis, herpesvirus infections).

In one sample description of the use of bee venom therapy, a physician reported anecdotally that among 128 patients with a wide spectrum of illnesses, all but 11 appeared to improve (Klinghardt, 1990). (Of the 11 who did not improve, 1 was worse and 10 were unchanged.) This report is typical of anecdotal apitherapy reports that begin with stories of beekeepers recounting various health improvements after receiving accidental multiple stings from their bees. Klinghardt's patients had diagnoses of gout, rheumatoid arthritis, fibromyalgia, spinal strain or sprain, spinal disc injuries, postlaminectomy pain, bunion, postherpetic neuralgia, incomplete healing of a fractured bone, intractable pain from large burn wounds, osteoarthritis, ankylosing spondylitis, vertigo, and multiple sclerosis. Earlier, Steigerwaldt and colleagues (1966) reported improvement among 84 percent of 50 cases of arthritis in a controlled study.

In contrast, interest in bees has been sporadic in conventional medicine, focusing mainly on three areas unrelated to the therapeutic uses proposed above. These areas are (1) the danger of hypersensitivity reactions, including anaphylactic shock, from the sting of insects of the genus Apis; (2) the use of bee venom itself as immunotherapy for

Table 42.1. Analysis of Bee Venom

Component	Action	Effect on pain/painful joint
Hyaluronidase and isoenzymes	Depolymerizes hyaluronic acid (the "glue" of the body).	Allows other components of bee venom to penetrate deep into tissues, inside cells, and inside joints.
Compound X	Lowers surface tension of all fluids (surfactant).	"Wets" cell walls with bee venom, allows better penetration.
Phospholipase A (20% of venom)	Converts lecithin (from cell walls) into lyso-lecithin, which acts as emulsifier, causes hemolysis in high doses. Most toxic component of venom.	Emulsifies debris within joints and other tissues, increases local pain briefly; counterirritant.
Melittin—a major component of venom; a peptide containing 26 amino acids	Stimulates ACTH secretion in the pituitary (cortisol). Protects lysosomal membranes. Powerful antibacterial agent. Causes lysis of mast cells. Also may be membrane-active, superoxide-production-inhibiting enzyme.	Strong anti-inflammatory effect and long-acting. Short-acting histamine effects—increased capillary permeability, edema, temperature elevation, itching pain, increased vitality and sense of well-being.
Apamin—a peptide containing 18 amino acids	Stimulates central secretion of serotonin and dopamine. Blocks nerve signal crossings in periphery.	Increases central and peripheral nervous system pain threshold; decreased pain, increased sense of well-being.
Mast cell degenerating protein (also called peptide 401)	Strong anti-inflammatory action (approximately 100 times more than hydrocortisone).	Reduces inflammation and pain through local action on tissue inflammation.
Other components: Acid phosphatase, α-glucosidase, phospholipase B, several peptides	Inhibition of complement, kinines, proteases, substance P, and other effects.	Anti-inflammatory, pain reducing.

Source: Adapted from Klinghardt (1990).

allergic reaction to such stings, especially to prevent life-threatening anaphylactic reactions in adults; and (3) the danger of infants contracting botulism from ingesting raw honey—possibly one death every 2 to 5 years (Wyngaarden and Smith, 1988).

The modern movement promoting apitherapy is spearheaded by veteran beekeeper Charles Mraz of Vermont and physician Bradford Weeks of Washington State, assisted by other members of the American Apitherapy Society. They cite studies identifying various biological properties for semipurified fractions of bee venom and for more purified products to help explain the curative properties attributed to this venom. Table 42.1, adapted from Klinghardt (1990), summarizes these properties, which include pronounced anti-inflammatory, analgesic, and immunostimulatory properties.

The American Apitherapy Society contends that hypersensitivity reactions to bee venom therapy are very rare, occurring mostly from stings by related species but not by the honeybee. The procedures the society recommends include always testing a new patient first with a small amount of venom to look for possible allergic reactions and never using bee venom without an emergency beesting kit (containing epinephrine) available.

In practice, proponents say that the best results are obtained when there is a "good reaction"—considerable swelling and inflammation—at the site of sting. Mraz believes that the optimal means of delivering venom is through a hypodermic needle administered by a licensed physician. However, since most medical practitioners do not recognize the benefits of bee venom, practicing apitherapists almost always use "the original hypodermic needle developed by Mother Nature and the honeybee some 30 million years ago: the bee stinger." Procedures for obtaining and purifying venom have been developed, but of course this product in liquid or dried form costs more than using live bees.

The usual treatment involves stinging the patient at a specific site relative to the illness and repeating the stings over a period of time. For example, it is suggested that the venom be injected into arthritic patients at trigger points in a daily course of treatment that lasts 4 to 8 weeks. Proponents indicate that there are typical patterns of responsiveness, depending on the ailment. A 50-year-old patient with arthritis might note pain relief in 2 weeks, mobility in 3 weeks, and freedom from symptoms in 4 weeks (Weeks, 1994).

Research on bee venom has included studies of whole venom and venom products. For example, in the 1960s and 1970s, studies on bee venom to treat rheumatic diseases were conducted by William H. Shipman of the U.S. Navy Radiological Defense Laboratory, James

Vick of the Walter Reed Army Hospital Medical Research Center, and Gerald Weissman of New York University Hospital and their colleagues, with funding by private and public sources. One finding was that whole bee venom could suppress the development of an induced arthritis in rats, although it could not alleviate the illness after it had started (Zurier et al., 1973). Treatment with separate fractions of bee venom had no positive effect.

In later studies in which the components of bee venom were purified further, the various properties, such as anti-inflammatory and antibacterial activity (see table 42.1), began to be associated with specific materials.

In a more recent study (Kim, 1992), a randomized, controlled trial was conducted comparing true honeybee venom therapy with a "sham" product for 180 patients suffering from chronic pain and inflammation; solutions were injected twice weekly for 6 weeks. Significant posttreatment reductions in pain and inflammation were recorded in the true bee venom therapy group and were maintained at 6-month follow ups.

The American Apitherapy Society endeavors to coordinate information on bee venom research. Starting with 100 citations 12 years ago, when patients in his medical practice first interested him in the subject, Bradford Weeks, the society's president, has now acquired more than 12,000 case reports on persons treated with bee venom (Weeks, 1994). Together, these 12,000 reports are the basis for the ongoing National Multicenter Apitherapy Study. Approximately 200 physicians and 200 beekeepers voluntarily contribute reports.

At this time, the database for the multicenter study contains mostly anecdotal information, such as "I had an illness; I was stung by bees; my health improved." As Weeks notes, there is no proof in such reports that a person really had the specified illness and really improved because of the bee venom treatment.

The American Apitherapy Society would like to obtain research funds to improve the collection of both retrospective (past) information and prospective (future) data. Funding could provide research staff to search out medical records for proof of illness, training for research staff and bee venom therapists on how to gather data, and support for statistical analyses.

Meanwhile, the multicenter study has in its database some 1,300 reports on patients with multiple sclerosis (subjectively reporting increased sensation and bowel and bladder control), 2,800 with rheumatoid arthritis, and other groupings of data on such problems as gout, viral illnesses, and premenstrual syndrome—nearly 100 percent of 40 women being treated for premenstrual syndrome by apitherapy became symptom free, according to Weeks (1993).

In some ways, apitherapy is a classic alternative therapy. It has ancient roots and, although discarded by mainstream medicine, has survived in folk practice.

Iscador/mistletoe

Iscador is a liquid extract from the mistletoe plant (*Viscum album*) that has been used to treat tumors for more than 60 years (Hajto et al., 1990a). A complex mixture, iscador has two properties that are thought to make it effective against tumors. Iscador is cytostatic and sometimes cytotoxic—that is, it can stop cell growth, sometimes even killing cells. In addition, iscador has immunostimulatory properties, affecting the immune system. Two protein components of the mistletoe extracts appear to be the major active ingredients, viscotoxins and lectins (Jung et al., 1990).

The mistletoe lectins have been studied in more detail than the viscotoxins. In general, lectins are a group of sugar-containing proteins that are able to bind specifically to the branching sugar molecules of complex proteins and lipids on the surface of cells. Certain lectins have both cell-killing and immunostimulatory activity. Their toxic effect occurs because they can stop protein synthesis in cells.

Viscotoxins can kill cells but do not act on the immune system. They act by injuring cell membranes. Considering the toxic properties of both major active ingredients of mistletoe extracts, it is not surprising that mistletoe itself can be poisonous and that proponents of iscador provide cautions about how much to take.

One study examined a lectin from a proprietary mistletoe extract that has been reported to show ability to affect the immune system in rabbits (Hajto et al., 1989). When a tissue culture of certain white blood cells was exposed to this lectin, increased secretion of certain immune system products resulted, including TNF alpha and interleukins 1 and 6, which are cytokines (see the glossary). In turn, there was an increase in the number and activity of certain types of white blood cells. A corroborating increase was seen in cytokine levels in serum of patients after injection of lectin doses (Hajto et al., 1990b).

Both the cell-killing and the immunostimulatory activities of iscador could potentially affect tumor cells. Whether iscador is an appropriate treatment for cancer has been the subject of at least 46 published clinical studies (6 collective reports, 5 small historical studies, 9 large historical studies, 14 retrospective studies, 10 prospective studies, and 2 randomized studies), which were reviewed by Helmut Kiene (Kiene, 1989). None of the studies fit the format of a controlled, randomized, double-blind clinical trial. Kiene points out that such studies would be difficult to do because visible local skin irritations appear early in mistletoe treatments; thus both patient and doctor would know about the treatment.[8]

Of 36 studies that Kiene decided were evaluable, he reported that 9 showed positive, statistically significant effects against diverse cancers, including ovarian, cervical, breast, stomach (postoperative), colorectal, and bronchial cancers and liver metastases. Usually the effect was to lengthen the survival time of the patient, commonly measured as median or average survival time; in one study, a significant reduction in the use of painkillers and psychopharmaceuticals was observed (see the glossary). The reviewer noted that the effect of mistletoe therapy tended to appear in situations involving patients with advanced stages of disease rather than patients with less advanced illness.

The antitumor effects observed in these studies with people are supported by studies with animal tumors. Furthermore, except for skin irritations, few uncomfortable side effects are reported by patients. This finding contrasts with the discomforts associated with more traditional anticancer radiation treatments and chemotherapy.

Much of the previous research was conducted in Germany, and the lead organization for a new study is also based there. NCI's Physicians' Data Query index identifies this study as a Phase III randomized trial of adjuvant treatment with INFA (interferon alpha) versus INF-G (interferon gamma) versus mistletoe extract (iscador M) versus no further treatment following curative resection of high-risk stage I/IIB malignant melanoma.[9] A three-volume compendium of research papers on iscador, including translations of some from German, is available (Scharff, 1991).

Emmanuel Revici, a Romanian-born physician, is still practicing in New York City in his late nineties. (His license was suspended in November 1993, but that is being challenged.) Revici has developed an approach to illness (particularly cancers) that he calls biologically guided chemotherapy (Lerner, 1994; Revici, 1961). The basis of Revici's approach is a concept that disease involves a biological dualism. While in a healthy body anabolism and catabolism balance, in a diseased body their imbalance results in diseases that are either anabolic (see the glossary) or catabolic. Correspondingly, the way the diseased body responds to treatment differs depending on the type of imbalance. In their choices of therapies, physicians must therefore be guided by which condition predominates.

Revici ascribes the effects of tumor cells to lipid imbalances. If fatty acids predominate—a catabolic condition—the tumor tissues are described as having an electrolytic imbalance and alkaline environment. If, instead, sterols predominate—an anabolic condition—there is a reduction in cell membrane permeability, according to Revici.

The patients Revici determines to have a predominance of fatty acids are treated with sterols and other agents with positive electrical charges that can theoretically counteract the negatively charged fatty acids. If sterols are predominant, treatment is with fatty acids and other agents that can increase the metabolic activity of fatty acids. The determination of anabolic (rich in sterols) or catabolic (rich in fatty acids) character is based on a series of medical tests and judgments about body type. For example, a lean individual would be more likely to have a catabolic condition, and a rounded individual, an anabolic one; Revici also considers females more likely to have an anabolic character, and males, a catabolic one. Based on the various tests, an individualized chemotherapy program is designed for each patient with cancer. (This individualization makes it harder to conduct controlled studies of treatment effectiveness.)

Along with Revici's choice of type of lipid to administer, he may incorporate other materials, such as selenium, in his lipid envelope. According to his theory, the additional agent will be delivered ("guided") directly to the tumor site cause of the site's affinity for the selected lipid carrier. Because of this specificity, lower systemic drug toxicity is expected.

OAM has expressed interest in an evaluation of Revici's approach as a cancer treatment. Besides anecdotal reports concerning Revici's patients, one independent clinical trial was already conducted by Joseph Maisin, director of the Cancer Institute of the University of Louvain, Belgium. Although the results were never published, Maisin is reported to have written to Revici that dramatic improvements occurred in 75 percent of 12 terminal cancer patients. These improvements included tumor regression, disappearance of metastases, and cessation of hemorrhage.

Revici has applied his dualistic theory to other conditions besides cancer. He first developed therapies for different kinds of pain. Among the other conditions he is reported to have addressed are itching, insomnia, vertigo, migraine, radiation burns, osteoarthritis, rheumatoid arthritis, convulsions, postoperative bleeding, AIDS, ileitis, colitis, and drug addiction.

Future Research Opportunities

In general, alternative biological and pharmacological treatments are a rich area for investigation. At this time, further research would be helpful in the following specific approaches.

- **Antineoplastons.** These should have high priority. Antineoplastons could be investigated through best case series and patient outcome methodology.

- **Cartilage products.** Simone's offer to perform a prospective study on shark cartilage is now being followed up, aided by his receipt of IND approval from FDA in early 1994. In addition, an evaluation of bovine cartilage (Catrix) should be undertaken.

- **EDTA chelation therapy.** The study of EDTA as chelation therapy that was dropped in 1991 should be resumed. However, since it is unlikely that a sponsor can be found, as an alternative OAM should consider less costly ways of testing EDTA chelation therapy. One might be to assemble from the research of physicians currently using it a best case series of patients who have allegedly benefited from it for occlusive heart disease and related conditions. A prospective outcomes study should be undertaken as well.

- **Ozone.** The data suggest that ozone may have some effectiveness with AIDS. Whether or not that is true, ozone should be evaluated for public health reasons because of its wide use among people with AIDS. Whether ozone has any anticancer effects, either in laboratory situations or in living organisms, should also be investigated.

- **Immunoaugmentative therapy.** Because of previous lack of documentation, a best case series should be assembled from cases treated, focusing on such intractable conditions as mesothelioma. An attempt should be made to document at least 10 indisputable successes. If these cases prove valid, a prospective patient outcomes study should be undertaken with self-selecting U.S. patients who are attending the immunoaugmentative therapy clinics in either Freeport (the Bahamas) or Germany.

- **714-X.** 714-X should be investigated through best case reviews, field investigations, and, if warranted, clinical trials.

- **Hoxsey method.** The Hoxsey treatment should be investigated both because of numerous anecdotal accounts attesting to its effectiveness and because the formula contains the poisonous substance pokeweed and is therefore a public health concern. Outcomes research should be conducted on patients at the Bio-Medical Center in Tijuana to determine what results, if any, are being achieved and what side effects may occur.

- **Essiac.** Essiac is widely used throughout North America. An observational study of patients taking this medication should be arranged.

- **Coley's toxins.** These should have high priority. Investigation could be done either by reactivating the Temple University study or by sending an observation team to China (Guo Zheren, Coley Hospital, Beijing Children's Hospital, People's Republic of China) or to Germany (Dr. Klaus F. Kolmel, Gottingen, Germany). H.C. Nauts and staff members at the Cancer Research Institute have indicated an interest in helping with any evaluation.

- **MTH-68.** This should have high priority. It shows promise as an innovative, nontoxic medication for various kinds of cancer and viral diseases. A possible approach is to join with the Hungarian scientists to initiate Phase III trials of MTH-68/N-trials that are now awaiting financial arrangements.

- **Neural therapy.** The literature should be studied, and a best case series should be assembled from cases treated. An attempt should be made to document at least 10 indisputable successes. If these cases prove valid, a prospective patient outcomes study should be undertaken with self-selecting patients.

- **Apitherapy.** Because of lack of documentation, a best case series should be assembled from cases treated. An attempt should be made to document at least 10 indisputable successes for each ailment treated. If these cases prove valid, a prospective patient outcomes study should be undertaken with self-selecting patients.

- **Iscador/mistletoe.** A best case series should be assembled from cases treated. An attempt should be made to document at least 10 indisputable successes. If these cases prove valid, a prospective patient outcomes study should be undertaken with

641

self-selecting patients. The new multicenter European study should be monitored.

- **Revici's guided chemotherapy.** This should have high priority. A prospective clinical study of cancer patients should be evaluated.

Key Issues and Specific Recommendations

The following key issues and recommendations relate directly to the material in this chapter:

- Changes in regulations for FDA approval should be made if alternative pharmacological and biological treatments are to have a fair hearing.

- To prepare for innovative approaches, the director of OAM should work together with the FDA to develop a memorandum of understanding so that proposed trials that have been approved by OAM can proceed. FDA and State authorities should declare a moratorium on seizures, raids, import alerts, and licensing actions against physicians, researchers, and health care providers whose work has been chosen by OAM for evaluation. In 1992-93, the case of S.R. Burzynski was an urgent case in point (see the "Antineoplastons" section).

- In choosing specific treatments for testing, priority should be given to drugs and vaccines that address major causes of preventable death in the United States: cardiovascular disease, cancer, and AIDS. Priority should also be given to testing treatments that particularly show promise for safety and low costs. To gain public recognition and credibility, it is important that OAM achieve some clear successes.

Footnotes

1.   Prudden noted in his report that he was providing data only on the 31 patients who "took Catrix consistently and followed instructions completely." If the number of patients who stopped treatment are included (approximately another 60 patients), the recalculated response rates (approximately 30 percent responding and 20 percent complete) are still satisfactory. However, cancer therapy studies usually deal with one

type of cancer at a time, and Prudden's patients had at least nine different types.

2. Some other researchers are interested in ozone's ability to stimulate production of interferon (Bocci and Paulesu, 1991).

3. The quantity of CD4 cells, a type of white blood cell, usually decreases sharply as the condition of a patient with AIDS worsens.

4. Congressman Bedell previously had surgery and radiation treatment for prostate cancer. At public meetings and hearings, he attributes to 714-X the stopping of a recurrence of this cancer 2 years after surgery. (No medical confirmation of the recurrence has been provided publicly.)

5. Ward, P.S. 1988. History of Hoxsey Treatment (contract report for the Office of Technology Assessment).

6. For example, the Merck Manual (Berkow, 1992) indicates that "the presence of immunogenic surface structures on human neoplastic cells permits their recognition by immunocompetent host cells as well as their interaction with humoral antibodies."

7. Indeed, Patricia Ward notes in her research paper that the American Cancer Society listed Hoxsey's remedy in 1971 on its unproven methods list without citing any research basis for this listing. Coley's Toxins

8. However, such a study is not impossible. A control treatment could be used that also produced a (harmless) rash. However, as Kiene (1989) cautions, local irritants are immunostimulatory; it would be necessary to make sure that their actions were strictly local.

9. The protocol number is EORTC-DKG-80-1, and the NCI file entry was last modified in November 1993. The lead organization is the European Organization for Research on the Treatment of Cancer (EORTC) Melanoma Cooperative Group of Hamburg, Germany, with the first participant listed as UR. Kleeberg of Haematologisch-Onkologische Praxis Altona. More than 20 European centers are involved in this trial, including hospitals in Germany, Austria, Belgium, Estonia, France, and Switzerland. Revici's Guided Chemotherapy.

Chapter 43

Chelation Therapy

"If it sounds too good to be true, it probably is." That maxim may be particularly relevant when it comes to chelation therapy. Although the proponents of this treatment are true believers, they're also hungry for respectability from the medical establishment, which scoffs at the mere mention of the therapy.

For people with clogged arteries—particularly those who understandably yearn for an alternative to heart bypass surgery or angioplasty—chelation therapy, if it really works, would be nothing short of miraculous. After all, the promise of chelation therapy is that it can reverse arterial blockages, the same obstructions that can trigger heart attacks. No wonder up to 500,000 people with coronary heart disease have lined up to get this alternative treatment.

All Cleaned out?

Here's the theory behind chelation therapy: In the procedure, patients receive intravenous infusions of a chemical called EDTA (ethylenediaminetetraacetic acid), usually along with vitamins, iron supplements, and trace elements.

In the bloodstream, EDTA works something like a magnet, clutching onto metals and minerals—including calcium in atherosclerotic plaques—and excreting them from the body through the urine, As calcium is cleared from the arteries, the blood can flow more freely,

---

with the hope of relieving angina (chest pain) and intermittent claudication (discomfort in the legs related to poor circulation).

Burton Goldberg, publisher of *Alternative Medicine Digest* and author of *Alternative Medicine Guide to Heart Disease*, describes chelation therapy as "a bit like gently scrubbing the inside of approximately 60,000 miles of arteries, veins, and capillaries." That's why people are willing to put up with a little inconvenience to give chelation therapy a try.

Show Us the Evidence

The FDA has given its approval to EDTA, but not for heart disease. Instead, it has received the government's sanction for the treatment of lead poisoning—nothing else.

When it comes to atherosclerosis, the evidence just isn't there yet. "In my view, we need more research," says Isadore Rosenfeld, M.D., author of Dr Rosenfeld's *Guide to Alternative Medicine*. "I don't recommend chelation therapy to my patients because I'm not satisfied that its effectiveness has been documented."

Not surprisingly, proponents of chelation therapy disagree. In a study in the *Journal of Advancement in Medicine* (a publication of a pro-chelation association), investigators analyzed 19 chelation studies involving more than 22,000 patients and concluded that about 87 percent of them experienced "measurable improvement" with chelation therapy.

But critics insist that most of those studies haven't met rigorous scientific criteria. A 1997 review article by researchers at the Department of Complementary Medicine at England's Postgraduate Medical School in Exeter, published in the journal *Circulation*, found that the cumulative results of well-designed studies "clearly and conclusively" indicated that chelation therapy produced improvements in the disease that were no more significant than a placebo.

According to the British researchers, chelation therapy is associated with "considerable risks and costs" and "should now be considered obsolete."

A number of mainstream health organizations—including the American Heart Association (AHA), the American College of Cardiology, and the American College of Physicians—have agreed that chelation therapy is unproven. An AHA position paper states that "there have been no adequate published trials using currently approved scientific methodology to support this therapy."

646

But even some physicians who align themselves with that point of view haven't completely closed the door. "Patients in my practice claim to have benefited from it," says Dr. Rosenfeld. "These are patients with angina or with peripheral vascular disease who have refused conventional surgical intervention, have opted to go with chelation therapy, and say they feel better."

However, he adds, "when I've looked for that improvement, either with a treadmill, test or an angiogram, hoping to find physical changes in the involved blood vessels, I haven't been able to document it. Even so, I think there are enough people taking it, and enough doctors doing it, to warrant further research. I don't think we ought to abandon it."

Meanwhile, some pro-chelation doctors insist that their patients have enjoyed other benefits, including preventing and treating Alzheimer's disease, cancer, diabetes complications, thyroid problems, psoriasis, and multiple sclerosis.

What to Expect

Each intravenous treatment lasts from 90 minutes to three hours, and doctors, may recommend at least three infusions per week. In a typical course of therapy, patients receive a total of 30 to 50 treatments, at a cost totaling $3,000 to $4,000.

Choosing a Practitioner

Some cardiologists do practice chelation therapy, despite the thumbs-down positions of the cardiology and heart associations. You'll need to take it upon yourself to check the person's credentials and experience. Also, contact the American Board of Chelation Therapy for a referral.

Safety Concerns

Until more research is conducted, Dr. Rosenfeld advises sticking with traditional therapies, which could save your life. But if you aren't a candidate for treatments, such as heart bypass surgery or angioplasty, then chelation therapy can be considered.

Even though current doses of EDTA are lower than they once were, concerns remain about side effects that have been reported in the, past, from headaches and nausea to rarer but still worrisome problems such as kidney damage, heart arrhythmias, anemia, blood clots, and bone marrow impairment.

Critics of chelation therapy point out that calcium is only one of many substances that make up plaques so that even though EDTA may escort calcium, out of the body, this process won't make much of a dent in the coronary blockages.

Here's another factor to consider. According to Dr. Rosenfeld, one fear is that the calcium devoured by chelation therapy may come, more from the bones than the arterial plaques. If that's true, the tradeoff for the hope of clearer arteries may be thinner bones, osteoporosis, and hip fractures—not exactly a small price to pay for an unproven therapy.

For More Information.

American Board of Chelation Therapy
1407-B N. Wells Street
Chicago, IL 60610
(312) 266-4639

American College for Advancement in Medicine
2321 Verdugo Drive
Suite 204
Laguna Hills, CA 92653
(714) 583-7666

American Heart Association
7272 Greenville Avenue
Dallas, TX 75231-4596
(800) 242-8721

Part Nine

Additional Help and Information

Chapter 44

Glossary

adiposity: the state of being fat.

adjustment: the chiropractic adjustment is a specific form of direct manipulation of joint (articular) areas, using either long or short leverage techniques with specific contacts. It is characterized by a dynamic thrust of controlled velocity, amplitude, and direction (see thrust). Colloquially referred to as "bone cracking."

adrenergic: activated by, characteristic of, or secreting adrenaline (scientific name, epinephrine) or similar substances that constrict blood vessels and raise blood pressure, preparing the body for "fight or flight."

adrenochrome: a red oxidation product of epinephrine that slows the blood flow because of its effect on capillary permeability. It is currently being tested as a psychomimetic drug (a drug that imitates natural substances that can affect a person psychologically).

allergic rhinitis: hay fever; significant nasal drainage and inflammation of the eyes in susceptible subjects, caused by inhaling allergens (usually pollens).

allopathy substitutive therapy: a therapeutic system in which a disease is treated by producing a second condition that is incompatible

Extracted from NIH Publication No. 94-066. December 1994.

651

with or antagonistic to the first. May be used to describe Western medicine as currently practiced.

amide: an organic compound in which the hydroxyl (-OH) of a carboxyl group (-COOH) of an acid has been replaced by the nitrogen-containing group -NH2. For example, O=C-NH2.

amine: an organic compound containing nitrogen, equivalent to replacing one or more atoms of hydrogen in ammonia by an organic hydrocarbon. For example, -NH2.

amyotrophic lateral sclerosis: a disease marked by progressive degeneration of the nerve cells that conduct electrical impulses, leading to degeneration of the motor cells of the brain stem and spinal cord and resulting in a deficit of motor skills among other symptoms; it usually ends fatally within 2 to 3 years. Also called Lou Gehrig's disease.

anabolism: constructive metabolic processes in which new substances are built.

anaphylaxis: a major type of allergic reaction to a substance, resulting in difficulty breathing and followed usually by shock and collapse of the blood system.

angina pectoris: a spasm with sudden chest pain, accompanied by a feeling of suffocation and impending death, most often due to lack of oxygen to part of the heart wall, and caused by excitement or activity.

angiography: the study of the cardiovascular system (heart and blood) by radioscopy after the introduction of a contrasting material, such as radioactive iodine, into the body.

anthropology: the study of human beings and their origin in relation to social, cultural, historical, environmental, and developmental aspects.

antioxidant: A compound that prevents oxidation of substances, particularly lipids, in food or in the body. Antioxidants are especially important in preventing the oxidation of polyunsaturated lipids in the membranes of cells. An antioxidant is able to donate electrons to electron-seeking compounds such as free radicals (see below). This in turn reduces electron capture and, thus, breakdown of unsaturated fatty acids and other cell components by oxidizing agents.

antipsychotic drug: a substance effective in the treatment of psychosis, a severe type of mental disorder involving total disorganization of the personality.

apoenzyme: the protein portion of an enzyme that can be separated from any cofactor but needs the cofactor present to function properly as an enzyme.

arrhythmia: any variation from the normal rhythm of the heartbeat.

ascorbyl palmitate: a derivative of vitamin C that is being tested as a preventive agent.

atherosclerosis: A buildup of fatty material in the arteries, including those in the heart.

autism: a condition characterized by preoccupation with inner thoughts, daydreams, fantasies, delusions, and hallucinations; egocentric, subjective thinking lacking objectivity and connection with reality; a disorder of currently unknown origin characterized by such activities.

benzopyrene: a highly carcinogenic organic chemical that is produced when carbon compounds are incompletely burned.

bind: an increasing resistance to motion in the problem area (in manual therapy the practitioner uses feedback obtained by touching the problem area to guide the medical procedure). See also ease.

bioelectromagnetics: the scientific study of interactions between living organisms and electromagnetic fields, forces, energies, currents, and charges. The range of interactions studied includes atomic, molecular, intracellular up to the entire organism.

biofeedback: the process of furnishing an individual with information, usually in an auditory or visual mode, on the state of one or more physiological variables such as heart rate, blood pressure, or skin temperature; it often enables the individual to gain some voluntary control over the physiological variable being sampled.

biofield: a massless field (not necessarily electromagnetic) that surrounds and permeates living bodies and affects the body. Possibly related to qi. See qi.

bioflavonoid: a generic term for a group of anti-oxidant compounds that are widely distributed in plants and involved in animals in maintaining the walls of small blood vessels in a normal state. See flavenoids.

biogenesis: Thomas Huxley's theory that living matter always arises by the agency of preexisting living matter. The opposing theory is spontaneous generation.

biomechanics: the study of structural, functional, and mechanical aspects of human motion.

biophoton: a small amount of electromagnetic energy emitted by molecules in living organisms. Biophoton emission is associated with processes, such as mitosis (cell division), and possibly with the vibrations of certain large molecules; It may also be used to communicate information over relatively large distances, as the firefly does.

biorhythm: the cyclic occurrence of body processes, such as in daily, or circadian, rhythm. Other rhythms may be monthly or yearly.

biostatistics: the science of applying statistics in biology, medicine, and agriculture.

botanical medicine: another term for herbal medicine.

carbohydrate: A compound containing carbon, hydrogen, and oxygen atoms: most are known as sugars, starches, and dietary fiber.

cardiac catheterization: the passage of a small fluid-gathering tube through a vein in the body into the heart to gather blood samples, to measure internal blood pressure, or to obtain other intra-cardiac information.

catabolism: destructive metabolic processes in which substances are broken down.

catecholamine: chemical messengers, such as dopamine and norepinephrine, that stimulate various receptors in the sympathetic and central nervous systems in the body.

catechu: an extract from the heartwood of the Asian catechu tree that contains catechin, a crystalline, contraction-causing chemical. Formerly used as an antidiarrheal agent.

cell proliferation: growth by the reproduction of similar cells.

cellular metabolism: the sum of the chemical processes of a cell, including the transformation of sugars into energy and related processes.

cervical dysplasia: deviations in the cells that cover the uterine cervix, which may begin as unusual increased cell growth and progress to the loss of the unique characteristics of a cell; tends to lead to a tumor.

chakra: one of the areas of rotation in the biofield, first elaborated in ancient Indian metaphysics.

chelation: formation of a complex molecule involving a metal ion and two or more polar groupings of a single molecule. Chelation can be used to remove an ion from participation in biological reactions, causing a change in the reaction.

chemopreventive: the attempt to prevent disease through the use of chemicals, drugs, or food factors, such as vitamins.

chemotherapy: treatment of disease by chemical compounds selectively directed against invading organisms or abnormal cells.

chiropractic science: the investigation of the relationship between structure (primarily of the spine) and function (primarily of the nervous system) in the human body.

chiropractic practice: a discipline of the scientific healing arts concerned with the development, diagnosis, treatment, and preventive care of functional disturbances, disease states, pain syndromes, and neurophysiological effects related to the status and dynamics of the locomotor system, especially of the spine and pelvis.

cholecystectomy: surgical removal of the gall bladder.

chronic hepatitis: a persistent inflammation of the liver.

chronic fatigue syndrome: an illness characterized by long periods of fatigue, often accompanied by headaches, muscle pain and weakness, and elevated antibody titers to some herpes viruses. The cause or causes are unknown.

circadian: a phenomenon being, having, characterized by, or occurring in approximately 24-hour periods or cycles (as of biological activity or function).

clairsentience: the ability to use touch to sense subtle variations in the biofield.

clairvoyance: the ability to perceive things that are out of the range of normal human senses.

closed system: a field or system that does not react with other fields or anything outside that system.

cochlear reflex: a contraction of the cochlea—a spirally wound tube that forms part of the inner ear—when a sharp, sudden noise is made near the ear.

cofactor: a non-protein chemical that is not an enzyme in its own right but must be present for an apoenzyme (i.e., the protein component of the enzyme) to function.

collagen: an insoluble, fibrous protein that occurs in bones as the major portion of the connective tissue fibers. Yields gelatin and glue on prolonged heating with water.

complementary medicine: another term for alternative medicine; frequently used in Europe.

congenital: something that exists at, and usually before, birth.

corpus callosum: the mass of white matter in the brain that connects the two hemispheres, linking the "creative" (or left-brained) side with the "raw intelligence" (or right-brained) side.

coumarin: an odorous material found in tonquin beans, sweet clover, and woodruff; used for scenting tobacco and as an anticoagulant to prevent excessive blood clotting.

cryosurgery: the application of extreme cold to destroy tissue.

cyclotron resonance: the resonant coupling of electromagnetic power into a system of charged particles undergoing orbital movement in a uniform magnetic field.

cytokine: a generic term for various small proteins that are released by cells and that act as intercellular communicators to elicit an immune response. Examples include the interferons and the interleukins.

cytokinesis: the contraction of a belt of cytoplasm, bringing about the separation of two daughter cells during cell division in animal tissues.

cytotoxicity: the degree to which a chemical is toxic, or lethal, to a cell, such as how toxic a chemotherapy agent may be to cancer cells.

Delphi method: a consensus procedure in which participating experts are polled individually and anonymously, usually with self-administered questionnaires. The survey is conducted over a series of "rounds." After each round, the results are elicited, tabulated, and reported to the group. The Delphi process is considered complete when there is convergence of opinion or when a point of diminishing return is reached.

diabetes mellitus: a disorder of metabolism in which the lack of available insulin causes an excess of sugar in the blood and urine, as well as excessive thirst and loss of weight. Various long-term problems can result.

diagnosis: the art of distinguishing one disease from another; the use of scientific and skillful methods to establish the cause and nature of a person's illness.

diet: All of the foods a person consumes either on a daily basis or on average over a period of time.

dietetics: the study and regulation of the diet.

direct technique: any manual medical method or maneuver that engages and passes through and beyond an area of increasing tissue or joint motion resistance, commonly called a "direct barrier." (Physical penetration of the body surface is not involved.).

dosimetry: the process of measuring doses of radiation (e.g., x rays).

double-blind: a term pertaining to a clinical trial or other experiment in which neither the subject nor the person administering treatment knows which subjects are receiving actual treatment and which are receiving a placebo.

dysfunction: a term used in medicine to describe abnormal, impaired, or incomplete functioning of an organ or part.

dysmenorrhea: a condition characterized by difficult and painful menstruation.

ease: a region of decreasing resistance to movement. In manual therapy the practitioner uses feedback obtained by touching the problem region to guide the medical procedure. See bind.

echocardiography: a method of graphically recording the position and motion of the heart walls or the internal structures of the heart and neighboring tissue by the echo obtained from beams of ultrasonic waves directed through the chest wall.

eczema: an inflammatory skin condition characterized by itching and the secretion of liquids from subdermal pockets of pus and water.

electroencephalogram (EEG): a recording of the electrical potentials on the skull generated by currents emanating spontaneously from nerve cells in the brain.

electromagnetic field: the force or energy associated with electromagnetic interactions, charges, and currents. EM fields include electrostatic, magnetostatic, radiation, induction, vector-potential, and scalar-potential fields, and Hertz and Fitzgerald potentials. The EM field is usually said to comprise two components: an "electric field" and a "magnetic field." However, according to apparently well-established theorems (e.g., Maxwell's equations), these two components are closely coupled and not truly independent of each other.

electromagnetic radiation: one type of EM field, namely, an oscillating EM field that has free motion in space at a distance from its source.

electromagnetism: the magnetism produced by an electric current.

electrophysiology: the study of the mechanisms and consequences of the production of electrical phenomena in the living organism.

electropollution: EM fields produced by sources that may have harmful effects on humans, such as electric power transmission and radio transmission.

electrosurgical excision: surgical removal of an organ or tissue by electrical methods.

embolism: the blocking of a blood vessel, usually by a blood clot or thrombus originating from a remote part of the circulatory system.

emission tomography: a computer-constructed image of the body, created by measuring radioactive presences in the body.

end play: discrete, short-range movements of a joint, independent of the action of voluntary muscles, determined by springing each vertebra or extremity joint at the limit of its passive range of motion; also called "joint play."

endocrine: a material that is secreted internally in the body, most commonly through the bloodstream rather than through the various ducts; of or pertaining to such a secretion.

endorphin: any of three compounds found naturally in the brain that may have adrenaline-like effects, such as a burst of energy or an analgesic effect.

endoscopy: visual inspection of any cavity of the body by means of an endoscope (an instrument to examine the interior of a hollow cavity inside the body, such as the bladder).

enzymes: proteins that catalyze many biochemical reactions, necessary in all life forms. A compound, usually a protein, that speeds the rate of a chemical reaction but is not altered by the chemical reaction.

epidemiology: the medical study of the incidence, distribution, and control of disease in a population; the conditions controlling the presence or absence of a disease or pathogen.

esophageal motility: the muscular movements of the esophagus, the tube that carries food from the mouth to the stomach. Orderly and rhythmic esophageal motility is necessary for swallowing; any disorder in this process may result in pain and dysfunction.

ethnobotany: the science of plants in relation to ethnic groups of humans.

etiology: the medical study of causes of disease.

faith healing: healing that occurs because of the patient's belief in a supernatural being or the healer.

fascia: a sheet of fibrous tissue that envelops the body beneath the skin; it also encloses muscles and groups of muscles, and separates their several layers or groups.

fatty acid: A principal component of fats and oils. A fatty acid is composed of a chain of carbon and hydrogen atoms with an acid group at one end. Examples include stearic acid (a saturated fatty acid), oleic acid, monounsaturated fatty acid, and linoleic acid (a polyunsaturated fatty acid).

fibromyalgia: a poorly understood illness characterized by fibrous muscular pain.

fibrositis: an inflammation of fibrous tissue.

flavonoids: a large group of metabolic byproducts of mosses and other plants, based on 2-phenylbenzopyran (a particular type of organic compound with a ring structure); for example, the chemicals that give yellow, red, and blue colors to plants.

forensic: evidence or material gathered for or used in legal proceedings or in public debate.

free radical: a molecule or atom in which the outermost ring of electrons is not complete, making it extremely chemically reactive.

Short-lived form of compounds with an unpaired electron in the outer electron shell. Because free radicals have an electron-seeking nature, they can be very destructive to electron-dense areas of cells, such as DNA and cell membranes.

galvanic skin response: a change in the electrical resistance of the skin, recorded by a polygraph; widely used as an index of autonomic (involuntary) nervous system reactions.

gastroenteritis: an inflammation of the mucous membrane of the stomach and the intestines.

gauss: a unit of magnetic flux density. In colloquial terms, the strength of a magnetic field is specified in terms of gauss; for instance, the strength of a typical household magnet that holds papers on a refrigerator is about 200 G.

glycyrrhetinic acid: a derivative of vitamin A that is being tested for its disease preventive activity.

Hawthorne effect: the observation that experimental subjects who are aware that they are part of an experiment often perform better than totally naive subjects.

heavy metal: a metal of high atomic number; may be used to measure electron density in electron microscopy; high concentrations of heavy metals can harm plant and animal growth.

hematology: the medical specialty that pertains to the anatomy, physiology, pathology, symptomatology, and therapeutics of blood and blood-forming tissues.

Hertz (Hz): the unit of measure used to specify the frequency of complete waves of electromagnetic radiation, such as light, radio waves, and x rays; expressed as cycles per second. These waves take on the property of a sinusoid (see sinusoidal). Table 14.1 in the "Bioelectromagnetics Applications in Medicine" chapter shows the electromagnetic spectrum ranging from 0 Hz to over 10^{20} Hz.

heuristic: anything that encourages or promotes investigation; that which is conducive to discovery.

high sense perception: a system of diagnosis based on clairsentience and clairvoyance.

hippocampus: a particular part of the gray matter of the brain; in humans, it extends from the olfactory lobe to the posterior end of the cerebrum.

homeopathy: an alternative medical system that treats the symptoms of a disease with minute doses of a chemical. In larger doses, the compound would produce the same symptoms as the disease or disorder that is being treated.

homeostasis: the maintenance of a static, constant, or balanced condition in the body's internal environment; the level of physiological well-being of an individual.

humoralism, humorism: an ancient theory that health and illness are related to a balance or imbalance of body fluids or "humors."

hydrocortisone: a complex chemical secreted by the human adrenal cortex which has life-maintaining properties and is important to sustaining blood pressure and the balance of fluids and electrolytes in the body.

hydrotherapy: treating a disease with water, externally or internally.

hypercholesterolemia: an excess of cholesterol in the blood.

hyperlipidemia: an excess of lipids (fatty components, such as cholesterol or triglycerides) in the blood.

hypertension: a persistent state of high arterial high blood pressure.

hypothalamic-pituitary-adrenocortical axis: the interaction involving chemical and neuronal signals between the hippocampus, pituitary gland, and the cortex (outer layer) of the adrenal glands, with significant impact on the body's state of health.

iatrogenic: an illness, injury, disease, or disorder induced inadvertently by physicians or their treatments.

662

ichthyosis: a group of skin disorders characterized by increased or aberrant development of keratin, resulting in noninflammatory scaling of the skin.

immunocompromising: anything that interferes with the healthy function of the immune system.

impedance: the state of resistance in electrical circuits.

incontinence: the inability to control one or both excretory functions (i.e., defecation and urination).

indirect technique: any manual medical method or maneuver that engages and passes through and beyond an area of decreasing resistance, commonly called an "indirect barrier." (Physical penetration of the body surface is not involved.).

indole: a type of nitrogen-containing organic compound with a double ring structure; a breakdown product of the amino acid tryptophan and related biologically active compounds.

infrasonic energy: energy waves transmitted at a frequency lower than the frequency at which humans are normally aware of sound.

innate intelligence: the intrinsic biological ability of a healthy organism to react physiologically to the changing conditions of the external and internal environment.

innate: something that inborn or hereditary.

interferon: one of a group of small immune system stimulating proteins produced by viral-infected cells or by noninfected white blood cells; it is used as an anticancer agent in some clinical trials because of its ability to inhibit further viral replication.

interleukin: one of a group of small proteins that are involved in communication among white blood cells and that activate and enhance the immune system's disease-fighting abilities.

internal validity: the certainty that the treatment or regimen under study, rather than something else, is responsible for producing study results.

irritable bowel (spastic colon) syndrome: a condition characterized by sudden, involuntary contractions of the colon.

ki: the Japanese term for qi.

kinesthetic senses: the senses by which movement, weight, and position are perceived; commonly used to refer specifically to the perception of changes in the angles of pints.

L-dopa: the naturally occurring form of the amino acid dopa, which is a precursor of epinephrine and other biologically active compounds. It is used in the treatment of Parkinson's disease.

leukocytes: a group of blood cells that have a nucleus but lack hemoglobin and that are involved in fighting disease; also known as "white blood cells.".

limbus: a general term for describing border structures, such as the limbic region of the brain.

lipid: A compound containing an abundance of carbon and hydrogen, little oxygen, and sometimes other atoms. Lipids include fats, oils, and cholesterol.

lipids: a generic term for organic compounds based on fatty acids, such as fats, waxes, fat-soluble vitamins, and steroids.

lipoprotein: A compound found in the bloodstream containing a core of lipids with a shell of protein, phospholipid, and cholesterol.

local healing: biofield healing that uses the practitioner's hands on the subject's body.

lymph: a clear, transparent, or yellowish-opaque liquid found in the vessels of the lymphatic system; this liquid returns proteins and other substances from tissues to the blood.

lymphatic system: the system of the lymph, including the lymph nodes, and the vascular channels that transport lymph.

lymphocyte: a white blood cell formed in lymphatic tissue, in normal adults, lymphocytes comprise approximately one-quarter of the white blood cells.

macronutrients: Compounds, such as fats, proteins, and carbohy-drates, that must be broken down or metabolized by the body to ob-tain energy or basic building material.

macrophage: a class of white blood cells, found in tissues, that are scavengers. Macrophage can wander the system or migrate to points of infection in the body.

magnetic resonance imaging: the use of nuclear magnetic reso-nance of protons to produce proton density maps or images of tissues or organs in the human body.

magnetite: a spinel (metal oxide) of iron (Fe_3O_4); a naturally occur-ring magnet.

manipulation: a term used in connection with the therapeutic ap-plication of manual force. Spinal manipulation, broadly defined, in-cludes all procedures in which the hands are used to mobilize, adjust, manipulate, apply traction, massage, stimulate, or otherwise influ-ence the spine and nearby (paraspinal) tissues with the goal of posi-tively influencing the patient's health.

materia medica: a collection of descriptions of products that are usable medically as drugs. In homeopathy, substances are included that may not be in the official pharmacopoeia (drug registry), as are descriptions of how to physically prepare the substances as drugs.

mental healing: a process whereby one individual endeavors to bring about the healing of another by using conscious intent, without the intervention of any known physical means. The term is often used synonymously with spiritual healing.

meridian: In Asian traditional medicine, the body has a channel with 12 portions, or meridians, which loop through the body in an endless circuit, connecting the principal organs and other body parts. The meridians are said to carry ching qi, which regulates the relationship between, and the functioning of, the various body structures.

meta-analysis: a method for combining the results of several or many studies to see if the combined results provide significant information that was not obtainable by examining individual studies.

metabolism: the sum total of the chemical and physical changes constantly occurring in a living body.

metaphysics: the branch of philosophy that systematically investigates first causes and the ultimate nature of the universe. Such investigations are generally of insubstantial elements and are outside physics, thus difficult to measure.

metastasis: the movement of cancerous cells in the body from a primary site to a distant site, usually through the blood or lymph system, with the subsequent development of secondary cancers.

micronutrients: Minerals and vitamins that are required for proper functioning of the body. These often act as cofactors or coenzymes in enzymatic processes.

mobilization: the process of making a fixed part movable; a form of manipulation characterized by nonthrust, passive joint manipulation.

modulation: the change of amplitude or frequency of a carrier signal of given frequency.

molecular biology: the study of the structure and function of macromolecule in living cells.

morbidity: the state or condition of being diseased, for an individual or community.

mortality: the death rate within a given population.

motion palpation: a term used in connection with using touch to diagnose passive and active segmental joint ranges of motion.

motor hand: the hand the practitioner uses to induce passive movement in the subject. See bind.

mucosal: a term for cells of or pertaining to the mucous membrane, a tissue layer that lines various tubular cavities of the body, such as the viscera, uterus, and trachea.

multivariate analysis or multivariate statistical treatment: a method of statistical analysis that employs several measurements of various characteristics on each unit of observation.

musculoskeletal manipulation: a hands-on procedure to physically correct or reset abnormalities of joint muscle and connective tissue function.

mutagenic: an agent that causes change or induces genetic mutation in the DNA of cells.

myocardial infarction: a sudden shortage of arterial or venous blood supply to the heart due to blockage or pressure; it may produce a sizable area of dead cells in the heart.

myofascial: of or relating to the sheets of fibrous tissue (that is, fasciae) that surround and separate muscle tissue.

necrosis: death of cells or groups of cells in a living body.

neurodegenerative disease: a disease that involves deterioration in the function and form of nerves and related structures. Alzheimer's disease and multiple sclerosis are examples.

neuropeptide: a small chain of linked amino acids with neurological activity.

neurotransmitter: a chemical messenger used by nerves.

neutrophil: a granular white blood cell having a nucleus with three to five lobes connected by slender threads of chromatin and cytoplasm containing fine, inconspicuous granules.

nocebo: effects a toxic or negative placebo event.

noetic: a thought process based on pure intellect or reasoning ability, (e.g., a noetic doctrine).

noninvasive: not involving physical penetration of the skin (e.g., a noninvasive diagnostic or therapeutic technique).

nonlocal: something that occurs at a distance; in physics a nonlocal effect is a form of influence that is unmediated, unmitigated, and immediate. Nonlocal healing is healing that occurs at a distance.

nutrients: Chemical substances in food that nourish the body by providing energy, building materials, and factors to regulate needed chemical reactions in the body.

nutrition: The biological science of nutrition includes the processes by which the organism ingests, digests, absorbs, transports, metabolizes, and excretes food substances. Nutrition as a science and discipline also includes areas such as food policy, dietary behaviors, agricultural practices, cultural and anthropological aspects of food, etc.

oncology: the study of all aspects of cancer.

open system: a system that interacts with other fields or systems, giving off or receiving energy or materials. The opposite is a closed system.

orthomolecular medicine: a system of medicine aimed at restoring the optimal concentrations and functions at the molecular level of certain substances normally present in the body, such as vitamins.

osteopathic: a system of therapy that emphasizes normal body mechanics and manipulation to correct faulty body structures.

otitis media: inflammation of the middle ear.

oxidation: the addition of oxygen to a compound or the removal of electrons from a compound.

p-value: the probability that the observed outcome of a particular experiment is due to random chance. Also known as uncertainty level.

Paleolithic: of or belonging to the period of human culture beginning with the earliest chipped stone tools, about 750,000 years ago, until the beginning of the Mesolithic period, about 15,000 years ago.

palpation: the physical examination of the body using touch.

paradigm: an explanatory model, especially one of outstanding clarity; a typical example or archetype.

parapsychology: the field of study concerned with the investigation of evidence for paranormal psychological phenomena, such as telepathy, clairvoyance, and psychological phenomena, such as psychokinesis.

pathogen: any disease-producing microorganism or substance.

pathogenesis: the cellular events and reactions and other pathologic mechanisms occurring in the development of disease.

pathology: the medical study of the causes and nature of disease and the body changes wrought by disease.

pellagra: a clinical syndrome due to deficiency of niacin, characterized by inflammation of the skin and mucous membrane, diarrhea, and psychic disturbances.

peptide: any of various amides that are derived from two or more amino acids when the amino group of one acid is combined with the carboxyl group of another; peptides are usually obtained by partial breakdown of proteins.

peroxidation: the process by which enzymes activate hydrogen peroxide and induce reactions that hydrogen peroxide alone would not effect.

person-years: a unit of time used in various statistical measurements of the aggregate effects of agents or events on people, as in epidemiology.

phagocyte: a cell (e.g., a white blood cell) that characteristically engulfs foreign material and consumes debris and foreign bodies.

pharmacology: the science that deals with the origin, nature, chemistry, effects, and uses of drugs.

pharmacopeia: a book describing drugs, chemicals, and medical preparations, especially one issued by an officially recognized authority and serving as a standard for the preparation and form of drugs; a collection or stock of drugs.

phenomenology: the study of phenomena; in psychiatry, it is the theory that behavior is determined by the way the person perceives reality rather than by external reality.

physics, classical: the branch of physics that studies mechanics and electromagnetism. It includes kinetics, optics, hydraulics, aerodynamics, and astrophysics.

physics, quantum: the branch of physics that deals with atomic and subatomic particles.

placebo: an inert substance that is given to the control group of patients in a blinded trial. A placebo is used to distinguish between the actual benefits of the medication and the benefits the patients think they are receiving.

platelet: a disk-shaped structure found in the blood of all mammals, chiefly known for its role in blood coagulation.

plethysmography: the recording of the changes in size when an organ or other structure is modified by the circulation of blood through it.

polarity: the differences between portions of a biofield, similar to the polarity or directionality of magnet fields; a form of manual healing that incorporates this feature.

positron emission tomography: a form of diagnostic imaging that makes use of the electromagnetic energy transitions of "excited" molecules to indicate changes in the function of tissues under investigation.

postoperative: something that occurs after a surgical operation.

potentized: in homeopathic pharmacy, a substance that is prepared by dilution while the diluting fluid is being agitated in a standard fashion; widely believed by practitioners to impart additional medical value to higher dilutions.

propranolol: a chemical that decreases heart rate and output, reduces blood pressure, and is effective in the preventive treatment of migraine.

proprioceptive: stimuli produced by movement in body tissues. Proprioceptive nerves are the sensory nerves in muscles and tendons that detect such movements.

prospective studies: Studies in which subjects are enrolled prior to their having developed the endpoint (i.e., condition or disease) of interest, and they are often followed until they develop such endpoints. Examples of prospective studies include clinical trials, in which some study subjects are given an investigator-imposed intervention, and cohort or panel studies, which usually do not include investigator-imposed intervention.

psoriasis: a chronic disease of the skin in which red scaly papules and patches appear, especially on the outer aspects of the limbs.

psychic healing: a term for biofield and mental healing, used especially in England.

psychogenic: anything that is produced or caused by psychic or mental factors rather than by organic factors.

psychoneuroimmunology: the study of the roles that the mind and nervous system play in various phenomena of immunity, induced sensitivity, and allergy.

psychopathology: the medical study of the causes and nature of mental disease.

psychosomatic medicine: the branch of medicine that stresses the relationship of bodily and mental happenings, and combines physical and psychological techniques of investigation.

pulmonary: anything pertaining to the lungs.

qi (chi, ki): in Eastern philosophies, the energy that connects and animates everything in the universe; includes both individual qi (personal life force) and universal qi, which are coextensive through the practice of mind-body disciplines, such as traditional meditation, aikido, and tai chi.

qigong (qi gong): the art and science of using breath, movement, and meditation to cleanse, strengthen, and circulate the blood and vital life energy.

quantum domain: the atomic and subatomic dimension dealt with in the science of quantum physics.

Raynaud's disease/phenomenon: a disorder characterized by intermittent, bilateral attacks in which a restriction of blood flow occurs in the fingers or toes and sometimes the ears or nose. Severe paleness, a burning sensation, and pain may be brought on by cold or emotional stimulation; these symptoms sometimes are relieved by heat. The condition is due to an underlying disease or anatomical abnormality.

reduction: any chemical process in which an electron is added to an atom or an ion, or an oxygen is removed. The opposite process is oxidation.

retrospective studies: Studies undertaken to determine whether those with and without a particular disease or condition differ according to past exposures. Examples of such studies include case-control studies and retrospective cohort studies.

rheumatoid arthritis: a chronic inflammation of the joints, which may be accompanied by systemic disturbances such as fever, anemia, and enlargement of lymph nodes.

sacrum: the part of the vertebral column (backbones) that is directly connected with or forms a part of the pelvis; in humans it consists of five united vertebrae.

secretory immunoglobulin A (IgA): the predominant immune system protein in body secretions such as oral, nasal, bronchial urogenital, and intestinal mucous secretions as well as in tears, saliva, and breast milk.

sensing hand: the hand used by the practitioner in manual therapy to detect changes (see bind); the sensing hand is used to assess the subject's increasing and decreasing resistance to the passive motion demands of the practitioner's motor or operating hand.

serial t- or z- tests: various types of statistical measurements that are used to determine whether data have significance.

serotonin: a naturally occurring body chemical that can cause blood vessels to contract; it is found in various animals, bacteria, and many plants. Serotonin acts as a central neurotransmitter and is thought to be involved in mood and behavior.

short leg: an anatomical, pathological, or functional leg deficiency leading to dysfunction.

sinusitis: the inflammation of any of the air-containing cavities of the skull, which communicate with the nose.

sinusoidal: of, relating to, shaped like, or varying according to a sine curve or sine wave, which is a waveform of single frequency and infinite repetition in relation to time.

sleep latency: the interval before sleep.

sociogenic: anything arising from or imposed by society.

somatic dysfunction: impaired or altered function of related components of the somatic system (the skeleton, joints, and muscles; the structures surrounding them; and the related circulatory and nerve elements).

somatic: pertaining to or characteristic of the body; distinct from the mind.

spiritual energy: energy that comes from a supernatural being or the cosmos.

structural diagnosis (osteopathic): an osteopathic physician's use of hands and eyes to evaluate the somatic system, relating the diagnosis of somatic dysfunction to the state of a patient's total well-being, according to osteopathic philosophy and principles.

subatomic: something pertaining to the constituent parts of an atom.

subluxation: a situation in which two adjacent structures involved in joints have an aberrant relationship, such as a partial dislocation, that can cause problems either in these and related joints or in other body systems that are directly or indirectly affected by them.

symptomatology: the study of symptoms.

syndrome: the signs and symptoms associated with a particular disease or disorder.

synergistic: entities working together or cooperating to produce a positive effect greater than the sum of the contributing individual entities.

systemic review: a method of analyzing a group of scientific studies that may individually be weak, producing results with more significance than the individual studies may have.

theosophy: a doctrine concerning a deity, the cosmos, and the self that relies on mystical insights by unusually perceptive individuals; it teaches that its practitioners can master nature and guide their own destinies.

thromboembolism: an obstruction of a blood vessel with clotting material carried by the bloodstream from the site of origin to plug another vessel.

thrombus: an aggregation of blood factors that creates an obstruction; more severe than a clot.

thrust: the sudden manual application of a controlled directional force on a suitable part of the patient's body, the delivery of which effects an adjustment (see adjustment).

transcranial electrostimulation: a method of clinical treatment involving electrical stimulation of the brain through the skull.

transcutaneous electrical nerve stimulation: a clinical treatment modality involving electrical stimulation of nerves through the skin.

trigger points: specific points in the muscular and fascial tissues that produce a sharp pain when pressed; may also correspond to certain types of traditional acupuncture points.

triplet states: a state in which there are two unpaired electrons.

turnover: the movement of a substance into, through, and out of a place; the rate at which a material is depleted and replaced.

vascular system: the system formed by the blood vessels.

visceral: pertaining to the soft interior organs in the cavities of the body.

Chapter 45

Additional Resources

Advocacy and Patient Support Groups

Whether looking for an alternative therapy or checking the legitimacy of something you've heard about, some of the best sources are advocacy groups, including local patient support groups. These groups include:

American Cancer Society
1599 Clifton Road, N E.
Atlanta, GA 30329
(404) 320-3333
(1-800) ACS-2345
Website: http://www.cancer.org

Arthritis Foundation
1330 West Peachtree Street
Atlanta, GA 30309
404-872-7100
1 (800) 283-7800
Website: http://www.arthritis.org

National Multiple Sclerosis Society
733 Third Ave.
New York, NY 10017(c)3288
(1 (800) 344-4867
E-mail: info@nmss.org
Website: http://www.nmss.org

HIV/AIDS Treatment Information Service
P.O. Box 6303
Rockville, MD 20849-6303.
1-800-448-0440
TTY/Deaf Access: 888-480-3739
Fax: 301-519-6616
E-Mail: atis@hivatis.org
Website: http://www.hivatis.org

Federal Resources

Federal government resources on health fraud and alternative medicine are:

FDA (HFE-88)
5600 Fishers Lane
Rockville, MD 20857
888-322-4636
E-mail: webmail@oc.fda.gov
Website: http://www.fda.gov

National Center for Complementary and Alternative Medicine
PO Box 8218
Silver Spring, MD 20907
888-644-6226
TTY/TDY: 888-644-6226
Fax: 301-495-4957
Website: http://altmed.od.nih.gov/nccam/

U.S. Postal Inspection Service
(monitor products purchased by mail)
Office of Criminal Investigation
Washington, DC 20260-2166
Website: http://www.usps.gov/postalinspectors/

Federal Trade Commission
(regarding false advertising)
CRC-240
Washington, DC 20580
(202)382-4357
Website: http://www.ftc.gov

Other Resources

Other agencies that may have information and offer assistance include local Better Business Bureaus, state and municipal consumer affairs offices, and state attorneys general offices.

Acupressure

Acupressure Institute
1533 Shattuck Ave.
Berkeley, CA 94709
800-442-2232
510-845-1059
E-mail: info@acupressure.com
Website: http://www.healthworld.com/acupressure/index.html

American Oriental Bodywork Therapy Association
6801 Jericho Tpk.
Syosset, NY 11791
609-782-1616
Website: http://www.natural-connection.com/institutes/oriental_body work.html

Jin Shin Do Foundation for Bodymind Acupressure
366 California Ave., Suite 16
Palo Alto, CA 94306

Jin Shin Jyutsu, Inc.
8719 E. San Alberto Dr.
Scottsdale, AZ 85258
602-998-9331
Fax: 602-998-9335
Website: http://www.inficad.com/~jsjinc/

Acupuncture

American Academy of Medical Acupuncture
5820 Wilshire Boulevard
Suite 500
Los Angeles, CA 90036
323)937-5514
Fax: 323-937-0955

American Association of Acupuncture and Oriental Medicine
433 Front St.
Catasauqua, PA 18032
(610) 266-1433
Fax: 610-264-2768
E-mail: AAOM1@aol.com
Website: http://www.aaom.org

National Commission for the Certification of Acupuncturists
11 Canal Center Plaza
Suite 300
Alexandria, VA 22314
703-548-9004
Fax: 703-548-9079
E-mail: info@nccaom.org
Website: http://www.nccaom.org

Alternative Medicine

American Association of Naturopathic Physicians
601 Valley Street, Ste. 105
Suite 322
Seattle, WA 98109
206-298-0126
Fax: 206-298-0129
Website: http://www.naturopathic.org

American Holistic Health Association
Suzan Walter, President
P.O. Box 17400
Anaheim, CA 92817-7400
714-779-6152
E-mail: ahha@healthy.net
Website: http://ahha.org

American Holistic Medical Association
4101 Lake Boone Trail,
Suite 201
Raleigh, NC 27606
Website: http://www.ahmaholistic.com

Bastyr University
14500 Juanita Dr. NE
Kenmore, WA 98028-4966
425-823-1300
Fax: 425-823-6222
Website: http://www.bastyr.edu

National College of Naturopathic Medicine
11231 SE Market St.
Portland, OR 97216
503-499-4343
Website: http://www.ncnm.edu/index.htm

Aromatherapy

Aromatherapy Seminars
117 N. Robertson Blvd.
Los Angeles, CA 90048
1-800-677-2368
310-276-1156

National Association for Holistic Aromatherapy
PO. Box 17622
Boulder, GO 80308-7622
415-564-6785
1-800-566-6735
Fax: 415-564-6799

Pacific Institute of Aromatherapy
P.O Box 6842
San Rafael, CA 94903
(415)479-9121
415-479-0614

Ayurveda

American Institute of Vedic Studies
PO Box 8357
Santa Fe, NM 87504-8357
505-983-9385
Fax: 505-982-5807
Website: http://www.vedanet.com/

Ayurvedic Institute
1131 Menaul NE
Albuquerque, NM 87112
505-291-9698
Website: http://www.jumbomall.com/shops/aurveda/

American Board of Chelation Therapy
1407 N. Wells Street
Chicago, IL 60610
(312)266-4639
Fax: 312-266-3658

American College for Advancement in Medicine
2321 Verdugo Drive, Suite 204
Laguna Hills, CA 92653
(714)583-7666
E-mail: acam@acam.org
Website: http://ww.acam.org/index.html

American Heart Association
7272 Greenville Avenue
Dallas, TX 75231
(800)242-8721
Website: http://guidetohealth.com/lnk/link2.html

Chiropractic

American Chiropractic Association
1701 Clarendon Boulevard
Arlington, VA 22209
(703) 276-8800
Website: http://www.amerchiro.org/index.html

Essence Therapy

The Flower Essence Society
P.O. Box 459
Nevada City, CA 95959
1-800-736-9222; 530-265-9163
Fax: 530-265-0584
E-mail: mail@flowersociety.org
Website: http://www.flowersociety.org
An organization that studies and promotes the therapeutic use of
flower remedies/essences.

Herbal Therapy

American Association of Naturopathic Physicians
601 Valley Street, Ste. 105
Suite 322
Seattle, WA 98109
206-298-0126
Fax: 206-298-0129
Website: http://www.naturopathic.org

American Botanical Council
P.O. Box 144345
Austin, TX 78714-4345
(512) 926-4900
Fax: 512-926-2345
E-mail: abc@herbalgram.org/
Website: http://www.herbalgram.org/index.html

The American Herbalists Guild
PO Box 70
Roosevelt, UT 84066
435-722-8434
Fax: 435-722-8452
E-mail: ahgoaffice@earthlink.net
Website: http://www.healthy.net/herbalists/Index.html

Herb Research Foundation
1007 Pearl, #200 F
Boulder, CO 80302
(303) 449-2265; 800-748-2617
Fax: 303-449-7849
E-mail: info@herbs.org
Website: http://www.herbs.org/index.html

Homeopathy

Homeopathic Educational Services
2124 Kittredge Street
Berkely, CA 94704
(510) 649-0294
Fax: 510-649-1955
E-mail: mail@homeopathic.com
Website: http://www.homeopathic.com

International Foundation for Homeopathy
PO Box 7
Edmonds, WA 98020
425-776-447
Fax: 425-776-1499
E-mail: ifh@nwlink.com
Website: http://www.healthy.net/pan/pa/Homeopathic/ifh/

National Center for Homeopathy
801 N. Fairfax St., Suite 306
Alexandria, VA 22314
703-548-7790; Fax: 703-548-7792
E-mail: nchinfo@igc.org
Website: http://www.homeopathic.org

National College of Naturopathic Medicine
11231 SE Market St.
Portland, OR 97216
503-499-4343
Website: http://www.ncnm.edu/index.htm

New England School of Homeopathy
356 Middle St.
Amherst, MA 01002
413-256-5949; Fax: 413-256-6223
E-mail: nesh@nesh.com
Website: http://www.nesh.com/main.html

Hydrotherapy

Desert Springs Therapy Center
66705 E. Sixth St.
Desert Hot Springs, CA 92240
760-329-5066; Fax: 760-251-6202
E-mail: dsrtspgt@gte.net
Website: http://www.tagnet.org/desertspringstherapy/

Uchee Pines Institute
30 Uchee Pines Rd., Suite 75
Seale, AL 36975-5702
334-855-4764; Fax: 334-855-9014
Website: http://www.sdamall.com/ucheepines/index.html

Imagery

The Academy for Guided Imagery
P.O. Box 2070
Mill Valley, CA 94942
1-800-726-2070
E-mail: strategicvisions@usa.net
Website: http://www.healthy.com/university/profess/schools/edu/imagery/index.html

Biofeedback Certification Institute of America
10200 West 44th Ave, Ste. 310
Wheatridge, CO 80033
(303)420-2902
Fax: 303-422-8894

Center for Mind/Body Medicine
5225 Connecticut Avenue, NW
Suite 414
Washington, DC 20015
(202) 966-7338
Fax: 202-966-2589
E-mail: cmbm@mindspring.com
Website: http://www.healthy.net/cmbm/center.htm

Center for Mindfulness Stress Reduction
University of Massachusetts Medical Center
55 Lake Avenue North
Worcester, MA 01655
(508) 856-2656
Website: http://www.ummed.edu/main/experts/expert40.htm

Mind/Body Medical Institute
Division of Behavioral Medicine
Beth Israel Deaconess Medical Center
Harvard Medical School
110 Francis Street
Suite 1A
Boston, MA 02215
(617) 632-9530
E-mail: webmaster@mcmc.net
Website: http://www.mcmc.net/mbmi.htm

Massage

American Massage Therapy Association
820 Davis ST., Suite 100
Evanston, IL 60201-4444
(847) 864-0123; Fax: 847-864-1178
Website: http://www.amtamassage.org

Associated Bodyworks and Massage Professionals
28677 Buffalo Park Rd.
Evergreen, CO 80439-7347
800-458-2267
Fax: 303-674-0859
E-mail: expectmore@abmp.com
Website: http://abmp.com

National Certification Board for Therapeutic Massage and Bodywork
8201 Greensboro Drive, Suite 300
Maclean, VA 22102
(800) 296-0664: (703) 610-9015; Fax: 703-610 9005
E-mail: mswiscoski@ncbtmb.com
Website: http://www.ncbtmb.com

Reflexology

International Institute of Reflexology
32 Priory Road
Portbury, Bristol BS20 7TH

Laura Norman and Associates Reflexology Center
41 Park Ave., Suite 8A
New York, NY 10016
1-800-Feet First
Fax: 532-4504
E-mail: reflexologist.com@cwixmail.com
Website: http://www.lauranormanreflexology.com

Reflexology Research
P.O. Box 35820
Albequerque, NM 87176
1-800-713-6711
Website: http://www.reflexology-research.com

Relaxation and Meditation

Association for Transpersonal Psychology
P.O. Box 3049
Stanford, CA 94305
650-327-2066
Website: http://www.igc.org/atp/

Institute of Noetic Sciences
475 Gate Five Road, Suite #300
Sausalito, CA 94965
415-331-5650
800-383-1394 (membership)
Fax: 415-331-5673
E-mail: membership@noetic.org
Website: http://www.noetic.org

Sound Therapy

American Music Therapy Association
8455 Colesville Road, Suite 1000
Silver Spring, Maryland 20910
301-589-3300
Fax: 301-589-5175
Website: http://www.musictherapy.org

Vitamin and Mineral Therapy

American College for Advancement in Medicine
23121 Verdugo Drive, Suite 204
Laguna Hills, CA 92653
E-mail: acam@acam.org
Website: http://www.acam.org/

Yoga

American Yoga Association
PO Box 19986
Sarasota, FL 34276
941-927-4977
Fax: 941-921-9844
E-mail: YOGAmerica@aol.com
Website: http://users.aol.com/amyogaassn/

Himalayan International Institute of Yoga Science and Philosophy
R.R. 1, Box 400
Honesdale, PA 18431
1-800-822-4547

International Association of Yoga Therapists
20 Sunnyside Ave, Suite A-243
Mill Valley, CA 94941-1928
415-332-2478
Fax: 415-381-0876

Rocky Mountain Institute of Yoga and Ayurveda
P.O. Box 1091
Boulder, CO 80306
303-443-6923
Website: http://www.boulderwellness.com/rmiya/rmiya.html

Index

Index

Page numbers followed by 'n' indicate a footnote. Page numbers in *italics* indicate a table or illustration.

E

ease, defined 658
 see also bind
East Earth Herb Inc. 365
Ebers Papyrus, Middle East medicine
 286
Echinacea (purple coneflower) 5, 93,
 94, 280, 297, 311, 323, 349, 372
echocardiography, defined 658
Eckhardt, Sandor 629
Eclipta alba 306
economic concerns
 alternative treatments 38
 biofeedback 552–53
 meditation 538–39
 psychotherapy 534–35
ECT *see* electroconvulsive therapy
 (ECT)
eczema, defined 658
EDTA chelation therapy 617–19, 640
education
 acupuncture schools 57
 chiropractic 414–15
 diet and nutrition 237–39, 248–49
 health care providers 240–43
 environmental medicine 101
 physician-centered model 10
Education, US Department of 510
 massage therapy profession 421
education levels
 alternative medicine patients 21,
 26–27
 illness 521
EEG *see* electroencephalogram (EEG)
Eeman, L. E. 447
effleurage, depicted 470
Einhorn, Alfred 630
Eisenberg, David 9, 10, 26, 28
elderly
 health fraud 35
 music therapy 563
Elderly, Nutrition Program for the 236
elders, powwowers 107
electric current treatments
 see also electrostimulation devices;
 transcutaneous electrical nerve
 stimulation (TENS)

electric current treatments, continued
 acupuncture 59
 tumors 34
electroacupuncture 5, 144, 159–67
 see also acupuncture
electroconvulsive therapy (ECT) 189
electroencephalogram (EEG), defined
 658
electroenephalography, described 142
electromagnetic fields 5
 see also bioelectromagnetics (BEM)
 biomedical effects 146–48
 defined 658
 described 134–37
electromagnetic radiation, defined
 659
electromagnetic spectrum, described
 136
electromagnetism
 defined 659
 homeopathy 73
electromyography, described 142
electrophysiology, defined 659
electropollution, defined 659
electroretinography, described 142
electrostimulation devices 5
electrosurgical excision, defined 659
ELF *see* extremely low frequency
 (ELF)
elimination therapy, Ayurveda 66
Emblica officinalis 307
embolism, defined 659
EM fields *see* electromagnetic fields
emission tomography, defined 659
emmenagogue, defined 345
emodin 625
emollient, defined 345
empacho 114, 115
*The Encyclopedia of Traditional Chi-
 nese Medicine Substances (Zhong
 yao da ci dian)* 288
endocrine, defined 659
endogenous fields, described 135
endorphins
 acupuncture 162
 defined 659
 imagery 164
 massage therapy 425
endoscopy, defined 659

hierarchy of resort, described 42
high-density lipoproteins *see* HDL
(high-density lipoproteins)
high sense perception, defined 662
Hildebrandt, G. 88
Hilsden, Robert 371, 374
hippocampus, defined 662
Hippocrates 127, 256, 399, 419, 437,
471, 481
Hippocratic injunction 12
Hirshberg, Caryle 527
Hispanic Americans, health practices
25, 43
see also Latin American rural practices
HIV/AIDS Treatment Information
Service 676
Hoffer, Abram 189, 190
Hoku points, acupuncture 164–65,
167
holism
biofield 439
described 12
Holistic Aromatherapy, National Association for 679
Holistic Health Association, American 678
Holistic Medical Association, American 678
holistic medicine 34
see also Ayurveda
Holistic Nurses Association, American 442
Holmes, Sue 260
home births 8
Homeopathic Educational Services
681
homeopathic medicine 4, 45, 71–83
FDA regulation 78–81
history 43, 77–78
naturopathic medicine 92–93
research 74–77
statistics 72, 82
treatment, described 81–82
Homeopathic Pharmaceutical Association, American 82
*Homeopathic Pharmacopoeia of the
United States* 72, 73
Homeopathic World 384

homeopathy 22n1
anthroposophically extended medicine 86, 89
cultural diversity 29
defined 662
flower essence therapy 384
materia medica 665
potentized substance, defined 670
research 16
resource information 681–82
Homeopathy, International Foundation for 682
Homeopathy, National Center for
contact information 682
homeopathic practitioners listing
82
professional training courses 72
Homeopathy, New England School of
682
homeostasis
defined 662
environmental medicine 98
Homer 471
Homewood, Earl 413
hops (*Humulus lupulus*) 351
hospital births 8
Hospital for Sick Children 219
Hospital Practice 588
Howard, John 412, 413
Hoxsey, Harry 624
Hoxsey method 624–25, 641
huang lian see coptis rhizome
huang qin see baical skullcap root
Huang Ti Nei Ching Su Wen 55, 436
Hufford, David J. 21, 30
Humana Inc. 359–60
humoralism, defined 662
humorism, defined 662
humor therapy 4
Huna 442
Huneke, Ferdinand 631
Huss, Magnus 116
Huxley, Aldous 582
Huxley, Thomas 654
Hyde, E. 499
Hydrastis 93
hydraulics 670
hydrocortisone, defined 662
hydrogen peroxide 5

Seventh-Day Aventist diet 221, 223–27
714-X 623–24, 640
shamanic healing 109
shamanism 4
  described 106–7
  South America 29
Shao, X. 474
shark cartilage 32, 614
Shaw, George Bernard 582
Shear, M. J. 628
sheep sorrel 626
Sheffield University 482
sheng di huang see foxglove
shengjiang see ginger
SHEN therapy 443, 444
shepherd's purse (*Capsella bursa-pastoris*) 354
Sherman Antitrust Act, chiropractic
  profession protection 21
shiatsu 430, 495–502
*Shiatsu: Japanese Massage for
  Health and Fitness* 501
Shiatsu: The Complete Guide 501
Shiatsu Society
  morning sickness study 500
  training and regulation 502
shield fern *see* dryopteris root
Shi Ji 55
Shipman, William H. 635
short leg, defined 673
sialogogue, defined 345
Siberian ginseng (*Eleutherococcus
  senticosus*) 350
sick building syndrome, environmental medicine 96, 103
Sila 438
Silybum marianum see milk thistle
similimum, defined 73
Simone, Charles 616, 640
Simpson, George Gaylord 520
sing (healing ceremonial) 110–12
single remedy, homeopathic medicine
  78
sinusitis, defined 673
sinusoidal, defined 673
sleep latency, defined 673
slippery elm (*Ulmus rubra*) 354, 627
Small Business Administration 418
Smith, Bob 116

SmithKline Beecham 364
Smolensky, Michael 588
snake venom 36
sociogenic, defined 673
sociologists, alternative health practices 28
Socrates 471
Sofroniou, P. 501
Sokol, Gerald 589, 590, 591
Solfvin, Jerry 571
somatic, defined 673
somatic dysfunction, defined 673
somatovisceral disorders 416–17
sorrel 626
sound therapy 4
  see also music therapy
  resource information 685
spas 36
spastic colon syndrome, defined 664
Speech and Drama, Central School of
  583
Sperry, Roger 12
Spiegel, David 532
Spiess, G. 631
spinal manipulation
  chiropractic 481–83
  cultural diversity 29
  described 665
spinel, described 665
spiritual energy, defined 673
spiritual healers 107
  statistics 41
spiritual healing 25, 525–27
  see also faith healing; religion
  described 665
spiritual values 11
spontaneous generation theory 654
*Spontaneous Remission: An Anno-
  tated Bibliography* 527
sports massage 423
spreading phenomenon, environmental medicine 99
Stalker, Nancy 361
Stanwick, Michael 597
star of Bethlehem (*Ornithogalum
  umbellatum*) 395
"Statistical Inquiries into the Efficacy
  of Prayer"(Galton) 571
Stehlin, Isadora B. 38, 83, 591

Health Reference Series
COMPLETE CATALOG

AIDS Sourcebook, 1st Edition

Basic Information about AIDS and HIV Infection, Featuring Historical and Statistical Data, Current Research, Prevention, and Other Special Topics of Interest for Persons Living with AIDS, Along with Source Listings for Further Assistance

Edited by Karen Bellenir and Peter D. Dresser. 831 pages. 1995. 0-7808-0031-1. $78.

"One strength of this book is its practical emphasis. The intended audience is the lay reader . . . useful as an educational tool for health care providers who work with AIDS patients. Recommended for public libraries as well as hospital or academic libraries that collect consumer materials." — *Bulletin of the MLA, Jan '96*

"This is the most comprehensive volume of its kind on an important medical topic. Highly recommended for all libraries." — *Reference Book Review, '96*

"Very useful reference for all libraries." — *Choice, Oct '95*

"There is a wealth of information here that can provide much educational assistance. It is a must book for all libraries and should be on the desk of each and every congressional leader. Highly recommended." — *AIDS Book Review Journal, Aug '95*

"Recommended for most collections." — *Library Journal, Jul '95*

AIDS Sourcebook, 2nd Edition

Basic Consumer Health Information about Acquired Immune Deficiency Syndrome (AIDS) and Human Immunodeficiency Virus (HIV) Infection, Featuring Updated Statistical Data, Reports on Recent Research and Prevention Initiatives, and Other Special Topics of Interest for Persons Living with AIDS, Including New Antiretroviral Treatment Options, Strategies for Combating Opportunistic Infections, Information about Clinical Trials, and More; Along with a Glossary of Important Terms and Resource Listings for Further Help and Information

Edited by Karen Bellenir. 751 pages. 1999. 0-7808-0225-X. $78.

Allergies Sourcebook

Basic Information about Major Forms and Mechanisms of Common Allergic Reactions, Sensitivities, and Intolerances, Including Anaphylaxis, Asthma, Hives and Other Dermatologic Symptoms, Rhinitis, and Sinusitis, Along with Their Usual Triggers Like Animal Fur, Chemicals, Drugs, Dust, Foods, Insects, Latex, Pollen, and Poison Ivy, Oak, and Sumac; Plus Information on Prevention, Identification, and Treatment

Edited by Allan R. Cook. 611 pages. 1997. 0-7808-0036-2. $78.

Alternative Medicine Sourcebook

Basic Consumer Health Information about Alternatives to Conventional Medicine, Including Acupressure, Acupuncture, Aromatherapy, Ayurveda, Bioelectromagnetics, Environmental Medicine, Essence Therapy, Food and Nutrition Therapy, Herbal Therapy, Homeopathy, Imaging, Massage, Naturopathy, Reflexology, Relaxation and Meditation, Sound Therapy, Vitamin and Mineral Therapy, and Yoga, and More

Edited by Allan R. Cook. 737 pages. 1999. 0-7808-0200-4. $78.

Alzheimer's, Stroke & 29 Other Neurological Disorders Sourcebook, 1st Edition

Basic Information for the Layperson on 31 Diseases or Disorders Affecting the Brain and Nervous System, First Describing the Illness, Then Listing Symptoms, Diagnostic Methods, and Treatment Options, and Including Statistics on Incidences and Causes

Edited by Frank E. Bair. 579 pages. 1993. 1-55888-748-2. $78.

"Nontechnical reference book that provides reader-friendly information." — *Family Caregiver Alliance Update, Winter '96*

"Should be included in any library's patient education section." — *American Reference Books Annual, '94*

"Written in an approachable and accessible style. Recommended for patient education and consumer health collections in health science center and public libraries." — *Academic Library Book Review, Dec '93*

"It is very handy to have information on more than thirty neurological disorders under one cover, and there is no recent source like it." — *RQ, Fall '93*

Alzheimer's Disease Sourcebook, 2nd Edition

Basic Consumer Health Information about Alzheimer's Disease, Related Disorders, and Other Dementias, Including Multi-Infarct Dementia, AIDS-Related Dementia, Alcoholic Dementia, Huntington's Disease, Delirium, and Confusional States; Along with Reports Detailing Current Research Efforts in Prevention and Treatment, Long-Term Care Issues, and Listings of Sources for Additional Help and Information

Edited by Karen Bellenir. 524 pages. 1999. 0-7808-0223-3. $78.

Arthritis Sourcebook

Basic Consumer Health Information about Specific Forms of Arthritis and Related Disorders, Including Rheumatoid Arthritis, Osteoarthritis, Gout, Polymyalgia Rheumatica, Psoriatic Arthritis, Spondyloarthropathies, Juvenile Rheumatoid Arthritis, and Juvenile Ankylosing Spondylitis; Along with Information about Medical, Surgical, and Alternative Treatment Options, and Including Strategies for Coping with Pain, Fatigue, and Stress

Edited by Allan R. Cook. 550 pages. 1998. 0-7808-0201-2. $78.

". . . accessible to the layperson."
— *Reference and Research Book News, Feb '99*

Back & Neck Disorders Sourcebook

Basic Information about Disorders and Injuries of the Spinal Cord and Vertebrae, Including Facts on Chiropractic Treatment, Surgical Interventions, Paralysis, and Rehabilitation, Along with Advice for Preventing Back Trouble

Edited by Karen Bellenir. 548 pages. 1997. 0-7808-0202-0. $78.

"The strength of this work is its basic, easy-to-read format. Recommended."
— *Reference and User Services Quarterly, Winter '97*

Blood & Circulatory Disorders Sourcebook

Basic Information about Blood and Its Components, Anemias, Leukemias, Bleeding Disorders, and Circulatory Disorders, Including Aplastic Anemia, Thalassemia, Sickle-Cell Disease, Hemochromatosis, Hemophilia, Von Willebrand Disease, and Vascular Diseases; Along with a Special Section on Blood Transfusions and Blood Supply Safety, a Glossary, and Source Listings for Further Help and Information

Edited by Karen Bellenir and Linda M. Shin. 554 pages. 1998. 0-7808-0203-9. $78.

"Recent and recommended reference source."
— *Booklist, Feb '99*

"An important reference sourcebook written in simple language for everyday, non-technical users. "
— *Reviewer's Bookwatch, Jan '99*

Brain Disorders Sourcebook

Basic Consumer Health Information about Strokes, Epilepsy, Amyotrophic Lateral Sclerosis (ALS/Lou Gehrig's Disease), Parkinson's Disease, Brain Tumors, Cerebral Palsy, Headache, Tourette Syndrome, and More; Along with Statistical Data, Treatment and

Rehabilitation Options, Coping Strategies, Reports on Current Research Initiatives, a Glossary, and Resource Listings for Additional Help and Information

Edited by Karen Bellenir. 481 pages. 1999. 0-7808-0229-2. $78.

Burns Sourcebook

Basic Consumer Health Information about Various Types of Burns and Scalds, Including Flame, Heat, Cold, Electrical, Chemical, and Sun Burns; Along with Information on Short-Term and Long-Term Treatments, Tissue Reconstruction, Plastic Surgery, Prevention Suggestions, and First Aid

Edited by Allan R. Cook. 604 pages. 1999. 0-7808-0204-7. $78.

Cancer Sourcebook, 1st Edition

Basic Information on Cancer Types, Symptoms, Diagnostic Methods, and Treatments, Including Statistics on Cancer Occurrences Worldwide and the Risks Associated with Known Carcinogens and Activities

Edited by Frank E. Bair. 932 pages. 1990. 1-55888-888-8. $78.

"Written in nontechnical language. Useful for patients, their families, medical professionals, and librarians."
— *Guide to Reference Books, '96*

"Designed with the non-medical professional in mind. Libraries and medical facilities interested in patient education should certainly consider adding the Cancer Sourcebook to their holdings. This compact collection of reliable information . . . is an invaluable tool for helping patients and patients' families and friends to take the first steps in coping with the many difficulties of cancer."
— *Medical Reference Services Quarterly, Winter '91*

"Specifically created for the nontechnical reader . . . an important resource for the general reader trying to understand the complexities of cancer."
— *American Reference Books Annual, '91*

"This publication's nontechnical nature and very comprehensive format make it useful for both the general public and undergraduate students."
— *Choice, Oct '90*

New Cancer Sourcebook, 2nd Edition

Basic Information about Major Forms and Stages of Cancer, Featuring Facts about Primary and Secondary Tumors of the Respiratory, Nervous, Lymphatic, Circulatory, Skeletal, and Gastrointestinal Systems, and Specific Organs; Statistical and Demographic Data; Treatment Options; and Strategies for Coping

Edited by Allan R. Cook. 1,313 pages. 1996. 0-7808-0041-9. $78.

"This book is an excellent resource for patients with newly diagnosed cancer and their families. The dialogue is simple, direct, and comprehensive. Highly recommended for patients and families to aid in their understanding of cancer and its treatment."
— *Booklist Health Sciences Supplement, Oct '97*

"The amount of factual and useful information is extensive. The writing is very clear, geared to general readers. Recommended for all levels."
— *Choice, Jan '97*

Cancer Sourcebook, 3rd Edition

Basic Consumer Health Information about Major Forms and Stages of Cancer, Featuring Facts about Primary and Secondary Tumors of the Respiratory, Nervous, Lymphatic, Circulatory, Skeletal, and Gastrointestinal Systems, and Specific Organs; Along with Statistical and Demographic Data, Treatment Options, Strategies for Coping, a Glossary, and a Directory of Sources for Additional Help and Information

Edited by Edward J. Prucha. 800 pages. 1999. 0-7808-0227-6. $78.

Cancer Sourcebook for Women, 1st Edition

Basic Information about Specific Forms of Cancer That Affect Women, Featuring Facts about Breast Cancer, Cervical Cancer, Ovarian Cancer, Cancer of the Uterus and Uterine Sarcoma, Cancer of the Vagina, and Cancer of the Vulva; Statistical and Demographic Data; Treatments, Self-Help Management Suggestions, and Current Research Initiatives

Edited by Allan R. Cook and Peter D. Dresser. 524 pages. 1996. 0-7808-0076-1. $78.

". . . written in easily understandable, non-technical language. Recommended for public libraries or hospital and academic libraries that collect patient education or consumer health materials."
— *Medical Reference Services Quarterly, Spring '97*

"Would be of value in a consumer health library. . . . written with the health care consumer in mind. Medical jargon is at a minimum, and medical terms are explained in clear, understandable sentences."
— *Bulletin of the MLA, Oct '96*

"The availability under one cover of all these pertinent publications, grouped under cohesive headings, makes this certainly a most useful sourcebook."
— *Choice, Jun '96*

"Presents a comprehensive knowledge base for general readers. Men and women both benefit from the gold mine of information nestled between the two covers of this book. Recommended."
— *Academic Library Book Review, Summer '96*

"This timely book is highly recommended for consumer health and patient education collections in all libraries."
— *Library Journal, Apr '96*

Cancer Sourcebook for Women, 2nd Edition

Basic Consumer Health Information about Specific Forms of Cancer That Affect Women, Including Cervical Cancer, Ovarian Cancer, Endometrial Cancer, Uterine Sarcoma, Vaginal Cancer, Vulvar Cancer, and Gestational Trophoblastic Tumor; and Featuring Statistical Information, Facts about Tests and Treatments, a Glossary of Cancer Terms, and an Extensive List of Additional Resources

Edited by Edward J. Prucha. 600 pages. 1999. 0-7808-0226-8. $78.

Cardiovascular Diseases & Disorders Sourcebook, 1st Edition

Basic Information about Cardiovascular Diseases and Disorders, Featuring Facts about the Cardiovascular System, Demographic and Statistical Data, Descriptions of Pharmacological and Surgical Interventions, Lifestyle Modifications, and a Special Section Focusing on Heart Disorders in Children

Edited by Karen Bellenir and Peter D. Dresser. 683 pages. 1995. 0-7808-0032-X. $78.

". . . comprehensive format provides an extensive overview on this subject."
— *Choice, Jun '96*

". . . an easily understood, complete, up-to-date resource. This well executed public health tool will make valuable information available to those that need it most, patients and their families. The typeface, sturdy non-reflective paper, and library binding add a feel of quality found wanting in other publications. Highly recommended for academic and general libraries. "
— *Academic Library Book Review, Summer '96*

Communication Disorders Sourcebook

Basic Information about Deafness and Hearing Loss, Speech and Language Disorders, Voice Disorders, Balance and Vestibular Disorders, and Disorders of Smell, Taste, and Touch

Edited by Linda M. Ross. 533 pages. 1996. 0-7808-0077-X. $78.

"This is skillfully edited and is a welcome resource for the layperson. It should be found in every public and medical library."
— *Booklist Health Sciences Supplement, Oct '97*

Congenital Disorders Sourcebook

Basic Information about Disorders Acquired during Gestation, Including Spina Bifida, Hydrocephalus, Cerebral Palsy, Heart Defects, Craniofacial Abnormalities, Fetal Alcohol Syndrome, and More, Along with Current Treatment Options and Statistical Data

Edited by Karen Bellenir. 607 pages. 1997. 0-7808-0205-5. $78.

"Recent and recommended reference source."
— Booklist, Oct '97

Consumer Issues in Health Care Sourcebook

Basic Information about Health Care Fundamentals and Related Consumer Issues, Including Exams and Screening Tests, Physician Specialties, Choosing a Doctor, Using Prescription and Over-the-Counter Medications Safely, Avoiding Health Scams, Managing Common Health Risks in the Home, Care Options for Chronically or Terminally Ill Patients, and a List of Resources for Obtaining Help and Further Information

Edited by Karen Bellenir. 618 pages. 1998. 0-7808-0221-7. $78.

"Recent and recommended reference source."
— Booklist, Dec '98

Contagious & Non-Contagious Infectious Diseases Sourcebook

Basic Information about Contagious Diseases like Measles, Polio, Hepatitis B, and Infectious Mononucleosis, and Non-Contagious Infectious Diseases like Tetanus and Toxic Shock Syndrome, and Diseases Occurring as Secondary Infections Such as Shingles and Reye Syndrome, Along with Vaccination, Prevention, and Treatment Information, and a Section Describing Emerging Infectious Disease Threats

Edited by Karen Bellenir and Peter D. Dresser. 566 pages. 1996. 0-7808-0075-3. $78.

Death & Dying Sourcebook

Basic Consumer Health Information for the Layperson about End-of-Life Care and Related Ethical and Legal Issues, Including Chief Causes of Death, Autopsies, Pain Management for the Terminally Ill, Life Support Systems, Insurance, Euthanasia, Assisted Suicide, Hospice Programs, Living Wills, Funeral Planning, Counseling, Mourning, Organ Donation, and Physician Training; Along with Statistical Data, a Glossary, and Listings of Sources for Further Help and Information

Edited by Annemarie S. Muth. 630 pages. 1999. 0-7808-0230-6. $78.

Diabetes Sourcebook, 1st Edition

Basic Information about Insulin-Dependent and Noninsulin-Dependent Diabetes Mellitus, Gestational Diabetes, and Diabetic Complications, Symptoms, Treatment, and Research Results, Including Statistics on Prevalence, Morbidity, and Mortality, Along with Source Listings for Further Help and Information

Edited by Karen Bellenir and Peter D. Dresser. 827 pages. 1994. 1-55888-751-2. $78.

"... very informative and understandable for the layperson without being simplistic. It provides a comprehensive overview for laypersons who want a general understanding of the disease or who want to focus on various aspects of the disease." *— Bulletin of the MLA, Jan '96*

Diabetes Sourcebook, 2nd Edition

Basic Consumer Health Information about Type 1 Diabetes (Insulin-Dependent or Juvenile-Onset Diabetes), Type 2 (Noninsulin-Dependent or Adult-Onset Diabetes), Gestational Diabetes, and Related Disorders, Including Diabetes Prevalence Data, Management Issues, the Role of Diet and Exercise in Controlling Diabetes, Insulin and Other Diabetes Medicines, and Complications of Diabetes Such as Eye Diseases, Periodontal Disease, Amputation, and End-Stage Renal Disease; Along with Reports on Current Research Initiatives, a Glossary, and Resource Listings for Further Help and Information

Edited by Karen Bellenir. 688 pages. 1998. 0-7808-0224-1. $78.

"Recent and recommended reference source."
— Booklist, Feb '99

Diet & Nutrition Sourcebook, 1st Edition

Basic Information about Nutrition, Including the Dietary Guidelines for Americans, the Food Guide Pyramid, and Their Applications in Daily Diet, Nutritional Advice for Specific Age Groups, Current Nutritional Issues and Controversies, the New Food Label and How to Use It to Promote Healthy Eating, and Recent Developments in Nutritional Research

Edited by Dan R. Harris. 662 pages. 1996. 0-7808-0084-2. $78.

"Useful reference as a food and nutrition sourcebook for the general consumer."
— Booklist Health Sciences Supplement, Oct '97

"Recommended for public libraries and medical libraries that receive general information requests on nutrition. It is readable and will appeal to those interested in learning more about healthy dietary practices."
— Medical Reference Services Quarterly, Fall '97

"With dozens of questionable diet books on the market, it is so refreshing to find a reliable and factual reference book. Recommended to aspiring professionals, librarians, and others seeking and giving reliable dietary advice. An excellent compilation." *— Choice, Feb '97*

Diet & Nutrition Sourcebook, 2nd Edition

Basic Consumer Health Information about Dietary Guidelines, Recommended Daily Intake Values, Vitamins, Minerals, Fiber, Fat, Weight Control, Dietary Supplements, and Food Additives; Along with Special Sections on Nutrition Needs throughout Life and Nutrition for People with Such Specific Medical Concerns as Allergies, High Blood Cholesterol, Hypertension, Diabetes, Celiac Disease, Seizure Disorders, Phenylketonuria (PKU), Cancer, and Eating Disorders, and Including Reports on Current Nutrition Research and Source Listings for Additional Help and Information

Edited by Karen Bellenir. 650 pages. 1999. 0-7808-0228-4. $78.

Digestive Diseases & Disorders Sourcebook

Basic Consumer Health Information about Diseases and Disorders that Impact the Upper and Lower Digestive System, Including Celiac Disease, Constipation, Crohn's Disease, Cyclic Vomiting Syndrome, Diarrhea, Diverticulosis and Diverticulitis, Gallstones, Heartburn, Hemorrhoids, Hernias, Indigestion (Dyspepsia), Irritable Bowel Syndrome, Lactose Intolerance, Ulcers, and More; Along with Information about Medications and Other Treatments, Tips for Maintaining a Healthy Digestive Tract, a Glossary, and Directory of Digestive Diseases Organizations

Edited by Karen Bellenir. 325 pages. 1999. 0-7808-0327-2. $48.

Disabilities Sourcebook

Basic Consumer Health Information about Physical and Psychiatric Disabilities, Including Descriptions of Major Causes of Disability, Assistive and Adaptive Aids, Workplace Issues, and Accessibility Concerns; Along with Information about the Americans with Disabilities Act, a Glossary, and Resources for Additional Help and Information

Edited by Dawn D. Matthews. 600 pages. 1999. 0-7808-0389-2. $78.

Domestic Violence & Child Abuse Sourcebook

Basic Information about Spousal/Partner, Child, and Elder Physical, Emotional, and Sexual Abuse, Teen Dating Violence, and Stalking, Including Information about Hotlines, Safe Houses, Safety Plans, and Other Resources for Support and Assistance, Community Initiatives, and Reports on Current Directions in Research and Treatment; Along with a Glossary, Sources for Further Reading, and Governmental and Non-Governmental Organizations Contact Information

Edited by Helene Henderson. 600 pages. 1999. 0-7808-0235-7. $78.

Ear, Nose & Throat Disorders Sourcebook

Basic Information about Disorders of the Ears, Nose, Sinus Cavities, Pharynx, and Larynx, Including Ear Infections, Tinnitus, Vestibular Disorders, Allergic and Non-Allergic Rhinitis, Sore Throats, Tonsillitis, and Cancers That Affect the Ears, Nose, Sinuses, and Throat, Along with Reports on Current Research Initiatives, a Glossary of Related Medical Terms, and a Directory of Sources for Further Help and Information

Edited by Karen Bellenir and Linda M. Shin. 576 pages. 1998. 0-7808-0206-3. $78.

"Overall, this sourcebook is helpful for the consumer seeking information on ENT issues. It is recommended for public libraries."
— *American Reference Books Annual, '99*

"Recent and recommended reference source."
— *Booklist, Dec '98*

Endocrine & Metabolic Disorders Sourcebook

Basic Information for the Layperson about Pancreatic and Insulin-Related Disorders Such as Pancreatitis, Diabetes, and Hypoglycemia; Adrenal Gland Disorders Such as Cushing's Syndrome, Addison's Disease, and Congenital Adrenal Hyperplasia; Pituitary Gland Disorders Such as Growth Hormone Deficiency, Acromegaly, and Pituitary Tumors; Thyroid Disorders Such as Hypothyroidism, Graves' Disease, Hashimoto's Disease, and Goiter; Hyperparathyroidism; and Other Diseases and Syndromes of Hormone Imbalance or Metabolic Dysfunction, Along with Reports on Current Research Initiatives

Edited by Linda M. Shin. 574 pages. 1998. 0-7808-0207-1. $78.

"Recent and recommended reference source."
— *Booklist, Dec '98*

Environmentally Induced Disorders Sourcebook

Basic Information about Diseases and Syndromes Linked to Exposure to Pollutants and Other Substances in Outdoor and Indoor Environments Such as Lead, Asbestos, Formaldehyde, Mercury, Emissions, Noise, and More

Edited by Allan R. Cook. 620 pages. 1997. 0-7808-0083-4. $78.

"Recent and recommended reference source."
— *Booklist, Sept '98*

"This book will be a useful addition to anyone's library."
— *Choice Health Sciences Supplement, May '98*

". . . a good survey of numerous environmentally induced physical disorders . . . a useful addition to anyone's library."
— *Doody's Health Science Book Reviews, Jan '98*

". . . provide[s] introductory information from the best authorities around. Since this volume covers topics that potentially affect everyone, it will surely be one of the most frequently consulted volumes in the *Health Reference Series*." — *Rettig on Reference, Nov '97*

Ethical Issues in Medicine Sourcebook

Basic Information about Controversial Treatment Issues, Genetic Research, Reproductive Technologies, and End-of-Life Decisions, Including Topics Such as Cloning, Abortion, Fertility Management, Organ Transplantation, Health Care Rationing, Advance Directives, Living Wills, Physician-Assisted Suicide, Euthanasia, and More; Along with a Glossary and Resources for Additional Information

Edited by Helene Henderson. 600 pages. 1999. 0-7808-0237-3. $78.

Fitness & Exercise Sourcebook

Basic Information on Fitness and Exercise, Including Fitness Activities for Specific Age Groups, Exercise for People with Specific Medical Conditions, How to Begin a Fitness Program in Running, Walking, Swimming, Cycling, and Other Athletic Activities, and Recent Research in Fitness and Exercise

Edited by Dan R. Harris. 663 pages. 1996. 0-7808-0186-5. $78.

"A good resource for general readers."
— *Choice, Nov '97*

"The perennial popularity of the topic . . . make this an appealing selection for public libraries."
— *Rettig on Reference, Jun/Jul '97*

Food & Animal Borne Diseases Sourcebook

Basic Information about Diseases That Can Be Spread to Humans through the Ingestion of Contaminated Food or Water or by Contact with Infected Animals and Insects, Such as Botulism, E. Coli, Hepatitis A, Trichinosis, Lyme Disease, and Rabies, Along with Information Regarding Prevention and Treatment Methods, and a Special Section for International Travelers Describing Diseases Such as Cholera, Malaria, Travelers' Diarrhea, and Yellow Fever, and Offering Recommendations for Avoiding Illness

Edited by Karen Bellenir and Peter D. Dresser. 535 pages. 1995. 0-7808-0033-8. $78.

"Targeting general readers and providing them with a single, comprehensive source of information on selected topics, this book continues, with the excellent caliber of its predecessors, to catalog topical information on health matters of general interest. Readable and thorough, this valuable resource is highly recommended for all libraries."
— *Academic Library Book Review, Summer '96*

"A comprehensive collection of authoritative information." — *Emergency Medical Services, Oct '95*

Food Safety Sourcebook

Basic Consumer Health Information about the Safe Handling of Meat, Poultry, Seafood, Eggs, Fruit Juices, and Other Food Items, and Facts about Pesticides, Drinking Water, Food Safety Overseas, and the Onset, Duration, and Symptoms of Foodborne Illnesses, Including Types of Pathogenic Bacteria, Parasitic Protozoa, Worms, Viruses, and Natural Toxins; Along with the Role of the Consumer, the Food Handler, and the Government in Food Safety; a Glossary, and Resources for Additional Help and Information

Edited by Dawn D. Matthews. 339 pages. 1999. 0-7808-0326-4. $48.

Forensic Medicine Sourcebook

Basic Consumer Information for the Layperson about Forensic Medicine, Including Crime Scene Investigation, Evidence Collection and Analysis, Expert Testimony, Computer-Aided Criminal Identification, Digital Imaging in the Courtroom, DNA Profiling, Accident Reconstruction, Autopsies, Ballistics, Drugs and Explosives Detection, Latent Fingerprints, Product Tampering, and Questioned Document Examination; Along with Statistical Data, a Glossary of Forensics Terminology, and Listings of Sources for Further Help and Information

Edited by Annemarie S. Muth. 574 pages. 1999. 0-7808-0232-2. $78.

Gastrointestinal Diseases & Disorders Sourcebook

Basic Information about Gastroesophageal Reflux Disease (Heartburn), Ulcers, Diverticulosis, Irritable Bowel Syndrome, Crohn's Disease, Ulcerative Colitis, Diarrhea, Constipation, Lactose Intolerance, Hemorrhoids, Hepatitis, Cirrhosis, and Other Digestive Problems, Featuring Statistics, Descriptions of Symptoms, and Current Treatment Methods of Interest for Persons Living with Upper and Lower Gastrointestinal Maladies

Edited by Linda M. Ross. 413 pages. 1996. 0-7808-0078-8. $78.

". . . very readable form. The successful editorial work that brought this material together into a useful and understandable reference makes accessible to all readers information that can help them more effectively understand and obtain help for digestive tract problems."
— *Choice, Feb '97*

Genetic Disorders Sourcebook

Basic Information about Heritable Diseases and Disorders Such as Down Syndrome, PKU, Hemophilia, Von Willebrand Disease, Gaucher Disease, Tay-Sachs Disease, and Sickle-Cell Disease, Along with Information about Genetic Screening, Gene Therapy, Home Care, and Including Source Listings for Further Help and Information on More Than 300 Disorders

Edited by Karen Bellenir. 642 pages. 1996. 0-7808-0034-6. $78.

"Provides essential medical information to both the general public and those diagnosed with a serious or fatal genetic disease or disorder." — *Choice, Jan '97*

"Geared toward the lay public. It would be well placed in all public libraries and in those hospital and medical libraries in which access to genetic references is limited." — *Doody's Health Sciences Book Review, Oct '96*

Head Trauma Sourcebook

Basic Information for the Layperson about Open-Head and Closed-Head Injuries, Treatment Advances, Recovery, and Rehabilitation, Along with Reports on Current Research Initiatives

Edited by Karen Bellenir. 414 pages. 1997. 0-7808-0208-X. $78.

Health Insurance Sourcebook

Basic Information about Managed Care Organizations, Traditional Fee-for-Service Insurance, Insurance Portability and Pre-Existing Conditions Clauses, Medicare, Medicaid, Social Security, and Military Health Care, Along with Information about Insurance Fraud

Edited by Wendy Wilcox. 530 pages. 1997. 0-7808-0222-5. $78.

"Particularly useful because it brings much of this information together in one volume."
— *Medical Reference Services Quarterly, Fall '98*

"The layout of the book is particularly helpful as it provides easy access to reference material. A most useful addition to the vast amount of information about health insurance. The use of data from U.S. government agencies is most commendable. Useful in a library or learning center for healthcare professional students."
— *Doody's Health Sciences Book Reviews, Nov '97*

Healthy Aging Sourcebook

Basic Consumer Health Information about Maintaining Health through the Aging Process, Including Advice on Nutrition, Exercise, and Sleep, Help in Making Decisions about Midlife Issues and Retirement, and Guidance Concerning Practical and Informed Choices in Health Consumerism; Along with Data Concerning the Theories of Aging, Different Experiences in Aging by Minority Groups, and Facts about Aging Now and Aging in the Future; and Featuring a Glossary, a Guide to Consumer Help, Additional Suggested Reading, and Practical Resource Directory

Edited by Jenifer Swanson. 536 pages. 1999. 0-7808-0390-6. $78.

Heart Diseases & Disorders Sourcebook, 2nd edition

Basic Consumer Health Information about Heart Attacks, Angina, Rhythm Disorders, Heart Failure, Valve Disease, Congenital Heart Disorders, and More, Including Descriptions of Surgical Procedures and Other Interventions, Medications, Cardiac Rehabilitation, Risk Identification, and Prevention Tips; Along with Statistical Data, Reports on Current Research Initiatives, a Glossary of Cardiovascular Terms, and Resource Directory

Edited by Karen Bellenir. 600 pages. 1999. 0-7808-0238-1. $78.

Immune System Disorders Sourcebook

Basic Information about Lupus, Multiple Sclerosis, Guillain-Barré Syndrome, Chronic Granulomatous Disease, and More, Along with Statistical and Demographic Data and Reports on Current Research Initiatives

Edited by Allan R. Cook. 608 pages. 1997. 0-7808-0209-8. $78.

733

Infant & Toddler Health Sourcebook

Basic Consumer Health Information about the Physical and Mental Development of Newborns, Infants, and Toddlers, Including Neonatal Concerns, Nutritional Recommendations, Immunization Schedules, Common Pediatric Disorders, Assessments and Milestones, Safety Tips, and Advice for Parents and Other Caregivers; Along with a Glossary of Terms and Resource Listings for Additional Help

Edited by Jenifer Swanson. 600 pages. 1999. 0-7808-0246-2. $78.

Kidney & Urinary Tract Diseases & Disorders Sourcebook

Basic Information about Kidney Stones, Urinary Incontinence, Bladder Disease, End Stage Renal Disease, Dialysis, and More, Along with Statistical and Demographic Data and Reports on Current Research Initiatives

Edited by Linda M. Ross. 602 pages. 1997. 0-7808-0079-6. $78.

Learning Disabilities Sourcebook

Basic Information about Disorders Such as Dyslexia, Visual and Auditory Processing Deficits, Attention Deficit/Hyperactivity Disorder, and Autism, Along with Statistical and Demographic Data, Reports on Current Research Initiatives, an Explanation of the Assessment Process, and a Special Section for Adults with Learning Disabilities

Edited by Linda M. Shin. 579 pages. 1998. 0-7808-0210-1. $78.

"Readable . . . provides a solid base of information regarding successful techniques used with individuals who have learning disabilities, as well as practical suggestions for educators and family members. Clear language, concise descriptions, and pertinent information for contacting multiple resources add to the strength of this book as a useful tool." — *Choice, Feb '99*

"Recent and recommended reference source."
— *Booklist, Sept '98*

Liver Disorders Sourcebook

Basic Consumer Health Information about the Liver and How It Works; Liver Diseases, Including Cancer, Cirrhosis, Hepatitis, and Toxic and Drug Related Diseases; Tips for Maintaining a Healthy Liver; Laboratory Tests, Radiology Tests, and Facts about Liver Transplantation; Along with a Section on Support Groups, a Glossary, and Resource Listings

Edited by Joyce Brennfleck Shannon. 600 pages. 1999. 0-7808-0383-3. $78.

Medical Tests Sourcebook

Basic Consumer Health Information about Medical Tests, Including Periodic Health Exams, General Screening Tests, Tests You Can Do at Home, Findings of the U.S. Preventive Services Task Force, X-ray and Radiology Tests, Electrical Tests, Tests of Blood and Other Body Fluids and Tissues, Scope Tests, Lung Tests, Genetic Tests, Pregnancy Tests, Newborn Screening Tests, Sexually Transmitted Disease Tests, and Computer Aided Diagnoses; Along with a Section on Paying for Medical Tests, a Glossary, and Resource Listings

Edited by Joyce Brennfleck Shannon. 691 pages. 1999. 0-7808-0243-8. $78.

Men's Health Concerns Sourcebook

Basic Information about Health Issues That Affect Men, Featuring Facts about the Top Causes of Death in Men, Including Heart Disease, Stroke, Cancers, Prostate Disorders, Chronic Obstructive Pulmonary Disease, Pneumonia and Influenza, Human Immunodeficiency Virus and Acquired Immune Deficiency Syndrome, Diabetes Mellitus, Stress, Suicide, Accidents and Homicides; and Facts about Common Concerns for Men, Including Impotence, Contraception, Circumcision, Sleep Disorders, Snoring, Hair Loss, Diet, Nutrition, Exercise, Kidney and Urological Disorders, and Backaches

Edited by Allan R. Cook. 738 pages. 1998. 0-7808-0212-8. $78.

"Recent and recommended reference source."
— *Booklist, Dec '98*

Mental Health Disorders Sourcebook, 1st Edition

Basic Information about Schizophrenia, Depression, Bipolar Disorder, Panic Disorder, Obsessive-Compulsive Disorder, Phobias and Other Anxiety Disorders, Paranoia and Other Personality Disorders, Eating Disorders, and Sleep Disorders, Along with Information about Treatment and Therapies

Edited by Karen Bellenir. 548 pages. 1995. 0-7808-0040-0. $78.

"This is an excellent new book . . . written in easy-to-understand language."
— *Booklist Health Science Supplement, Oct '97*

". . . useful for public and academic libraries and consumer health collections."
— *Medical Reference Services Quarterly, Spring '97*

"The great strengths of the book are its readability and its inclusion of places to find more information. Especially recommended." — *RQ, Winter '96*

". . . a good resource for a consumer health library."
— *Bulletin of the MLA, Oct '96*

"The information is data-based and couched in brief, concise language that avoids jargon. . . . a useful reference source."
                                    — *Readings, Sept '96*

"The text is well organized and adequately written for its target audience."
                                    — *Choice, Jun '96*

". . . provides information on a wide range of mental disorders, presented in nontechnical language."
— *Exceptional Child Education Resources, Spring '96*

"Recommended for public and academic libraries."
                            — *Reference Book Review, '96*

Mental Health Disorders Sourcebook, 2nd Edition

Basic Consumer Health Information about Anxiety Disorders, Depression and Other Mood Disorders, Eating Disorders, Personality Disorders, Schizophrenia, and More, Including Disease Descriptions, Treatment Options, and Reports on Current Research Initiatives; Along with Statistical Data, Tips for Maintaining Mental Health, a Glossary, and Directory of Sources for Additional Help and Information

Edited by Karen Bellenir. 600 pages. 1999. 0-7808-0240-3. $78.

Ophthalmic Disorders Sourcebook

Basic Information about Glaucoma, Cataracts, Macular Degeneration, Strabismus, Refractive Disorders, and More, Along with Statistical and Demographic Data and Reports on Current Research Initiatives

Edited by Linda M. Ross. 631 pages. 1996. 0-7808-0081-8. $78.

Oral Health Sourcebook

Basic Information about Diseases and Conditions Affecting Oral Health, Including Cavities, Gum Disease, Dry Mouth, Oral Cancers, Fever Blisters, Canker Sores, Oral Thrush, Bad Breath, Temporomandibular Disorders, and other Craniofacial Syndromes, Along with Statistical Data on the Oral Health of Americans, Oral Hygiene, Emergency First Aid, Information on Treatment Procedures and Methods of Replacing Lost Teeth

Edited by Allan R. Cook. 558 pages. 1997. 0-7808-0082-6. $78.

"Unique source which will fill a gap in dental sources for patients and the lay public. A valuable reference tool even in a library with thousands of books on dentistry. Comprehensive, clear, inexpensive, and easy to read and use. It fills an enormous gap in the health care literature."   — *Reference and User Services Quarterly, Summer '98*

"Recent and recommended reference source."
                                    — *Booklist, Dec '97*

Osteoporosis Sourcebook

Basic Consumer Health Information about Primary and Secondary Osteoporosis, Juvenile Osteoporosis, Related Conditions, and Other Such Bone Disorders as Fibrous Dysplasia, Myeloma, Osteogenesis Imperfecta, Osteopetrosis, and Paget's Disease; Along with Information about Risk Factors, Treatments, Traditional and Non-Traditional Pain Management, and Including a Glossary and Resource Directory

Edited by Allan R. Cook. 600 pages. 1999. 0-7808-0239-X. $78.

Pain Sourcebook

Basic Information about Specific Forms of Acute and Chronic Pain, Including Headaches, Back Pain, Muscular Pain, Neuralgia, Surgical Pain, and Cancer Pain, Along with Pain Relief Options Such as Analgesics, Narcotics, Nerve Blocks, Transcutaneous Nerve Stimulation, and Alternative Forms of Pain Control, Including Biofeedback, Imaging, Behavior Modification, and Relaxation Techniques

Edited by Allan R. Cook. 667 pages. 1997. 0-7808-0213-6. $78.

"The text is readable, easily understood, and well indexed. This excellent volume belongs in all patient education libraries, consumer health sections of public libraries, and many personal collections."
                    — *American Reference Books Annual, '99*

"A beneficial reference."
            — *Booklist Health Sciences Supplement, Oct '98*

"The information is basic in terms of scholarship and is appropriate for general readers. Written in journalistic style . . . intended for non-professionals. Quite thorough in its coverage of different pain conditions and summarizes the latest clinical information regarding pain treatment."   — *Choice, Jun '98*

"Recent and recommended reference source."
                                    — *Booklist, Mar '98*

Pediatric Cancer Sourcebook

Basic Consumer Health Information about Leukemias, Brain Tumors, Sarcomas, Lymphomas, and Other Cancers in Infants, Children, and Adolescents, Including Descriptions of Cancers, Treatments, and Coping Strategies; Along with Suggestions for Parents, Caregivers, and Concerned Relatives, a Glossary of Cancer Terms, and Resource Listings

Edited by Edward J. Prucha. 587 pages. 1999. 0-7808-0245-4. $78.

Physical & Mental Issues in Aging Sourcebook

Basic Consumer Health Information on Physical and Mental Disorders Associated with the Aging Process, Including Concerns about Cardiovascular Disease, Pulmonary Disease, Oral Health, Digestive Disorders, Musculoskeletal and Skin Disorders, Metabolic Changes, Sexual and Reproductive Issues, and Changes in Vision, Hearing, and Other Senses; Along with Data about Longevity and Causes of Death, Information on Acute and Chronic Pain, Descriptions of Mental Concerns, a Glossary of Terms, and Resource Listings for Additional Help

Edited by Jenifer Swanson. 660 pages. 1999. 0-7808-0233-0. $78.

Pregnancy & Birth Sourcebook

Basic Information about Planning for Pregnancy, Maternal Health, Fetal Growth and Development, Labor and Delivery, Postpartum and Perinatal Care, Pregnancy in Mothers with Special Concerns, and Disorders of Pregnancy, Including Genetic Counseling, Nutrition and Exercise, Obstetrical Tests, Pregnancy Discomfort, Multiple Births, Cesarean Sections, Medical Testing of Newborns, Breastfeeding, Gestational Diabetes, and Ectopic Pregnancy

Edited by Heather E. Aldred. 737 pages. 1997. 0-7808-0216-0. $78.

"A well-organized handbook. Recommended."
— *Choice, Apr '98*

"Recent and recommended reference source."
— *Booklist, Mar '98*

"Recommended for public libraries."
— *American Reference Books Annual, '98*

Public Health Sourcebook

Basic Information about Government Health Agencies, Including National Health Statistics and Trends, Healthy People 2000 Program Goals and Objectives, the Centers for Disease Control and Prevention, the Food and Drug Administration, and the National Institutes of Health, Along with Full Contact Information for Each Agency

Edited by Wendy Wilcox. 698 pages. 1998. 0-7808-0220-9. $78.

"Recent and recommended reference source."
— *Booklist, Sept '98*

"This consumer guide provides welcome assistance in navigating the maze of federal health agencies and their data on public health concerns."
— *SciTech Book News, Sept '98*

Rehabilitation Sourcebook

Basic Consumer Health Information about Rehabilitation for People Recovering from Heart Surgery, Spinal Cord Injury, Stroke, Orthopedic Impairments, Amputation, Pulmonary Impairments, Traumatic Injury, and More, Including Physical Therapy, Occupational Therapy, Speech/Language Therapy, Massage Therapy, Dance Therapy, Art Therapy, and Recreational Therapy, Along with Information on Assistive and Adaptive Devices, a Glossary, and Resources for Additional Help and Information

Edited by Dawn D. Matthews. 512 pages. 1999. 0-7808-0236-5. $78.

Respiratory Diseases & Disorders Sourcebook

Basic Information about Respiratory Diseases and Disorders, Including Asthma, Cystic Fibrosis, Pneumonia, the Common Cold, Influenza, and Others, Featuring Facts about the Respiratory System, Statistical and Demographic Data, Treatments, Self-Help Management Suggestions, and Current Research Initiatives

Edited by Allan R. Cook and Peter D. Dresser. 771 pages. 1995. 0-7808-0037-0. $78.

"Designed for the layperson and for patients and their families coping with respiratory illness. . . . an extensive array of information on diagnosis, treatment, management, and prevention of respiratory illnesses for the general reader."
— *Choice, Jun '96*

"A highly recommended text for all collections. It is a comforting reminder of the power of knowledge that good books carry between their covers."
— *Academic Library Book Review, Spring '96*

"This sourcebook offers a comprehensive collection of authoritative information presented in a nontechnical, humanitarian style for patients, families, and caregivers."
— *Association of Operating Room Nurses, Sept/Oct '95*

Sexually Transmitted Diseases Sourcebook

Basic Information about Herpes, Chlamydia, Gonorrhea, Hepatitis, Nongonoccocal Urethritis, Pelvic Inflammatory Disease, Syphilis, AIDS, and More, Along with Current Data on Treatments and Preventions

Edited by Linda M. Ross. 550 pages. 1997. 0-7808-0217-9. $78.

Skin Disorders Sourcebook

Basic Information about Common Skin and Scalp Conditions Caused by Aging, Allergies, Immune Reactions, Sun Exposure, Infectious Organisms, Parasites, Cosmetics, and Skin Traumas, Including Abrasions, Cuts, and Pressure Sores, Along with Information on Prevention and Treatment

Edited by Allan R. Cook. 647 pages. 1997. 0-7808-0080-X. $78.

". . . comprehensive easily read reference book."
— *Doody's Health Sciences Book Reviews, Oct '97*

Sleep Disorders Sourcebook

Basic Consumer Health Information about Sleep and Its Disorders, Including Insomnia, Sleepwalking, Sleep Apnea, Restless Leg Syndrome, and Narcolepsy; Along with Data about Shiftwork and Its Effects, Information on the Societal Costs of Sleep Deprivation, Descriptions of Treatment Options, a Glossary of Terms, and Resource Listings for Additional Help

Edited by Jenifer Swanson. 439 pages. 1998. 0-7808-0234-9. $78.

"Recent and recommended reference source."
— *Booklist, Feb '99*

Sports Injuries Sourcebook

Basic Consumer Health Information about Common Sports Injuries, Prevention of Injury in Specific Sports, Tips for Training, and Rehabilitation from Injury; Along with Information about Special Concerns for Children, Young Girls in Athletic Training Programs, Senior Athletes, and Women Athletes, and a Directory of Resources for Further Help and Information

Edited by Heather E. Aldred. 624 pages.1999. 0-7808-0218-7. $78.

Substance Abuse Sourcebook

Basic Health-Related Information about the Abuse of Legal and Illegal Substances Such as Alcohol, Tobacco, Prescription Drugs, Marijuana, Cocaine, and Heroin; and Including Facts about Substance Abuse Prevention Strategies, Intervention Methods, Treatment and Recovery Programs, and a Section Addressing the Special Problems Related to Substance Abuse during Pregnancy

Edited by Karen Bellenir. 573 pages. 1996. 0-7808-0038-9. $78.

"A valuable addition to any health reference section. Highly recommended."
— *The Book Report, Mar/Apr '97*

". . . a comprehensive collection of substance abuse information that's both highly readable and compact. Families and caregivers of substance abusers will find the information enlightening and helpful, while teachers, social workers and journalists should benefit from the concise format. Recommended."
— *Drug Abuse Update, Winter '96-'97*

Women's Health Concerns Sourcebook

Basic Information about Health Issues That Affect Women, Featuring Facts about Menstruation and Other Gynecological Concerns, Including Endometriosis, Fibroids, Menopause, and Vaginitis; Reproductive Concerns, Including Birth Control, Infertility, and Abortion; and Facts about Additional Physical, Emotional, and Mental Health Concerns Prevalent among Women Such as Osteoporosis, Urinary Tract Disorders, Eating Disorders, and Depression, Along with Tips for Maintaining a Healthy Lifestyle

Edited by Heather Aldred. 567 pages. 1997. 0-7808-0219-5. $78.

"Handy compilation. There is an impressive range of diseases, devices, disorders, procedures, and other physical and emotional issues covered . . . well organized, illustrated, and indexed."
— *Choice, Jan '98*

Workplace Health & Safety Sourcebook

Basic Information about Musculoskeletal Injuries, Cumulative Trauma Disorders, Occupational Carcinogens and Other Toxic Materials, Child Labor, Workplace Violence, Histoplasmosis, Transmission of HIV and Hepatitis-B Viruses, and Occupational Hazards Associated with Various Industries, Including Mining, Confined Spaces, Agriculture, Construction, Electrical Work, and the Medical Professions, with Information on Mortality and Other Statistical Data, Preventative Measures, Reproductive Risks, Reducing Stress for Shiftworkers, Noise Hazards, Industrial Back Belts, Reducing Contamination at Home, Preventing Allergic Reactions to Rubber Latex, and More; Along with Public and Private Programs and Initiatives, a Glossary, and Sources for Additional Help and Information

Edited by Helene Henderson. 600 pages. 1999. 0-7808-0231-4. $78.

Health Reference Series Cumulative Index

A Comprehensive Index to 42 Volumes of the Health Reference Series, 1990-1998

1st ed. 1,500 pages. 1999. 0-7808-0382-5. $78.